The Encyclopedia of Common Diseases

By The Staff
of Prevention Magazine

Compiled and Prepared By:

Charles Gerras, Executive Editor

E. John Hanna, Senior Editor

John Feltman, Associate Editor

Joan Bingham, Joseph Golant,
    Anne Moyer, Assistant Editors

Library of Congress Cataloging in Publication Data

The encyclopedia of common diseases.

Includes index.
1. Medicine, Popular. I. Gerras, Charles.
II. Prevention.
RC81.A2N43   616'.003   75-35754
ISBN 0-87857-113-2 hardcover
ISBN 0-87857-150-7   deluxe

20   19   hardcover
20   19   deluxe

Printed in the United States of America on recycled paper

Contents

Introduction

The world of science as it relates to health has moved rapidly since the publication of the first edition of *The Encyclopedia of Common Diseases*. In the '60's alone, hearts were transplanted, the Pill passed into common usage, scores of environmental causes of cancer were identified, nutritional therapy for emotional disturbances earned new respect and hundreds of other changes in our attitudes toward disease became commonplace. In terms of health, the years since World War II have brought the civilized world into a whole new era.

The rapidity with which this new era in medicine has developed explains why the material in this edition is more than 75 percent new. Some subjects, such as crib death and venereal disease, did not appear in the original at all. Others, such as Emotional and Nervous Disorders and Back Ailments, have been greatly expanded. Some sections, particularly those on the heart and cancer, are books in themselves.

Each disease section has been carefully researched for the latest information and all medical and scientific conclusions are based on reports from the most respected of the world's medical and scientific journals.

Obviously, in the face of serious illness no book, however thorough it might be, can take the place of a consultation with a physician. However, the informed patient understands, more readily, the symptoms of his illness and the aims of the treatment. Furthermore, he is prepared to ask the doctor the right questions and volunteer important information that can help in his treatment.

Every person is responsible for his own health. He must learn how his body works and what can threaten its functioning. The person who identifies these threats and tries to avoid them is taking the most important steps there are in battling disease. This book outlines these steps in a useful, understandable manner.

The underlying philosophy of *The New Encyclopedia of Common Diseases* is "natural is best." This means that when there is solid scientific evidence that drugless, non-surgical treatments have proven effective, they are emphasized.

Of course, some ailments allow no time for experimentation with home remedies. For example, pneumonia, heart attack or appendicitis demand immediate medical attention. The miraculous advances medical science has made show to their best advantage at such times. But as a rule, health comes from the way people live, not from doctors and hospitals. This book is a blueprint for better, more healthful living.

Section 1
Alcoholism

1. Bad Diet Can Cause Alcoholism
2. Megavitamin Therapy Salvages Alcoholics
3. Magnesium Helps To Control The D.T.'s (Delirium Tremens)
4. Food Addiction Related To Alcoholism

1. Bad Diet Can Cause Alcoholism

Alcoholics Anonymous has helped some people solve their drinking problems; for others, it hasn't brought results. Fortunately, there are nutritional measures which have been used successfully to treat compulsive drinking. Best of all, they can be employed in the privacy of your own home.

There is a close relationship between nutritional deficiencies and the use of alcohol. Dr. Roger J. Williams, University of Texas biochemist, and one of our country's leading nutritionists, has noted that although alcoholics tend to have a poor diet (often through neglect), the reverse situation also applies: bad diet creates alcoholics.

"It is our opinion that the disease of alcoholism is *essentially a disease of one's appetite* and insofar as this is true, it probably can be consistently prevented by the application of nutritional knowledge," Dr. Williams wrote in his classic work, *Alcoholism: The Nutritional Approach* (University of Texas Press, 1959). "The role of individuality in body chemistry must be recognized, as well as the fact that no individual person can be sure, in advance, that he does not have the potentiality of becoming an alcoholic. Any young person who finds himself or herself liking alcohol or its effects very much, or who has any tendency to become intoxicated, should be on his guard, always, at all times."

Dr. Williams has been studying the problem of alcoholism and nutritional disorders for many years, and he arrived at this conclusion after intensive studies and research. He noted that alcohol contains large amounts of carbohydrates and *no* vitamins or minerals—thus making it very difficult for the body to utilize the carbohydrates found in the alcohol. If an individual persists in his drinking habit, the alcohol consumed uses up the vitamins and minerals being stored in the liver for carbohydrate processing.

In his studies and experiments, Dr. Williams used rats extensively as his experimental animals in an effort to determine why people drink excessively. "There is no question whatever that the tendency of experimental animals to drink alcohol is influenced most remarkably by the composition of food they get," wrote Dr. Williams. He explained that the deficiency of the B complex vitamins caused by drinking alcohol, in turn, caused an even greater need for glucose. In addition, the lack of the B complex vitamins induced malfunctioning of the liver. Both contributed to liver injury and interfered with its repair. This liver injury, Dr. Williams said, may also contribute to the craving for alcohol.

To clarify what Dr. Williams means: by drinking, an individual has given himself a deficiency in a number of important B vitamins. This makes it impossible to convert glucose into its storage form (which is glycogen). Being unable to convert surplus glucose and thus remove it from the bloodstream until needed, the liver is failing to function properly and the sugar piles up in the blood. The body then combats this glucose excess by releasing extra insulin into the bloodstream. Later, when the body needs more glucose, the liver is unable to supply it. Hypoglycemia—low blood sugar—becomes chronic. Lacking glucose, energy is low and the brain does not function properly, and the alcoholic feels that the quick energy he gets from alcohol is the only thing that will set him right. He may actually feel, as many alcoholics do, that he will die if he does not get a drink quickly.

From his studies with rats, Dr. Williams confirmed the theory that a B complex deficiency manifests itself as a disorder in the body's appetite mechanism. He went further to state that "body wisdom becomes body foolishness," as the rat, because of the irregular appetite mechanism, craved alcohol instead of craving good food.

Human Diet Makes Rats Alcoholics

Even more to the point, perhaps, was a study conducted at Loma Linda University in California in 1967. Instead of artificially manipulating the diet, Dr. U. D. Register experimented with feeding rats the kind of diet that is common among people in the United States. The experiment conducted was performed to see if an individual's normal diet of food and drink affects the rate of alcohol consumption. Dr. Register and his colleagues believe there is such a relationship.

A popular, but poor quality U.S. diet consisting of hot dogs, spaghetti, meat balls, sweet rolls and soft drinks was given to

3

these rats. They were also given the choice of drinking either ten percent alcohol or water. This popular diet was compared to the standard food prepared in the laboratory such as the corn-soy-alfalfa diet—and a control "milk-vegetable" diet.

It was found that the rats being fed the popular diet consumed 12.8 ml. of alcohol per 100 gm. body weight per week, as compared to the rats on the milk-vegetable control diet who were consuming 2.3 ml. of alcohol. Adding coffee to the popular diet doubled the alcoholic consumption, and when the diet was augmented with both coffee and spices (such as cloves and mustard) the alcohol consumption of the rats was 46 ml. per week.

After continuing the popular U.S. diet for 10 weeks, the rats were switched to the control diet. During the first week, the drinking level dropped to 3.8 ml. and within three weeks, most of the rats had completely stopped drinking. Indicative of how strong the relationship to diet is, when the "popular diet" was resumed once again, the rats returned to the previous level of alcohol consumption.

Dr. Register concluded his report by stating that the deficiencies resulting from the lack of the vitamin B complex family may account for the basic dependence that the drinker has on alcohol. Without these vitamins, humans become quite confused, irritable, unstable, and are unable to adjust to many stressful situations. He also stated that the combination of a "poor quality," yet popular U.S. diet, combined with coffee and spices, "may lead a person to turn to alcohol as an anesthetic or a poor solution to the increasing problems facing him in his complex life."

Therefore, one can't say that an alcoholic is a person who simply won't "pull himself together" and stop drinking. He is unable to stop drinking—just as he can't stop using air and water. A definite physiological craving has been created for alcohol by a deficiency of the vitamins of the B complex, according to these study results.

A number of doctors including Cecelia Rosenfeld, M.D., of Los Angeles, have reported success in treating the alcoholic patient with diets used for hypoglycemia. What is this diet? Dr. Sam E. Roberts in this book, *Exhaustion: Causes and Treatment* (Rodale Press, 1967), discusses it quite thoroughly. The diet consists of meats, fresh eggs, and fruits. Coffee and cigarettes are absolutely forbidden—and even unprocessed coarse carbohydrates such as whole potatoes and whole grain bread are to be taken only in small amounts. The consumption of vitamins and minerals is encouraged, especially vitamin B, from brewer's yeast and desiccated liver tablets.

Year by year, as additional evidence keeps mounting, we are compelled to believe that this diet is the best possible approach to alcoholism. It is sometimes hard to convince alcoholics of this, but every drinker should fortify his diet with very substantial amounts of all the B vitamins. Not only will he repair his obvious malnutrition—he might even stop drinking.

2. Megavitamin Therapy Salvages Alcoholics

In treating alcoholism in humans, many physicians have obtained good results with megavitamin therapy. Operating on the theory that certain people, independent of social or psychological stresses, are predisposed to alcoholism because of a biochemical flaw, they use massive doses of vitamins as harmless chemicals to balance the body's faulty chemistry.

Whatever this biochemical flaw is, research indicates that it is closely related to the biochemical flaw associated with schizophrenia. In fact several scientists have established a strong link between schizophrenia and alcoholism. These scientists who are associated with the American Schizophrenia Foundation estimate that from 20 percent to 40 percent of all alcoholics are schizophrenic. The heartening news is that these alcoholics respond favorably to the same therapies which have been helping many schizophrenics to end the war with their own souls—the niacin therapy developed by Dr. Abram Hoffer of Saskatchewan, Canada, and Dr. Humphrey Osmond of Princeton, N.J.

Dr. Abram Hoffer and Dr. Osmond have reported the successful treatment of schizophrenia, long considered the incurable scourge of mankind, with massive doses of niacin (B_3), vitamin C, B_6 and other vitamins—sometimes called the megavitamin therapy. Their studies were reported in the *British Journal of Psychiatry* (July, 1968).

Schizoid Tendencies Shown

What does this have to do with alcoholism? Drs. Hoffer and Osmond have also developed the HOD (Hoffer Osmond Diagnostic) test or *Symptometer Test* to determine schizophrenic tendencies. When this test has been given to alcoholics as it was at Guest House, a rehabilitation center for alcoholics in Michigan, it was found that as many as 40 percent showed the same perceptual disorders as do those who are suffering with schizophrenia. It was decided to test the megavitamin treatment on them

6

to see if it would work on alcoholism as it had with schizophrenia. The results were so dramatic that many who for years were chained to John Barleycorn are now back with their loved ones living useful lives with no lost weekends.

The value of the HOD as a diagnostic tool was established when it was found to corroborate the results of another diagnostic test—a biochemical mauve factor test which made it possible to distinguish biochemically ill psychiatric patients from others. Those who have the mauve factor, maintain Dr. Hoffer and Dr. Osmond, have a disease they call malvaria, whether they are diagnosed as neurotic, alcoholic, pseudoneurotic or retarded.

Further evidence of the effectiveness of this megavitamin therapy on alcoholism has been reported by Dr. Russell F. Smith, medical director of Michigan State Boys' Training School. Dr. Smith conducted a study in which he treated 507 alcoholics with massive vitamin B_3 therapy. "On an average of 6 grams of this well known, common, cheap vitamin a day," Dr. Smith reported in the newsletter of the American Schizophrenia Foundation (Oct. 1968), "87 percent of our group of hard core, treatment resistant, difficult alcoholics derived benefit."

Niacin Surpasses Other Therapies

Comparing these results with other therapeutic agents commonly used in the treatment of alcoholics, Dr. Smith said, "B_3 far surpassed them in effectiveness. This comparison becomes more effective," he pointed out, "when we remember that many drugs today used in the treatment of alcoholism have a high potential for abuse and for suicide. When the niacin therapy is used instead, these serious risks become virtually nonexistent—a great advantage indeed."

Dr. Smith said that in his opinion "B_3 far surpasses other therapeutic agents commonly used in the treatment of alcoholics." Most dramatic are the number who have maintained continued abstinence from alcohol since beginning niacin therapy. A college instructor in English, for instance, who had not taught a complete term in the last five years, has now completed one successful year of teaching on a dose of 12 grams of niacin daily. A 40-year-old painter had a schizoid background and a drinking history dating back to age 11. On a dose of 12 grams of niacin, and steadily decreasing amounts of antidepressants, he is now completing the first seven months of sobriety in 29 years.

Dr. Smith feels that niacin may be intimately involved in the physiology of alcohol tolerance. Some patients who began to drink again reported a loss of tolerance to large quantities of alcohol. Many reported being able to drink only roughly one half pint before becoming drowsy, very intoxicated, or falling asleep. Massive niacin therapy would seem to influence some of the basic physiologic mechanisms that underlie the alcoholic disease itself.

Dr. David Ramon Hawkins, director of the North Nassau Mental Health Center, completed an extensive study of 315 schizophrenics at his out-patient clinic. Seventy of the patients had alcoholism as well. They scored high on the HOD test. The majority of the patients had had previous treatment or hospitalization, some up to 12 years. Psychotherapy or psychoanalysis for periods ranging to 20 years was common. "Some of the patients' families had spent up to $150,000 on years of expensive treatment which had been to no avail," Dr. Hawkins said.

All of the patients were put on a massive dosage of vitamins B_3 and C as well as phenothiazine and pyridoxine (vitamin B_6).

Blood Sugar Control Helps

It is interesting to note that all patients were also placed on a hypoglycemic diet (low in carbohydrates, high in proteins and medium in fats—frequent small meals rather than three large meals). Patients were encouraged to keep coffee-drinking to a minimum and to maintain a regular, daily physical exercise program.

Improvement was dramatic, "71 percent," Dr. Hawkins reported. The greatest response to treatment was made by the patients with alcoholism plus schizophrenia. "This treatment approach was found to be extremely economical and within the reach of every family," Dr. Hawkins pointed out.

The prognosis of patients with the combination of schizophrenia and alcoholism has hitherto been quite grave and has exhausted many families, financially as well as emotionally. The chances for recovery from schizophrenia while still actively drinking are almost nil, Dr. Hawkins reported. "By treating their schizophrenia with megavitamin therapy and simultaneously pushing them into A.A., our results were extremely good. I have never seen so many patients and their families pleased. Since we started using this new approach we have closed our out-patient shock unit. Hardly any of these patients needs to be hospitalized any more. The whole attitude of the patients and their families is so overwhelmingly different there is no comparison with the previous situation."

In the megavitamin therapy, vitamins are used not as vitamins but as harmless and very useful chemicals, to balance the faulty body chemistry. They are used in much larger dosages than the daily vitamin requirement, sometimes a thousand times larger. Besides B_3, several other vitamins are used in the megavitamin therapy: vitamin C, pyridoxine (B_6), B_1, B_{12}, and vitamin E.

Dr. Russell F. Smith, whose report was cited earlier, notes that ascorbic acid, for instance, was not a part of the original treatment plan to test the merits of the niacin therapy. During the study however, some patients complained of sustained weakness, dry skin, occasional rashes or odd dietary cravings. Realizing that massive B_3 acts as a drug and not as a vitamin (drugs deplete vitamin C) and that the high consumption of nicotine and coffee common to alcoholics can cause depletion of vitamin C, they tested the urine of these patients and found all evidence of urinary excretion of ascorbic acid had ceased. When there is no urinary excretion, the body is operating on insufficient vitamin C.

These patients were placed on increasing doses of vitamin C until excretion occurred. At that point (average dose 1000 mg. daily) all the side-effects disappeared.

One might conclude, Dr. Smith observed, that with massive niacin therapy, certain imbalances will have to be defined and compensated. The megavitamin therapy attempts to compensate for these imbalances and, together with the hypoglycemic diet (low in carbohydrates, high in protein), is helping many schizophrenics and alcoholics to realize their potential for full, happy, creative lives.

3. Magnesium Helps To Control The D.T.'s (Delirium Tremens)

A major stumbling block to full recovery—the withdrawal syndrome known as *delirium tremens* (the DT's)—has also proven curable through nutritional treatment. The symptoms of this medical syndrome are hallucinations, uncontrollable tremors called "the shakes," the inability to sleep and a sort of waking stupor in which such basic knowledge as the year and the place is lost. The DT's are not directly caused by alcohol. They are a withdrawal syndrome, occurring when the alcoholic tries to stop drinking. The naked fear they cause is more than a psychological condition. Realistically, the end result of *delirium tremens* is death in 10 to 15 percent of those who suffer it.

In 1967, Dr. Edmund G. Flink, chairman of medicine at West Virginia University's medical school conducted a series of experiments with sufferers of alcoholism and concluded that the alcoholic, both through poor diet and because alcohol tends to deplete the tissues of magnesium, is highly prone to develop a magnesium deficiency. When he has such a deficiency, his efforts to stop drinking will result in the terrible symptoms that are characteristic of both *delirium tremens* and simple magnesium deficiency. So unendurable are these symptoms that they make it impossible for many to end their alcoholic habit. But simple improvement in the amount of magnesium in the alcoholic's system can end the symptoms and make it much more possible for him to break his deadly habit. Nor is it even necessary for him to receive the mineral by injection. A diet containing high magnesium foods, or a plain oral supplement such as dolomite tablets, will serve to restore the magnesium balance and diminish the horrors of *delirium tremens*.

Later studies of patients immediately after withdrawal from alcohol provide "further evidence" of significant depletion of magnesium in alcoholics, reported Dr. John E. Jones of West Virginia University Medical Center in an article in *Medical Tribune* (July 11, 1968). The severity of withdrawal symptoms when alcohol is removed often matches the lowered magnesium levels in the patient.

In the experiment, seven chronic alcoholic patients who had suffered nervousness or delirium on withdrawal of alcohol got large doses of magnesium on the first and second day after withdrawal, and two others got their magnesium on the sixth to tenth day. Though no significant retention of magnesium was noted in any of seven normal non-alcoholic control patients following doses of the same amounts of magnesium, Dr. Jones found that all but one of the alcoholic patients retained the magnesium.

4. Food Addiction Related To Alcoholism

While compulsive eaters must learn to scrutinize their diets for what may be the cause of their food addiction, nobody has to tell the alcoholic that his problem is that he drinks too much, even if he takes only one sip of his favorite, spirited beverage. But now it appears that in many cases of alcoholism the tendency to reach for yet another drink is caused less by the "need" for alcohol, than by the craving for the native food from which the alcoholic beverage is distilled, according to a report by Dr. Theron G. Randolph which appeared in *Health News and Views* (Spring issue, 1971).

Most of us know about sugar addicts, or hypoglycemics, who continually eat cake, candy or ice cream, which causes their blood sugar level to soar, and make them feel fine for the moment. Before much time has elapsed, however, their blood sugar level nosedives, and their desire for more sugar returns, only stronger. A similar response is unwittingly experienced by many people to foods other than sugar—foods such as corn and other grains which are the basic ingredients used in the making of commercial whiskey and beers, noted Dr. Randolph.

Dr. Randolph cogently argued that problem drinking for some people may be the result of a form of food addiction. But unlike ordinary food addiction, the disease of alcoholism is exacerbated greatly because the alcohol increases the severity of the withdrawal symptoms and the ensuing desire for more of the same drink by acting as a "vehicle" to speed the native material through the walls of the gastrointestinal tract into the body.

Dr. Randolph reported the case of a former alcoholic who suffered withdrawal symptoms after he ate a food containing wheat starch. The doctor kept him off this food for five days after that, then returned it to his diet once again. When he ate the wheat a second time, the reformed alcoholic felt dizzy, light-headed and uncoordinated, and developed inflamed nasal passages. "It's the most amazing thing," the former alcoholic commented, "to have a hangover when I have not had a drink for 26

12

months. Even the anxiety complex and the remorse are dead ringers for the way I used to feel. Why should I be remorseful after eating wheat?"

The answer, noted Dr. Randolph, is that his reaction to wheat starch was but a recurrence of his reaction to the malt-wheat-rye blend in the whiskey which he had formerly drunk in great quantity. He turned out to be sensitive to wheat in any form. Following this incident, Dr. Randolph checked the diets of 40 problem drinkers, and learned that they were sensitive to roughly the same foods that were the raw products of their beverages. "Sensitivity to corn, malt-wheat-rye, grape and potato," Dr. Randolph reported, "were encountered in that order of frequency. It is well known that alcoholic beverages consumed in this country are derived from foods in approximately the same order."

Yet you can suffer the withdrawal symptoms of an alcoholic without touching a drop of booze if you slip into the advanced stages of food addiction, such as that caused by eating quickly-absorbed, refined foods in frequent doses. Even before the saturation point is reached "beyond which intake cannot be increased," noted Dr. Randolph, you could experience "the clinical phenomenon of drunkenness . . . , the development of binge-like thirsts and appetites, all features of the hangover, 'black outs,' acute depressions and even a condition clinically indistinguishable from so-called pathological intoxication" if you become a far-gone food addict.

Section 2
Allergy

5. An Allergy May Be What's Ailing You

Every time that Henry cuts the lawn with his gas mower, he gets a severe headache. His wife says that she feels sure his problem is psychosomatic—because he is overweight and really needs the exercise.

Each time Max beats the rug for Alice, he breaks out in huge beads of perspiration, and begins to cough and wheeze. "Yeah," Alice observes, "your asthma always gets you when there's work to be done."

Hal loves to cook. But whenever he spends all day Sunday getting a big meal ready for guests, he develops a severe headache. Hal is so nauseated by the time the meal is prepared, that he has to go out for a breath of air before he can face his guests at the dinner table.

Henry thinks his doctor is crazy for dropping by to see what kind of lawn mower he uses. Max laughs at the suggestion that his allergy may be to household dust. Hal couldn't possibly afford to get rid of the gas range in the kitchen, the gas furnace and the gas water heater! Are the doctors losing their minds these days?

"No, indeed," says Dr. Marshall Mandell, ecologic-allergist at the New England Foundation for Allergic and Environmental Diseases in Norwalk, Connecticut. Such allergies to gasoline engines, gas appliances, household dust, and many other common offenders do occur, he says.

One Person In Ten Suffers From Allergy

Almost one out of every ten Americans—or approximately 20 million—suffer from one allergy or another, according to the Allergy Foundation of America. The symptoms may be so severe as to be totally incapacitating, or so minor as to merely cause inconvenience. Hay fever and asthma are two common forms of allergic reaction which are discussed in detail elsewhere in this book. But insomnia, restlessness, and a general feeling of fatigue and indifference, and other minor complaints once thought to be

16

exclusively psychosomatic, may also be indications of continued exposure to allergenic factors.

There is an old saw that we tend to avoid what is "bad" for us and to be drawn towards those things that are beneficial. But in the case of allergic reactions, research is showing some interesting new evidence that allergies can be addictive—that people may tend to go back again and again, like the alcoholic, to those very things which again cause them great harm.

Chain Smoker, Chocolate Addict Have Something In Common

Dr. Mandell bases his conclusions on the result of 125,000 separate "provocative" allergy tests, in which small amounts of potentially allergenic substances are injected, or placed under the tongue or on the patient's skin. If a reaction occurs, the patient does indeed have an allergy. Dr. Mandell speaks of the person, for instance, who is allergic to chocolate—and may never suspect his sensitivity! Why? Because in some cases, the substance which produces the allergic symptoms, also produces withdrawal symptoms. Just as the drinker who has overindulged gets a hangover as a withdrawal symptom, so the insomniac who gets choked up at 1 A.M. and starts wheezing may be reacting to some frequently eaten allergenic food. Perhaps he then eats some candy, or drinks some hot beverage containing chocolate, and immediately feels better. Why? Because his body has become addicted to the very substance which to him is poison.

The chain smoker is another example. Dr.Mandell believes that the truly compulsive smoker's body craves what will really harm him the most. Thus, in spite of health warnings and all the rest, he goes right on chain smoking because he finds it so difficult to give up his source of bodily as well as emotional satisfaction. The cigarette relieves his tension—makes him feel calmer, more relaxed. Similarly, chocolate can bring the chocolate addict relief from his symptoms.

Another kind of case is that of Jack Lamon. A businessman who commonly entertained many of his firm's potential customers, he was brought into the hospital in a catatonic stupor. At first it was thought to be a reaction to alcohol or drugs, but subsequent blood investigation showed that there was only a small amount of alcohol present, and no drugs could be elicited by chemical tests. The patient had no history of psychosis, and he had never shown such a reaction in the memory of his mother or his wife.

It was discovered that for the first time in his life Jack had eaten lobster thermador. However, the significance of this was not realized until a few weeks later when the same reaction took place. This time he had just eaten a dinner with lobster salad included in the menu.

Further testing revealed that Jack had several other severe chemical and food allergies, and when he avoided these substances, he had none of the severe reactions.

Bakers Allergic To Wheat

Allergies to wheat are very common among bakers and bakers' apprentices. One interesting clue which has led doctors to consider desensitizing "shots" as a means of overcoming allergies can be seen in the work of Dr. H. Herxheimer at the Asthma Polyclinic of the Free University of West Berlin. He has established that bakers' apprentices who show an initial sensitivity to wheat flour when first employed, may gradually lose his sensitivity over a period of one or two years. Others will show no sensitivity when employed, and later will develop these reactions.

Help is available for those who are sensitive to wheat flour. One note of warning, however, needs to be sounded. It is important for some people not to eliminate just wheat flour products from the diet. It may also be necessary to eliminate other cereals which may cause reactions in people whose bodies are building up sensitivity to wheat. Cereal grains found to cause allergic reactions in tests by Drs. Arthur Lietze and Albert Rowe, Sr. and Jr., were oats, corn, rice, millet and wild rice. Rye and sorghum did not cause strong enough reactions to be significant. However, barley extracts did appear to cause confusion in some patients.

It was found by Drs. Lietze, Rowe and Rowe that sometimes labels on foods failed to disclose the presence of barley or sorghums. They also discovered that breads containing less than 10 percent of wheat flour did not cause reactions. Just the label "wheat free" was no assurance, however. They found that several products thus labeled contained more than 10 percent wheat flour or gluten—the latter being an extract of wheat.

The solution? For those sensitive to wheat flour, there seems only one practical way out. Go back to home baking, using special recipes which most allergists have available for the asking.

Unrecognized Allergies Can Be Dangerous

Injections, infusions, or tube feedings may also contain substances to which people are allergic. If the allergies of an individual have already been established, it is important that relatives who accompany him for admission to a hospital or emergency clinic inform medical personnel of such sensitivities. Allergic persons should carry among their identification cards one on which their allergies are listed. This is especially important in the case of allergies to antibiotics or other drugs.

Frequently, allergies are mistakenly diagnosed as other illnesses. One 19-year-old man, cited by Dr. Mandell, was told by a world-famous clinic that his symptoms were due to a psychiatric problem. Another well-known clinic diagnosed his trouble as low blood sugar. However, tests indicated that his asthma, as well as numerous food allergies, was due to chemical susceptibility to certain additives, preservatives, and colorings commonly used in processed foods. Heavy perspiration, nasal congestion, and other allergenic symptoms appeared when small amounts of hydrocarbons were introduced by injection. In talking with him, the physician found that the young man's sports car had a leaky exhaust which might put fumes inside the car. When the condition was corrected in the automobile, many of the severe sensitivity reactions subsided.

Some people can help themselves by merely avoiding the substances to which they are allergic—as the person who responds to natural gas, and has a gas furnace and a gas range. These may be expensive appliances to replace, but such drastic measures will often pay for themselves many times over in reduced medical bills. It should be cautioned here, though, that this substitution should be made only when medical tests definitely indicate fuel gas is the offending substance.

In cases where substances cannot be eliminated—as with household dust, molds, common pollens, etc., injections of tiny amounts of these materials given over a period of time may desensitize the patient.

In the event that you or any member of your family may be experiencing symptoms that you suspect might be allergic in origin, you will be interested in the following table that Dr. Mandell presented to the Second Annual Convention of the International Academy of Metabology in New York City in March, 1973. The subjective symptoms and objective signs that have been elicited by provocation techniques may involve every body region or system. This is a list of the most common reactions induced by testing. It also indicates the symptoms and syndromes experienced by allergic individuals after exposure to foods, beverages, inhalants and a variety of chemicals. These symptoms are not always due to allergy, but they often are unrecognized, controllable (reversible) manifestations of allergy that are misdiagnosed as "idiopathic," "essential," "functional," "of unknown etiology," "of psychosomatic origin" or "a response to social stress."

Symptoms Induced By Provocative Testing

1. *Skin:* Itching, burning, flushing, warmth, coldness, tingling, sweating on back of neck, etc. Hives, blisters, blotches, red spots, "pimples."
2. *Ear, nose, throat:* Nasal congestion, sneezing, nasal itching, runny nose, postnasal drip. Sore, dry, or tickling throat, clearing throat, itching palate, hoarseness, hacking cough. Fullness, ringing, or popping of ears, earache, intermittent deafness, dizziness, imbalance.
3. *Eye:* Blurring of vision, pain in eyes, watery eyes, crossing of eyes, glare hurts eyes; eyelids twitching, itching, drooping, or swollen; redness and swelling of inner angle of lower lid.
4. *Respiratory:* Shortness of breath, wheeze, cough, mucus formation in bronchial tubes.
5. *Cardiovascular:* Pounding heart, increased pulse rate, skipped beats, flushing, pallor, warm, cold, tingling, redness or blueness of hands, faintness, precordial pain.
6. *Gastrointestinal:* Dryness of mouth, increased salivation, canker sores, stinging tongue, toothache, burping, retasting, heartburn, indigestion, nausea, vomiting, difficulty in swallowing, rumbling in abdomen, abdominal pain, cramps, diarrhea, itching or burning of rectum.
7. *Genito-urinary:* Frequent, urgent, or painful urination; inability to control bladder; vaginal itching or discharge.
8. *Muscular:* Fatigue, generalized muscular weakness, muscle and joint pain, stiffness, soreness, chest pain, backache, neck muscle spasm, generalized spasticity.
9. *Nervous system:* Headache, migraine, compulsively sleepy, drowsy, groggy, slow, sluggish, dull, depressed, serious, crying; tense, anxious, stimulated, overactive, restless, jittery, convulsive, head feels full or enlarged, floating, silly, giggling, laughing, inebriated; unable to concentrate, feel-

ing of separateness or apartness from others, amnesia for words or numbers or names, stammering or stuttering speech.

What should the person do who suspects he may have some sort of sensitivity? His first step should be to seek competent medical advice from an allergy specialist.

6. Allergic? You Can't Trust Food Labels To List All Ingredients

One summer day in 1974, Jeffrey Shallit, 16, of Wynnewood, Pa., ate a piece of packaged cake. Moments later, he rushed into his parents' bedroom clutching his throat. It was closing up on him. His parents, knowing that Jeffrey was allergic to many foods, and ready for most emergencies, gave him an antihistamine. He broke out in a rash and began to wheeze. When two adrenalin shots failed to help, Jeffrey was rushed to the hospital where he was placed in an oxygen tent. Another adrenalin shot and intravenous solutions were administered, but it was touch and go for five hours. Finally, Jeffrey came around.

The underlying cause of Jeffrey's attack was a series of loopholes in food labeling regulations which permit hundreds of additives and food substances to be used in food products without declaration on the label. While Jeffrey was well aware of the fact that he was highly allergic to peanuts, the label on the cake he ate said not a word about peanuts. But when his father called the bakery, he discovered that the "vegetable shortening" mentioned was actually a mixture of peanut oil and cottonseed oil (*Philadelphia Evening Bulletin,* Aug. 16, 1974).

A Fatal Dish Of Ice Cream
But Jeffrey was luckier than 10-year-old Michael Grzybinski, of Dedham, Mass. Michael, like Jeffrey, was allergic to peanuts and knew it. In 1972, at a friend's house, he ate some ice cream called "Butterfinger," which had no ingredients listed on it except for a picture of a candy bar. Assuming there were no peanuts in it, Michael ate the ice cream.

Minutes later, he was dead, the victim of an extreme allergic reaction.

At the time, it was thought that Michael's tragic death would serve notice on the Food and Drug Administration (FDA) and food manufacturers that they had a responsibility to label manufactured food products completely and truthfully. As Michael's father commented at the time, "Michael's death will not go to waste" (*Boston Globe*, May 21, 1972).

But Jeffrey's experience shows that the food industry and its official regulators learned little from Michael's death.

In fact, present FDA regulations exempt food manufacturers from telling the consumer *any* of the ingredients they add to a multitude of food products. Other products need only list *some* of the ingredients. Even when there is a list of ingredients on a label, this may only be a *partial* contents disclosure.

Consumer Protection Becomes Consumer Confusion

The problem is basically this: The FDA has established a large number of so-called "standards of identity." The original—and quite valid—purpose of these standards was to ensure that certain manufactured food products which had become known to the consumer by common names would be substantially the same regardless of manufacturer. In other words, all mayonnaise, regardless of manufacturer, would contain the same basic ingredients because it would be derived from the same government-established recipe. However, the FDA has also ruled that ingredients in a great many products covered by a standard of identity need not be listed on the label.

Some ingredients may come under such broad headings as spices, flavors and colors, while others are simply not identified at all. As a result, consumers often cannot determine, for example, whether nuts or oat gum are contained in ice cream, whether lard is contained in jam, whether mustard is contained in mayonnaise, or whether Red Dye No. 2 is in any particular cake mix.

Even when ingredients are required to be in certain products, consumers often are not told by a label declaration of their inclusion. Examples of this include caffeine in cola beverages and egg yolks in mayonnaise.

The problem is made almost intolerable for the consumer because, while not *requiring* the listing of all ingredients, the FDA does *permit* the companies to list those ingredients they wish to. Thus, one often finds a list of ingredients on an ice cream label and a listing of six ingredients on a cola beverage. But these are lists of only those ingredients which the manufacturer *wants* to include along with those ingredients whose disclosure the FDA may require.

Foods That Can Fool You

The FDA has established standards of identity for the following foods or classes of foods, which means that they may have either mandatory or optional ingredients not mentioned on their labels:

Cacao products
Cereal flours and related products
Macaroni and noodle products
Bakery products
Milk and cream
Cheeses, processed cheeses, cheese foods, cheese spreads, and related foods
Frozen desserts
Food flavorings
Dressings for food
Canned fruits and fruit juices
Fruit pies
Fruit butters, fruit jellies, fruit preserves, and related products
Nonalcoholic beverages
Shellfish
Fish
Eggs and egg products
Oleomargarine, margarine
Nut products
Canned vegetables
Tomato products

Until such time as the FDA or Congress act, the situation will become progressively worse. It is bad ethically, but downright dangerous medically. As Dr. Vincent J. Fontana of New York University Medical Center has pointed out, a large number of allergic reactions could probably be prevented if all foods, beverages, and drugs contained complete and truthful ingredient labeling (*Family Practice News*, April 15, 1974).

Knowing what is in food is important to every consumer who is concerned about what he eats. It is especially vital to millions of Americans with allergies.

7. Food Additives—3,000 Unsuspected Allergens

Processed convenience foods are expensive. First you pay for the food itself. Second, you pay a premium because the manufacturer has gone to all the trouble of chemicalizing, packaging, and advertising the product. Finally, an additional bill for processed foods is handed exclusively to a certain unlucky group of shoppers—those who have allergies. Besides their cash, these people pay for their food in such coinage as coughing, itching, runny nose, swollen throat, swollen tongue, nasal polyps, asthma, skin lesions, belching, flatulence, hives, canker sores, constipation, painful joints, bleeding in the gut, and good old-fashioned headaches. All because of something called *food additives*.

If you're among the 22 million people who the Allergy Foundation of America says suffer seriously from allergies, or among the 100 million Americans who Howard G. Rappaport, M.D., and Shirley M. Linde, M.S., estimate have some allergic sensitivities (*The Complete Allergy Guide*, Simon and Schuster, 1970), this is but a taste of the calamities skulking in processed food. The list of symptoms mentioned above represents those which have been linked with *a single class of food additives*—flavorings. There are 13 classes all together.

But aren't there also natural foods which can cause allergies? Sure there are, potentially every one of them. The point is, once you find out you're allergic to raspberries, your problem is over. You just don't eat them any more. With processed foods, it's a different story, because you literally have no idea what you're eating. In all likelihood, your doctor doesn't either. The label on the container may say "Beef Stroganoff Mix" or "Fruit Cocktail," but the day after you serve it, you could put the same label on your overflowing garbage can and it would be about as accurate. The fact that the label may include in its list of ingredients (if it has one at all) things like "preservatives," "artificial coloring," and "antioxidants" is no help at all. There are no less than 33 different kinds of preservatives, 34 different food colorings, and

28 antioxidants. Which particular agents are being used in your so-called Beef Stroganoff or Fruit Cocktail is anybody's guess.

Russian Roulette In The Supermarket

The result is that allergy sufferers are playing Russian roulette every time they go shopping for processed foods. The odds against them are staggering.

At last count, the Food and Drug Administration had approved close to 3,000 additives for use in foodstuffs and beverages. Among them, besides the preservatives, coloring agents and antioxidants, are 45 sequestrants; 111 surface active agents; 36 stabilizers and thickeners; 24 bleaching and maturing agents; 60 buffers, acids and alkalies; 4 sweeteners; 117 nutritive supplements; 502 natural flavorings, and a whopping 1,610 synthetic flavorings. In addition, there are 157 "miscellaneous" additives, which include such items as texturizers, firming agents, and binders.

Sound like a lot to be gambling with? Actually, it's only the beginning, because a great many other additives are also injected into our foodstuffs as "secret formulas." As Dr. Ben F. Feingold points out, "These formulas for the most part are not available to the public" (*Annals of Allergy*, June, 1968). The manufacturer need not list them, need not even reveal them to a doctor treating an allergy victim near death. This is perfectly legal. In addition, there is the problem of these additives combining with each other or with bodily substances to create a whole new spectrum of bizarre allergens. According to the authors of *The Complete Allergy Guide*, Dr. Stephen D. Lockey has reported tracking down 30,000 additives so far in foods, beverages, and drugs. If that isn't enough, consider this: routine skin testing used by allergists is of little or no use in determining sensitivity to many food additives.

Allergic reactions to this galaxy of additives are not mere nuisances. Dr. Rappaport stated that one-third of all chronic diseases in children under 17 are caused by allergies, and that allergies are the most common cause of disability among schoolchildren. "Allergy victims spend an estimated $135 million for medicines and another $100 million for injections. Allergic patients require an average of *three times* as many medical visits as those with other types of illnesses." How many actually die each year as a result of allergies? Dr. Rappaport puts the figure at "many thousands."

Yellow Dye Can Cause Asthma

All this suffering caused by food additives should come under the heading of "criminal negligence."

Yet virtually none of the products containing these additives are accurately labeled. When was the last time you saw a bottle of soda pop that said on the label "contains Red No. 2" or "contains Yellow No. 5"? Yet the latter additive, also known as tartrazine, has been reported to cause severe intractable asthma (Chafee and Settipane, "Asthma Caused by F. D. & C. Approved Dyes," *Journal of Allergies,* 1967). Keep in mind that these are just coloring additives. Consider the whole population, the profusion of concealed chemicals in the food supply, and you get some idea of the magnitude of the crime involved in using, but not identifying, food additives.

All the thousands of these additives, by the way, are classified as "intentional" and are approved by the FDA. The matter of contamination by such substances as hormones, antibiotics, and pesticides is a different kettle of synthetic fish, but just as rotten as far as the allergy sufferer is concerned.

What about simply forcing the manufacturers to list the additives on the label? Allergy victims and doctors have been pleading for years to get such a ruling. But you can forget that one too: manufacturers are allergic to labeling.

The solution is obvious. If you want to avoid needless allergies, as well as a host of other debilitating conditions, don't eat processed foods. There isn't any dish you can't make at home that won't come out fresher, tastier, more nutritious, and probably less expensive than commercially-prepared foods. The cost of a grinder, blender, a couple of natural food cookbooks, and a few extra pots and pans isn't much when you consider your shopping bill will be less. And just think of all those hives, headaches and doctor bills you may be avoiding.

8. For About One-In-Four, Children And Chocolate Don't Mix

There are numerous foods that are possible sources of allergy in children. One of the worst, however, and yet one that we seem to hear the least about, is cocoa in all its forms. Children most commonly eat it as chocolate candy or as chocolate syrup in milk. Both these forms are no less dangerous than any other form of cocoa.

A special danger presented by chocolate is that it both tastes delicious to almost everyone and is habit-forming, in precisely the same sense as coffee and cigarettes are habit-forming. Children allergic to milk or to wheat cereals will frequently develop an aversion toward such foods. They will not drink milk or eat bread under any circumstances. But once they have grown accustomed to chocolate, they go on wanting it in spite of asthma attacks and other allergic symptoms the chocolate may produce.

When you consider how often nursery school and kindergarten teachers will distribute chocolate candy to their charges with no awareness of the harm they might be doing, and when you consider that the allergic child who will refuse a glass of milk every time will be more inclined to accept the piece of candy, then it can be seen that this particular allergen may well deserve to be considered the most dangerous of all.

We cannot really blame the teacher or the friendly neighbor who unthinkingly offers a child a piece of chocolate. How often do you recall seeing any warning at all that cocoa and chocolate are potentially dangerous foods? Yet in a September, 1966, article in the *Annals of Allergy*, Joseph H. Fries, M.D., of Nassau Hospital, Long Island, New York, listed the following allergic reactions of children to eating chocolate:

Chills
Vomiting
Itching mouth
Abdominal pain

Chest wheeze
Cough
Clogged nose
Sneezing
Eczematous eruption of the skin
Itching
Hives
Sores around the mouth

Three Of Every Four Allergic Children Vulnerable

Nor are such reactions to chocolate scarce, as one might think from the utter lack of publicity given to the dangers of this sweet. As reported in his *Annals of Allergy* article, Dr. Fries took 100 consecutive records of allergic children who had come to his hospital for testing. Taking them just as they come in order, with no attempt at selection, made this an excellent random sample from which to draw conclusions. Of the 100 records he examined, 76 of the children were found to react allergically to chocolate. And this is a very good indication that of all allergic children, we can expect three-quarters to react with one or more of the symptoms listed above when they eat this delicious but inherently troublesome food.

The frequency of the chocolate allergy was a surprise even to Dr. Fries, a practicing pediatrician who might have been expected to be aware of the problem. But obviously, this material has somehow managed to remain unknown even to the experts.

Perhaps the trouble lies in the very deliciousness of chocolate. We don't like to think that anything we really enjoy could be harming us, and doctors are as human as the rest of us in that respect.

Chocolate Contains A Powerful Stimulant

Yet even if the child is not allergic to chocolate, the simple fact is that chocolate contains the alkaloid theobromine, which is used medically as a heart stimulant. Theobromine is recognized as a frequent cause of gastrointestinal distress, and is as dangerous for a child as caffeine or nicotine. Parents who would not think of permitting their children to drink a cup of coffee or smoke a cigarette are every day unknowingly giving them equally stimulating and habit-forming alkaloid theobromine every time they give them chocolate candy, cocoa or chocolate milk.

If you have been giving chocolate to your child, can you stop it now? You certainly should, but you won't find it easy. In the words of Dr. Fries, "Whereas with many other allergenic foods an instinctive dislike exists and there is a willingness on the part of the child to avoid them, no such helpful dislike is seen with chocolate . . . . Even in the occasional instances I have observed of fairly severe physical disturbances (abdominal pain, vomiting, nausea) associated with ingestion of chocolate, the child still welcomes it."

Theobromine is closely related chemically to caffeine, according to Dr. Fries. "Analogy suggests habituation to the alkaloid," he says. "Such habituation would explain in part the devotion one sees to chocolate ingestion."

Carob Makes An Excellent Substitute

All in all, once you have made up your mind to stop your child's chocolate eating, you will not find it easy sledding. The child will go on demanding his candy and probably refuse to understand that it is bad for him. Dr. Fries suggests that instead of outright deprivation, you offer a substitute. "There have appeared on the market confections made from carob bean (St. John's Bread), the fruit of the carob tree," he says. "These mimic to a remarkable degree the appearance, the texture, and most important, the taste of chocolate. Carob is a legume of low allergenic potential." And he suggests that your best chance of actually breaking your child of the chocolate-eating habit is to substitute confections made with carob. These are frequently available using honey or molasses as a sweetener, rather than sugar. If you make up your mind to eliminate chocolate from your home, you will have no difficulty in finding carob substitutes that are not only just as good, but are actually far better in taste as well as in nutrition.

9. The Pulse Test For Allergy

Suppose you suspect that you are one of those individuals who is allergic to one or more substances that will not be revealed by the skin patch test allergists normally administer.

Is there anything you can do for yourself to discover food and possible chemical substances that you should be avoiding for the best health?

According to the late Arthur F. Coca, M.D., whose classic work, *The Pulse Test,* has been reprinted in paperback by Arco Publishing Company, if you can develop some skill in taking your own pulse accurately, that is the only tool you need to uncover your own allergies.

Pulse Speeds During Attacks

One of the most prominent allergists in the country, Dr. Coca made his original discovery about allergy and pulse rate when his wife had a heart attack. Two heart specialists gave her five years to live . She began to notice that further attacks came after eating certain very common foods. At the same time Dr. Coca discovered that her pulse always became faster when she ate these foods. So he began in his practice to use this means of determining which foods caused allergies in his patients.

In his wife's case the heart attacks did not recur. And probably more astounding even than this, other complaints disappeared, too, when she stopped eating foods to which she was allergic. (She had suffered from many minor symptoms—indigestion, heartburn, hives, neuralgia, tiredness, dizziness, constipation, nasal stuffiness and so forth.)

Putting to work in his own practice what he had learned from his wife's experience, Dr. Coca quickly found that he could relieve his patients of many diseases simply by having them avoid foods that raised their pulse rate. He tells us in his book that there are three steps necessary to provide proof that the foods are actually the exciting cause of the disorders. First, many of the patients had not one but several distressing symptoms, all of which disappeared when they avoided foods to which they were allergic. Second, in most instances, all the former symptoms could be produced at will simply by eating the forbidden food again, and third, without exception, the pulse rate was increased when these foods were eaten.

Here are two samples from Dr. Coca's case histories: A woman of 70 was overweight and troubled with neuralgia, constipation, colds and fatigue. By the pulse-rate test, she was found to be allergic to nine foods. As long as she avoided these foods her symptoms disappeared, and in the bargain she lost 35 pounds of weight. A young man who suffered from epilepsy found that he was allergic to four different kinds of food. After experiencing no seizures for three months, he deliberately ate one of the offending foods and, next morning, had another seizure.

How To Get Started

Here is an outline of Dr. Coca's pulse-testing technique.

Begin by recording carefully everything that you eat at every meal for about a week. In addition, take your pulse at the following times each day during the week: before rising (in a lying down position before you get out of bed in the morning), just before each meal, three times (at 30 minute intervals) after each meal and again just before going to bed. This is a total of fourteen pulse counts each day.

Now, how do you take your pulse? Dr. Coca says, "The most convenient spot is at the wrist an inch and a half above the base of the thumb. Place the left hand (if you are right-handed) in the lap with the palm facing up. Then place the first two fingers of the right hand on the wrist so that their average distance is about an inch and a half from the base of the thumb, and three quarters of an inch from the end of the wrist. . . .

"When counting your pulse, have a watch or a clock with a second hand close in view. Pick up the pulse with the fingertips and wait until the second hand reaches 60. Then count on the next pulse-beat and continue counting the beats until the second hand has made a complete circuit and returned to 60 which will make the completion of the minute. The number of the pulse-beats counted in one minute is the pulse rate."

Look For Wide Variations

It does not matter whether you stand or sit for making the tests, but be consistent—do either one or the other for all tests. If the highest pulse count that you get every day for a week is not over

84 and if it is the same each day, you are probably not allergic to any food. On any given day the range from the lowest count to the highest count will probably not be more than 16 beats.

A count greater than 85 points to food allergy.

If the highest count varies more than two beats from day to day you are certainly allergic. That is, if on Monday you should have a count of 72, on Tuesday 78, Wednesday 76, Thursday 71.

If your rates seem to indicate that you are not allergic to any food you ate on a particular day, but on the other days the jump from high to low is great or there is a count above 84, then it is wise to eat again for several days the same foods you had on the non-allergenic day, adding to it only one food at a time, to see if you can locate the offending food that way.

Smoking complicates the whole picture. Dr. Coca's own patients had to give up smoking while they were doing the tests. There are many people who are allergic to no food, but are allergic to tobacco.

Finding Your Specific Allergens

Now, suppose you have discovered that, according to your pulse test, you are probably allergic to something you eat every day (and it seems that most food allergies involve some common everyday kind of food). How do you go about finding out which one it is?

Give yourself a couple of free weekends, when your time is your own, and you can experiment to your heart's content. Eat nothing for dinner on Friday night. Next morning, begin your tests by eating one everyday kind of food at a time and taking your pulse just before eating and at half hour intervals after eating this single food. You might first eat a slice of bread, let's say. Next you might take a boiled egg, do the three pulse tests at half-hour intervals after eating it, then try another food, and so forth. Dr. Coca says that ten or twelve single foods can thus be tested in a weekend.

Dr. Coca tells us that in general the pulse rate does not fluctuate greatly in the average person during usual daily activities, so you needn't worry that a change in rate is due to stress or strain rather than the food you eat. However, there are, of course, some activities that do increase the pulse. We suggest that on days when you are doing your first pulse testing you follow your usual activities. Don't decide to learn a new dance step, put a new roof on the porch, take up long distance running or something equally violent. Special exertion to which you are not accustomed can easily raise your pulse.

In a chapter entitled "Almost Miraculous Case Histories," Dr. Coca tells of his own patients suffering from diabetes, ulcers, eczema, hemorrhoids, overweight, epilepsy and hives, whose health was restored as soon as they discovered and eliminated the offending foods. A physician and his wife, both diabetics, found that they were allergic to cereals. After they had eliminated cereals from their meals they found that they could eat foods generally forbidden to diabetics, with no increase in their blood sugar levels. Of course for the rest of their lives they had to make certain they ate nothing that contained any grain substance.

Another patient suffering from eczema found that he was allergic to cereals, oranges, honey, fowl, lamb, a popular shaving cream and soap powder. Cutting out the use of all these eliminated his eczema and at the same time brought his blood pressure down from 140 to 120.

A chemist with stomach ulcers found that he was allergic to milk, after he had lived for some time on milk alone at his doctor's suggestion. He was allergic to only that one food and after he cut it out, he had no more trouble with his stomach.

10. A Sting Is Serious Business If You're Allergic

It is estimated that only about 30 Americans a year die from stings of *Hymenoptera* (bees, hornets, yellow jackets, wasps and fire ants). The venom they release can act as an allergen in sensitive people or as a poison when there are frequent stings in a short time. But it is the relatively few persons with a true allergy who get the worst of it—a bad case of hives all over the body, or wheezing, dizziness, stomach cramps, diarrhea, vomiting and faintness. A few get a tightness in the throat and suffer slight respiratory symptoms. Joints may become swollen and painful.

For most of us a bee sting causes a painful swelling at the site of the sting, which disappears after several hours. If you get more of a reaction than that you should make very certain that where bees are, you aren't.

The worst thing about the *Hymenoptera* is that there are so many of them. A sensitive person can't really be sure that he won't be confronted with a bee or wasp when he's out on a summer day. And they often sting with little or no provocation. The only member of the *Hymenoptera* family that seems to "think twice" about stinging is the honey bee. For him, to sting is to die, since the stinger and the venom sac remain in the victim, causing the bee fatal abdominal injury. A honey bee encountered as it works among the flowers won't sting unless provoked. But hornets and yellow jackets are easily disturbed and will sting literally at the drop of a hat, especially near their nest-building activity. Their stings are sharp, painful and quick to bring serious results in allergic people.

Beekeepers Develop Immunity

Researchers from the State University of New York at Buffalo kept an extensive history of 45 beekeepers, hoping to throw some light on bee sting immunity for help in treating sensitive individuals. Two of the men reported 1,000 to 2,000 bee stings a week, but the average number was 50 to 100 times a week. Blood tests showed that almost all of the beekeepers had built up immunity.

Persons with other allergic disorders are the ones most likely to be allergic to the stings of bees and other insects. Anyone who suspects an unusual allergy to stings should have skin tests by a physician to pinpoint the allergenic insect. The desensitization injections can be given. The treatment involves concentrations of venom injected in minute amounts until a tolerance is built up in the patient. Venom extracts available are: the honey bee, bumble bee, wasp, hornet, yellow jacket, red ant and fire ants. Serious reactions are halted by this treatment in about 97 percent of cases.

Emergency kits are also available for sensitive persons. Such a kit might include a hypodermic syringe with adrenalin, an adrenalin inhaler, a tourniquet and antihistamine tablets. An injection of adrenalin is the best way to counteract shock, according to the Allergy Foundation of America. The tourniquet is used to stop the spread of venom (application of ice to the sting site also helps). The inhaler helps to combat spasms in the bronchial tubes. The antihistamines sometimes help to counter inflammation.

Some Simple Rules For Avoiding Stings

The best way to combat dangerous stings is to prevent them. Here is a check list for discouraging bee stings:

Keep the garbage can clean and covered. Any kind of food attracts bees and wasps.

Gardening in any but well-turned patches of earth is dangerous for a sensitive person. Hornet nests are hard to spot in shrubs that are being trimmed, and yellow jacket nests often lie in lawns and underbrush.

Do you wear brightly colored billowy clothing in the warm months? It's the very thing that attracts insects. So do sweet smelling cosmetics and hair sprays. These things make you resemble a flower and bees love flowers.

Don't move wood or logs in empty lots or in the woods. These are typical locations for wasps' nests. If you shake up a wasp's home, you can expect him to retaliate.

Don't go barefoot, and don't let your children go barefoot on unfamiliar territory, unless you are willing to risk a sting on the bottom of the foot.

If you do get stung, get rid of the stinger at once by scraping, not pressing, it off with your fingernail. The longer the stinger stays in your skin, the more venom it releases into your body. It takes two or three minutes for the stinger to empty. If the insect doesn't lose his stinger, knock him off the skin quickly.

Remember, bees don't take kindly to interference in their regular routine. If you see a bee, move out of range if you can. If you can't get away, don't thrash about. Try to remain calm. Don't make sudden movements. They can make a bee sense that he is in danger, and that's when instinct tells him to sting. He might kill you.

Section 3
Anemia

11. Understanding Iron Deficiency Anemia

Iron deficiency is the single most common cause of anemia in the world. Afflicting all nations, it is epidemic in such countries as India, Vietnam and Bangladesh. But although a deficiency of iron is epidemic among the people of impoverished countries, what has not been generally recognized is that iron deficiency is also quite common in the United States.

Writing in the *Journal of the American Medical Association* (March 13, 1972), Dr. Clement A. Finch, a noted authority on iron metabolism, estimated that 25 percent of the women and infants in this country are deficient in iron—about one out of every four. That may not be an epidemic, but it's an alarming number! Because in America, where plenty of iron is available, risking one's health by becoming iron deficient is a little like starving to death in a food warehouse.

Iron Builds Healthy, Red Blood

The cause of iron deficiency anemia is a combination of the limited amount of iron which can be absorbed from the modern diet, and the occurrence of blood loss. But before looking closer at the symptoms, causes and prevention of iron deficiency, let's take a look at what iron does in maintaining your health.

In all, a normal adult's body contains four or five grams of body iron. Women have less than men: they are smaller and they lose iron periodically for much of their lives. Thus, a 40-year-old woman, the mother of two children, would normally have a total body iron content of four grams. This is not a lot of elemental iron: hardly a thimble full.

Even though you don't have steel girders circulating in your vessels, iron is still the most important element in your body. That's right, iron is the most valuable substance in the body, and not just in humans but throughout the animal kingdom! Why? Because animal life could not go on without iron.

Most of your body iron—about three of the four grams—is found in the red blood cells, as an essential component of

40

hemoglobin. There it acts as postmaster general of the circulation, carrying oxygen from the lungs to the tissues. A small amount of iron is found in muscle, and trace amounts serve in the enzyme systems of the cells. The remaining iron, about one gram, or a fourth of the total, is called *storage iron,* because it's not really in use. Stored in the liver, spleen and bone marrow, it's in reserve in case the body needs it. Storage iron is a buffer, a "spare tire" to keep from running out of this precious substance. Once your storage iron is used up, the symptoms of iron deficiency anemia are not far away, especially if you continue to take in less iron than you need.

Anemia Causes Extreme Fatigue

You might suspect, hearing how varied and important are the functions of iron, that many different symptoms could result from its deficiency. You'd be right. Probably the most common symptom is fatigue. We all get tired, but the fatigue of iron deficiency anemia is one of extreme dead-tiredness. A patient who was iron deficient remarked that when she walked she had the feeling that an elephant was perched on each of her shoulders. Another said that she was okay for about the first five steps she took, but then her shoes felt like they weighed 25 pounds and got heavier with each step. Needless to say, they were happy to rid themselves of the elephants and weighted shoes by correcting the iron deficiency.

Rapid heartbeat upon even the slightest exertion is a symptom of iron deficiency, as is moderate swelling of the ankles and face. In long-standing cases, the fingernails turn brittle, lose their luster and begin to curve sharply downward at the tip of the nail. The skin, too, may change. It may lose its normal stretchability and become thick and dry. The linings of the mouth and eyes may turn from a healthy pink to a pale or sallow color. The tongue may become sore, and have a slick, shiny red appearance. Nervousness, headache and loss of appetite are common symptoms of iron deficiency.

Sometimes iron deficiency is accompanied by bizarre cravings. A group of patients written up in the *Annals of Internal Medicine* (September, 1968) knew when they were becoming iron deficient because each would develop a ravenous appetite for ice. One patient ate it by the five-pound block, and her husband took her to the doctor because he couldn't get any sleep. Her crunching of ice all night kept him awake. Sure enough the lady was iron deficient, and after appropriate treatment her craving for ice disappeared.

Why does iron deficiency occur? Because people don't get enough from what they eat to make up for the losses of iron by the body. Iron balance works like a checking account at the bank. There are certain bills that must be paid—the rent, groceries, utilities—and if you don't put enough money into the bank to cover these expenses, your account will become deficient and the bank will waste no time letting you know.

Absorption Is The Key

In general, there are two ways you can fail to get enough iron in your diet. You may not be eating foods that are rich in iron, or you may not absorb enough of the iron you do eat. Let's talk about the latter, poor absorption, first.

Normally, the body can absorb *at most* only about 10 percent of the iron it gets in food. This is enough to supply your needs if you eat the right foods and don't lose an excessive amount of blood. Meat, fish and fowl are rich in iron. Green vegetables, sun-dried raisins, brown rice, wheat germ and fruit contain good portions of iron.

But one of our problems in getting enough iron from the diet is that modern processing of foods as well as some cooking methods take out much of the iron before it reaches us. White bread, for example, said to be "iron-enriched," actually contains no more iron than would normally be obtained from whole wheat bread without any enrichment. More important, the organic iron naturally present in whole wheat is better absorbed than the inorganic iron with which refined flour is enriched.

Another cause of poor iron absorption is an inadequate production of hydrochloric acid by the stomach. Hydrochloric acid is necessary to convert dietary iron into an absorbable form. The content of hydrochloric acid in the stomach decreases as people grow older, which may play a role in the iron deficiency of elderly persons.

Lack of iron absorption may result from chronic diarrhea or even the regular taking of laxatives, because the iron is simply not absorbed when food is flushed through the intestine at a faster than normal rate. Diseases of malabsorption, such as sprue and celiac disease, are accompanied by poor absorption of iron.

Of course, you have to eat the right iron-containing foods to have any chance at all to absorb iron and avoid anemia. A lot of ordinary folks simply don't eat enough of the right foods to satisfy their bodies' need for iron.

In infants who are iron deficient, a poor diet is almost always the cause. In the book, *Iron Metabolism* (Little, Brown & Company) by Dr. T. H. Bothwell and Dr. Finch, the authors point out that a child's blood volume triples in the first year of life, and a lot of iron is required to make all those new red blood cells. The increased need for iron continues at least until the time of puberty. Babies not only should be fed at the breast or with an iron-enriched formula, they should be started on meat-containing baby foods at the age of three months.

Vitamin C Aids Iron Absorption

No matter how much iron you get in your diet or from some iron preparation, that mineral is useless to you unless it is absorbed. It is estimated that even under the best circumstances, only 10 percent of the iron that is consumed is utilized by the body. There are several teammates which iron insists upon before it will play the blood game. One of these is vitamin C. In fact, severe anemia is one of the symptoms of scurvy, a condition which results from prolonged depletion of vitamin C stores. The importance of vitamin C to the absorption of iron was highlighted by Emil Maro Schleicher, Ph.D., director of hematology at St. Barnabas Hospital in Minneapolis, who noted in the February, 1970 issue of *Minnesota Medicine* that "while clinicians may be aware that iron salts such as ferrous sulfate and ferrous gluconate are effective hematinics (blood builders) they may not fully appreciate the reason for compounding ferrous salts with ascorbic acid."

Dr. Schleicher treated 30 female patients, age 14 to 42, who suffered from iron deficiency in the blood plasma due to excessive internal bleeding. He gave each patient one tablet twice daily containing 200 milligrams of ferrous fumarate (another iron salt) and 600 milligrams of ascorbic acid. Iron deficiency "was alleviated within 60 days."

It is possible that the vitamin C partnership with the iron may have served to correct a malabsorption syndrome. Twenty-one of the patients were examined a year after therapy was discontinued. All of them experienced normal menstrual discharges, and blood tests revealed that their iron stores remained normal.

In another study, reported in the *American Journal of Clinical Nutrition,* April, 1968, by Dr. Paul R. McCurdy of Georgetown

University School of Medicine and Dr. Raymond J. Dern of Loyola University Stritch School of Medicine, vitamin C was proved unquestionably to enhance iron absorption. McCurdy and Dern found that with doses of ferrous sulfate ranging from 15 to 120 mg., ascorbic acid in 200 to 500 milligram amounts nearly doubled the absorption of the iron. At every dosage level of iron, they found that 500 milligrams of ascorbic acid was better than 200 milligrams.

When taking vitamin C to boost iron absorption, you've got to take enough. It has been shown that what is considered a normal intake of vitamin C by the National Research Council—"from 10 to 50 milligrams"—had no effect whatsoever on the absorption of iron. This was demonstrated in earlier Scandinavian studies by H. Brise and L. Halberg. It took at least 200 milligrams of the vitamin to initiate absorption of iron while the best possible absorption was achieved with doses of 500 milligrams. Using 500 milligrams, it was found that 1.88 times as much iron—nearly twice as much—was absorbed. Thus, it is possible to administer less iron and secure greater absorption by adding vitamin C to the iron compound.

Copper, too, in minute amounts, is essential for the best absorption of iron. C. A. Elvehjem and W. C. Sherman, writing in the *Journal of Biological Chemistry* (98, 309-1932) tell us that while the body can assimilate iron without copper, it cannot utilize iron for hemoglobin regeneration unless copper is included in the diet. One of the best sources for copper as well as for iron is liver.

Women Need More Iron Than Men

Just as infants and children need more iron than adults, women need more iron than men—twice as much. The reason is that women lose iron in the menstrual cycle, pregnancy and childbirth. One pregnancy may deplete a woman of almost a gram of iron—unless she takes adequate iron supplements. Between the ages of about 15 and 45, a woman loses an average of one-third of a gram of iron each year in the menstrual bleeding. A third of a gram per year for 30 years equals 10 grams of iron. Considering that her *total body iron* at any given time is about four grams of iron, the loss of 10 grams cannot be taken lightly! Disastrous results don't occur, however, because the 10 grams of iron are lost over such a long period of time. A woman can absorb enough extra to make up for it—if she takes good care of herself. Many women are in a precarious state of iron balance because their iron stores have been used up and not replaced.

"The Disease Of Virgins"

Iron deficiency anemia in young girls was noted long before this age of opulent supermarkets. A dramatic, severe form that once plagued many teenage girls is called chlorosis, or the green anemia. It was usually caused by an inadequate iron intake, excessive early menstruation, and deficits of other nutrients such as protein, says Dr. William D. Snively in his book, *Sea of Life* (David McKay, 1969). The first report of this ailment came from a European physician, Dr. Johannes Lange, way back in 1554. Dr. Lange called the ailment "the disease of virgins" because most of the patients he saw were virgins. He believed that all that was needed to cure the disease was for the virgin to marry. Actually, iron deficiency anemia had nothing to do with virginity. It simply occurred frequently in young girls because of their early menstrual problems and their tendency to eat improperly. Dr. Lange described the symptoms of the green anemia in a most accurate manner. He wrote ". . . her face is sadly paled, the heart trembles with every movement of her body, and the arteries of her temples pulsate, and she is seized . . . with shortness of breath . . . her stomach loathes food and particularly meat, and the legs especially at the ankles become edematous at night . . ."

In the spring of 1965, the U.S. Department of Agriculture obtained one-day diet records from members of families included in the Household Food Consumption Survey. The average daily iron intake of over 5,000 girls and women from 15 to 54 years of age was about 11 milligrams. When the data was broken down, there was no striking difference according to the level of income. Nor did it matter whether the girl was a Southern belle or a Northern yankee. In all income groups and in both the North and South, girls 15 to 17 years of age consumed less iron per 1,000 calories than did women 35 to 54 years of age.

Over the past years, more recent surveys have consistently shown that girls consume an average iron intake of about 10 to 11 milligrams per day. Thus they are getting only 55 to 60 percent of the recommended dietary allowance which is 18 milligrams a day for all females from 11 to 50 years of age.

What To Do If Anemia Strikes

The best way to stay ahead of iron deficiency anemia is to eat a diet rich in iron. This is nature's way, and no one has yet come up with anything better. Since meat is the best source of iron, two good servings of meat should be eaten every day. Liver, a highly nutritious food, is rich in iron. So are apricots, wheat germ and molasses. Whole wheat bread and whole grain cereal are additional good sources of iron. Set them on your table, and when buying food, purchase whole grain or iron-enriched flour products in preference to non-enriched ones. When preparing food, keep in mind that the more it is cooked the less iron will be available. It isn't necessary to eat the meat rare, but couldn't you eat it medium rather than very well done? Also, favor broiling over frying in the preparation of meat.

Your doctor will probably prescribe ferrous sulfate or ferrous gluconate. Iron compounds are, of course, necessary for the frankly anemic. Bear in mind, however, that a large dose or even an average dose can cause gastrointestinal irritation, according to the *Merck Index*. Ferrous gluconate causes less distress than the sulfate.

However, by adding 500 mg. of vitamin C, your doctor may well get good results with less of the compound, and thus lessen the incidence of digestive disorders that are frequently associated with iron therapy.

Ferrous compounds can also be destructive of vitamin E, which is sorely needed by the anemic because it conserves oxygen. If you must build up your blood or your daughter's quickly and cannot wait for the relatively slower—though safer—process of replenishing iron stores through eating iron-rich foods, separate the times when you take your iron and vitamin E by twelve hours. Try taking your iron in the morning and your E after dinner. This does not hold true for natural organic iron in foods. The iron in foods does not cancel out vitamin E.

By all means, include iron-rich foods in your diet and in your daughter's. But since teenage girls have notorious eating habits and tend to eat and run, your very best insurance against iron deficiencies would be to give her several tablets of desiccated liver several times a day, every day of the month. Desiccated liver is a good source of natural iron plus the B vitamins that are so necessary to the manufacture of sufficient hydrochloric acid, which helps utilize both the iron and vitamin C.

Once a girl has become anemic, therapy is a tricky matter. Sometimes enriching her diet with liver and other iron-rich foods will pull her out of it. Sometimes therapy via food alone will not work. This is for your physician to decide.

Far better to prevent iron deficiency in the first place.

12. You Need Vitamin E To Prevent Anemia

The red cells in the blood stream have an important job to do, a job that only they can perform—carrying oxygen-bearing hemoglobin to every cell in the body. They have been specially designed to do that one job and do it well. Without them and their life-giving oxygen, our cells would "starve" and die.

But red cells don't go on working forever. After about 120 days they break up and their hemoglobin is lost. Fortunately, however, not all of the red cells expire at the same time. The turnover that does take place, although seemingly on a grand scale, is perfectly normal, biochemist Isaac Asimov reassures us: "If our average adult has 25,000,000,000,000 (twenty-five trillion) red cells altogether and 1/125 (or 0.8 percent) of them break up each day, then 200,000,000,000, (two hundred billion) are being destroyed daily, or 2,300,000 each second. Of course, this should not be at all disturbing. The body can, and does, replace the quantity being broken down as fast as they are being broken down" (*The Living River*, Abelard Schuman).

But such a happy state of equilibrium doesn't always prevail. Sometimes the red cells quit prematurely. They disintegrate in the bloodstream before their time is up. The bone marrow can't replace them fast enough, and the result is *hemolytic anemia.* Iron supplements, recommended for some forms of anemia, won't help here; iron is vital to the formation of hemoglobin-rich cells, but the problem now is one of cell longevity, not quantity. There may be plenty of iron on hand to manufacture hemoglobin, but if that hemoglobin and the red cell that contains it meet an early end, it won't be doing your body much good.

Vitamin E Preserves Red Cells
Research findings reported in *The American Journal of Clinical Nutrition* (April, 1971) indicate that only vitamin E can keep these red cells on the job until they reach "retirement age."

The link between vitamin E and the health of red blood cells was demonstrated by Drs. Patrick J. Leonard and Monty S.

Losowsky of the Department of Medicine, St. James's Hospital, Leeds, England. They selected eight patients with vitamin E deficiency, as indicated by low plasma vitamin E levels and the abnormal susceptibility of their red cells to hemolysis (breakdown) by hydrogen peroxide in the test tube. (This hemolysis test is a standard diagnostic procedure for detecting vitamin E deficiency in man.)

To find out just how long the subjects' red cells were holding up, they were "labeled" with tiny amounts of radioactive chromium and reinjected into the bloodstream. Then, by measuring the rate of disappearance of the radioactivity, the researchers could tell just how fast the tagged red cells were being destroyed.

After a three-day wait to allow for an initial rapid loss of radioactivity from the cells, blood samples were taken at regular intervals. The radioactivity was measured, and the results plotted on a graph. Normally, the injected chromium could be expected to lose half of its radioactivity every 25 days, but in this case the chromium half-life for all eight subjects averaged out to only 19.2 days. This could mean only one thing: Their red cells were breaking down much too soon.

Aware that "in vitamin E deficiency, the red cell is known to be abnormally fragile in the response to hydrogen peroxide," the doctors decided to try vitamin E therapy. After an interval of from five to 15 days, they began giving the subjects a daily dose of alpha tocopherol (vitamin E)—200 milligrams orally and 100 mg. by injection.

They didn't have long to wait for results. In from one to four days, the plasma vitamin E level shot up to normal or above in all eight subjects, remaining "significantly higher" than before treatment in all but one.

But even more startling was the abrupt change in the plotted curves of the falling radioactivity. Following the start of vitamin E therapy and coincident with the attainment of normal plasma vitamin E levels, the rate of radioactivity loss in five of the eight subjects dropped markedly—the chromium-tagged red cells were no longer disappearing as fast. In fact, the half-life of the radioactive chromium was now averaging 24.9 days, well within the normal range. Somehow, the vitamin E was protecting the red cells, allowing them to survive longer. As Leonard and Losowsky put it, the results could only be interpreted as "suggesting a direct effect of circulating tocopherol . . . in maintaining the integrity of the red cells," resulting in "an actual improvement in red cell survival."

Mechanism Is Not Yet Certain

How does vitamin E promote the health and long life of the red cells? Many scientists have suggested that because the vitamin is a natural antioxidant in the body, it protects the cells by preventing the formation of hydrogen peroxide. In the absence of vitamin E, they explain, some of the essential fatty acids in our diets—notably linoleic acid—are permitted to combine with oxygen and form hydrogen peroxide, a known destroyer of red cells. In fact, the rate of formation of hydrogen peroxide in the blood has been used as an index of vitamin E deficiency.

Other researchers have suggested that without enough vitamin E, there may be a greater fragility of the outer membrane of the red cells, resulting in more frequent ruptures and the spilling of valuable hemoglobin. Or perhaps certain intracellular enzymes needed for membrane integrity are more readily oxidized in the absence of vitamin E. Whatever the case, vitamin E's protective effect on the red cells cannot be denied, even if the exact mechanism has yet to be agreed upon by scientists.

Particularly in the case of premature babies born with vitamin E deficiency and accompanying anemia, doctors have successfully employed vitamin E therapy, even after iron supplementation has failed. Four California investigators, Drs. J. Ritchie, M. Fish, V. McMasters and M. Grossman, gave 75 to 100 I.U. of vitamin E to five of seven premature infants. Even though the babies were on a commercial formula supplemented with 15 to 30 mg. of iron daily, their anemia failed to respond until vitamin E was added to their diet. Then, after a few days, their plasma tocopherol levels rose, their red cell survival time lengthened and the anemia was corrected (*The New England Journal of Medicine,* November 28, 1968).

Both in the test tube, and then in the babies, vitamin E had stopped the accelerated destruction of red cells. "The critical factor in both circumstances is that there must be, in the fluid bathing the erythrocytes (red cells), a level of tocopherol adequate to protect the red cells from oxidative damage and resultant hemolysis," the doctors concluded.

Deficiency Often Unidentified

But how common is this vitamin E deficiency anemia? Apparently it is much more widespread than generally suspected. As the four researchers cautioned, "The frequency with which this syndrome is observed will depend on the level of awareness of its existence, and the care with which it is sought. Some of the manifestations such as anemia, puffy eyes and firm legs with shiny skin, not unusual in premature infants and often called 'physiologic' or 'characteristic of prematures,' may prove in many cases to represent vitamin E deficiency."

In fact, thousands of premature infants have died—and may still be dying—because a vitamin deficiency is the last thing most doctors will look for when confronted with illness. Even with vitamin E deficiency well established by now as a cause of anemia in the newborn, we wonder how many doctors have learned about it—and how many hastily turned to another page in their medical journal rather than read an article about a vitamin.

Similar findings were reported three years earlier by two pediatricians at the University of Pennsylvania Hospital in Philadelphia. Drs. Lewis A. Barness and Frank A. Oski told a meeting of the American Pediatrics Society in May, 1965, that "A vitamin E deficiency appears to be a common nutritional disturbance that manifests itself as a hemolytic anemia in the premature infant of low birth weight."

The pair successfully corrected the condition in eight infants at the university hospital in an average time of 10 days, with vitamin E taken by mouth. "Vitamin E, unlike other nutrients, does not readily cross the placental barrier to nourish the fetus," Dr. Oski reported. Thus, infants often start out in life with low stores of the vitamin: serum tocopherol levels of newborns are only about one-fifth maternal blood levels. Faced with such a situation, the expectant mother would be well advised to increase her intake of the nutrient to make sure the infant gets enough. She should also nurse the new child, if possible. Mother's milk is an excellent source of vitamin E.

Premature infants aren't the only ones likely to suffer from hemolytic anemia, however. Back in the late 1960's, astronauts on Gemini orbital missions in outer space were returning to Earth with the same malady. It was found that the oxygen atmosphere aboard their spacecraft led to faster consumption of vitamin E, exposing the red cells to damage from hydrogen peroxide. In 1969, vitamin E supplements were added to the astronauts' diets and the problem cleared up.

You and your family may never be exposed to the same kind of risks and demanding situations as the astronauts, but the evidence is mounting that the amount of vitamin E in your diet can make the difference in protecting you from hemolytic anemia. And with the nutrient readily available from wheat germ oil, sunflower seeds and natural supplements, it hardly seems worth the risk to not get enough. Especially in the case of infants, expectant mothers and those with a history of anemia.

13. Pernicious Anemia

The word "anemia" brings to mind someone who is pale, listless, weak and devoid of spirit and energy. Actually, the word comes from the Greek and means literally "not-blood" or "lacking in blood."

There are so many different kinds of anemia that even the experts get them confused sometimes, so it is not surprising that we laymen find ourselves baffled, if we try to thread our way through the maze of terminology—aplastic, cytogenic, idiopathic, lymphatic, myelogenous, macrocytic, hypochromic. These are only some of the terms used to describe various kinds of anemia. The one we are concerned with here is pernicious anemia, one of the macrocytic anemias.

Symptoms Are Unusually Severe

Anemia is a deficiency of blood or a deficiency in the number of red blood corpuscles or a deficiency in the hemoglobin (red) content of the corpuscles. In macrocytic anemias, the body, trying desperately to provide enough red blood, produces abnormally large corpuscles. Hence the term *macrocytic*, which means "large cell." The laboratory technician, looking at a sample of blood in a microscope, can diagnose the pernicious anemia victim, for the corpuscles are few and very large.

Symptoms of pernicious anemia are: lack of hydrochloric acid in the stomach, an inflamed tongue and frequently, changes in the nervous system, all the way from painful neuritis to actual degeneration and destruction of parts of the spinal cord. The pernicious anemia patient lacks coordination of muscles, sways visibly when he stands with eyes closed, loses his sense of position, may become spastic, or have spasms. In addition, he suffers from upset stomach, extreme paleness, shortness of breath and indescribable fatigue.

Not a pleasant picture, is it, especially when you recall that before 1926 practically all cases of pernicious anemia had a fatal ending? No one knew what to give so that the red blood corpuscles would regenerate themselves and return to normal size. No medicine could relieve the symptoms. No amount of rest could relieve the terrible fatigue.

In 1926, researchers Whipple, Minot, and Murphy were successful in using liver to treat pernicious anemia. In some ways this was an unwieldy method of treatment. Patients rebelled against eating the enormous amounts of liver that were necessary. There must be something in liver that could be isolated, scientists thought, and used by itself. Years of patient effort brought to light the magic "something"—vitamin B_{12}, which was first tried on a pernicious anemia patient in 1948.

Some Facts About Vitamin B_{12}

So powerful a substance is the pure, crystalline vitamin B_{12} that, we are told, one heaping tablespoonful of it has the blood-regenerating power of 28,000 tons of raw liver. It is 10,000 times as strong as the most potent liver extract—the most effective medicine per unit of weight ever discovered. Is pernicious anemia, then, caused by the patient not getting enough vitamin B_{12} in his food? Partly. But it also appears to be more complicated than that. Even if there is enough vitamin B_{12} in his food, pernicious anemia will occur if there is something lacking in the tissues or secretions of his stomach. What is this "something"? It is called the "intrinsic factor," meaning something that occurs only in the stomach itself which cannot come from anything "extrinsic" or outside the stomach.

Normal stomachs secrete enough of this factor to get the vitamin B_{12} out of the foods in which it occurs—animal foods, mainly, such as meat, organ meats, eggs, milk. Pernicious anemia patients cannot make use of the B_{12} because they lack this mysterious "factor."

The main point we want to make about pernicious anemia is simply this—there is no need for anyone to suffer from this disease these days. Vitamin B_{12} can be injected by a physician. By injecting it, he can be sure that it is going to be used by the patient's body. Giving it by mouth may not be successful until, by trial and error, he discovers whether there is an intrinsic factor in the patient's stomach or whether the vitamin B_{12} is excreted unchanged rather than being used. More often than not, the doctor gives the intrinsic factor by mouth, along with the vitamin. This preparation is made from material taken from an animal's stomach.

Sometimes people who apparently have pernicious anemia do

not respond to treatment with vitamin B_{12} with or without the intrinsic factor. In cases like this it seems that another B vitamin, folic acid, will often bring results. That's because a deficiency of folic acid can cause a megaloblastic anemia very similar to the B_{12} related disease.

Likely Candidates For Folate Deficiency

Women taking the Pill are especially at risk. Both sequential and non-sequential types of oral contraceptives have been found to cause folate deficiency which sets the stage for this kind of anemia.

Seven young women between the ages of 21 and 39 whose diets, incidentally, were considered eminently satisfactory, were nevertheless treated at the University of Florida between September, 1968 and April, 1969 for megaloblastic anemia. These women suffered with anemia in spite of the fact that they had plenty of iron and plenty of B_{12} in their blood. However, they had low folate levels. Five of these patients showed a brisk response to orally administered folic acid (250 micrograms per day), and this was followed by rapid improvement in their anemia and a remission of associated symptoms. (Folic acid is usually not included in synthetic vitamin preparations.) In two other patients, cure of the megaloblastic anemia followed withdrawal of the oral contraceptives.

Megaloblastic anemia frequently strikes women during pregnancy also. Dr. Mason Trowbridge, Jr. of Bangor, Maine, project director of the Eastern Maine General Hospital's Pernicious Anemia Detection Program, worked hard to educate doctors, other health professionals and the public on the vital need for folic acid in pregnancy. Writing in the *Journal of the Maine Medical Association* (December, 1964), Drs. Trowbridge, George O. Chase, a pathologist, and Anders T. Netland, an obstetrician, discussed a number of cases of anemia in late pregnancy. They pointed out that "Folic acid deficiency must be considered in well-to-do private patients and not just the poor. Our cases do not bear out the statement that anorexia, gastrointestinal disturbances, and failure to maintain weight are essential factors." They stated that if there is any doubt about the anemia in question, the physician could prescribe both folic acid and vitamin B_{12}, since B_{12}-deficiency anemia can then be ruled out at a later date.

Overcooking Destroys Folic Acid

All green vegetables are rich in folic acid. In fact the name folic is derived from the Latin "folium" meaning leaf. But folic acid is greatly diminished in greens that have been out of the garden for any length of time and allowed to stand at room temperature. And the vitamin is heat soluble and water soluble, so you cannot depend on overcooked vegetables for any appreciable amount.

At a London Symposium on anemia and gynecology held in 1967, a Dutch physician challenged his hosts with the startling fact that nearly all known cases of megaloblastic anemia in pregnant women come from English-speaking countries. As reported in *Medical News*, April 7, 1967, Dr. F. I. de Vries of Amsterdam went so far as to call this type of anemia "the English disease," and he was supported by colleagues from Hungary, Belgium, and Portugal. Delegates from Australia and North America agreed that its incidence is as high in their countries as it is in Britain.

The doctor's thesis went straight to the point. He suggested that the methods of vegetable cookery preferred by English-speaking people destroy all the folic acid in the food. Under such conditions the added strain of pregnancy can bring on megaloblastic anemia.

This theory is borne out in an article by Dr. Victor Herbert in the *American Journal of Clinical Nutrition* (September, 1968). Dr. Herbert states that megaloblastic anemia characteristic of folic acid deficiency is seldom seen in the Chinese people. He suggests that this is probably due to their high intake of leafy vegetables which are only slightly cooked in little or no water.

The fact remains that by using any or all of these substances, liver, liver extract, vitamin B_{12} and the intrinsic factor, and folic acid if it is necessary, these so-called macrocytic anemias can be overcome, rapidly, inexpensively and without any danger at all to the patient. For, of course, liver and the B vitamins are not drugs which may be dangerous in large amounts—they are food. And certainly anemia is a disease of malnutrition.

14. Sickle Cell—The Inherited Anemia

The story of sickle cell anemia is a medical detective story, and it provides a striking example of a fundamental but almost totally neglected truth about disease and inherited nutritional requirements.

In the U.S. today, it is estimated that up to 10 percent of the 22,000,000 Americans of African descent carry the sickle cell trait. Of these, 50,000 have sickle cell anemia—a painful and terrible disease, leading to early death by hardened sickled (or bent) red blood cells clogging circulation and thus depriving tissues of oxygen. The anemia factor is involved because sickled cells have an abnormally short life and the blood thus becomes deficient in red blood cells.

Individuals who inherit the sickle cell trait from one parent only (and therefore carry only one "defective" gene) are usually free of the disease—though, as *Medical World News* points out (December 3, 1971)—it is now known that unusual oxygen deprivation, as in anesthesia, can trigger a sickle cell crisis in these normally symptom-free carriers. In contrast, those who inherit the trait from both parents, carrying two "defective" genes and a high proportion of red blood cells susceptible to sickling, are constantly vulnerable to the slightest drop in oxygen value. At any time, crisis may develop and death threaten.

Typically, the American approach to the problem has been a search for a drug treatment for the disease. Researchers have been experimenting with the substance cyanate as an anti-sickling agent. Cyanate, believed to be non-toxic, is a relative of the well-known poison, cyanide. Dr. Anthony Cerami and colleagues at Rockefeller University and Cornell University Medical Center reported at the April, 1972, annual meeting of the Federation of American Societies for Experimental Biology, that in experimental studies cyanate proved effective and safe in treating sickle cell anemia patients over a six-month trial period. Earlier, in test tube studies, the researchers had established that cyanate irreversibly inhibits sickling of red blood cells drawn from sickle cell anemia patients.

To the laymen, it is always baffling how a research team determines which particular chemical (out of thousands) to test as a possible new medication. In the case of cyanate, Dr. Cerami gives us the fascinating background, which also provides a clearer picture of what a genetic "defect" actually means in terms of the structure of molecules in body cells.

Pinpointing A Molecular "Error"

It was in 1950 that Linus Pauling first demonstrated that sickle cell patients had abnormal hemoglobin (the oxygen-carrying substance in red blood cells). Subsequently investigators were able to pin down exactly what the abnormality consisted of: in the two protein chains that form part of the hemoglobin molecule, a single amino acid (out of a total of nearly 600) was replaced by a different amino acid. The normal human gene dictates the uptake of the amino acid, glutamic acid, to fill a particular spot in one of the two protein chains of hemoglobin, while the gene in the sickle cell individual dictates the uptake of the amino acid, valine, for this position.

This small difference could make a big difference in how the red blood cell behaves. Because of the chemical difference between the two amino acids, it was postulated that (under conditions of oxygen reduction) the abnormally positioned valine could form bonds with adjacent hemoglobin, building up a long abnormal hemoglobin chain which would distort the cell into the sickle shape.

All this was very exciting scientifically—precise identification of the gene-caused molecular "error" and a reasonable hypothesis of how the slight difference in molecular structure could cause the disease. But it was of no help at all to sickle cell anemia sufferers. No matter how well understood scientifically, what could they do about an inherited gene that promotes sickness and death?

Cyanate Breaks The Sickling Bond

Clinically-oriented investigators decided to take off from the theoretical foundations established by molecular scientists. They searched for a substance that might break the protein bond that presumably tied the hemoglobin molecules together and caused the abnormal "sickling." A research team, reporting in 1971, tried urea, a well-known protein denaturant (or bond-breaker), and came up with initially promising results. However, Dr. Cerami and his associates reasoned that the urea itself was unlikely to be effective, since so much of it inevitably would be cleared from the bloodstream by the kidneys, which normally pass their waste product into the urine. Possibly, the researchers thought, the effective agent might be the cyanate which is present in urea solutions.

Cyanate has indeed proven to be an effective agent in test tube studies and in experimental use with patients. If no unexpected side-effects turn up in long-term therapy, then cyanate would appear to be the specific need of all who carry the sickle cell trait—most especially, of course, those who inherit the gene from both parents.

However, as Dr. Cerami points out, cyanate would have to be administered for the life of the patient. The body is constantly manufacturing new red blood cells to replace those that die, and each new batch would have to get its protection from sickling by the presence of adequate cyanate.

Now that's the kind of discovery the drug manufacturers love—a drug the patient has to take for his entire life. Fortunately for the Afro-Americans who inherit the sickle trait, however, some investigators believe the remarkable absence of sickle cell anemia in Africa might point to a better way—as we'll see in the next chapter.

Sickle Cell Protection In Native Foods?

Many thousands of years ago in the malaria-ridden regions of Africa, a genetic change (or mutation) occurred and eventually spread through inheritance to millions of tribesmen. This inherited characteristic, known as the sickle cell trait, bestowed resistance against the ravages of malaria. It survived and spread because it was beneficial.

For thousands of Afro-Americans, the trait is no longer beneficial. We have seen that it is responsible for a particularly damaging and life-shortening form of anemia. But the situation is different in modern Africa. As Robert G. Houston reports in an article in the *American Journal of Clinical Nutrition* (November 26, 1973), in Africa the sickle cell trait is carried by an estimated 25 percent of a susceptible population of nearly 300 million. Based on the probability of inheritance from both parents, several millions could be expected to have sickle cell anemia. Yet the fact is the disease in Africa is rare.

"In the entire quarter century of 1925 to 1950, less than 100 cases of sickle cell anemia had been reported in Africa for all age groups," Houston reports, citing the findings of A. B. Raper (*Journal of Tropical Medicine*, 53:49, 1950). More than two decades after Raper's account, A. G. Motulsky, writing in the *New England Journal of Medicine* (288:31, 1973), and other researchers continue to puzzle over the discrepancy—the very great difference between the number of Africans who "ought" to have sickle cell anemia and the number who actually do.

As Houston puts it in his article, "The evidence suggests the existence in Africa of an inhibiting environmental factor on the clinical manifestations of the disease."

In America, a substance has been identified—cyanate—which, if taken for life, might be expected to provide lifelong protection against these same "clinical manifestations of the disease."

Mr. Houston, who is associated with the Foundation for Mind Research, Pomona, New York, has put together these two sets of facts from the two sides of the Atlantic and pursued the question which must inevitably occur to a nutrition-oriented investigator: Is cyanate, or its precursors, a component of the native African diet? Are Africans protected, through the foods they eat, by the very same substance that Afro-Americans on an American diet must take as a drug?

Diet Made The Difference

The author's findings on traditional African foods indicate that the answer to these questions is "yes." The two richest known food sources of thiocyanate (from which cyanate is broken off by enzyme action in the red blood cell) are yams and the African plant, cassava. (Cassava is the plant from which tapioca is manufactured in the U.S., but it is not known whether thiocyanate value remains high after processing.) Both yams and cassava are staples in the African household, commonly stored and used in the concentrated form of flour.

Additionally, says Houston, certain precursors of thiocyanate are provided in Africa's other two staple foods, millet and sorghum. These precursors are the nitrilosides or vitamin B_{17}—sugary cyanide-containing molecules, which are broken down to yield thiocyanate by enzymes widely present in body tissue. (One of the nitrilosides, as you may know, is amygdalin, which is found in apricot seeds and provides the active principle in the controversial anti-cancer agent, Laetrile.)

Africans on their native staple diet, Houston calculates, are provided daily with as much cyanate as the cyanate dose found effective by American researchers treating sickle cell anemia. The typical U.S. diet, on the contrary, is markedly deficient in both thiocyanate and its precursors. Africans probably get 1,000 milligrams or more of thiocyanate a day, Houston says, whereas the amount ingested by Afro-Americans probably rarely exceeds 25 mg.

In view of all these facts, Houston proposes that the disease, sickle cell anemia, be characterized as "a genetically determined nutritional deficiency anemia involving dependence on cyanate precursors." Just as scurvy occurs only in vitamin C deficiency and pellagra develops when there's a deficiency of niacin, so sickle cell anemia (under this interpretation) could develop in susceptible individuals only if there were a dietary deficiency of nutrients that provide adequate cyanate.

Good News For Black Americans

This could be wonderful news indeed for the more than two million Afro-Americans who carry the sickle cell trait. The black community in the U.S. might well want to support a program of government research funds to test the dietary approach, food development making thiocyanate-rich staple foods conveniently available, and a popularization of native natural foods of African ancestors. And, though the final proof is not yet in, it would certainly make good sense for an individual family in which the trait occurs to bring yams and cassava (perhaps in the form of tapioca) and millet and sorghum into the daily eating pattern. Cabbage also has nitrilosides which yield a relatively high quantity of thiocyanate—though nowhere near the amount contained in yams and cassava.

But this information is important not only to black Americans but to all of us. It is a demonstration we can all take to heart of the correctness of Dr. Melvin Page and a few other nutritionists who have long been insisting that "ethnic" food—food that has been eaten through many generations by any particular racial strain—is of prime health importance to that strain. The theory, in a nutshell, is that "ethnic" foods either have been eaten because they possessed special survival value, or in the course of being chosen over the centuries by a particular group that has been adapting to them, have come to be of special importance to that group. The more we learn, the more we realize how correct that viewpoint is.

Section 4
The Appendix

15. Your Appendix And Its Function

15. Your Appendix And Its Function

Just what the function of the appendix is in the human body is not known. Many physiologists suggest that it might be left over from some evolutionary process. One experimenter was convinced that the appendix is a blood-forming organ. He had been studying the effects of radiation on living things and found that radiation victims are likely to die of anemia because the blood-building powers of the bone marrow are damaged. However, experiments with rabbits showed that when the spleen and appendix of the animal were protected with a lead shield, the animal survived what would normally be a fatal overdose of X-ray. It was deduced from this that the spleen and appendix make enough blood to enable the damaged tissues to recover.

The reason that a seemingly insignificant organ, little bigger than the index finger and similar in shape, can cause such misery is that it sometimes becomes blocked by foreign matter or infected. The infection grows until the entire organ is a cylinder of infection, and then the symptoms begin. When laxatives are taken as a means of relieving the distress which follows, they encourage peristaltic action (that wave-like motion of the intestines which pushes fecal matter through and out of the body) and this causes a pressure on the full and rigid appendix, often forcing it to burst.

How Appendicitis Acts

Acute appendicitis attacks are sudden and give little forewarning. Typically, a case will follow this pattern: the patient will quite suddenly find that he has a terrible stomachache. The pain will be generalized throughout the entire abdominal area. Gradually it will concentrate in the lower right portion of the abdomen. Though the pain is usually much more intense, the distress the patient suffers is much like constipation. (It is for this reason that the dangerous temptation to use a laxative presents itself.) Strangely, in spite of the pain and general stress on the body, a high fever is not one of the early symptoms of appendicitis.

When a doctor sees the patient, he will check for tenderness at the expected site of the pain by touching the abdomen. He will note that the abdominal muscles are rigid. A blood count will usually show a high number of white blood cells, which have been called out by the body to fight the illness. These are the usual warnings of appendicitis, but doctors agree that the presence of these signs is no guarantee that the appendix is really the problem, nor does the absence of several of them mean that appendicitis can be ruled out.

Problems Of Diagnosis

One of the complicating factors in diagnosing appendicitis is the type of person it happens to. Most victims are under 30 and as many as 25 percent are under 14. The symptoms of appendicitis—bellyaches, nausea, vomiting, constipated feeling—are rather common in children. And trying to get any definite information out of a frightened and crying child who is in pain is nearly impossible.

If the appendix of an elderly person acts up, the problem of diagnosis is complicated once more. Such people are often inclined to disregard even severe pain, their stomach muscles are often so weak that the characteristic rigidity is not apparent, or the symptoms are masked by any number of other old age disease conditions. Because of this unfortunate resistance to accurate diagnosis, almost all suspected appendicitis cases are operated on as soon as possible.

Natural Foods And Appendicitis

In *The Causation of Appendicitis,* Dr. A. Rendle Short remarks that vegetarians are relatively immune to appendicitis. Several of our other sources suggest too that the meat in the diet might be responsible for appendicitis. This idea probably finds its roots in statistics which show wartime figures of appendicitis incidence to be below those of other times. Of course, meat was scarce during World War II, but so were sugar, canned goods and other refinements of the modern diet. It is possible that the scarcity of the many really harmful foods was responsible for the downgrade of appendix problems, rather than the lack of meat.

Sluggish elimination, and the lack of fresh, unprocessed foods which can cause it, appear to be a possible cause of appendicitis. Eating foods that are as close to their natural state as possible is a good defense against this disease of civilization. A high percentage of cellulose, or "roughage," foods in the daily diet will keep alimentary channels open. Such foods as cabbage, asparagus, apples, cauliflower, carrots, peas and onions are excellent for this purpose.

Is The Appendix Really A Useless Left-Over?

For years doctors have considered the appendix to be a vestigial organ, that is, one used by man in some earlier stage of his history, but no longer of any apparent physiological use. The only thing the appendix could do, according to the medical consensus, is become inflamed, causing painful appendicitis. For years the surgeons rule of thumb has been to remove the appendix if operating near it. However, several doctors have warned that the appendix, as well as other parts of the body not yet credited with specific functions, may indeed have a vital purpose today, and that removing a healthy appendix may lower the body's resistance to invading disease organisms.

The growing case against unnecessary surgery, particularly the offhand removal of parts of the body thought to be vestigial, was strengthened by a report from the Medical College of Ohio at Toledo. A study involving the case histories of 1,165 patients revealed that almost 67 percent of patients who had developed cancer of the bowel before they reached 50 years of age had had their appendixes removed.

Women who had had prior appendectomies were more susceptible than men, noted Dr. George Padanilam, assistant resident in surgery at the medical college, who reviewed the clinical histories and raised the possibility that the appendix may help protect its owner from cancer.

Including patients of all ages, 28 percent of those suffering carcinoma of the bowel were missing their appendixes. Dr. Padanilam called this information "statistically significant" compared with the percentage rate of appendectomies in other types of cancer and in people who had experienced heart attacks.

Dr. Padanilam reported that "the appendix could produce antibodies against viruses responsible for carcinoma of the colon," and appealed to fellow surgeons to think twice before removing the mysterious organ that is often called vestigial. Until the relationship of the appendix to cancer can be defined more clearly, he said, doctors should not remove a normal appendix while operating in that area of the body. The practice, known as incidental appendectomy, could be especially unfavorable to young people, Dr. Padanilam concluded.

An Immunologic Organ?

This is not the first time that a physician has related appendectomy to subsequent development of cancer. In February of 1966, Dr. Howard R. Bierman of the Institute for Cancer and Blood Research, an affiliate of Loma Linda University, told a meeting of the American College of Surgeons that "the human appendix may be an immunologic organ whose premature removal during its functioning period permits leukemia and other related forms of cancer to begin their development."

According to his studies of hundreds of cancer patients, 84 percent had had their appendixes removed in the early part of their lives. Only 25 percent of the non-cancer patients studied by Dr. Bierman were missing their appendixes.

Dr. Bierman developed his theory on the basis of two studies, the first one of patients seen in private practice and the second taken from postmortem records. In 122 private patients with proven lymph cancers and leukemias, the incidence of previous appendectomy was 28.7 percent. The group of postmortem patients showed almost the same rate of appendectomy, 29.9 percent. The average age for appendectomy was 24.2 years. The average diagnosis of cancer in these same persons was made at 46.7 years, some 22 years later.

Of the 549 cases who died from various types of cancer, 34.8 percent had had their appendixes removed. The percentage in the non-cancer group was 23.4. A remarkably high incidence of appendectomy also appeared with cancer of the colon, ovaries and breast. For example, almost half of the 74 cases with cancer of the colon and the rectum had had their appendixes removed.

Dr. Bierman admitted that his findings were inconclusive, but he believed that they did support the argument that the appendix has a function. The current practice of removing a functioning normal appendix, particularly before the age of 30, should be discontinued, said Dr. Bierman.

Dr. J. R. McVay, Jr., working independently, reported in *Cancer* (July, 1964) that there was an unusual incidence of appendectomies in patients who had died of cancer of the colon. In analyzing 914 postmortems, Dr. McVay found 229 cases with cancer of the colon, and of these 18.3 percent had lost their appendixes. In 198 patients with other cancers, the appendectomy rate was significantly less, 12.6 percent.

Dr. McVay's studies indicated that the colon, and to a lesser degree, the lung, breast, cervix, stomach and pancreas, may all be dependent on the appendix for some degree of anti-cancer protection. It has been suggested that the tissue of the appendix may have some protective function against cancer-causers by supplying a protective layer of antibodies. Other experiments have indicated the possibility that the appendix secretes a protective material that is effective against a wide variety of foreign antigens.

All Lymphoid Organs Resist Infection

Lymphoid tissue, which appears in the appendix, is also present in the thymus, the spleen and the tonsils. These tissues are recognized as interceptors of infectious organisms. Lymphoid tissues collect in the appendix where the number of lymph follicles reaches a peak in people between the ages of 10 and 20. After 30 there is an abrupt reduction to less than half the number of follicles, and it tapers off to only a trace after age 60. This phenomenon is also repeated in the tonsils, presumably because the body's major threats from infectious diseases occur in early life.

The tonsils, and often the adenoids too, have also fallen victim to unnecessary surgery. For years swollen tonsils and often healthy ones, have been removed for the mistaken purpose of preventing future throat infections and even colds. The operation is usually of no value.

Some years ago Dr. David C. Poskanzer of Harvard Medical School's Departments of Preventive Medicine and Neurology, suggested that appendectomies and tonsillectomies may be implicated with multiple sclerosis (MS), a disease of the nervous system. In an article in *The Lancet* (December 18, 1965), Dr. Poskanzer said that incidence of prior tonsillectomy was studied in a control group of 240 MS patients, using their spouses and their brothers and sisters closest in age for comparison study. Results showed that patients had a "significantly higher" tonsillectomy-rate than their comparison group.

When appendectomy comparisons were made between patients and their spouses, the MS patients had a more significant number of operations performed. Although Dr. Poskanzer said no ready explanation is available, the tendency toward increased risk of multiple sclerosis after appendectomy mainly involved male patients.

Dr. Poskanzer suggested that some infective agent (germ or virus) originating outside the body played a role in the causation of multiple sclerosis. He believed that whatever it is, it may well be active in childhood many years before the development of the disease, and kept in dormancy by the lymphoid system which includes the tonsils, adenoids and appendix.

The body's lymphatic system, of which these organs are a part, is relatively unknown. One thing that is known about it, however, is that it plays a decisive role in the body's defense against invading organisms. In fact, it is the very thing that often interferes with skin grafts and organ transplants by rejecting the foreign part unless it is toned down by X-rays and drugs.

Section 5
Arthritis

16. Diet Can Control Arthritis

The secretary was in her early 20's but her career held little promise, even though she had the right credentials. One look at her hands told the story: the joints of her fingers were swollen to the point that she could no longer work without suffering the excruciating pain of rheumatoid arthritis.

Doctors had given her little hope. She could continue taking her aspirin and other drugs, they said. Maybe there was an operation in her future. But hope? There was no real hope at all.

It was in this condition that the young woman reported to a clinic in Desert Hot Springs, California, operated by Dr. Robert Bingham, an orthopedic surgeon who has been treating arthritis for many years.

"She was perhaps typical of many of the patients that we see here," Dr. Bingham recalls. "She had no place else to go. Her disease was getting worse, not better. And no one offered the slightest bit of hope to her."

But Dr. Bingham did, and he accepted her at his clinic. The result: "Within six weeks after treatment started, the swelling in her hands had gone down. And by three months, there was no trace of her arthritis."

A miracle? Magic? Some secret, as yet unknown treatment? No.

Dr. Bingham cured the young woman's arthritis strictly with diet, a treatment which many—if not all—conventional medical authorities scorn as totally without merit.

Despite Dr. Bingham's apparent success using diet to treat arthritis (over a period of 16 years), the Arthritis Foundation, which is the major fund-raising and research-sponsoring organization in the United States, has published a *Handbook for Patients* in which there is a section on diet. It asks: "Can Diet Help?"

The handbook says that except for gout (a form of arthritis), "There is no such thing as an 'arthritis diet.' While a special diet may be prescribed by a physician to maintain good health or to correct some specific deficiency," the manual continues, "diet is never the focal point of treatment. It should be remembered, however, that good nourishment is essential to good health and that a person who is either over- or under-weight can often benefit by proper diet."

So much for diet—at least from the "official" spokesman for those suffering from arthritis. But if researchers and scientists such as Dr. Bingham had not cast off the yoke of conventionality, thousands upon thousands of people would never have received any help at all. And this applies to other areas of research besides arthritis.

Nation's Worst Crippler

Arthritis is the nation's greatest crippler. The center of the painful and disabling attack is on the joints and the vast network of connective tissue that holds the body together. Rheumatoid arthritis, the most ravaging form of this condition, can be so painful that even the touch of a bed sheet is agony for its victims. Among the more than 80 different rheumatic conditions that threaten health are osteoarthritis, gout, lupus, spondylitis, scleroderma and a vast group of arthritic diseases categorized as rheumatism.

The Arthritis Foundation estimates that more than 13 million Americans are afflicted by some form of this condition with a quarter of a million more becoming victims of the disease every year.

Arthritis almost defies categorization. It can strike anyone at any age—as witnessed by the secretary mentioned earlier. On the other hand, it concentrates its crippling effect mainly in the 20-to-45-year-old age bracket. For some unknown reason, rheumatoid arthritis attacks three women for every man. On the other hand, gout and rheumatoid spondylitis (an inflammation of the vertebrae) attack 90 percent more men than women.

The human suffering from these conditions is awesome; the cost in dollars and cents almost impossible to estimate. For example, figures show that arthritis sufferers lose an estimated 115 million days a year from work, a figure equivalent to 470,000 persons out of work for the entire year. This means more than a billion and a half dollars in lost wages each and every year.

In this context, any help that can be offered the arthritic is of great value. And although the nutritional approach doesn't have all the answers, there is enough known to make it worth trying.

Dr. Bingham's Approach To Arthritis

"No person who is in good nutritional health develops rheumatoid or osteoarthritis," says Dr. Bingham. With the help of a computer and a nutritional analysis program, he carefully examines the dietary history of each patient, identifying those nutrients which seem to be either deficient or excessive.

The patient with rheumatoid arthritis, Dr. Bingham points out, has a history of not getting enough food, not getting enough of the right kinds of food, and is usually nervous, tense, anxious, over active, has poor resistance to infection and has a history of chronic inflammatory or infectious diseases.

The patient with osteoarthritis, on the other hand, has frequently had too much to eat, but the worst kinds of foods—refined flour substances, too many sweets, and fats.

For the patient with osteoarthritis, the most common dietary modification required is to increase the protein and calcium intake and add supplemental vitamins, trace minerals and anabolic hormones.

Since these patients are usually overweight, Dr. Bingham suggests increased protein in the form of fortified low fat milk or dairy products which also provide well-absorbed calcium. Other forms of calcium which he suggests are oyster shell tablets (six a day) or six bone meal tablets a day. Vitamin D is very important for osteoarthritis patients. Dr. Bingham recommends 1,000 I. U. from natural sources like halibut liver oil together with 25,000 units daily of vitamin A. This is the treatment phase. For prevention, he suggests half of this amount.

A radical change in dietary habits is usually necessary to bring about improvement in the rheumatoid arthritic patient. Here is a typical program as suggested by Dr. Bingham:

1. Confine the patient to bedrest, 16 hours a day.
2. Increase water consumption to 8 or more glasses a day.
3. Gradually decrease all drugs to the minimum the patient can take without too much pain. Reduce and slowly eliminate all corticosteroid medications.
4. Place on a high protein diet.
5. All foods possible are eaten fresh, raw, natural—using a grinder or blender if necessary.
6. Eliminate tobacco, alcohol, refined carbohydrates and saturated fats.
7. Prescribe vitamins, minerals, hormones, and enzymes.

Raw Foods Are Recommended

Since patients with rheumatoid arthritis are usually deficient in protein and in vitamin C, Dr. Bingham recommends 2,000 mg. of natural vitamin C each day and three glasses a day of raw milk, which supplies both protein and calcium. Raw milk is preferable, he says, because it contains an anti-stiffness factor which is destroyed by pasteurization. Where raw milk is not available, pasteurized is acceptable.

Dr. Bingham emphasizes that "it is important to keep the principles in mind that to preserve the natural food intact including proteins and amino acids which have not been damaged by heat, hormones and enzymes which have not been altered by cooking, drying, storage or preservation, and vitamins in the highest biological efficiency, the foods must be as fresh and ripe as possible, grown by organic methods, free of residues of poisonous pesticides and fertilizers and delivered and prepared in as natural and palatable a form as possible."

Alcohol, refined carbohydrates, and saturated fats are eliminated from the diet. Smoking is prohibited. All foods are eaten fresh and raw to the greatest possible extent. He urges his patients to eat lots of raw vegetables, fresh fruit, milk, butter, eggs, fish and cheese. Those patients who are overweight are strongly urged to reduce, but to be careful to get enough protein by eating dairy products, poultry, fish and meats, as well as nuts, whole grains and seeds. A grinder and a blender are often beneficial in maximizing the use of such fresh, natural foods, he notes.

Of course, as a Board-certified orthopedic surgeon, Dr. Bingham brings to the care of his patients other approaches than the purely nutritional. For example, many patients are ordered to get a great amount of bed rest. They are gradually weaned from drugs to the greatest possible extent. He has also found that the dry warm desert climate and the use of deep pool, natural, hot mineral waters are valuable. Supervised exercise, hot wax baths and hot packs and ultrasound may also be indicated and prescribed in some cases.

While most doctors discourage initiative on the part of their patients, Dr. Bingham has found that the most improvement resulted when intelligent and well-motivated patients cooperated by studying and learning as much about good nutrition as they could to help in the management of their own arthritic problems.

In fact, the only failures have occurred in patients who would not learn or could not accept a new dietary plan, or who would not give up certain habits such as alcohol, tobacco, and the overuse of pain-relieving, tranquilizing and hyponotic drugs, which have detrimental metabolic effects.

If your doctor has told you that diet has nothing to do with your arthritis, consider this comment from one of Dr. Bingham's patients: "Good nutrition is the only thing that has helped me." Another said, "I started getting better when I changed my diet." And another said, "Why didn't my other doctors tell me these things about food and nutrition?"

We do not recommend that you attempt to treat yourself for either form of arthritis. Treatment is too complicated and varied to be covered in this brief section, and really must be professionally supervised.

What we do recommend is that the arthritic look for a doctor who is aware of what nutrition can do in avoiding permanent crippling and pain. Everyone who follows the principles of good nutrition and sane living improves his chances of avoiding arthritis in the coming years.

17. Is Arthritis A Deficiency Disease?

Even though attempts to treat arthritis and related troubles by nutritional means have been rather limited so far, the results have been exceptionally promising, believes Dr. Roger J. Williams, the famous biochemist who was the first man to identify, isolate and synthesize pantothenic acid.

In his book, *Nutrition Against Disease* (Pitman Publishing Corporation, 1971), Dr. Williams says that injuries, infections, allergic reactions, and psychological stresses may all play a part in the cause of arthritis, but the most probable underlying cause, poor nutritional environment for the cells and tissues involved, has been largely neglected.

Dr. Williams says that many of the difficulties associated with arthritic disease stem from poor lubrication by the synovial fluid, which is produced in our bodies by living cells from raw materials furnished by food. He maintains that if any mineral, amino acid, or vitamin is in deficient supply, or if the cells are poisoned by bacterial toxins or allergens, this incapacitates the cells and can lead to poor lubrication, so that every movement brings friction and pain.

Dr. Williams notes that many arthritics are woefully deficient in the B vitamins, most notably niacin, pantothenic acid, folic acid, vitamin B_6 (pyridoxine), and others as well.

"The First And Best Step"

Dr. Williams does not contend that administration of the B vitamins will cure arthritis, but he calls them "a link" in the chain of evidence between poor nutrition and arthritis. And he sums up his approach to treating arthritis with the motto: "When in doubt, try nutrition first."

Dr. Robert Bingham, whose promising results using nutritional therapy are described elsewhere, obviously agrees whole-heartedly. Addressing the American Nutrition Society's annual seminar in Pasadena, California, in 1967, Dr. Bingham expressed fully and convincingly a point of view which he summed up in a quotation from the brilliant, pioneering dentist Weston A. Price:

"Applied nutrition in everyday life is the only way a human being may avoid arthritis and it is the first and best step for a patient to take to treat his arthritis."

It is impossible to dispute Price's findings, which have since been confirmed by dozens of independent studies, that wherever there is a group of isolated people, whether primitive or otherwise, whose diet is abundant in natural unprocessed foods and sufficiently varied to supply all necessary nutrients, there is not a single case of arthritis to be found. This in itself is not conclusive proof, since the way of life of such isolated and usually primitive people is different in many respects besides diet from that of more civilized and arthritic people. But Dr. Bingham points out that to any specialist in disorders of bone it is apparent that nutrition plays a major role.

"Diseases of the bones and joints which are due to deficiencies in a single nutritional factor are many. They include scurvy, a vitamin C deficiency; osteoporosis, from lack of calcium and protein; neuropathy, from vitamin B complex deficiency; and degenerative joint disease due to a combination of nutritional deficiencies." Furthermore, he says, these same nutritional deficiencies open the door to many of the infectious diseases by lowering the natural resistance of the body to bacteria, viruses and parasites. This further emphasizes the relationship between nutrition and arthritis, because "secondary arthritis is often caused by diseases which interfere with the absorption, digestion and metabolism of certain vital nutritional factors." Such diseases include disturbances of the digestive system, food allergies, endocrine (glandular) diseases and the changes in body chemistry associated with the menopause and the aging processes of the body.

Significant Subclinical Deficiencies

Dr. Bingham notes that while gross nutritional deficiencies can be recognized by the medical practitioner, "subclinical deficiencies, usually too small to be detected by ordinary means, usually multiple in their existence and occurring over a period of years may bring on more subtle changes in the bones and joints and result in degenerative bone and joint disease. This used to be considered a disease of old age, but in our era of 'civilized foods' with its increased use of nutritionally poor foodstuffs we are seeing this condition in more and more young people and are not surprised to find it in the 30's and 40's where our medical authorities taught us to expect it in the 60's and 70's."

Once arthritis has developed, not all patients can be helped by nutritional or any other means, in Dr. Bingham's opinion. However, he does feel that the major portion of the medical profession would be amazed to learn how many arthritics can be helped by nutritional measures. It is in the area of prevention of arthritis, however, that he believes truly good nutrition coupled with a healthful life can be completely successful.

The Nutrients Involved

Dr. Bingham has attempted to isolate the specific factors that enter into resistance to arthritis, and lack of which permit the disease to develop:

"First is under-nutrition. This is usually the result of ignorance, neglect and poverty." By examination and analysis of children suffering from an early form of rheumatoid arthritis he finds that the deficiencies involved are "deficiencies in vitamin C, the B complex vitamins, calcium, vitamin D and iron. Iron deficiency anemias are found in 10 to 15 percent of both the younger and older groups. Poor iron absorption from deficiencies in the B complex vitamins, gastric acidity and the trace minerals associated with iron are found . . . . In spite of the fact that generations ago vitamin D deficiency was so well recognized that all children were given cod-liver oil, today the propaganda about 'good wholesome food' and dependence on intermittent administration of multiple vitamins has increased the number of cases we have seen with vitamin D deficiencies and rickets. The reliance of some families on prepared milk and processed foods has so decreased their natural vitamin C content that in some areas, particularly in Canada, vitamin C is now added to evaporated milk."

Dr. Bingham believes over-nutrition is the second great problem. "Our sedentary occupations, more riding in automobiles than walking, (and) foods high in sugar, starches and fats have produced an overweight population, particularly in women and older people. The human digestive system, being naturally lazy, absorbs these simple types of foods more quickly and completely than it does the proteins which may or may not be in normal supply. As a result the average older person is deficient in bone and muscle protein, bone calcium, good joint cartilage and is overweight with excessive fat deposited in the tissue, the body organs and the arteries. Osteoarthritis or degenerative arthritis of the joints is basically a disease of poor circulation of the joints. The increased weight and increased fat associated with arteriosclerosis provides a basis for gradual joint destruction before the patient is aware that much of this has occurred.

"Third, environmental dangers to nutrition, such as pesticides in foods impaired by smog and even radioactive fallout are becoming hazards which must be carefully watched and studied."

Finally, it has been said that there is a "rheumatoid personality," and Dr. Bingham grants that severe mental and emotional distress can lead to the crippling disease. But here again, he demonstrates, it comes down to nutritional disorder.

"Nutritionists know that nervous and mental and emotional stress interfere with appetite, digestion, absorption of food, the choices of food, nutritional habits and dietary patterns. Emotional stress exerts a control on the glands of internal secretion, particularly the thyroid, adrenals and pituitary, and they play an important role in bone and joint metabolism. Naturally, any disturbance in the nervous and emotional function of a person produces biological changes which can affect the bones or joints."

Dr. Bingham maintains that not only is arthritis preventable through good nutrition, but arthritis is also curable.

There are specific nutrients which have been identified as helpful agents in treating arthritis. One dietary approach appeared in the July, 1959, issue of the *Journal of the National Medical Association*. It described a special regimen restricting water intake and included the administration of fish liver oil on a fasting stomach. The two authors, Dr. Charles M. Brusch and Dr. Edward T. Johnson of the Brusch Medical Center in Cambridge, Massachusetts, studied over a hundred cases of arthritis, osteoarthritis and rheumatoid arthritis.

The two doctors restricted the caloric intake of their patients to between 1,800 and 2,400 calories a day. They limited the patients' daily water intake, confining it to one hour before breakfast. But whole milk and soup at room temperature were permitted at meals. The cod liver oil was taken either at bedtime or one or more hours before breakfast, but at least one-half hour after the water intake. Completely eliminated from the diet were soft drinks, candy, cake, ice cream or any foods made with white sugar.

The two doctors reported that 92 percent of the arthritis patients responded to the dietary regimen within periods of two to twenty weeks. This consisted, they said, of a marked reduction of pain and general improvement in well-being in the majority of patients. Objectively, they reported, there was diminished tissue swelling, improved range of motion and mobility, less fatigue, better complexion, improved luster of the skin, and increased mental alertness.

Important Role For Vitamin C

Vitamin C should play a prominent role in the "nutrition first" approach to arthritis. Drs. E. Abrams and J. Sandson reported in the *Annals of Rheumatic Disease* (23:1964) that synovial fluid—the lubricating fluid of the joints—becomes thinner, allowing easier movement, when serum levels of ascorbic acid are high. These findings fits in well with earlier work reported by Dr. L. C. Cass and associates in the journal *Geriatrics* (Vol. 9, 1954). Cass found that elderly persons, particularly those in institutions, eat very little fruit and have correspondingly low levels of vitamin C. More significantly, when chronic arthritis patients were given massive doses of vitamin C every day, they reported that the pain was less and they had improved appetite and a new sense of well-being.

Dr. W. J. McCormick of Toronto reported in the *Archives of Pediatrics* (April, 1955) that he gave massive doses of vitamin C in injections and orally in a number of cases of rheumatic fever. "The patients made rapid and complete recovery in three or four weeks without cardiac complication." The usual hospital treatment may go on for three or four months, with cortisone or aspirin being given and a high rate of heart complications. Dr. McCormick has also given massive doses of vitamin C in cases of "incipient arthritis"—that is, arthritis which is just beginning—with "similarly favorable results."

What does he mean by "massive doses"? From one to ten grams daily; that is, in terms in which one buys natural vitamin C products, from 1,000 milligrams to 10,000 milligrams a day.

So despite the fact that most medical authorities are loathe to admit it, nutrition does—or at least can—play an extremely important part in the treatment (and perhaps prevention) of arthritis. Admittedly, the mass of available research is confusing, because many different approaches have been at least partially successful. But remember that there are some 80 different rheumatic conditions, and there is no reason to believe that all of them have the same cause or the same cure.

18. Pantothenic Acid Against Arthritic Pain

In 1974, there appeared in England a daring new paper, well-reasoned, well-documented, and convincing, that goes a long way toward unraveling the mystery of arthritis and explaining why proper diet is a better safeguard and treatment than any drug treatment yet devised. The paper is a monograph published by E. C. Barton-Wright, D. Sc., F. R. I. C., F. I. Biol., entitled "Arthritis: A Vitamin Deficiency Disease," and makes a strong argument that a deficiency of pantothenic acid induces arthritis in the human being.

The word pantothenic is derived from Greek and means "from everywhere." The vitamin was so named by its discoverer, Dr. Roger Williams, who found that it occurs in practically all foods. He later came to regret his choice of name, however, when he found that because the vitamin is so widespread, physicians and nutritionists tend to assume that deficiencies of it are impossible. In fact, though, the vitamin is quickly destroyed by heat and therefore much of it is lost in cooking while practically all of it is destroyed by large-scale food processing. Thus, while it is true that one can get a good supply of pantothenic acid simply by concentrating on eating raw foods every day, for most people who eat everything cooked and most foods highly processed as well, a sufficient supply of pantothenic acid is unlikely.

Chemical assays of the pantothenic acid values of foods have found that the vitamin is very well supplied by yeast, desiccated liver, alfalfa (which very few people ever eat) and fresh eggs (which are avoided by more and more people). Otherwise, even among raw foods, you have to eat widely and well to get much pantothenic acid into your system.

Yet pantothenic acid is vital to human life. It is an essential element in the body's formation of coenzyme A, which is a part of the Krebs cycle, the process by which the acid by-products of energy production are converted to carbon dioxide and water and removed from the body. To the extent that this removal of wastes is not performed efficiently, lactic acid is formed and deposited in the muscle tissues where it induces fatigue. If the function were stopped completely, the result would be death.

The vitamin is essential to the proper functioning of the adrenal glands. An induced deficiency causes hemorrhages in those all-important glands and their quick degeneration. A lesser deficiency interferes with their smooth functioning and reduces their ability to produce cortisone and the other important hormones of the adrenal cortex.

A deficiency of pantothenic acid retards the formation of bone while at the same time it induces excessive calcification in the joints. It also calcifies and hardens cartilage. These symptoms, broadly speaking, are the symptoms of osteoarthritis, which is by far the most common form of arthritic diseases.

Dr. Barton-Wright has been investigating the relationship between pantothenic acid and arthritis since about 1960. He stumbled on it accidentally in the course of using royal jelly (a secretion of the honey bee which is very rich in pantothenic acid) in an attempt to protect mice against leukemia. The attempt was a complete failure, he admits, but in the course of wide-ranging investigations made at that time, it was found that the blood of arthritics always has less than normal values of pantothenic acid. The normal value was considered anything above one microgram per milliliter of whole blood, while any value below .95 micrograms was associated with some arthritis, and below .50 micrograms, sufferers "were in every case severely crippled and in two cases bedridden."

Capsules Brought Pain Relief

Once convinced that there was a relationship between low blood levels of pantothenic acid and arthritis, Dr. Barton-Wright and his associate, Dr. W. A. Elliott, initiated some clinical trials. "In the first trial, 20 patients . . . were injected intramuscularly in the buttock with 50 milligrams of calcium pantothenate at pH 4.6. This was found to give temporary alleviation after seven days treatment." The further use of the vitamin, however, brought about no further improvement and it was decided that the vitamin alone could not be the entire answer. Eventually, after a great deal of experimentation, it was found that capsules containing a formulation based on pantothenic acid but also containing sebacic acid (a crystalline dicarboxylic acid) and cysteine (a crystalline amino acid) were remarkably successful. "Four capsules were administered before breakfast and after 14 days all patients were free from pain, inflammation subsided and they were able to carry out their normal activities."

Barton-Wright is the first to acknowledge, of course, that such a study is far from conclusive. He would like to see others extend and check out his studies. But Barton-Wright himself is convinced that it is pantothenic acid that plays the key role in preventing arthritis and probably in treating and controlling it as well.

There is no doubt that one of the inevitable phenomena of arthritis is low blood levels of pantothenic acid. Such low levels could, of course, arise because of some metabolic defect in the absorption of the vitamin or because the individual person has an inordinately high requirement for it.

Whatever the problem, it is compounded by the fact that modern diets provide very little pantothenic acid. And the amounts of this nutrient we do get are easily depleted—even in healthy individuals.

Barton-Wright points out that "the substance is thermolabile, and especially sensitive to dry heat, and large amounts are destroyed in toasting and roasting food, and as far as vegetables are concerned it dissolves in the cooking water, and in fact, as much as 66 percent may be lost in this way."

Yet that is only the beginning. It should be remembered that the two most important functions of pantothenic acid are the production of adrenal cortical hormones and the synthesis of coenzyme A. Therefore, if you use more energy for any reason, whether it be giving the house a thorough cleaning, or working around the garden, or doing a better and more energetic job at work, then you are inescapably using up more pantothenic acid in the course of your activity. If you are worried about anything; if you go in for competitive sports; if you are in love and in hot pursuit of your beloved; or if you are just perpetually anxious about your ability to meet the mortgage payments and still go on eating, you are being subjected to unusual stress. Any kind of illness also subjects you to stress. In fact, just about everything in life except living a purely vegetable existence puts stress upon you and puts added requirements upon your adrenal glands to produce the hormones that control and regulate your reactions. And so you use up more pantothenic acid.

In view of all the ways there are of losing pantothenic acid, Barton-Wright believes that, "this vitamin is required in human diet in comparatively large amounts; at least 25-50 milligrams daily." Compare these figures with the average daily intake of the average American diet: 4.5 milligrams of pantothenic acid per 2,500 calories.

In other words, the average person who does not eat more than 3,000 calories a day and usually less, should be getting some 40 or 45 milligrams a day more pantothenic acid than he actually is now in order to be sure that he is getting enough.

Value Of Raw Foods Confirmed

Where are you going to get the extra pantothenic acid? Not from the ordinary vitamin B-complex supplement which either contains no pantothenic acid at all or contains it in ridiculously small quantities. If you take brewer's yeast, however, you can obtain four milligrams for each gram of yeast that is taken. An equal amount can be obtained from desiccated liver. A single egg will provide five or six milligrams of the vitamin. And beyond that, it is still important to eat a salad every day or substitute some other raw or very lightly cooked vegetables in order to be sure of obtaining from the diet as much pantothenic acid as you actually require.

In other chapters, we described the dietary aspects of the quite successful arthritic treatment of Dr. Robert Bingham of Desert Hot Springs, California. We stated that all foods are eaten fresh and raw to the greatest possible extent. Dr. Bingham urges his patients to eat lots of raw vegetables, fresh fruit, milk, butter, eggs, fish and cheese. It is obvious, on examining the preceding, that the diet Dr. Bingham urges on his patients is one unusually high in pantothenic acid, as well as in all other vitamin and mineral nutrients.

But such a diet alone is not the entire story, in the opinion of Dr. Bingham. Just so, Dr. Barton-Wright acknowledges that while pantothenic acid alone will relieve the pain of arthritis, it is not curative. If you are already arthritic, you cannot hope that pantothenic acid alone is going to improve your condition very much, if at all, even though there is good reason to believe that a sufficiency of this vitamin will keep healthy people from ever becoming arthritic.

Probably the best hope that any large number of arthritics may actually be able to overcome their disease, lies in the willingness of the medical profession to extend Dr. Barton-Wright's studies and fully test his results, and perhaps ultimately make available to patients his compound based on pantothenic acid but including other materials that he found first in royal jelly.

If he has done nothing else, Dr. Barton-Wright has given us a new and deeper understanding of why it is that fresh foods, preferably eaten raw, are so superior nutritionally to the most tempting and sophisticated substitutes that the food processing industry can offer.

19. Nutritional Buffers Arthritics Can Use Against Aspirin And Steroids

The person suffering from arthritis would give practically anything to get even temporary relief from his agony. Yet despite billions spent on research, no one has yet found a better control of arthritic pain than aspirin. The medical profession is in agreement that while you can try a lot of different things to relieve the pain of arthritis—such as gold salts, phenylbutazone, antimalarial drugs, indomethacin, or cortisone and related steroid drugs—by far the most successful weapon against its torment is common aspirin, no doubt because of its analgesic, or pain-killing effect. While aspirin may not help the condition, it does make life bearable for millions of people who have arthritis.

Arthritics Need More Vitamin C

Any doctor will tell you that when you take aspirin for arthritis, however, you do not take it the same way you might if you wanted to relieve a headache with that drug. If you take aspirin for a headache, you stop taking it when the pain goes away. Not so when you are on aspirin therapy for arthritis. For then you must take aspirin at regular intervals throughout the day, and continue to take it even when the pain subsides. But there is one other aspect of aspirin therapy for arthritis that your physician may never have heard about, and therefore hasn't told you. It is this: if you must take aspirin regularly to relieve the pain of arthritis, you should also be taking supplementary vitamin C to relieve some of the side effects of high-dosage aspirin treatment.

San Francisco researchers Marvyn A. Sahud and Richard J. Cohen of the University of California's Department of Medicine and the Paul M. Aggeler Memorial Hematology Research Laboratory reported in the May 8, 1971, issue of *The Lancet* that patients who took 12 or more aspirin tablets per day over a long period of time to relieve the pain of arthritis were found to have significantly lower blood platelet and plasma levels of ascorbic acid (vitamin C) than patients who supplemented a high dosage of aspirin with that vitamin.

According to the report, "It appears that a high dosage of aspirin in patients with rheumatoid arthritis is associated with tissue ascorbic acid depletion. Administration of supplemental ascorbic acid to rheumatoid patients receiving a high dosage of aspirin as primary therapy seems warranted."

The researchers selected 34 patients who had rheumatoid arthritis and 48 healthy subjects to serve as controls. The patients were split up into five groups according to the sort of therapeutic regimen they had followed for the treatment of arthritis for three months prior to the experiment. Seven of them had taken a high dosage of aspirin, that is, twelve or more tablets per day; seven others had taken a high dosage of aspirin plus corticosteroid drugs; ten of them had taken fewer than 12 aspirin per day; eight had taken a high dosage of aspirin supplemented by vitamin C; and the remaining two patients had been on indomethacin therapy.

All Drugs Depleted Vitamin C

When blood samples were taken of the 34 patients and 48 controls, and measured for concentrations of ascorbic acid in blood plasma and in platelets, the results showed that ascorbic acid levels of both plasma and platelets were below normal in patients who had taken high doses of aspirin with or without corticosteroids, and even lower in those patients on indomethacin therapy, while the ascorbic acid levels of both platelets and plasma were within the normal ranges measured in the control subjects for patients who supplemented high doses of aspirin with vitamin C.

The report said that regardless of how severe the arthritis was in the individual patients, "The major determinant of reduced ascorbic acid concentration in platelets appears to have been the daily dosage of aspirin." Sahud and Cohen added that, "It seems reasonable that patients receiving large doses of aspirin for the treatment of rheumatoid arthritis should take vitamin C supplements."

Aspirin can also cause dangerous internal bleeding. Dr. James Roth, professor of Gastroenterology at the University of Pennsylvania Graduate School of Medicine, demonstrated in 1963 that aspirin makes 60 to 70 percent of all people bleed internally no matter what the form of the aspirin. The usual loss is about a teaspoon or so of blood, and occasionally a patient loses as much as three ounces internally. Sometimes, according to Roth, the result of aspirin intake may even be a severe hemorrhage.

Damaged kidneys examined over a two-year period at the South African Institute for Medical Research disclosed that of 300, eight percent were damaged by aspirin. Dr. Cyril Abrahams told a conference of rheumatism, arthritis and allied disorders that the amounts of analgesics taken by some of these patients over periods varying from three to 22 years were "tremendous." *Medical Tribune* (November 21, 1968) reported that some had taken the equivalent of some 60,000 tablets (20 kilograms), though damage can result from as little as one kilogram (3,000 tablets) of analgesics.

Further illustration of the complications that can arise with prolonged use of aspirin was provided in a report by three scientists from the National Institute of Arthritis and Metabolic Diseases. They described two cases of rheumatoid arthritis to the American Rheumatism Association meeting in 1961 that were mistakenly diagnosed as gout, because of characteristically high levels of uric acid in the patients' blood. Treatment with colchicine, a standard gout remedy, brought no results. Further investigation disclosed that the high uric acid levels had been caused by aspirin taken to relieve joint pain, not by gout at all.

Of course, the pain of arthritis is usually too severe and crippling to ignore; and if your physician has put you on aspirin therapy for arthritis to reduce pain and inflammation in your joints, presumably he knows your case best. But if you are suffering from arthritis, we do urge you to at least take a lot of vitamin C in conjunction with the therapy.

Steroids Have Nasty Effects Too

In addition to aspirin, doctors who treat victims of severe arthritis almost invariably prescribe some form of cortisone (a steroid drug) to ease the pain, and get the patient back on his feet. Cortisone is a substance derived from the adrenal glands, which have a lot to do with maintaining resistance to disease. Human beings, and animals as well, have these glands. ACTH (used as a drug, too) is a substance made from the pituitary, or master gland of the body. When ACTH is injected, it stimulates the adrenal glands to produce cortisone. When cortisone was first tried out on arthritis patients, results were astonishing. Pain disappeared, a sense of well-being and a good appetite returned.

However, it was soon admitted that improvement stopped as soon as treatment stopped, so cortisone was no cure. In addition, it was found that in many cases extremely serious aftereffects ensued.

Patients might be disturbed mentally. They might develop abnormally round faces and abnormal growths of hair. ACTH might bring about diabetes or high blood pressure. Then, too, any slight infection becomes a menace to the patient taking these drugs, for he is not aware of the infection. If it should be something serious, it can develop into a fatal disease rapidly, while the patient, delighted that he feels so well, overexerts himself and courts disaster.

No one knows exactly how these side effects come about, but we do know that glands powerfully influence all the activities of the body. Taking a hormone, any hormone, is bound to disturb the delicate balance among the glands and bring abnormalities. Cortisone and ACTH, as well as any other drugs affecting glands, should never be taken except under strictest supervision, so that side effects can be detected early.

Doctors know that the relief won't last, and they know that serious consequences—addiction, increased susceptibility to serious infection, dangerous mental changes—are common in those on cortisone. They know, too, that one of the most predictable problems associated with heavy cortisone use is "steroid ulcers."

In a discussion of this very special type of ulcer, R. Menguy, writing in the *American Journal of Digestive Diseases* (December, 1967), says "Steroid ulcers appear to have certain characteristics which differentiate them from the ordinary 'garden variety' of peptic ulcer." Their most dangerous characteristic is the lack of symptoms. They often appear without the usual manifestations of ulcer distress—no pain, no digestive discomfort, no warning blood. Add the fact that these ulcers have a high incidence of hemorrhage and perforation, and it is clear that a patient with a steroid ulcer can be next to death before he knows what hit him.

Perhaps the most remarkable thing about Dr. Menguy's article is that it had to be written at all. More than fifteen years before, the *Journal of the American Medical Association* (December 15, 1951) described studies in Boston with ACTH injections given daily for three to four weeks to arthritis patients whose stomachs were normal when therapy was begun. In each of the cases, stomach secretions rose to the levels found in cases of active ulcers. Cortisone brought similar results. One young man on ACTH six months for arthritis developed an ulcer as a direct result of the drug. His ulcer hemorrhaged fatally.

Vitamin B$_{12}$ Can Help

Fortunately, there is evidence that such side-effects can be avoided. Three Rumanian researchers announced in *Archives Internationales de Pharmacodynamie et de Therapie* (Sept., 1965) that vitamin B$_{12}$ neutralizes the ulcer-causing effect of cortisone in experimental animals. Hadnagy, Biro and Kelemen discovered that sometimes B$_{12}$ improves glucose tolerance in patients using cortisone. Where cortisone inhibits the regeneration of the liver in rats, vitamin B$_{12}$ stimulates this regeneration and can counteract the damaging effect of the cortisone.

Also, when vitamin E is added to the diet, response to standard procedures for treating arthritis is quicker and the need for powerful drugs like cortisone decreases or is eliminated entirely, the Japanese Rheumatism Society was told at its annual convention (*Modern Nutrition*, February, 1967). Drs. Takefumi Morotomi and Sadao Kira, of the University of Medicine at Kyoto, Japan, conducted a study of 50 patients who were receiving a form of cortisone, with additional vitamin E in 150 milligram to 160 milligram doses daily, and most of the patients were able to reduce the steroid dose from 30 milligrams to nine milligrams or less within nine weeks. Among other advantages, the side-effects of the steroid were reduced markedly.

A typical case involved a 29-year-old housewife with arthritis of the elbows, arms, fingers and legs who improved on very high steroid doses, but lost ground when attempts were made to reduce dosage. Using the weakened steroids alone, she scarcely was able to walk. When vitamin E was added, just 3 milligrams of the steroid was enough to keep her active to the point of folk dancing and bicycle riding.

20. An Amino Acid Shows Promise In Relieving Rheumatoid Arthritis

A new line of research has produced evidence that a very ordinary nutrient—the amino acid histidine, a component of almost every protein we eat—is an effective and safe therapy for patients with rheumatoid arthritis.

The new treatment, which was first described at a meeting of the American Federation for Clinical Research in Washington, D.C., late in 1969, is based on an unorthodox theory about the origin of the disease. Unlike many researchers in this field, the investigator—Dr. Donald Gerber, associate professor of medicine at State University of New York Downstate Medical Center—believes that the cause of rheumatoid arthritis is related to metabolism. Metabolism is the process by which the body synthesizes (and also breaks down for production of energy) the complex structures it needs from nutrients that circulate in the bloodstream. The clue that led Dr. Gerber to the metabolism theory was the finding (originally made in European research laboratories) that rheumatoid arthritis patients have a deficiency of histidine in their bloodstreams. Their serum histidine concentration averages about 28 percent below that of normal people.

Now, it is virtually impossible that faulty diet could be blamed for the histidine insufficiency in rheumatoid arthritis patients. We ingest histidine with other amino acids when we consume protein—and other protein components would also be in short supply if faulty eating habits were responsible. But the fact is that shortage of this one amino acid—and this one only—is specific to people with rheumatoid arthritis. Histidine level is actually a gauge of the disease's progress; the more severe the condition, Dr. Gerber says, the lower the histidine level.

So we come to the question: Could rheumatoid arthritis be caused by a faulty metabolism that diminishes this nutrient to below tolerable levels, resulting in disease? And, if so, how does

93

the mechanism work? What is histidine's function in maintaining healthy joints?

Answers to these questions are yet to be found. But, as Dr. Gerber told a reporter for *Medical World News* (February 13, 1970), he is confident that his clinical findings in the histidine treatment of rheumatoid arthritis patients will cast light on the cause of the disease.

All Symptoms Alleviated

Dr. Gerber's carefully controlled investigation of histidine treatment involved 59 patients, all with definitely diagnosed rheumatoid arthritis, and many of them severely affected. Patients took histidine by mouth, the amount prescribed varying with the severity of the disease (and the extent of histidine deficiency in the serum). The average was three grams a day. While the study was still in progress, Dr. Gerber reported on results already achieved, with patients taking the supplemental histidine for as long as 11 months.

The improvement noted in the patients' condition is described by *Medical World News* as "at least equal to that obtained from gold therapy—without the side effects often encountered with the metallic agent." Not all the patients responded equally well, but on the average they felt better. They had less morning stiffness, and found that they could cut down their usual medication, such as aspirin and cortisone.

As for objective measurements of improvement: despite their reduction of usual medication, patients taking histidine increased their walking speed by an average six seconds for every 50 feet; their grip strength (indicative of the strength of wrist and fingers) was increased by 30 mm. of mercury; and their blood sedimentation rate (indicative of the extent of inflammation) was substantially reduced.

Of all these measurements, Dr. Gerber says, the most convincing is the fall in sedimentation rate. This blood test, which is used to determine the extent of pathological condition in disease, is something that cannot be influenced by the patient's own attitude. Thus, he might make an extra effort to strengthen his grip or speed up his walking, but the blood test is strictly outside his control.

Dr. Gerber does not call his treatment a "cure." Of 18 patients who were tested by taking them off the medication, 14 got worse—though there was lingering benefit, since the onset of deterioration didn't begin till some five months after they stopped taking histidine. The indication is that histidine treatment must be maintained indefinitely, which would make it a "control."

At the least, histidine has been shown a beneficial treatment for the relief of symptoms and one that is free from the recognized dangers of traditional medication. As *Medical World News* put it, "No side effects were encountered at any time." The reason for this clean record will suggest itself immediately to informed readers: Histidine is a nutrient, not a foreign chemical taken into the body. So, though the long term effects of the new therapy are yet to be judged, we can be reasonably sure that the safety factor is there.

At the best, Dr. Gerber says, histidine may halt future ravages. Many of his patients were already severely damaged, and histidine could not be expected to repair what had been forever destroyed. But could histidine actually prevent the disease from advancing, if administered early enough before irreversible damage occurred? Dr. Gerber believes that is possible, though there is no proof as yet.

As a caution against the assumption of "cure," Dr. Gerber notes that the "rheumatoid factor" (present in the serum of most rheumatoid arthritis patients) is not affected by the histidine treatment. This mysterious substance, which is believed to be involved in the active disease process, is not destroyed by histidine but remains in the patient's blood.

The Rheumatoid Factor

Scientists are in wide disagreement about the significance of the rheumatoid factor (RF). It is known to be an antibody, with an immune reaction to altered or denatured gamma globulin (which is also an antibody). So, however they may differ in their disease theories (viral theory, metabolic theory, autoimmune theory, and others), rheumatoid arthritis researchers are nevertheless in agreement that this disease must in some way be related to the immune mechanism. Every theory has to reckon with this fact.

In his work with histidine, Dr. Gerber has performed laboratory tests showing that in the test tube this amino acid will suppress the denaturization of gamma globulin. In other words, histidine seems to provide protection against an RF reaction that may be a key factor in the disease process.

The metabolic theory of rheumatoid arthritis is not the "in" thing in scientific centers today. The current emphasis in many laboratories is on tracking down a possible virus that may be the initiating cause. This approach fits into the orthodox medical philosophy: find a virus and make a vaccine and you've got the problem licked!

In the meantime, patients continue to be treated with drugs that they and their physicians know cannot cure but can do much harm. Often the patient has very little choice; if the pain and swelling in his joints are not eased with medication, he has trouble moving around, but if he becomes inactive, his condition deteriorates rapidly. As all rheumatoid arthritis patients and their families know, the worst moments come after a full night's rest in bed. A test of how the disease is progressing is how long it takes the patient to "work off" his early morning disability.

Now that a reputable physician in a leading university medical center has demonstrated the therapeutic value of a harmless nutrient, we would like to think that rheumatoid arthritis patients everywhere will benefit from this discovery at an early date. However, histidine in purified pharmaceutical doses, such as would be prescribed by a physician, is not yet available except on an experimental basis to research clinicians.

If you are afflicted with this disease, histidine therapy may prove the answer to your problem. Ask your doctor to keep abreast of developments so that you can benefit at the earliest possible moment. As for the present, the best solution is to include as much histidine in your diet as possible.

Concentrate on protein foods. A high protein intake will, of course, automatically give you a large quantity of amino acids, since these are what protein is composed of. The amino acid, histidine, is present in almost every protein. Foods particularly rich in histidine include whites of eggs, meat, fish, wheat germ, soybean meal, brewer's yeast and peanut flour.

21. Rheumatoid Arthritis Linked To Gluten Intolerance

In Melbourne, Australia, thirty patients at the Alfred Hospital, all suffering from "incurable" rheumatoid arthritis, were treated with an experimental drugless treatment that consisted of controlled diet. Twenty of them had striking remissions of the disease. At the time the new treatment was reported on in the *Medical Journal of Australia* (August 1, 1964), the remissions had been maintained for substantial periods by all, in some cases for as long as 18 months.

This was rheumatoid arthritis, the agonizing inflammation of the joints that has received the attention of thousands of very fine doctors, and for which nearly every known drug has been attempted as a treatment in the hope of stumbling on something that would bring relief. The best they've done up to now is to secure temporary remission with the cortical steroid hormones (cortisone, ACTH, etc.) at the cost of subsequent damage to the bone. And after a few months of steroid treatment, the stiffness returns and the pain is as bad as ever. Therefore, even though only twenty patients out of a total of 30 secured seemingly permanent remissions, this 66 percent success by dietary means alone takes on enormous significance.

What was this astonishingly beneficial diet? Simply a high protein diet with vitamin supplements and the one added feature that all gluten was rigorously eliminated.

Low-Grade Protein

Gluten is the incomplete protein substance that is formed when water is added to wheat. It has a special sticky, rubbery quality that provides a perfect trap for carbon dioxide bubbles formed in the baking process, so that bread containing gluten rises and makes the high loaf with which we are all familiar. Present to a lesser extent in rye, but entering the diet of most people chiefly through wheat products, it is gluten that makes breads, cakes and other wheat-containing foods problematic for some people.

As much is indicated in the *Australian Medical Journal* reported by Dr. R. Shatin, the physician who conducted the experiment. After pointing out that the cereal grains, which were introduced into man's diet comparatively late in human history, represented a radical change of diet that "confronted man's metabolism with an historic challenge," Dr. Shatin states: "The pathogenesis of rheumatoid arthritis, as put forward in this concept, rests on the inherited susceptibility . . . which can be activated by the environmental factor, gluten . . . into a primary and fundamental lesion-enteropathy."

His theory, to put it in simpler language, is that an inherited inability to metabolize gluten leads to a malfunction of the intestine (such as occurs in celiac disease) and that this in turn causes rheumatoid arthritis. It obviously does not cause it in all people, or everyone who eats wheat or rye would be suffering from this vicious ailment.

If future researchers demonstrate conclusively that Dr. Shatin is right, it may ultimately be found that many cases of rheumatoid arthritis can be eliminated by removing gluten from the diet. Dr. Shatin does not consider this incomplete cereal protein the only responsible element, however. He points to other factors "such as infection, trauma or drugs acting on the small intestine." But two-thirds of his patients secured remissions on the gluten-free diet.

Possible Mechanism

Why should the inability to digest and absorb gluten lead to the development of rheumatoid arthritis?

We can find two clues in the laboratory tests that are used to diagnose the illness. First, the *Merck Manual* tells us that "a moderate hypochromic, normocytic anemia not responsive to iron almost always is present during the active stages." This indicates that an active attack of rheumatoid arthritis is somehow associated with the rapid destruction of the red blood cells from a cause that is not associated with iron deficiency. This is a condition that is determined in the laboratory by the rate of erythrocyte sedimentation, which is to say the rate at which a sediment of dead cells is thrown off when blood is whirled in a special instrument.

A study on the effect of diet on erythrocyte sedimentation rate was published in August, 1964, in the *Journal of the Alabama Medical Association*, by E. Cheraskin and W. M. Ringsdorf, Jr., the noted researchers of the University of Alabama Medical Center. Making a double-blind study of 84 male dental students, these investigators found that both abnormally high and abnormally low rates of decay of the red blood cells could be corrected in a few days' time by a diet that eliminated carbohydrate and added 40 grams a day of a high grade protein supplement. By eliminating carbohydrate from the diet, Cheraskin and Ringsdorf inevitably eliminated all gluten, which is found only in the carbohydrate foods, which include the cereal grains. And it is entirely possible that it is the elimination of the gluten, rather than the undifferentiated carbohydrate, that did the trick of bringing the rate of reproduction and death of the red blood cells to normalcy.

Dr. Shatin believes that in many people, selected by their own heredity, the inability of the intestine to absorb gluten leads to the establishment of antibodies. And if we check the *Merck Manual* for the laboratory findings that establish rheumatoid arthritis, sure enough we find that an abnormal gamma globulin, which is to say an abnormal type of systemic antibodies, is found in 60 to 70 percent of rheumatoid arthritis cases.

It is Dr. Shatin's concept that every time gluten is eaten, the body rushes gamma globulin to the intestine to fight it just as it would fight any infection. One result is a constantly inflamed condition of the intestine and Dr. Shatin believes that this chronic inflammation spreads out and is carried into the joints, producing the condition of rheumatoid arthritis.

Hereditary intolerance to gluten is not universal. Your doctor can perform a simple diagnostic procedure—called the d-xylose tolerance test—to determine your reaction to gluten. If it is positive, gluten may have been inflaming your intenstine all your life and the condition will seem perfectly normal to you. But later in life, you may find that you have rheumatoid arthritis or some other type of chronic inflammation. Why take such a chance?

22. Sunlight For Arthritis Relief

Crippled by arthritis in his hips, Dr. John Ott of Lake Bluffs, Illinois, moved to Sarasota, Florida, in the hope that prolonged sunbathing would help his condition. He was able to walk only with a cane and faced the prospect of having to wear metal braces in order to stand upright. Clad in sunglasses and trunks he sunbathed day after day on the Sarasota beach—and found no benefit at all in the exposure.

One day his sunglasses were accidentally broken. The arthritic continued to go out on the beach without them, though the glare troubled his eyes. Within a few days he believed that he could notice a dramatic improvement in his condition. When he was able to throw away his cane, he was certain.

"The weather had been nice for several days," as Dr. Ott recalls the incident in his book, *My Ivory Cellar*, "and there was some light work outside that I was doing as best I could with my cane in one hand. Suddenly I didn't seem to need the cane ... My hip hadn't felt this well for three or four years. I began walking back and forth a mile. I ran into the house and up the stairs two at a time to tell my wife."

X-Rays Show Real Improvement

Linking his arthritis improvement to the full spectrum of the sunlight reaching his eyes, Dr. Ott set up his own continuing therapy in outdoor spectacle-less living; he also moved his office to a corner of the plastic greenhouse, which he had built to allow the sun's ultra-violet rays to reach his plants. When X-rays of the hip later confirmed that his improvement was "real"—in fact, "surprising and most unusual" in the words of his doctor—Ott reflected: "For six months I had been imagining I felt better, and it was a great relief to have those X-ray pictures and examination confirm my imagination!"

The arthritic condition had been improved by sunlight, but not as is generally thought by the action of sunlight on the skin. It was by acting on the system through the eyes, he now felt, that the sunlight had vastly benefited his health.

It may turn out to be the good fortune of millions of arthritics that the man who had this experience is also an expert in the field of optics. Dr. Ott is the original developer and pioneer of time lapse photography, a technique by which natural progressions that are too slow for careful observation can be photographed and projected as a continuous motion picture. If you saw the Walt Disney film "Secrets of Life," you saw a picture of the actual development and growth of a pumpkin plant from seed to mature melon. That was time lapse photography, and it was done by Ott.

Such special photographic studies, very often for medical purposes (such as photographing the development of a cancer cell) have been Ott's life work. When he had reason to believe that the action of sunlight on the unshielded eye had brought him such great improvement in the supposedly hopeless and untreatable condition of arthritis, he was well equipped to investigate further. The first step in his investigation was a check of the sunglasses he had worn, to determine which portions of the natural sunlight had been filtered out by them. The answer, it turned out, was that the glasses had filtered both the ultraviolet and the long infrared rays of the sunlight.

Pituitary And Pineal Glands

The next step was a check on the medical literature. There was little to be found, but there was one research scientist—Dr. Richard Wurtman—who had done a great deal of work in the area. An associate professor of endocrinology at Massachusetts Institute of Technology, Dr. Wurtman had formerly been at the National Institutes of Health where he had intensively investigated the effect of light on the pituitary and the pineal glands, finding that both these glands of the brain were stimulated by ultraviolet light entering the eye. Both these glands are key glands in the entire endocrine structure of the human being. Not only do they play their own roles in control of such basic functions as growth and maturation, but their hormone secretions also control the activities of entire systems of other glands. Their health and activity are universally understood to be vital to the health and activity of the entire body. And while we know of no studies that can show a direct relationship between these glands and arthritis, the lack of such studies might well be precisely the reason why no specific cause for arthritis has yet been discovered.

Certainly we have the subjective evidence of many thousands of arthritics that they have been benefited by exposure to sunlight. And for the fact that many thousands of others have received absolutely no benefit from long periods of baking in the sun, we now have a rational explanation for the first time. While exposing their bodies they may have been shielding their eyes with sunglasses and thus actually preventing the benefits they might have received if they had gone about fully clothed, but without any glass between their eyes and sunlight.

Glass Filters Ultraviolet

"Life on earth evolved under the full spectrum of natural sunlight, ranging from short ultraviolet wave lengths on one end to long infrared rays on the other," says Ott. "Too much of either extreme is harmful, but certain amounts of both are essential." He points out that window glass and indeed any type of glass will block out up to 99 percent of the ultraviolet light. This means that not only sunglasses, but also ordinary clear eyeglasses will keep the eyes from receiving the potential benefits of the full spectrum of sunlight.

He proposed a method, which he follows himself, to overcome this deprivation: (1) stay outdoors as many hours a day as you can (without your glasses), since completely unhindered natural light is the best preventive; (2) substitute ultraviolet-transmitting plastic for glass (which screens out ultraviolet) in your windows and in your spectacles; (3) for indoor lighting, use a new type of full spectrum fluorescent bulb specially designed to mimic natural light both in invisible ultraviolet emission and in the distribution of color bands of the visible spectrum. This is Vita-Lite, a product of the Duro-Test Corporation, North Bergen, N.J. Vita-Lite, unlike sunlamps which expose you to dangerous concentrations of ultraviolet, emits these rays in a concentration as safe as outdoors in the shade.

Before anyone starts exposing his eyes to strong sunlight, however, he should consider the following warnings:

Proceed With Caution

To quote Dr. Ott in a *New Scientist* article (February 4, 1965), "Skin cancer is thought by many to be directly associated with excessive exposure to sunlight, and it is generally acknowledged that it is the ultraviolet part of the spectrum that is to blame. A number of different ailments of the eye are also related to excessive exposure to ultraviolet in sunlight. . ."

Sunlight is powerful. Be very cautious about it. Never look directly into the sun. It is in no way necessary to your efforts.

Indirect and reflected sunlight are just as good—perhaps better—so long as there is nothing actually preventing the ultraviolet rays from entering the eye. Sunlight on the body in small, reasonable amounts is an activator of vitamin D and an improver of health. But the amounts must be small. An excess can stimulate or cause skin cancer. Never expose yourself to sunlight long enough to cause painful burning. Any discomfort associated with the exposure means you are getting too much. And if your skin has no exposure at all, but you just take off your glasses for short periods of time while out in the sun, you will be getting the benefits that Dr. Ott recommends.

The safest method, and all that one really requires, is to spend several hours a day outdoors *in the shade,* leaving the eyes unshielded and exposed to natural daylight.

If you suffer from arthritis and want to try Dr. Ott's method, we certainly hope it will work for you. We see no chance that it will do you any harm.

23. Bursitis Cases Benefit From Vitamin B₁₂

Bursitis gets its name from the bursa, or pocket, into which the round or ball end of a bone fits to form a movable joint. There is a buffer surface of fluid and tissue to give these bones an easy, frictionless movement. If this tissue becomes inflamed or the fluid thickens, or calcium deposits form, bursitis is the result.

Actually there are 140 such pockets, or bursae, in the body, but the one that seems to give the most trouble is located at the shoulder joint. This one is technically named the subdeltoid bursa. Bursitis is so common here that many people assume bursitis to mean a painful shoulder joint and nothing else. And "painful" is the word. Every movement of the shoulder or arm causes friction, which is translated into almost unbearable pain. Bursitis can be an occupational hazard. Baseball players, orchestra leaders, violinists and others who work the arm very hard, or hold it for long periods of time in difficult positions, experience it so frequently that it is often called "glass arm" or "tennis elbow."

The habitual use of one arm more than the other, as required in many occupations which are more functional than artistic can lead to bursitis. The tailor who sews and irons with one arm continually or a factory worker who uses the same arm in working a lever for an entire day—these people are left open to trouble by the limitations of their jobs. It is useless to suggest that these people switch to using the other arm or hand, for they will remind you that they lose efficiency this way. However, they should make an effort to balance the work both sides accomplish by using the unfamiliar side in things that require less efficiency—opening doors, holding a book, lifting a chair, brushing the teeth, combing the hair, and so forth. Try to give the "busy" arm a chance to rest a bit.

In spite of the similarity of symptoms, a painful shoulder is seldom true arthritis, unless the patient has exhibited a tendency toward the disease by showing it in other joints of the body. True arthritis of the shoulder occurs in only five percent of all cases of arthritis.

Treatments Commonly Used

The medical profession has developed several standard methods of treatment for bursitis. Most of the ideas sound a good deal like the measures taken against arthritis. For relief of pain, one is advised to keep the limb immobile by putting it in a sling that will keep it slightly raised. If that fails, doctors prescribe painkillers from aspirin to demerol, as well as hydrocortisone, injections into the nerves to block the pain and surgery to scrape out the joint. Everything and anything is tried, and oftentimes the cure turns out to be worse than the affliction.

Diet is rarely mentioned as a possible treatment for bursitis and its related problems. However, the question was brought up rather obliquely in an article by Dr. N. W. Paul, abstracted in the *Journal of the American Medical Association* for November 30, 1957. In a report on 314 patients with so-called "tennis elbow" (Dr. Paul prefers to call it radiohymeral bursitis), evidence was found that the primary cause was neither injury nor occupation but a metabolic disturbance. In other words, the body either isn't using its food efficiently, or it isn't getting the proper food in the first place. This inability of the body to use its food properly is reduced to two possible causes by the author: either nervous or hormonal disturbance. To correct this, he orders all emotional tension and stimulants to the nervous system be reduced. Physical therapy is not suggested—and an antipurine diet is recommended. This diet is based upon Dr. Paul's theory that too much uric acid is present in the blood stream, as in gout, and that foods containing this acid should be discontinued.

Vitamin B$_{12}$ Is The Answer

An article appeared in *Industrial Medicine and Surgery*, June, 1957, by Dr. I. S. Klemes, Medical Director of the Ideal Mutual Insurance Company and J. C. Penney Company in New York City, which supports this view. Dr. Klemes treated subdeltoid bursitis (shoulder bursitis) with vitamin B$_{12}$ with great success. His theories on vitamin B$_{12}$ were supported by an article from the *Journal of the American Medical Association* (June, 1956) in which the authors noted these facts about folic acid and vitamin B$_{12}$. "Vitamin B$_{12}$ and folic acid both seem to be essential in the synthesis of nucleoproteins. . . . . It seems certain that vitamin B$_{12}$ is of importance in the metabolism of nervous tissue, although the mechanism of its action is not known. . . . . Vitamin B_{12} has proved effective in relieving the pain of trigeminal neuralgia in a significant proportion of patients."

A Convincing Case History

Dr. Klemes gave several case histories to illustrate the effectiveness of vitamin B_{12} in dealing with bursitis. A typical one involved an executive who was encountered as he rested, baking under an infrared lamp in the hot summer. He was there at his own request. He had all the clinical signs of acute subdeltoid bursitis—pain and marked restriction in movement of the shoulder, plus tenderness over the bursa. The patient refused to have an X-ray and was not favorable to a series of vitamin B_{12} injections. When he returned three days later, he was in such pain that he agreed to the procedure suggested to him before.

X-rays showed an appreciable amount of callus in the subdeltoid bursa. He experienced relief within a few hours after the first injection of vitamin B_{12}. The relief continued steadily and in five days the man was symptom–free. He was able to move his arm above shoulder level. X-rays taken six weeks later showed definite absorption of callus, and there was no return of symptoms; functional restoration remained complete.

This course of treatment was effective for Dr. Klemes in all types of bursitis cases. He reported only three cases failed to respond. Certainly it is worth trying in place of cortisone, nerve blocks and surgery! The relief is rapid. Calcium deposits, if any, are absorbed. There are no side effects and over-dosage is almost impossible. There is no definite site for the injections and they are given as follows: daily doses of 1 cc. or 1000 mcg. of vitamin B_{12} for seven to ten days; then three times per week for two or three weeks; then one or two a week for two or three weeks, depending upon clinical indications. Also important is the fact that the treatment is relatively inexpensive compared with X-ray and hormone treatments.

Readers not yet plagued by bursitis might save themselves from the problem by regularly eating foods rich in the elements which are said to make bursitis disappear, foods rich in B vitamins. These are brewer's yeast, wheat germ, liver (desiccated liver or whole) and other organ meats.

24. If You Have Gout, Try Cherries

If the devilish torment of gout or arthritic pain is cramping your toe, your fingers, or your ear lobe, try eating cherries. It may or may not help, but of one thing you can be certain—it won't hurt. And that's a lot more than can be said for many of the nostrums for arthritis prescribed by the medical fraternity.

Why cherries seem to help the gouty patient, no one seems to know, and none of the big foundations are trying to find out.

But according to Ludwig W. Blau, Ph.D. whose big toe at one time gave him so much torment that he was confined to a wheelchair, it was a bowl of cherries that changed his life. The family had gone out and he was left alone with his crippling gout. He got hungry and manipulated his wheelchair over to the icebox. Almost every food which met his hungry gaze was too high in the amino acid purine for his restricted gouty diet, except the cherries. So he ate one, two, three and polished off the whole bowl. The next morning, miracle of miracles! The pain in his foot was practically gone! Could the cherries have brought him this great good fortune? Just in case, he continued to eat at least six cherries every day. He was soon out of the wheelchair and free of pain. Then one day he had to make a business trip out of town, and forgot all about the cherries. Within a few days, he felt as though he was in purgatory. The devil was stabbing his big toe with a screwdriver and turning it without mercy. Doctor Blau went back to his cherries and went on enjoying life, eating six to eight cherries every day.

When Dr. Blau reported his first experience with cherries to his own physician, remarkably the doctor did not laugh. He started doing some checking on his own. Soon there were 12 case histories of people whose gout or arthritis had been helped by either eating cherries or drinking cherry juice. Dr. Blau wrote them up in *Texas Reports on Biology and Medicine* (Vol. 8, No. 3, Fall, 1950). The cherries did not seem to be effective against the rheumatoid type of arthritis—only the gouty type. But some people with rheumatoid arthritis reported relief by drinking cherry juice, probably because they had both types of arthritis at the same time and the relief they experienced was caused by the clearing up of their gouty arthritis.

A thoroughgoing scientist, Dr. Blau offered apologies in his article for the dearth of clinical and laboratory data and control. He felt, nonetheless, that it was proper to publish the information available so that "it might offer a merciful measure of relief to the hundreds of thousands of American victims who suffer the agonizingly painful torture that drives many to thoughts of suicide."

Research Agencies Won't Investigate

In the intervening years, Dr. Blau has been trying, without success, to get foundation funding for research into the mystery of the relationship between cherries and the metabolic malfunction that results in gout. The possibility of any food's offering relief for a specific ailment is far removed from the thinking of the leading research scientists, whose opinions shape the grants of the foundations. There is plenty of money for drug research, but none to study food therapy.

When the national office of the Arthritis Foundation was asked about Dr. Blau's discovery, a spokesperson replied that as of 1975, no studies involving cherries for gout had been undertaken and none were planned.

Instead, physicians continue to rely upon drug therapy as the only treatment for gout. According to the Arthritis Foundation, one of these, colchicine, "is an extremely powerful drug and the amount needed to control an attack of gout is about the same as the amount that will cause abdominal cramps and diarrhea." A new drug, allopurinol, can cause skin rashes and vomiting as well as diarrhea and abdominal pain. That warning is found in the 1975 edition of the *Physicians' Desk Reference*.

Probenecid is another drug commonly used to overcome and prevent the accumulation of uric acid in the body. This drug increases the excretion of uric acid by the kidneys and hence over a period of time depletes the body of its abnormal stores.

According to the *Physicians' Desk Reference*, probenecid can cause headache, gastrointestinal symptoms, nausea, vomiting and urinary frequency; also dermatitis pruritus (itchy skin) and a host of other uncomfortable symptoms including aplastic anemia.

Besides these medications, the orthodox treatment for gout includes a strict dietary control. Foods which are highest in purines are those which are highest in good protein values: meats, especially the organ meats, fish, fowl, some beverages and vegetables and all whole grain cereals.

But, according to Dr. Blau, the whole rationale for a low purine diet and for elimination of uric acid needs a searching review.

Uric Acid And Achievement

For one thing, there are many studies which indicate that such personal characteristics as drive, achievement and leadership are positively associated with the level of uric acid in the serum.

In 1959 Stetten and Hearon studied the relationship between serum uric acid concentration and army intelligence tests in 817 inductees. The relationship between high serum uric acid and high intelligence was statistically significant (*Perspectives of Biological Medicine* 2:185-196, Winter, 1959).

"A tendency to gout is a tendency to the executive suite," according to biochemist George Brooks and social psychologist Ernst Mueller. Higher than average uric acid content in the blood, the Michigan researchers report, is associated throughout history with a high level of intellectual attainment (*Journal of the American Medical Association*, February 7, 1966).

In order to check their theory, Brooks and Mueller gave 113 University of Michigan professors thorough physical and psychological examinations. They found that those with a higher than average uric content in their blood scored significantly higher than the rest in such qualities as drive, leadership and achievement.

It is highly possible, Brooks and Mueller indicate, that uric acid serves as a stimulant to the higher cortical (reasoning) center of the brain.

This being so, why would anyone want to decrease his uric acid? Because it can lead to painful gout, many believe. But researchers have tended to discount urates as a cause of pain because similar uric blood levels also occur in patients with other diseases, and in people free of disease. "The mere presence of high uric acid in the blood is not enough to cause gout; its salts must be precipitated in and around the joints, and this does not always happen in individuals who have a high content of uric acid in the blood," says Dr. Roger J. Williams (*Nutrition Against Disease*, Pitman, 1971).

As long as the uric acid remains in the blood, it may be a stimulus to higher achievement but it has no effect on your big toe. It is when the uric acid is not metabolized normally, that it comes out of solution and turns into crystals that can drive you up the wall.

And that's where the cherries seem to come in. According to Dr. Blau, cherries do not hasten the excretion of uric acid, they simply prevent crystallization. Since high blood uric acid and high I.Q. are partners, he says, we have no business trying to reduce the level of serum uric acid. But if we can prevent crystallization, that is a different story. Dr. Blau has found that he can have his high I.Q., and he can handle purines in his diet and suffer no gouty pain at all, so long as he continues to eat cherries. He reported that all kinds of cherries, fresh or canned, are equally effective. One patient, he said, eats only red sour cherries; others eat the sweet, and some mix sour with the sweet. One patient, nearly 60-years-old, ate cherries for a little over a month before she obtained relief. However, in all other cases relief was obtained in less than 10 days.

Even though in some cases blood analyses showed higher than normal uric acid, no attacks of gouty arthritis were reported after eating cherries.

Cherry Juice Works Too

Eight years after Dr. Blau's revelations, some gout-sufferers in Sturgeon Bay, Wisconsin, participated in a test of cherry juice. "Outstanding results were reported," according to an article in *Food Field Reporter* (November 10, 1958) which disclosed that several local dentists were suggesting cherry juice to their patients and one of them found it useful for the treatment of pyorrhea.

"There is no definite scientific data on just how the juice aids in relieving pain caused by diseases where improper balance of calcium is evident," said the *Food Field Reporter*, "but it is believed that it may be the pigment in the cherries that brings relief."

Cherries contain several pigments, but they also contain more calcium than phosphorus, which makes for a good balance, quite a lot of potassium (191 mg. to 100 grams), and very little sodium (2 mg. to 100 grams). Sour cherries especially are a wonderful source of vitamin A—as many as 1000 international units per 100 grams. The sweet cherries on the other hand have only 110 units to 100 grams. Both the sweet and the sour have traces of thiamine, riboflavin, niacin and ascorbic acid (vitamin C). The sweet cherries have more calories than the sour but both are comparatively low in calories (58 calories for the sour cherries and 70 calories for the sweet per 100 grams).

At the core of the problem of gout is ". . . an enzyme deficit," says J. P. Seegmiller in the book, *Gout* (Grune and Stratton, 1967, p. 38). "The enzyme uricase which is responsible for converting the sparingly soluble uric acid to much more soluble allantoin, is absent in all members of the widely divergent species—man, birds, and reptiles. As a result, uric acid rather than allantoin becomes the end product of purine metabolism. The remarkably inefficient renal excretion of uric acid in man causes the human species to have the highest serum urate concentration and thereby makes the whole species in a sense heir to the gout."

Is it possible that the common, ordinary cherry contains the enzyme which helps to convert uric acid to a more soluble substance? This is only a theory. It has never been scientifically analyzed. And the chances of its being tested by any of the big research organizations are slim. Yet there are other ways of collecting at least statistical evidence.

Results In Three Days

If you suffer the agony of gouty arthritis why not try it yourself? You might be one of the lucky ones like Mr. Smarra of Hermine, Pa. whose wife reported:

"My husband has been bothered for almost a year and the only thing that would relieve him was a trip to the doctor to have the fluid removed from his knee and a shot of medicine. The last time he made the trip to the doctor, the office was so packed he came home thoroughly disgusted.

"The next Sunday we saw the article about cherries and gout. We had some sour cherries in our freezer and he has been eating a dessert dish of them at lunch and dinner. Within three days the swelling was down and the stiffness was gone. He is still eating the two dishes daily and his knee is a lot better for the first time in a year."

Try to get organically-grown fresh cherries to do yourself the most good. In this respect sour cherries may be your best bet. No other fruit tree is so free of insect and disease problems as the sour cherry tree. It grows in a wide variety of soils and is hardly ever damaged by cold weather or late frost. Don't let the name sour cherries mislead you as to their flavor. The Montmorency cherries do turn red about a week before they are fully ripe and if you taste them at that time you might pucker up. But if you taste the fruit when it is fully ripe, you will find they are deliciously sweet, and even more flavorful than sweet cherries. Sweet cherries are much harder to grow. They require suitable soil and are troubled by a number of insect pests. The commercial variety may harbor many more toxic residues from insecticides.

Why not try cherries or cherry juice as a treatment for your gout or arthritic pain? It is certainly a most pleasant treatment without an undesirable side effect, and who knows? Maybe you will be among those who found that in spite of gouty arthritis, life can be a bowl of cherries.

25. How Personality Influences The Development Of Arthritis

Betty Aldrich is in her late forties, married and the mother of two children. Like many other married women, she feels that life is nothing but a series of quarrels with her husband, problems with the children, frustrations with bills, meals and household chores.

The way Betty sees it, she has given unselfishly of herself from the very first day of her marriage 15 years ago—and in exchange has received nothing but abuse. Her husband is hypercritical, thoughtless and inconsiderate. Many are the nights Betty cries herself to sleep while George watches the late show.

When disagreements develop, Betty does not argue. She keeps her feelings bottled up inside and broods over them for days.

In addition to the problems with her family and with herself, Betty Aldrich also has a physical problem. Recently she began suffering from a severe case of arthritis. It has grown rapidly more severe, and she is now partially crippled by it. Medical therapy has not helped.

Betty's story is sad, but not unique. In recent years researchers have begun to recognize a definite relationship between certain personality types and the development of arthritis.

Early in 1967 George F. Solomon, M.D., an assistant professor of psychiatry at Stanford University, announced his then far-out theory that arthritis, with all of its physical pain and physical deformities, could actually be related in some way to a "negative" personality.

One of the few men to share Solomon's view at that time was Dr. Sidney Cobb of the Institute for Social Research at the University of Michigan. Cobb studied 97 couples and concluded that wives are more likely to develop rheumatoid arthritis if there is continual bickering in their marriages than if the relationship is less strained.

Except for scattered reports like this, the literature on arthritis and the mind is virtually nonexistent. In May of 1968, the same Dr. Solomon who pioneered in the field made a more detailed report on it. He presented his views at the Second Conference on Psychophysiological Aspects of Cancer before the New York Academy of Sciences.

An Auto-Immune Disease?

Solomon is one of many researchers who believe that arthritis is an auto-immune disease. That is, it is related to the body's own immunity system. When foreign bodies such as bacteria or viruses enter the body, the system sends out antigens to meet the invaders. When the antigens clash with the foreign bodies, they produce antibodies, the actual substances which surround and destroy the invaders. In arthritis, it is possible that antibodies are never produced against the invading viruses, so those viruses lodge in the joints to cause trouble. Another theory is that the antibodies are produced, but are unable to differentiate between the enemy viruses and the healthy cells. As a result, they destroy both. According to this theory, the body's own defense system causes arthritis.

Solomon believes in the first theory. He suggests that certain emotional patterns may affect hormonal balance, and, in turn may lower a person's ability to produce antibodies against viruses or whatever else the cause of arthritis may be.

To support his theory, Solomon referred to the work of a fellow researcher, Dr. R. H. Moos. He told the New York Academy of Sciences:

"Moos' review of the literature of over 5,000 patients with rheumatoid arthritis found that investigators agreed that arthritics, when compared with various control groups, tend to be self-sacrificing, masochistic, conforming, self-conscious, shy, inhibited, perfectionistic. . . ."

Following the issuance of the Moos report, Solomon teamed up with Moos to conduct a further investigation. He chose a group of women and gave them the Minnesota Multiphasic Personality Inventory, a test designed to probe the basic personality make-up of people.

Pattern Of Repression

The results were persuasive. Unlike most others, the women with arthritis who took the test were invariably nervous, tense, worried, moody, depressed, concerned with what they considered rejection from their mothers and strictness from their fathers. Instead of having occasional outbursts of anger such as most people experience, the arthritic women inhibited any expression of emotion. They showed tendencies to comply and to be subservient. They had a great need for security, were shy and introverted.

Solomon then carried out another study including "rheumatoid factor" as an element to test the relationship between arthritis and personality.

A good deal of interest has been generated of late concerning the role "rheumatoid factor," a substance found in the blood of rheumatoid arthritics, plays in the development of the disease. Solomon attempted to find out by comparing two groups of healthy female relatives of rheumatoid arthritic patients, one group having, and the other lacking rheumatoid factor in their blood.

His study showed that if it is true that the rheumatoid factor plays a part in development of arthritis, it is equally true that the state of emotional health is also important. The healthy relatives who had the rheumatoid factor were more frequently well-adjusted and with positive outlooks on life. Those healthy women who suffered from anxiety, depression, low self-esteem, alienation, fear and worry were—fortunately—lacking in the rheumatoid factor. This perhaps explains why they were not suffering from arthritis.

Solomon concludes, "It seemed as if the occurrence of psychic disequilibrium (emotional upset) in the presence of rheumatoid factor might lead to overt rheumatoid disease. . ." If a person is physically healthy, he says, but possesses the rheumatoid factor, he must make sure he maintains psychological health as well if he is to avoid arthritis.

Personality Affects Outcome As Well

While carrying on the study, Solomon made another discovery—accidentally. He found that certain women seemed to improve with medical care, while others grew progressively worse and ended up crippled just as Betty Aldrich did. This, too, according to Dr. Solomon, was at least partly the result of personality. Solomon says a progressive worsening of an arthritic condition is caused by "unsuccessful ego adaptation." What he means is this:

When people are faced with emotional or psychological changes, they react to them in many different ways. For example, when embarrassed, one person may routinely react by laughing.

Another may become angry. Another may simply shrug. The way we adapt to various situations in order to save face is called "ego adaptation." Each of us has a whole set of ego adaptations. The healthy person chooses positive adaptations, but the arthritic, according to Solomon, reacts negatively. When embarrassed, the arthritic will probably keep his feelings bottled up inside and will brood over the embarrassment for days or weeks. Solomon's study suggested that the people who are lacking in satisfactory ego adaptation are the ones who grow progressively worse with arthritis, eventually ending up crippled.

A Summary Of Previous Research

Actually, Dr. Solomon wasn't the first researcher to put his finger on this problem. An article in the *Canadian Medical Association Journal* (September 15, 1957) reported that rheumatoid arthritis is a "stress disease and represents a maladaptation of psychobiological stress."

The authors discuss previous research and study along these lines, and summarize the findings of the preceding 20 years. Briefly, here are their findings. In 1935, a study showed that arthritics seemed to try to escape from emotional conflicts through physical function. A study involving 32 patients, in 1935, led the observer to note that "a fairly severe emotional disturbance of one kind or another had been present before any sign of rheumatoid arthritis." This doctor (Thomas) also remarked that, in general, he had found that sexual adjustment of rheumatoid arthritics was inadequate.

A very common emotional mark in rheumatoid arthritics was noted by Halliday in 1937 and 1942: rheumatoid arthritics show a definite restriction of emotional expression, as well as strong elements of self-sacrifice. This impression is backed up by a 1954 study which concluded that rheumatoid arthritis seems to follow events which upset the balance between aggressive impulses and their control. For example, let's say a man is unhappy in his job, but knows that he must keep it for the sake of his family's welfare. His resentment against his circumstances might never be spoken outright, but repressing it might lead to arthritis.

It seems to be of major significance in supporting the emotional stress and arthritis theory to note that there is a relative absence of arthritis among those who are actually adjudged insane. It would seem that these people have given up the struggle to control the repressions and frustrations which are believed to manifest themselves in arthritis.

These brief summaries were contained in the above mentioned Canadian journal as a preface to the detailed description of a similar study. Eighteen arthritis patients were observed. The problem was to get 18 non-arthritics whose background was as similar as possible, to act as controls. The solution lay in using the brother or sister of the patient, as close in age as possible, and of the same sex if that were possible. This procedure also would eliminate hereditary differences. The age of the subjects ranged from 20 to 60 years.

All of the people, both arthritics and non-arthritics, used in the study were interviewed by a social worker to determine their environmental background, both in the past and at present. They each spent from three to ten hours with a psychiatrist, who attempted to acquire an accurate picture of their individual personalities and mental attitudes. And finally, all were given objective psychological tests.

The general findings of the examinations were these: In childhood the arthritic patients had shown impulsiveness and love of strenuous activity—sports and games, etc. The brothers and sisters of these people showed an opposite tendency in childhood; they were quiet, shy and obedient, sometimes envying the boisterousness of their brother or sister.

As adults, these characteristics reversed themselves in the people observed. The arthritics had restrained their activity in games and sports (not necessarily due to invalidism), as though answering some inner compulsion. They were obsessed with the need to be tidy and punctual, etc. Any aggression they'd shown as children was now replaced with self-sacrifice and forgiving attitudes.

And what of the non-arthritic brothers and sisters? Of course you've guessed it: they became aggressive, full of self-confidence and free of shyness as adults.

Triggered By Major Life Changes

Another study on the same subject was outlined in the August 15, 1957, issue of the same periodical, the *Canadian Medical Association Journal*. Studies of 43 rheumatoid arthritis patients yielded some interesting generalizations. For example, a majority of the patients associated the onset of the disease with the death of a spouse, separation from a spouse, prolonged separation from a family or leaving home to become established—all situations which carried in them the elements which could be woven into great emotional stress. Add to this the traits of immaturity, dependence, concealed hostility and excessively insistent cooperation in everything, and you have a picture of the average arthritic in this study.

This information does not imply that any person to whom such unfortunate things happen will end as a rheumatoid arthritic. Most persons who lose parents, who end an unhappy marriage in divorce or separation, or who meet with frustration in beginning a career do not find themselves victims of this disease. Somehow or other they must have accumulated inner resources to battle against such a breakdown. Even though the trigger of stress was pulled, it did not bring a physiological breakdown.

How much arthritis is actually caused by our emotions? Nobody can answer that question. But one point that can be made with some assurance is that arthritis is directly related to a defeatist outlook. The person who sees nothing but the storm clouds and never glimpses the silver lining is the kind of person most likely to get arthritis.

26. Is The Way You Sleep Causing Neuritis?

Sometimes doctors overlook the obvious in treating patients who have arthritic-type pain or discomfort around the joints. J. I. Rodale discovered this truth for himself in a very personal way, and in the following section he outlined a common-sense approach to relief that is just as useful today as the day it was written:

Many years ago, I began to experience neuritic pains in the hands, arms and shoulders. There would be dull twinges and pains, and I found it extremely difficult to don my overcoat. If I raised my arms above a certain level, the pain would increase. I couldn't turn my head without experiencing pain in the neck and shoulders. I would get up in the morning with a feeling in the shoulders and neck as if someone had sat on me all night, and my fingers had a numbness which made it difficult for me to tie my shoelaces.

The doctor diagnosed it as neuritis, but its cause had him baffled and, in spite of months of medical treatments of all kinds, including osteopathy, the painful condition persisted. As I look back now, I can see that in this doctor's practice, he specialized in finding cures, but never spent any time in seeking causes. He asked me no questions about my daily life and habits in order to come upon some clue that might lead to the answer. I just kept coming and he kept treating it, mainly with diathermy, but nothing happened.

A friend of mine had about the same symptoms that I did and every time we would meet we would swap talk about our condition.

The Cause Discovered

One night I discovered the cause of my trouble. It was about 3:00 A.M. when I suddenly awoke from a disturbed sleep. My entire arm was numb from shoulder to finger tips. In fact, it was practically paralyzed. I tried to think quickly and noticed that I had been sleeping with my head on the paralyzed arm. I became convinced that this habit was at the bottom of all my trouble. My own hard head had been digging down on my arm for hours.

I stayed awake for a long time, thinking and observing the action of my arms and head. I would watch my arm attempting to move upward so that it could be a pillow to my head, but I fought against it. It took about a week to win complete control over them, and after that, the habit was completely mastered. Never again did I sleep with my head on my arms and, miracle of miracles, the neuritis in my arms completely vanished.

I then went to see my friend who had the same condition I did, and when I related my experience to him, a light came into his eyes. He did not sleep with his head on his arms. In his case, it was a way he had of folding back his left arm in a v-shape and sleeping with his body pressing on it. He now cured himself of this habit, sleeping with his arm spread out in a relaxed way, and within a week his neuritic pains completely disappeared.

When I saw how simple it was to cure these two cases, I began to think of the hundreds of thousands of people who must be suffering from the same thing, and since, in questioning people, I found that a majority of them sleep with their head pressing on their arms, I figured that I had a job to do. I had to share my knowledge with as many persons as possible. So I wrote a book on the subject, *Sleep and Rheumatism*, as well as several magazine articles. As a result, hundreds of people have been cured of what I call pressure neuritis.

Medical Recognition Of The Idea

A doctor friend of mine, a phlebitis specialist in New York, was incensed when he received a copy of my book, and said to me at our next meeting, "Why do you meddle in such things? You are not a doctor."

To give you another reaction from a doctor, may I quote from a letter received from a woman who read my book:

"The doctor tells me that I have osteoarthritis. The pains I complained about—terrific headaches and pains from the back of the neck up and down to the lower back as well as between shoulders—completely disappeared after I arose and walked about for about a half hour. I asked my doctor (an M.D.) if it wasn't pressure pains. I suspected what your book confirmed. The doctor gave me some 'double talk' and said that the pain was due to adhesions, and he suggested 'radar' treatments. I went three times a week until your book opened my eyes. I was mad clean through. Why wasn't my doctor honest enough to tell me the pains were due to pressure exerted in sleep?

"I sent him your book and told him, 'I know and so does Mr. Rodale that osteoarthritis is incurable (degenerated bones cannot be restored), but I am glad to have been corroborated in my suspicion that my pains were pressure pains and I didn't need a doctor for that.' "

I make no comment except to say that my own cure has so far been in effect for over 16 years. Many others have had similar experiences. I have had hundreds of letters testifying to my method's efficaciousness in completely clearing up pressure neuritis.

Here is a typical case: One day I was in a broker's office and overheard the bookkeeper complaining to a customer's man that she had been having terrible pains in her arms and shoulders. "I have to go to my doctor this afternoon for vitamin B injections and I dread going," she said, "and tomorrow I am supposed to go to my dentist to have my teeth X-rayed. The doctor thinks that it might be infected teeth, and I might have to have all of them extracted."

I walked over to her and related my own experience. When I explained that possibly head pressure could be the cause of her own trouble, she was delighted to find an excuse for not going to the doctor or dentist. She at once admitted that she slept with her head on her arms. In about a week, that girl was as free of pain as a new-born baby, without the benefit of any vitamin B injections. Of course, not everyone who has pains in the arms and shoulders gets them from sleep pressures, but it is surprising how many cases do arise from this cause.

Some Additional Facts

The sleep neuritis comes from pressure on nerves, which damages them and from blood congestions caused by pressure on veins, but the amazing thing is how quickly the condition clears up when the sleep pressures are eliminated. You might ask: but how can I prevent myself from doing these things during sleep? The answer is that you begin by trying, and pretty soon your subconscious mind has learned a new set of sleeping habits. All you need do is to draw an imaginary line along your shoulders, and in sleep never let your arms go above that line. Keep your arms down at the sides and as relaxed as possible.

In Germany, a survey showed that practically 100 percent of

the population aged between 40 and 50 were afflicted with some form of arthritis or neuritis, but this, of course, included very mild cases. Ask any person over 60 and you will find that he is suffering from vague bodily pains and twinges. Many of these cases are due to pressures exerted in sleep, although I have also found that some of it is due to sleeping on soft mattresses, which cause the spine to curve downward. Most of these people continue to suffer because cures are usually attempted with medication, whereas the cause is purely a mechanical one.

Dr. Emanuel Josephson of New York City, who wrote a commentary on my book, said that pressures on the arm and shoulder during sleep can lead to bursitis. The cause is injury to the lubricating system of the shoulder. There is a delicate sac in the shoulder joint which is moistened by an oily fluid. Pressure on the shoulder muscle during sleep can in some cases cause a breakdown of its lubricating system, giving rise to a case of subdeltoid bursitis. Many of these cases are operated on.

Many a drunkard has fallen asleep in a hallway and, because there are no pillows handy, used his arm for that purpose. But when one is drunk, the circulation and forces of the body are at an even lower ebb than in ordinary sleep, so that when the man is suddenly awakened, his arm is so paralyzed that he can hardly move it. Such cases sometimes have to be hospitalized, and in the big cities, so many of them are brought into hospitals that this condition has been called Drunkard's Neuritis.

Yet, though the doctors have handled so many of these drunkards, and knew that it came from sleeping on their arms, they did not think to associate it with other cases of arm neuritis. You can search high and low in the medical profession and nary a word will you find that the head pressing on the arm in sleep is the cause of these thousands of cases of pressure neuritis.

Section 6
Asthma

27. What Makes Children Asthmatic?

In hundreds of thousands of homes across the United States, parents go to bed each night fully aware that they might be awakened in the hours before dawn by a child wheezing and gasping for breath. No matter how experienced they become in the ways of an asthmatic child, parents never really get over the terror of these moments. To forestall further asthma attacks, they will consult one doctor after another, move out of the state, buy expensive drugs and special foods. They reluctantly forbid their child to play outdoor games and veto the purchase of a family pet that could trigger future attacks.

The shortness of breath in asthma results when the bronchial passages become narrowed through exposure to some type of stress, either physical (an allergen) or psychological. Because the incidence of acute asthma has grown so alarmingly in recent years, the hunt for its cause and cure is even more earnest now than it ever was. Researchers have fanned out in a great variety of investigations: heredity, air pollution, food allergy, infections, emotional disturbances, family incompatibility, and dozens more. Every one of these shows some promise.

One interesting approach was reported by Dr. J. Aaron Herschfus in *The Allergic Patient* (January-February, 1967). Dr. Herschfus developed a method of pinpointing the pre-asthmatic child, in much the same way as doctors look for a pre-diabetic or incipient heart patient. He found that a family history of allergy is a major warning signal of a possible asthmatic condition in a child, especially when accompanied by frequently recurring colds, bronchitis, tonsillitis, or ear infections. Statistics prove that children with a positive family history of allergy have a higher incidence of asthma than those without such a history.

Early Eczema May Mean Asthma

At a meeting of the American College of Chest Physicians, Dr. Herschfus announced the unusual finding that infantile eczema (a skin rash) is predictive of asthma. One study showed that when eczema occurs in infants under three months of age, 40 percent of these children will develop asthma by the age of three years. There is also evidence that bronchial asthma is twice as likely to occur among children with severe eczema as it is in children with mild cases. If eczema is involved, dietary manipulation can be used as a control. Several foods are particularly implicated as likely allergens—including cow's milk, eggs, chocolate and wheat. Dr. Herschfus stated that when cow's milk was withheld from potentially allergic infants, only seven percent later developed asthma, compared with a control group in which 30 percent developed asthma.

The trouble in tracking down the cause of asthma in children is that the possibilities are so varied. A child is seldom allergic to just one thing. There can be any number of elements in this environment that trigger an attack either alone or in combination. One psychiatrist has written that the asthmatic child actually suffers from "an allergy to life."

Some doctors believe that almost half of all asthmatic conditions are due to food allergy. But other doctors are just as positive that asthma is rarely caused by food. They believe that the cause is largely emotional or hereditary.

An emotional response may be either subconscious or deliberate. Some children frankly admit that they can bring on an attack by breathing hard, coughing or running. When asked why, they confess that they do it to get out of doing something they don't want to do.

Maybe It's Mother

A report in the *Archives of General Psychology* (December, 1966) says that psychiatrists generally agree on the mother as one primary cause of childhood asthma. "Something in the mother's personality sets off a child's dark, hidden fears and anxieties," the theory goes. "This in turn produces allergic reactions in the child which constrict the bronchial tubes and make breathing difficult or even painful." When 14 psychiatrists, pediatricians and clinical psychologists got together and tried to describe the asthma-causing mother, they came up with some confusing conclusions: "On the whole, clinicians tend to agree that the asthmatogenic mother is concerned with her own adequacy, self-defensive, protective of others, sensitive to demands, in need of reassurance from others, irritable, and tends to feel guilty."

The trouble with this definition is that many parents of asthmatic children begin with none of these failings, but the anxiety of living with an asthmatic child is likely to produce undesirable personality traits in even a normal, well-adjusted person.

Attacks Triggered By Irritants In Air

Many cases of childhood asthma are associated with something over which the mother has no control—polluted air. Studies are bringing to light some sad facts about the ability of filthy air to cause allergic disorders so serious that the children have to be hospitalized to receive adequate care.

Research by Dr. Jerome Glaser (*Allergy in Childhood*, Charles C. Thomas, 1956) and by H. Arbeiter ("How Prevalent is Allergy Among United States School Children?" *Clinical Pediatrics*, 1967) shows that most allergies in children are already well established by six years of age. And chronic allergic disorders are linked, beyond a shadow of a doubt, with one of the most common long term ailments of our civilization—air pollution.

One of the first classic studies of air pollution and its allergy-prone victims was made in 1946. It involved American troops and their wives and children stationed in Yokohama, Japan. Researchers found a special form of asthma among the men, wives and children which they called Tokyo-Yokohama asthma, or T-Y asthma. These asthma cases originated in the heavily industrialized Kanto Plain, between Yokohama and Tokyo, and were clearly correlated with the high industrial air pollution level in the area. Although the disease did not have all of the usual asthma specifics, patients generally recovered if they were promptly removed from the area after being affected.

"A Study of the Epidemiology of Asthma in Children," (*Journal of Allergy*, June, 1967) by Leonard S. Girsh, M.D., Elliot Shubin, B.S., and Charles Dick, M.D., studied the correlation between atmospheric conditions, degree of air pollution and the number of patients seeking relief from upper respiratory and asthmatic symptoms. Dr. Girsh and his associates found that elevated barometric pressure and its attendant stagnation of the air doubles or triples asthma incidence. And when pollutants and dirt were trapped in the air—pollutants like oxides of nitrogen, sulfur and carbon and dust—the asthma rate increased nine times over.

A paper entitled "An Effect of Continued Exposure to Air

Pollution on Incidence of Chronic Childhood Disease" by Harry A. Sultz, M.D., and associates was presented at a 1969 meeting of the American Public Health Association. Dr. Sultz studied the incidence of both asthma and eczema in children under 16 years of age in the Buffalo, N.Y., area. All of the cases in the study were severe enough to warrant hospitalization.

In a nine year period, the researchers studied 617 hospitalized cases of acute asthma and another 165 hospitalized cases of eczema, the itchy, red skin rash that allergists now refer to as "the asthma of the skin."

The investigators found that the incidence of both diseases was highest when air pollution was at its peak.

Finally, it's worth emphasizing that there is one recurring element in the asthma puzzle that is within the control of every parent—diet. Certain foods are themselves allergenic, and in a household where the possibility of asthma is suspected, these foods should absolutely be excluded from the menu. Wheat and milk may not be the culprits in every case of asthma, but the search for troublemakers can profitably start here. These two foods, along with eggs and chocolate, are most frequently mentioned in discussions of childhood allergy and asthma. These few foods can easily be avoided with supplements introduced to replace any nutritional losses. Why take a chance on encouraging the appearance of respiratory misery in your child?

28. Your Asthma May Be A Symptom Of Hypoglycemia

If you suffer from asthma, your symptoms may be caused by a disturbance in your blood sugar regulating mechanism that is putting you in the ranks of the estimated fifty million people in this country with hypoglycemia—low blood sugar.

Such is the thesis put forward by two highly respected men, Carleton Fredericks, Ph.D., and Herman Goodman, M.D., who discuss the many manifestations of this disease in their book *Low Blood Sugar and You* (Constellation International, New York, 1969). One of the unexpected manifestations of hypoglycemia, they say, is allergic reaction—hay fever or asthma.

Maintaining that the accepted forms of medical treatment for asthma often fail to control the condition, Fredericks and Goodman cite the example of a small boy whose terrible asthmatic attacks made him gasp, "It takes all my strength to breathe."

The boy's many allergies to food had already been identified and the offenders removed from his diet, all to no avail. These restrictions did not reduce the number or severity of his attacks, but they did debilitate him. Milk products were denied him, thus depriving him of calcium, and he proved allergic to calcium supplements. In addition, his food allergies changed abruptly and without warning. Foods considered safe would suddenly trigger an asthma attack. Because of restrictions in his diet, the boy was retarded in growth. Both he and his parents lived in a constant state of anxiety. The boy repeatedly traveled the route from colds to bronchitis to severe asthmatic attack.

Constant Craving For Sugar And Salt

The child did show from the onset some symptoms suggestive of low blood sugar. He was constantly and ravenously hungry, particularly for starches and sugars. He grew pale and irritable if he could not satisfy his craving quickly. Beside his craving for sugar, he also had a craving for salt, which is a symptom of possible adrenal failure. According to Dr. J. W. Tintera, an authority on the subject of low blood sugar, inefficiency of the adrenal glands is common to both hypoglycemia and allergy.

These symptoms of low blood sugar were never considered in any of the examinations and case histories performed by the boy's doctors. In fact, when his parents suggested that the boy's craving for sugar and salt might indicate an abnormal sugar level, they were assured that these cravings were meaningless, that a high sugar intake is good for an asthmatic, that the boy did not have low blood sugar in spite of the fact that no sugar tolerance test was given.

Driven by the desperation that only parents can know as they watch their child struggle for every breath, they pursued their hunch until they found a medical nutritionist. He performed a six-hour glucose tolerance test which did indeed confirm the presence of severe hypoglycemia.

Sensible Diet Stopped The Wheezing

During the next six months, the child was placed on a strict hypoglycemic diet (high protein, high fat, low carbohydrate). He had two colds—the usual trigger to an attack of wheezing. But this time the dreaded asthma symptoms never appeared. His parents watched with joy as his sensitivities to foods, pollen, dust and bacteria faded. After six years, he was still free of asthmatic attacks.

The case of this one boy illustrates the wide chasm that exists between scientific knowledge and medical practice. The great majority of physicians in our country are not aware of the unbelieveable array of symptoms caused by low blood sugar. Many are not aware that unless a five- or six-hour glucose tolerance test is included in the medical check-up, the condition usually evades diagnosis. There are not many doctors today who look for hypoglycemia, and even fewer who recognize it as a cause of some asthmatic attacks.

While, as we saw in the previous chapter, there are many causes of asthma, low blood sugar seems to be the most neglected factor, one which deserves serious consideration.

According to Fredericks and Goodman, an allergy such as asthma is a "biochemical war within the body" which causes the release of histamine, a chemical which in excessive amounts is responsible for water-logged nose, swelling hives, itching skin, asthmatic chest, and watery eyes. No one knows why one person suffers with asthma and another does not. Low blood sugar could be the deciding factor in many cases.

Surprising Clues About Asthmatics

The same thought occurred to Dr. E. M. Abrahamson, who wrote *Body, Mind and Sugar* (Henry Holt & Co., New York, 1951).

Dr. Abrahamson's investigation went as follows: (1) Tests showed that asthmatics have a consistently low blood sugar. Reasoning from this point, it seemed to follow that diabetics (whose blood sugar is abnormally high) should not suffer from asthma. As Abrahamson notes, "Joslin, the great authority on diabetes, had a few patients who had suffered from asthma but lost it when they acquired diabetes." (2) Asthmatics have an excessive amount of potassium in their blood. Diabetics have a low level of potassium. (3) Asthmatics become worse when they eat excessive amounts of table salt. Diabetics can get along with less insulin when they take large amounts of salt. (4) Asthmatic attacks are especially dreaded because they occur most frequently at night after the patient has been asleep for several hours. In these early hours of the morning the blood sugar level is at its lowest. (5) Injections of glucose are sometimes given to asthmatic patients to relieve their attacks. This of course raises their blood sugar, relieving the attack. But it does not permanently help the asthma, because taking more and more glucose (or any other form of sugar) eventually results in a still further lowering of the blood sugar. (6) The drugs used for asthma such as morphine, amytal, ephedrine and adrenalin, all raise blood sugar levels. Can this be merely coincidental or is this the reason for their temporary effectiveness?

Testing the theory that low blood sugar may make one susceptible to asthma, Dr. Abrahamson put 12 asthma patients on a diet designed to prevent low blood sugar. All of them improved considerably. How then could he explain a patient who was being treated for asthma at the allergy clinic and was also taking insulin for her diabetes? This patient's asthma grew so much worse that she carried a hypodermic needle of adrenalin always with her and could not get through a day without several injections. A 6-hour test of her blood sugar revealed that for the first two hours after she took the prescribed dose of adrenalin, her blood sugar level soared to the diabetic range. Had the test been stopped then, it would have revealed just diabetes, resulting from a high blood sugar. But during the next four hours it fell far below the normal range and at once her asthmatic wheezing began again. In this unusual case the patient suffered from both high and low blood sugar at different times of the day, depending on when and what she had last eaten. The medicine she took for her diabetes made her asthma worse. The adrenalin she took for her asthma made her diabetes worse. She was given a diet which would bring her blood sugar to normal levels and both the diabetes and the asthma finally disappeared.

The answer to achieving a normal blood sugar is to eliminate those foods which bring about a sudden, but short, rise in the blood sugar. In general, these are sugars and simple starches and, as Dr. Abrahamson discovered with all his patients, caffeine, which gives you a "lift" by stimulating the Islands of Langerhans (a part of your pancreas) to produce insulin. As a result the blood sugar level drops too far and all kinds of symptoms can result. This persistently low blood sugar which, according to Dr. Abrahamson, is responsible for asthma and other allergies, is called "hyperinsulinism" meaning, simply, too much insulin.

29. Is A Change Of Climate The Answer To Asthma?

The course of recurrent bronchial asthma follows a fairly regular pattern and can usually be expected to act in the following manner: it acts up about every two to six weeks, with moderate to severe symptoms for one to three days, then diminishes within the next five days and disappears until the next full scale attack.

These attacks are not easy to take. The inability of the patient to take a good breath of air is one of the most common and alarming characteristics of an asthma attack. This is accompanied by coughing and wheezing and a fever that hovers between 100° and 104° F. for as long as four days. Couple this with loss of appetite, nausea and vomiting and you have some idea of the ordeal imposed by an attack of bronchial asthma.

Anyone who has ever seen an asthmatic in the throes of an attack has no difficulty in understanding the lengths to which he will go to escape these dreadful symptoms. Jobs are abandoned, businesses liquidated, whole families transplanted to the arid West or the crisp North in the hope that Dad or one of the kids can sleep at night or work a full day without the racking wheeze and cough that at once resembles choking and asphyxiation. It has become almost a cliché in medical movies or novels for the white-coated wise man to look kindly from behind his desk and say, "Young man, you need a change of climate. You must get away from here or I won't be responsible."

Many medical authorities are doubtful as to climates being able to work the miracles often attributed to it. In most cases of asthma they are convinced that allergy is the main culprit. A change of climate is suggested only as a last resort after patch tests and subcutaneous injections have failed to show a cause.

For those who have begun to eat a good diet and tried every medical suggestion to no avail, there is always the hope that a new location will have an atmosphere which is free from the offending irritant. This possibility alone will send thousands scurrying—some to the West to escape whatever it is that bothers them in Maine, others to the East Coast to escape Arizona's aridity.

The Effect Of Barometric Pressure

Insofar as climate can affect asthma, barometric pressure is considered to be the most acute cause. As far back as 1698, Floyer wrote that a drop in barometric pressure, resulting in excessive humidity, is injurious to the asthmatic. In an experiment reported in the *New York State Medical Journal* (January 15, 1957) by Dr. Harry Swartz, seven asthmatics, known to be sensitive to pollen, were confined in a room that had been made pollen-free. The following weather changes were then simulated: pressure fall, rise in humidity and heavy rain. By evening, all seven had asthma. A few days later the same group went into the room again. This time heavy rain was simulated, but no temperature variation or drop in pressure. None of the participants experienced any asthma symptoms. Pressure change was considered proven as the cause. As further evidence, many allergists consider pre-storm weather, with its marked pressure fluctuations, to be adverse to many asthmatics. This is not to say that it is a sure thing that an asthmatic will suffer from a quick pressure change—for many asthmatics are entirely independent of the barometer for their attacks—but those whose chest becomes tight and breathing labored for no apparent reason may find that they can predict their distress periods by keeping an eye on the barometer.

If sudden pressure changes are a bother, then the solution would appear to be a change of locale to a place whose barometric pressure is fairly constant. A few minutes with a good atlas or almanac should supply that information, or a request to the United States Weather Bureau would probably bring one barometric data for any place in the world.

Consideration Of Other Weather Factors

In the study of weather factors that affect asthma, Dr. Swartz also examined other elements such as wind, humidity, temperature and altitude. He found that, generally speaking, marked increases in humidity are bad for asthmatics. (Foggy atmospheres are considered almost intolerable—pity the poor Londoner!) However, one can suffer just as dreadfully from a lack of humidity. In hot desert areas, many asthmatics suffer just as desperately as those in moist atmosphere regions. The reason is that the desert dusts are highly alkaline and may act as bronchial irritants, thereby causing attacks.

Those asthmatics who are easy prey to temperature are legion, too. Some asthmatic victims react to heat and cold as others react to pollen or dust. This does not mean that it takes a hot summer day to make them wheeze, or a winter's morning that makes one's breath freeze. Any definite change in temperature—so long as it is noticeable—will bring on the symptoms. In this same category are those who are affected by the wind. Dr. Swartz tells of some people who suffer attacks merely by walking in a cold wind, even to the point of actually dying as a result. Though cold winds are most often named as dangerous, it has been noted that many asthmatics find that winds affect them if the wind comes from a certain direction! Of course, this phenomenon is partly explained by the fact that winds carry all types of potential irritants such as pollen, smoke, insects, dust particles, etc.

Sunlight—plain, simple sunlight—plagues many asthma sufferers so that bright, pleasant days actually force them to remain indoors.

Another classic test concerning asthma and atmosphere was reported in the *New York State Medical Journal* for November 15, 1953. This time guinea pigs were used as subjects. A group of these animals was made highly sensitive to pollen. When the guinea pigs were injected with high concentrates of pollen, there was almost no reaction so long as the atmospheric pressure was kept rising. But when the barometer was allowed to fall, the animals showed a response so severe that it was nearly always fatal. Again the point is made that the important factor was not any specific level to which the pressure rose or fell, but the very fact that there was a change at all.

Home Humidifier Can Cause Wheezing

Sometimes, asthma-like reactions can be triggered by the climate *inside* your house. If you are using a humidifier, for example, the unit must be kept clean. The water in some humidifiers provides an ideal breeding ground for certain molds which can cause unpleasant reactions in hypersensitive individuals.

The organisms which can grow in humidifiers (or air conditioners) are considered "city cousins" of the spores which cause a condition known as "farmer's lung." The latter is a respiratory ailment that stems from breathing microscopic mold organisms that breed in the warm, moist hay stored in barns.

Sometimes the source is dust coming from a building where animals, particularly birds, are kept. The spores cause chills, coughing, wheezing, and a shortness of breath within four to six hours of exposure. But in recent years, spores very similar to these have been found in heating, humidifying and air conditioning units in homes, factories and office buildings. Researchers from the Marshfield (Wisconsin) Clinic Foundation, under a grant from the National Heart and Lung Institute, investigated this problem.

Dr. F. J. Wenzel, executive director of the foundation, reported, "There is plenty of stuff in the water that will support the growth of these organisms, although it's hard to identify and run down the specific organisms that cause people to develop hypersensitivity pneumonitis. Often, a humidifier is the last thing a person thinks of when he gets sick."

Asked why it is that so few people seem to be bothered by this condition, Dr. Wenzel replied, "Some people get it and some don't. There is something different about the people who get the disease and we've got to try to find out what the difference is."

That opinion is shared by Dr. Jordan N. Fink, chief of the Allergy Department at the Veterans Administration Hospital in Milwaukee, and one of the authors of an article on this problem in *Annals of Internal Medicine* (80:501-504, 1974).

"We can't determine in advance who will be susceptible to the spores and who will not," Dr. Fink said. "I wish we could, but we can't at this time."

But he did go on to explain that the reaction that these few individuals develop to the spores is not an infection, and is not contagious. It's an allergic reaction.

He explained that some people, for unknown reasons, become sensitized to the spores when they first inhale them. They then become allergic to them and develop an immune response which can be overwhelming. When they inhale the spores again, they become ill. "And why? We don't know. That's what we are trying to work on here," Dr. Fink said.

If you are one of the few individuals who are affected in this way, you will know it by the flu-like symptoms you develop soon after exposure. If the symptoms disappear when you leave your house for a day or so, you know that something—perhaps the humidifier—in your house is causing the distress. If you have no symptoms, then there's no problem—you don't have the allergy.

From a practical point of view, Dr. Fink said in an interview with Associated Press in May of 1972, the best course of action is simple cleanliness.

"We do not advocate removal of home humidification systems," Dr. Fink said. Rather, he advocates "frequent cleaning and proper maintenance as the equipment manufacturers suggest."

An Ideal Spot For Asthmatics

Many years ago, a town in the foothills of the San Gabriel Mountains, Tujunga, California, enjoyed much publicity as an ideal spot for asthmatics. It was reported that 80 percent of adults and virtually all children who went there suffering from asthma, found relief. There were enthusiastic quotations from people who found relief during a brief visit to this haven, then moved there permanently, venturing out only in cases of dire necessity. And they were unanimous in their statements that they never had a recurrence of the wheezes and coughs since. One allergy specialist reported sending underprivileged asthmatic children to the area who were underweight, on restricted diets and suffering constant attacks. In the short space of a few weeks, they gained weight, took foods they could never eat before, and most remained free from any further seizures. This is quite a recommendation. But even Tujunga, we are sure, has failed for some.

If you think climate is what causes your asthma, try your best to recall or make note of the time of year it bothers you least, the type of day that allows you to be most comfortable. Do a little research and find out just where such a climate is general, then go there—for a visit. Stay a few weeks to see if it's the cure you hoped it would be. Wait until you're sure before you leave your house and job for a dream that may turn out to be the same nightmare you've been trying to get away from.

Section 7
Backache

30. Backache

For millions of people in this country, happiness would be a back that doesn't ache. Almost everyone who has reached middle age knows the excruciating pain of an aching back. Once considered mainly an affliction of manual laborers, the bad back syndrome has now solidly entrenched itself among the middle class and the affluent as well. In 1974 some two million new cases of back trouble were reported, bringing the total number of back pain sufferers in the United States at that time to a whopping seventy million people, or about one out of every three adults. Most doctors claim that, with the exception of respiratory diseases, back pain causes more people to visit doctors' offices every year than any other medical complaint.

The bulk of the backache complaints are chronic and occur in the lower back region near the bottom of the spine, generally known as the sacral and lumbar regions. An orthopedist will explain that a bad back pain may be the result of a damaged vertebra or joint, it can emanate from the cushion-like discs that separate the 24 detached vertebrae in the spine (nine vertebrae of the lower spine are naturally fused together), or it can emanate from the muscles that support the spine and central back region. While back injury can be sudden, stemming from things like auto accidents, lifting heavy weights, falls or quick unnatural movements, most bad backs, it is now generally agreed, are the culminating result of many facets of a person's life and the triggering incident is merely the last in long series of events.

Backache: A Problem Of Evolution

In an anthropological sense, it is the common belief of doctors and students of anatomy that man's back problems started when he began walking upright on two legs, forsaking the primordial locomotion of his earliest ancestors who walked on all fours. In the course of standing erect, the function of the spinal column had changed entirely, with a greater weight on the lower regions of the spine. According to H. Clements in his book *What to Do About a 'Bad Back' and Disc Trouble* (Drake Publishers, New York, 1972), this new vertical position "changed entirely the balance of the body, altering its support from four to two supports, at the same time placing greater strains on both the muscular and nervous systems. It also changed the function of weight-bearing, since the spine, no longer in the horizontal plane, found itself balancing its weight in the vertical one. Thus, the spine, once functioning as a beam, now had to adapt itself to the disadvantages of becoming a pillar, in which the spinal discs were detrimentally placed. Now, the whole weight of the head and the upper part of the body had to be transmitted through them, in addition to which they had to absorb the shocks which were now more obviously directed towards the brain and nervous system. The body had constantly to battle against the forces of gravity, a top heavy mass with the inadequacy of only two supports."

In the transformation to an upright posture, standing erect was not the only position which placed greater strain on the lower back region; sitting erect, without the help of the arms or external supports—a posture variation which came with man's ability to stand erect—placed tremendous new strain on the lower back region. Perhaps even more so, since, as man became more sedentary, he began to sit more and walk less, fitting much of his work and recreational environment to one of his favorite posture positions: sitting.

Current research into the ill-effects sitting has on chronic lower back trouble has indicated that in some instances, especially when deep cushioned chairs are used and the legs are propped up, sitting may put more of a strain on the lower back than standing. Reporting in the *Wall Street Journal* (May 28, 1972) on the conclusions of 12 years of studies at the University of California Medical Center at San Francisco, journalist Frederick C. Klein noted that "studies by Dr. James M. Morris and others there have shown that discs in the lower lumbar region— the major site of back pain—are subjected to greater pressure when an individual is sitting than when he is standing. This helps explain why so many persons in sedentary jobs come down with back ailments.

Strong abdominal muscles surrounding the lower sacral-lumbar region lessen the possibility of strain caused by ordinary, yet sometimes strenuous, exertions on the lower back region. "Exercises to firm up stomach muscles have become a key part of bad-back therapy, and overweight patients invariably are advised to slim down," reported Klein.

Pinning Down The Cause

Doctors persist in a never-ending battle over the basic cause of low back pain. Some adhere to the classic assumption that low back pain is almost always the result of an injury or faulty habits of posture; others espouse newer research which suggests that chronic back trouble is due to a degenerative disease that everyone has to some degree; still others, specifically psychiatrists, believe that a great deal of the chronic back trouble is psychosomatic in origin. The treatments themselves are just as varied in nature as the suspected causes, ranging from simple aspirin to surgery.

But from the mass of data collected and analyzed by orthopedic experts and medical researchers, there is probably no one common cause of chronic back problems; rather, backaches are due to an entire constellation of contributing factors. There is no simple cure or panacea for the chronic back problem. A positive change in a back condition usually calls for a change in life style, including diet, posture, sleeping and exercise habits.

In a segment of the CBS News program *60 Minutes* (Vol. VII, Number 7, February 16, 1975), entitled "Oh, My Aching Back," CBS correspondent Morley Safer reviewed the many treatments for bad back currently being employed by physicians, ranging from manual manipulation of the back to deadening the nerves in the nose to relieve back pain. Safer concluded by interviewing Dr. Hugo Keim, an orthopedic surgeon at New York's Columbia Presbyterian Medical Center. Mincing few words, Dr. Keim stated: "Most people come to a doctor with an unrealistic expectation. They have been abusing themselves, and by abusing I mean they've been over-eating and over-drinking— probably, and not exercising at all. They've let it kind of hang out too much, and they're in poor tone, poor shape. And this has been going on for 15, 20, 25 years. They have a job where they don't exercise at all. And so, after all these years of abuse, they now come to the doctor with back pain, but expect a pill or a shot or a laying on of the hands or something that's going to suddenly transform them into the youth that they were twenty years ago, and this doesn't always work. And they don't realize that what really is the key to the whole situation is that they must change their way of life."

31. Slipped Disc

Among the most prevalent of the incapacitating maladies affecting the back are lumbago (low back pain), sacroliac (hip-joint) strain, sciatica (pain radiating through the back of the thigh and leg caused by inflammation of the sciatic nerve) and herniated or "slipped" disc. The most painful of these back afflictions, slipped disc, involves the intervertebral discs, which act as cushions against vertical stress in the spinal column and control movement between the bones.

The body of the disc is made up of three parts: the top and bottom consist of tough fibers of cartilage that cement the disc to the bones immediately above and below; the sides of this human shock absorber are made up of tough layers of gristle and elastic tissue that allow compression and flexion when the spine is subjected to impact; and the innermost portion of the disc, known as the *nucleous pulposus*, is filled with a jelly-like material that gives the structure its elasticity. Surrounding the disc is a circular ligament which functions as a retaining wall to hold the flexible mass in proper position.

When weakness occurs in either the disc or its supportive ligaments, or when the disc is weakened and compressed beyond its normal capacity, it can be permanently damaged or ruptured. The result is that the disc protrudes or "slips" out of alignment and presses against the spinal nerves; thus the term "slipped disc." The name "slipped disc" is itself a misnomer since the disc does not actually "slip" from the vertebra at all; it becomes misaligned and presses against a delicate spinal nerve.

The discs can take great stress in the youthful body; they can be compressed in any direction with little difficulty since their composition is 88 percent water, making them extremely flaccid. But as a person grows older, the interior jelly-like material loses about 11 percent of its water making it less amenable to compression, and more vulnerable to stress.

As we grow older this loss of fluid from within the disc is considered normal; however, those who begin losing this precious fluid prior to middle age are probably suffering from a degenerative disorder of the disc itself. The reason why the outside casing of the disc should degenerate so easily at an early age, allowing buffering fluids to seep out, is still not clear.

Some researchers believe that a degeneration of collagen, the most abundant protein substance manufactured in our bodies and a major component of all connective tissue, may be at the core of the problem, since it is an integral component of the tough outer casing of the disc structure. According to the *Wall Street Journal* (July 21, 1967), Dr. Jerome Gross, a Harvard University researcher, was concerned about a "cross-linking mechanism" which holds the collagen molecules together in strengthening the disc. "In one series of tests he (Gross) induced a disease in rats and dogs that prevented the formation of these cross links and caused existing ones to break down. As a result, the animals' bones bent and their spines curved. Eventually, researchers hope they can find ways to prevent such a breakdown in men and thus perhaps curb degeneration of the spinal discs."

Slipped Disc Treatments

Many patients fail to achieve complete recovery from slipped discs even after several months' treatment with conventional measures such as pain-killing drugs, muscle relaxants, traction and bed rest on a hard mattress. They resign themselves to a painful future of nagging backache. However, there are some treatments that do help some people, and they vary greatly, depending upon whether it is a problem involving muscular ligaments surrounding the vertebrae or the actual skeletal surface itself. In each instance, the treatment should vary with the individual case. Some of the treatments include chiropractic manipulation of the backbone; elaborate exercise programs which strengthen the ligaments surrounding the discs; intensive therapies using penetrating heat and cold; sophisticated radiofrequency beams which destroy painful nerves near the misaligned discs; the ancient Chinese art of acupuncture; the injection of anesthetic-like substances into the vertebra; and, in the most extreme of circumstances, surgery.

According to an article in *The New York Times Magazine*, (February 3, 1974), there are basically three points physicians agree upon when it comes to the treatment of slipped discs. First, a backache victim who has no skeletal disorder absolutely does not need surgery. Second, even in cases where there is a skeletal disorder, most of these—up to 90 percent, say some authorities—still do not need surgery. Third, in the 10 percent (or thereabouts) of the skeletal disease cases that do require operation, there must be no snap decision by a knife-happy surgeon catering to an impatient patient. The decision to operate should be made only after consultation with both a neurosurgeon and an orthopedist, and only after a battery of searching tests has pinpointed the location and severity of the disorder.

Surgery for slipped disc may involve the elementary, yet risky, removal of bone fragments to alleviate the pain caused by the protruding disc or the removal of the entire disc itself. The latter procedure is called spinal fusion, or arthrodesis. This involves implanting bone chips, often taken from the patient's hip or thigh, at the site of the disc removal, thus joining the vertebrae in an immobile form of welded joint. The process may involve the fusion of more than one consecutive disc. Although this provides short-term relief for some patients, the procedure is frowned upon by many doctors since it may permanently restrict the victim's ability to twist or bend his back, and, as is often the case, the fusion will simply move the point of distress to another part of the spinal column. Until researchers develop a synthetic disc which will be able to adhere permanently to the vertebrae and retain sufficient elasticity, spinal fusion remains a controversial remedy—if, indeed, a remedy at all.

32. How To Protect Your Back

It is heartening to know that the chances of dying of a bad back are practically nil. It is also good to know that surgery is seldom required to cure a bad back. Only about one out of twenty people with bad backs will ever need an operation, says Dr. Leon Root, a New York orthopedic surgeon and co-author with Thomas Kiernan of the book *Oh My Aching Back* (David McKay, 1973).

These statistics bring little comfort to someone doubled over with a backache. However, there are steps you can take right now which can help you live a happy life without a backache, or if you do have one, will help you handle it with common sense, so that your first episode does not lead to a lifetime of agony.

According to Dr. Root, the great majority of back ailments could have been avoided at the very beginning through the application of a little practical knowledge and common sense when the first ache or spasm manifested itself.

Here are some suggestions that can prevent and often alleviate low back pain.

Standing

After you have been standing in one position for any length of time, the low back or hips tend to sag forward. This accentuates your swayback, straining and weakening the spine which can trigger a painful back condition.

You can help prevent this if you remember to keep one of your hips flexed. Do this by placing one foot on a stool or a step. If you are at the sink, place one foot on the edge of a pulled-out drawer. As long as one or both hips are flexed, the low back is not straining forward.

To find the correct standing position, do this: With your knees slightly bent, sit against a wall. Tighten your abdominal and buttocks muscles so that your back is flat against the wall from shoulder blades to buttocks. Holding this position, straighten your legs till you are in standing position. Now, maintaining this posture, walk around the room and back to the wall. Have you held the position? Keep trying.

Sitting

The Schering Corp., a pharmaceutical house, published a guide for low back pain patients in which they suggest that "A back's best friend is a straight-back chair. If you can't get the chair you prefer," they suggest, "learn to sit properly on whatever chair you get. In order to avoid forward slump when you are sitting try this: throw your head well back, then bend it forward to pull in the chin. This gesture will straighten the back. Now tighten abdominal muscles to raise the chest. Check your position frequently."

Once you have had back trouble, you would be wise to invest in a foot rest that will bring your knees up slightly higher than your hips, and use it whenever and wherever possible. If you should find yourself without such a foot prop, remember to cross one knee over the other. Switch legs frequently to avoid constriction of the blood circulation.

Get a hard seat for your automobile and sit close enough to the wheel while driving so that your legs are not fully extended when you work the pedals.

Lifting

Never lift anything heavy above the level of the elbows. You can easily lift an object off the floor by bending the knees and the hips without causing too much damage. But when you try to raise a heavy object higher than the waist, it is impossible to do it without arching in the back. This arching causes a strain.

If you're a woman, you should make it a rule never to lift a weight greater than 25 pounds. Men should limit themselves to lifting half their weight, less if they are overweight. When lifting objects from the floor, use your arms and legs as much as possible and your back as little as possible. To do this, always bend your knees to reach the object to be lifted, keeping your spine as straight as possible.

Choose A Mattress Cautiously

In the event of back pain, your best course is to consult with a doctor or orthopedist immediately. Chances are he will suggest getting into bed with a heating pad. When every move is a torment, that sounds like heaven. But what kind of a bed? Is the mattress firm enough to support your back and yet not so firm that it prevents your muscles from relaxing?

When we get down to basics, for a person with a bad back, a

mattress is perhaps the most important article of furniture in the whole house. The right choice of mattress might help to prevent that aching back in the first place. Do not presume that the firmer the mattress the better it is for you. A bed which is too hard can interfere with relaxation because it does not allow for the body to be cradled. This leaves unsupported hollows so that muscles cannot relax, reports Judith Hann, who surveyed bedding for bad backs (*New Scientist,* May 3, 1973).

A completely new type of mattress, now produced in England, combines differential areas of softness and hardness so that the spine can remain straight. Where the body protrudes—at the shoulders and hips—the mattress is much softer, with firm sections for the head, legs and the spinal area. In the U.S., several lines of mattresses which are firm, yet conform to the body's contours are available at various furniture and department stores.

Your weight has a great deal to do with the firmness of the mattress you should choose. The heavier you are, the firmer the mattress should be. Even if you use foam rubber, it comes in various degrees of firmness and you can find the right type.

A firm mattress is usually constructed with innerspring, foam, or other material. Innerspring mattresses are sold in a variety of sizes and degrees of hardness. Since the advent of the box spring, an almost infinite combination of mattress and spring firmnesses is available. For instance, one well-known department store chain offers sleep-set combinations ranging from a 220-coil mattress with matching springs 63 strong, to a super-firm 1250-coil mattress with a 108-coil support system. A wise shopper purchases no less than an 850-coil mattress with about 100 coils in the box springs for proper support.

Another wise choice may result in a compromise which involves the use of a one-inch thick foam "mattress topper" to cover an overly-firm innerspring set, giving the patient good support but providing a degree of support comfort. Another alternative, equally effective, is a dense latex foam mattress with a bed board, preferably ¾'' thick, inserted between springs and mattress. This allows the sleeper to rest without sagging, while avoiding the super-firmness of many bedding combinations. The purchaser, however, must be certain he is buying a densely-textured, natural foam rubber product. Some synthetics tend to break down easily, resulting in a sagging, bumpy surface within a short time.

33. Exercises You Can Do For A Better Back

Stories of people afflicted with crippling back pains when only reaching for a doorknob or tying their shoes are legion. Back pains caused by such simple body movements have rendered many patients literally immobile, fearful that any new gesture could put them in a bed—a hospital bed. Ironically, the padded chairs and mincing steps they adopt are nothing more than a prescription for more agony and debilitation.

Although there are many different medical approaches to curing a bad back, nearly all orthopedic specialists agree that this type of immobility is overwhelmingly one of the most common causes of back problems. Nature provided a great mass of powerful muscle to keep the discs of our spine in place. When these muscles are in good shape, they do the job masterfully. If muscles are permitted to atrophy through lack of use, the job must be taken over by a support garment. Eventually, even the garment loses its efficiency and a spinal fusion may be needed to keep everything in place. Whether muscles do the job, or a surgeon, is in most cases entirely up to the individual.

Exercise—the right kind—is more than a preventive for back problems. It is also the single best cure, not only infinitely less dangerous and painful than surgery, but actually, in many cases, more effective.

This is the considered opinion of an orthopedic surgeon, a doctor who is not afraid to operate on the spine when he thinks the situation calls for it. Dr. Arthur Michele, Professor and Chairman of the Department of Orthopedic Surgery at New York Medical College and Director of Orthopedic Surgery at five New York City hospitals, has done that often enough.

Dr. Michele is convinced that many of his patients would never have had to limp into his consulting room or be wheeled into his operating theater had they followed a simple exercise regimen he describes in his book *Orthotherapy* (M. Evans and Company, Inc., New York, 1971). Perhaps more to the point, because the average person isn't interested in his back muscles until they desert him, Dr. Michele says that his exercises are equally as potent as a cure—providing the spine has not become hopelessly degenerate. In fact, he says, after 35 years of orthopedic practice he is convinced that these exercises "can bring about what seem to be near-miracles."

The Muscle Responsible For Back Pain

Dr. Michele explains that the underlying cause of the majority of back problems involves an extraordinarily large complex of muscles in the lower back known as the *iliopsoas*. He describes it as "mainly a broad flat muscle in the lower back, but like an octopus, it has arms reaching out in many directions." Its lower segments are attached to the pelvis, hips, and thigh bones, while its upper extremities go to every vertebra in the lumbar area of the lower spine, and even up to the lower thoracic vertebrae in the mid-back. The *iliopsoas* causes the natural curve in the spine, controls the general posture, and is involved with the entire working of the back and hips.

All too often, one of the many arms of the *iliopsoas* is abnormally short—either because of birth anomaly, or more often, contraction resulting simply from lack of stretching and use. Because the arms of the *iliopsoas* have a grip on so many bones, joints, and vertebrae, a shortness in any one arm, Dr. Michele explains, can result in a large number of symptoms, whose site is not necessarily at the point of the underlying muscular problem. These typical symptoms, he says, include pain or stiffness of the spine, herniated (slipped) intervertebral disc, actual fracture of the spine or degenerative disorders of the spine, weakening and subsequent fracture of the thigh bone of older people (often mistakenly blamed on a fall), arthrosis of the knee, arthrosis of the hip, a pain in the chest and poor functioning of internal organs.

A 27-year-old woman whose husband was a doctor came to Dr. Michele complaining of severe aching of the knees, hips and lower back. During her menstrual period the pains were often so severe as to be disabling. Finally she began to have headaches. She had already been to a gynecologist and had been X-rayed, but no cause for her problems could be found.

"Her case history is a perfect progression of the symptoms which can result from muscle imbalance," Dr. Michele says. Her joint pains were caused by the imbalance bringing about an uneven distribution of her body weight. After following a regular exercise program, "most of her painful symptoms are gone," Dr. Michele reports.

Another patient, a woman of 25, had a severe pain in her shoulder radiating into her hand, a headache and a miserable backache that simply would not go away. "Ultimately I was able to trace her various symptoms, head and back pain to a rigid muscle in the hip . . . after six weeks of an exercise program, she was able to report for the first time in two years that she wasn't in pain," the orthopedic surgeon declares.

Some Exercises Can Be Harmful

The first thing to know about exercises for a bad back is that some of them—in fact *lots* of them—can do you more harm than good. Standing with legs straight and bending to touch toes is one of them. Push-ups are also bad for the back. Don't do sit-ups unless you use a curling motion with your feet free and your knees slightly flexed. In other words, don't do any of the exercises or calisthenics you used to do in gym class; nearly all of them can put you in traction.

Dr. Michele gives two basic series of exercises. The first series is designed for people whose backs are already in bad shape. The second series consists of exercises designed to maintain a back that is in good condition. Here are some exercises from the first series—for those people whose back muscles need some help. If you're currently under treatment, ask your doctor about these exercises.

If possible, set aside 20 minutes to a half hour, twice a day, for best results from these exercises. "Years of neglect, years of letting your muscles go unsupervised, cannot be atoned for in a few minutes of lackadaisical stretching every now and then," the physician counsels.

First, wear something that will not impede your movement in any direction. If you really want to get in the mood, don a leotard or sweat suit, but underwear, old slacks or pajamas are just as good. And take your shoes and stockings off. The exercises below are by no means a complete program, but they get to the heart of many muscular difficulties. In performing these exercises, it is important to warm up gradually and do the exercises in order, because the last ones act most directly on the *iliopsoas* itself.

The Neck And Shoulder Uncramper

Here's an exercise designed to relieve cramping and pain in the neck and shoulders. Stand with your feet slightly separated.

149

Bend forward with your arms and head hanging loosely. Bring your arms forward, up and back in a free-swinging circle. If it is more comfortable for you, swing just one arm at a time. Make from 50 to 300 continuous circles with your arms at least once a day. This exercise is good for loosening the muscles of the shoulders, shoulder blades and upper back. As the muscles stretch, you will be able to make larger circles, and accomplish the stretching with less repetition. (See Illustration A)

For An Ache In The Middle Back

Moving down the back, the next exercise is designed to work out the muscles of shoulder blades and middle back. It also helps correct any exaggerated forward or backward curvature of the spine.

Standing with your feet wide apart and body bent forward at the waist, clasp your hands behind you. Let the weight of your head and shoulders pull your torso forward. Now, remaining bent at the waist, lift your torso by raising your head and arching your back while pulling your shoulder blades sharply together. Hold this position for a fast count of 10. Then relax and let your body droop forward again. Repeat this movement 10 to 20 times whenever your upper back, neck or shoulders feel cramped. Otherwise, once or twice a day will suffice.

The Low Back Stretcher

This exercise is for stretching the low back and the hamstring muscles of the upper thighs. It accomplishes with orthopedic safety what the traditional toe-touching exercise was designed to do. Begin by sitting on the floor and putting your left leg out in front of you, toes straight up, and the leg swung over as far as possible toward your left side. Bend your right knee and bring the right heel in close to the crotch, keeping the left knee flat on the floor and holding your left hand in the small of your back. Sitting as erectly as possible, twist to the left until you're facing the outstretched left leg. Now reach out your hand and try to touch your left toes, bending from the hips. Bounce your torso up and down to loosen your muscles and get closer to your toes. Eventually, you should work up to 100 quick bouncing motions. At first, you may not get too close to your toes, and probably won't be able to do 100 repetitions, but keep at it. It will get easier every day. (See Illustration B)

The Knee-Chest Stretch

If you've ever been to an orthopedic specialist, chances are he told you to do this exercise.

Lie on your back on the floor with a pillow under your head and your knees bent. Keep your feet about 12 inches apart. Now grab your right knee with your right hand and pull it as close to your chest as you can. Bounce it toward your chest 20 to 50 times. Do the same with your other knee. To wind up, pull both knees up to the chest together and hold them as close to your chest as you can for the count of ten. (See Illustration C)

Relaxing Your Up-Tight Spine

Here's an exercise which is similar to one of the basic yoga exercises. Kneel on the floor with your knees about six or eight inches apart and bend forward from the waist, stretching your arms out over your head. Your elbows should be straight so that your forehead and lower arms and hands are actually resting on the floor. Being sure to keep your thighs perpendicular to the floor, press your chest down as far as it will go, all the way to the floor if possible. Hold it for a fast count of ten, then relax the chest but stay down there for another few seconds. Repeat as many times as you can in three minutes. This exercise stretches the hip joints, the entire spine, and the shoulder muscles as well: the perfect prescription for an up-tight back. (See Illustration D)

For Hip Muscles

The next exercise stretches the tight hip and thigh connector muscles, and increases the range of motion, thus facilitating correction of hip and thigh disalignment.

Stand at arm's length from a wall with your side to it. Place the flat of your hand on the wall for support, which you should be able to do without stretching. Now, bounce the hip facing the wall sharply toward the wall, so that your whole pelvis is jerked to the side. Repeat 20 to 50 times and then switch sides. If you can't do 20, do as many as you can without straining yourself (the same goes for all the other exercises). (See Illustration E)

And Finally . . . En Garde!

This next exercise gets right down to the *iliopsoas*. "This exercise is a critical one, as it stretches the *iliopsoas* and aids body flexibility and alignment," Dr. Michele comments.

Get into a fencer's thrust position, as illustrated. Place your right foot forward, bending your knees and stretching your leg as far in front of you as you can. Turn your right foot in slightly, but try to keep the left one pointing straight ahead, with the heel lifted. Holding your torso erect, bounce your torso backwards until a pull is felt in the groin. To help balance yourself, keep your left hand on your left hip and your right hand on your right thigh. Do 50 bounces and then repeat with the left foot forward. Dr. Michele urges doing this exercise "as many times in a day as you have time and strength for." (See Illustration F)

If you think you do not have enough time to do these exercises, realize how much easier it is to find a half hour, even in a busy day, than it would be to get any work done at all when you are wracked with the pain that comes when muscle imbalance continues uncorrected on its damaging course.

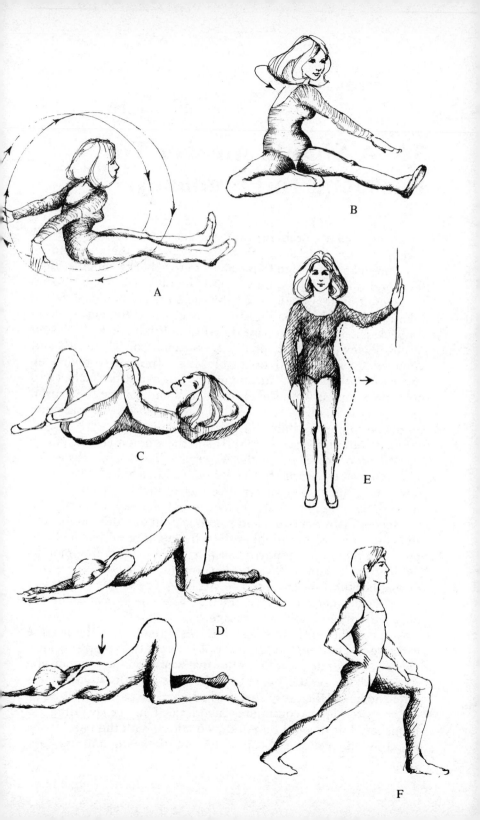

A

B

C

D

E

F

34. A Simple Answer To Backache In Pregnancy

Pregnancy has its problems, not the least of which is that old faithful misery, backache. Women going into their second or third pregnancies resign themselves to sore backs, much as they do to morning sickness, nerves and sleeplessness. They blame the weight of the developing baby, when they should really be blaming themselves. Bad posture was given as the main reason for backache in pregnancy by Mabel Lum Fitzhugh, R. P. T., and Michael Newton, M.D., of the Department of Obstetrics and Gynecology at the University of Mississippi. A woman who carries herself properly in pregnancy can avoid backaches and other problems as well. For example, in some women the painful circulatory difficulties that develop into varicose veins can often be traced to poor posture during pregnancy.

Most mothers can see themselves in the women Drs. Fitzhugh and Newton described in the *American Journal of Obstetrics and Gynecology* (April 15, 1963). Mrs. E. M., aged 27, was in her third pregnancy. She first noticed swelling leg veins in the seventh month of her first pregnancy, but she had no pain. With her second baby, swelling and pain began in the fifth month, and she could relieve the problem best by keeping off her feet and propping them up whenever possible. It took only three months for low back pain and varicose veins in both calves to show during her third pregnancy. The swelling was so severe that she wore elastic bandages during the day. Extreme pain at night was only partially relieved by massage.

At the end of six months, Mrs. E. M. agreed to try the posture exercise devised by the Mississippi University experts, because she was desperate for relief. After two weeks on the program she discarded the elastic bandages. At eight months (two months after she began the exercises) she had no more pain, night or day, except after long, continuous standing. The leg swelling diminished, but it could be reinduced, along with the pain, if she stood in a poor posture position for as little as one minute.

Another person in pain, Mrs. C. E., a 33-year-old mother of eight, came for consultation when she was six months pregnant with her ninth child. She complained of pressure pain in the lower abdomen for the previous month. This pressure had become increasingly severe with each pregnancy, but had never begun so early. Low back pain was another complaint. She began to educate herself to proper posture and she practiced faithfully because she said the exercise felt good. One month later she said she was free of abdominal and back pains. Mrs. C. E. had no recurrence through the rest of the pregnancy.

Little Time—No Equipment

What is the magnificent treatment that freed these women from a common ailment so many women come to expect with pregnancy? Drs. Fitzhugh and Newton call it the pelvic tilt exercise for posture correction. It takes only a minute or two to learn, requires no equipment and no time out from household chores. In fact, the doctors urged their patients to do the exercise in the kitchen, using the sink as a prop. That way they are encouraged to do it more frequently:

1. Stand about a foot and a half to two feet away from the sink—far enough to be able to bend forward at the hips and rest your hands on the edge of the sink with arms straight. Then raise your hips and relax your abdomen, increasing the sway in the small of your back.

2. Inhale, round your back, tuck your buttocks under and exhale. Keep knees slightly flexed during this maneuver to get full rotation of the pelvis.

3. Repeat the movement three times—first, raise the hips as you inhale, then tuck the buttocks under during exhalation.

4. Now drop your hands from the support and stand erect, trying to raise your breastbone straight up. The shoulders are relaxed, knees slightly flexed and the buttocks tucked underneath. Your weight will be evenly balanced on both feet.

Pregnant women are instructed to do this exercise about twelve times a day, or any time they approach the sink or a chair. They are also to stay conscious of maintaining a level pelvis standing or walking. The exercise itself takes little more time than it does to dry a dish.

The pelvic tilt aims to minimize the awkward bulk of pregnancy, and to balance the extra weight on all four sides of the body. This is the most favorable alignment. When poor posture spoils it, certain muscles are stretched out of line, while others are contracted tightly to maintain balance. The contracted muscles ache, and the stretched ones become useless.

In pregnancy some muscles are meant to stretch, particularly those in the abdominal wall being pushed out by the growing uterus. But the added weight and forward expansion of the abdomen mechanically increase the curvature in the lower part of the back. This stretches the abdomen further, and the muscles in the lower part of the spine tighten more, trying to keep the abdominal load from sinking still further.

Over-stretching the abdominal wall, together with the increased inward curve of the lower spine, tilts the whole pelvis forward, permitting the growing uterus to slide forward, far out of balance, and far away from the weight-bearing center of gravity in the body. Instead of being carried, the developing fetus merely hangs by the abdominal muscles, sling fashion. It is obvious that the woman who permits her abdomen to hang forward increases the strain on the muscles in her back and is asking for backache.

Align The Pelvis

The logical thing is to re-position the pelvis at a more level position, so that the center of gravity of the uterus is moved backward toward the body, and its weight borne more directly by the pelvic bone and the leg bones, instead of the stomach muscles. Do this, and the inward curve of the lower back automatically straightens; the pressure is off the lower back muscles. Result: no low back pain.

The shift in body weight depends partly on the slight flexing of the knees called for in the exercise. When the knees are extended straight out as they are likely to be when the stomach hangs forward and the lower back curves in, the stretch at the back of the knees grows stronger as the abdomen gets heavier. The tendency is to brace for a standing position by pushing back strongly at the knees. Just a light flexing of the knees is enough to reduce this hyper-extension and help to correct the position of the pelvis.

The patient is directed to bend over the sink because she achieves a greater degree of pelvic movement than she would if she tried the exercises standing erect. The low back muscles become more flexible, and this helps during labor and delivery. When buttocks are tucked under, the lower back muscles that hold the spine erect get some relief from the tension common to the sway-backed posture, when they actually support a good part of the uterus weight.

The tone of the abdominal wall is also improved by leaning forward. This position tightens the transverse muscles of the abdomen, changing them from a slack to a snug support. There is no effort involved in keeping the abdomen in good tone as long as the pelvis remains level and knees are slightly flexed.

Of course, the circulation in the lower legs improves with the knees relaxed. Standing with the back of the knees tightly stretched tends to compress the veins of the back of the knee and slow down the blood flow.

For many women, the price of poor posture in pregnancy is the need for potent, possibly dangerous drugs, and even surgery to relieve varicose veins and aching back. Here is a safe, effective solution to the problem. All the women who followed the simple exercises outlined here have had partial to complete relief in a few weeks.

The body is equipped with the muscles needed to avoid backache and abdominal pain in pregnancy. A wise, health-minded woman can insure the ease of her pregnancy by training herself to stand and walk with maximum natural comfort and minimal chance of injury.

35. What Causes Back Trouble During Menopause?

Osteoporosis, or porous bone, the disease which causes some aging persons to develop a stoop in the upper back, is one of the most frequently encountered causes of back trouble. The reversed curve in the lower back increases as the upper spine slumps forward. One of the chief causes of osteoporosis, says Drs. William Ishmael and Howard B. Shorbe, in their booklet *Care of the Back* (Lippincott, 1964), is the menopause. In fact many women date their pain in the back from the onset of the change of life.

Menopause causes a diminishing supply of estrogen in the female system. This leads to demineralization of the bone structure which is, of course, the condition called osteoporosis.

Porous bones, however, are *not* an inevitable part of growing older and you *don't* have to have osteoporosis just because you are going through the menopause—not if your nutrition is meeting the excessive stress which menopause places on your body's machinery.

The logical way to treat osteoporosis is calcium supplementation, according to one of America's top authorities, G. Donald Whedon, M.D., director of the National Institute of Arthritis and Rheumatic Diseases, who in October, 1967, delivered a memorial lecture to the medical faculty of the University of Ottawa entitled, "Recent Developments and Comprehension of Osteoporosis."

Dr. Whedon observed that "regardless of its multiple causes—osteoporosis is characterized by overactive resorption of bone, brought about by an insufficiency of calcium (whether due to a dietary deficiency, malabsorption, or excessive urinary loss) which stimulates parathyroid secretion." (The parathyroid is the gland whose hormone triggers the release of calcium from the bones.)

Calcium supplementation is effective only when the calcium is accompanied by enough phosphorus, magnesium and vitamin D to permit its ready absorption into the structure of the bone, and the most natural and effective calcium supplement is bone meal which contains not only calcium but phosphorus, magnesium and many important trace minerals.

Dr. Lewis Barnett, an orthopedic surgeon, pointed out that magnesium independently plays a very important role in the formation of hard, dense bone tissue. Dr. Barnett noted that groups of patients who drank water with high magnesium content continued to have hard, virtually unbreakable bones regardless of age, whereas other patients who got less magnesium and relatively fragile bones no matter how good their diet was otherwise.

Section 8
Bad Breath

36. The Many Causes Of Halitosis

36. The Many Causes Of Halitosis

One is almost forced to conclude, after reading the experts, that bad breath is an individual problem which cannot be solved by employing general measures. There is disagreement on what causes bad breath and more disagreement on how to treat it. Everyone does know that, while the condition itself is not harmful, it is a source of great embarrassment and concern to those who suffer with it.

Scientists have spent considerable time and effort in attempting to solve the problem. However, medical men generally agree that there is no one very effective way of controlling this unpleasant condition.

Among the possible causes of bad breath: certain incompatible bacterial flora in the mouth, constipation and infrequent bowel movements, gases absorbed from the intestinal tract and breathed out through the lungs. This last is considered the chief cause of this unpleasant problem. In overweight people, it is this problem that is more prevalent due to the additional number of blood vessels in which odorous debris can collect before being deposited in the lungs.

The *Journal of the American Medical Association* (March, 1960) named upper respiratory infections—colds—as an important causal factor. A coated tongue, gum infections and dental cavities were mentioned as common causes; so were menstruation, pregnancy and nervous tension. And don't forget smoking as a well-recognized cause of bad breath.

Of course, the most obvious step to be taken against bad breath is to be certain of the cleanliness of the mouth. Brush teeth properly and frequently to eliminate the collection of debris that can give off a foul odor.

Sometimes the most careful brushing fails to catch foods lodged in tight places between or behind the teeth. If foods frequently become entangled in what seem to be traps formed by the teeth, it is wise to consult a dentist about creating a less vulnerable surface. Denture plates, particularly those that cannot be removed for cleaning, sometimes are responsible for caught foods. Check dentures frequently and disinfect them with a cleansing solution daily.

Use dental floss to keep corners and crevices free of any odorous, decay-causing food remnants. Decayed teeth, themselves, are perhaps the most easily recognizable cause of bad breath.

When offensive breath persists in spite of good dental care and the usual mouthwashes and breath fresheners that are, after all, only palliative measures, then diet and digestion may be the culprits. No matter how good and nourishing one's diet, if the stomach does not contain enough hydrochloric acid, the food will not be digested, and therefore, not assimilated.

Acid is required to break down food, and when it is lacking in the stomach to any serious degree, unwanted bacteria grow and the result can be a putrid development of undigested food within the body, which can cause chronic bad breath. A doctor who recognizes the value of hydrochloric acid in the stomach could be consulted for guidance in correcting this problem by prescribing the proper amount of HCL for the system. There are tablets of hydrochloric acid betaine plus pepsin (the most effective form) available for just this purpose. But they should be used with caution.

Garlic has a reputation as the classic bad breath offender. But garlic odor on the breath does not always come from garlic. The *Journal of the American Medical Association* (February 4, 1974) reports that garlic-like breath odor may be attributable to exposure to selenium and tellurium. Many laboratory technicians are exposed to these dangerous chemicals, and the resulting garlic-like breath may be the forerunner of such symptoms as nausea, vomiting, lethargy and central nervous system disorders. Extreme and prolonged exposure can even cause death.

Some shampoos and many lipsticks contain small amounts of selenium as do rectifiers in television sets.

Anyone experiencing garlic-like breath without consuming garlic should search for possible exposure to selenium or tellurium.

In 1960, the work of Dr. Seizo Kawasaki, a Japanese researcher studying breath odors, was reported in *Dental Abstracts.* He used a group of female students, ranging in age from 20 to 22 years of age, to test his theory that the type of food one eats is responsible for the degree of odor on the breath. The food one eats causes a change in the chemistry of one's saliva, and a change in the odor of the breath is also due to this phenomenon, said Dr. Kawasaki. In the tests he conducted he found that, within three hours, the saliva is affected by the type of food eaten. The odor of the saliva is strongest after carbohydrates are eaten; it is somewhat less after protein foods are taken in; fat foods actually inhibit the odor.

According to Dr. Kawasaki, a component of saliva known as mucin is the cause of odor on the breath, and carbohydrates cause it to increase, while fats cause it to decrease. Protein foods are less likely than carbohydrates to give breath problems.

Certain chemicals can cause bad breath when they are present in the body. Among these are arsenic, lead, bismuth and methane. They are all food additives and are likely to be present in some part of what you eat every day. If bad breath plagues you, perhaps the processed foods you eat are responsible.

In an article in *Modern Medicine* (February 19, 1973) Dr. Walter C. Alvarez, M.D., stated, "The commonest cause of a really severe case of bad breath is a strong or painful emotion."

He based this statement on years of observation and study of the subject. Dr. Alvarez described the case of a woman who came to him with a cramped leg which she thought was paralyzed. Her breath was so bad he said he had to air out his office after she left. The next day he saw the woman again, but this time her leg was better, her fear was gone and her breath was sweet.

Another patient of Dr. Alvarez experienced foul breath every time her husband drove down a narrow, steep road in the California mountains. Within a few minutes of returning to level land her breath always became sweet again.

Because people who are distressed often have a fecal odor to their breath, Dr. Alvarez theorizes the smell may come from the colon through mesenteric veins into the liver. The severe emotional upheaval stops the liver's normal cleansing action so that the foul odor travels in the blood to the heart and lungs and out through the mouth.

Diabetes, according to Alvarez, can be another cause of bad breath.

Chances are that all of us will have bad breath one time or another. One billionth of an ounce of onion oil can be detected on the breath by the sense of smell. Garlic travels in the blood stream with such determination that it can be demonstrated on the breath of a newborn baby if the mother has eaten it shortly before delivery. There are many such pungent odors. Even pleasant ones sometimes take on a less desirable character when mixed with others. Aside from these, we all get foods stuck in our teeth, we all sometimes forget to—or can't—brush our teeth; we have coated tongues or sore throats; we suffer from indigestion or gas at some time. One healthful way to disguise unpleasant mouth odors is to chew parsley, long known for its power to neutralize breath odors, or pungently pleasant herbs such as mint, rosemary, basil or thyme. Chewing gum and lozenges, and other candy breath disguisers can harm the teeth and the system due to their artificial flavoring and sugar.

The greatest psychological inducement to the use of mouthwashes is the promise that they sweeten breath, but according to a statement in *Dental Abstracts*, "The quality of the breath can be improved more effectively by mechanical procedures than by cosmetic preparation. The use of a toothbrush lessens mouth odors for at least two hours, whereas the masking aroma of a dentifrice lasts only a half hour."

If bad breath persists, see a dentist or physician to be certain that no serious physical disorder is the cause.

Section 9
Bedwetting

37. You Can Do Something About Bedwetting

In *Medical Care of the Adolescent* (published by Appleton-Century-Crofts, Inc., 1968) urologist R. Richard Muellner, M.D., asserted that bedwetting (enuresis) plagues about 10 percent of five-year-olds and tends to disappear as children grow older. However, surveys show that one to three percent of 20-year-old servicemen suffer from enuresis.

Dr. Muellner stated that many cases of enuresis could be nipped in the bud by observant parents. "There is every reason to believe that the child of four who voids more frequently than usual during the day and has no greater bladder capacity than a child of two is a potential bedwetter." That is the time to start increasing a child's bladder capacity. Gently forcing fluids and urging longer waits after the first sensation of the need to void "might well prevent all the unhappy consequences of prolonged enuresis."

A full account of the problem and its treatment by a prominent British physician appeared in *Parents,* a British magazine, and is reprinted with permission.

Enuresis At Teenage
By William Moodie, M.D., F.R.C.P., D.P.M.

Most people think of enuresis as the habit some children have of wetting the bed long after most are dry by night. As a matter of fact, the word means loss of control of the bladder by day, or by night, or both, and it is by no means limited to young children. Many adolescents and adults are afflicted in this way, either constantly, or in times of stress.

It is looked upon as a shameful thing, so much so that sufferers are often too shy even to consult their doctor about it.

This is quite understandable, but it really should not be thought something to be ashamed of.

It is a symptom, and as such is just like a cough or a pain.

It is something that cannot be controlled at will, though it is thought of as something that ought to be overcome, and as childish.

If the loss of control occurs both by day and night, it is a sign of serious disturbance of the nervous system, and medical advice should be sought at once; but such cases are rare in comparison with those in which it happens only at night.

Usually the habit has existed from early life. It often results from overstrenuous toilet training. Perhaps a child has continued to be wet at night after the time that his mother thinks he "should know better" and so much pressure is brought to bear on the matter that it turns into a major issue, a cause of tension and anxiety in the household, or perhaps the child is blamed.

Anxiety in a child's mind is one of the surest ways of making the whole thing permanent. Of course, the child often does not show the anxiety, and adopts a "couldn't care less" attitude, but this is only his way of covering up his shame.

Boys and girls can both be enuretic and it is generally accepted that the age of five should be taken as the time when the average child is dry. Many are dry long before that, but it is as damaging to have a child dry too soon, as too late. If a child is over-trained and dry very soon, tension and anxiety too often appear in other disguises. Toilet training should be a steady and easy process. Then it is normal and leaves no ill effects.

The most common form of enuresis is bedwetting, and in the simple case and the commonest, it happens according to a certain pattern. In this article we shall discuss the symptom as it occurs over the age of 10.

Between five and 10, psychological factors play the greatest part in perpetuating the trouble, and these must be sorted out in each particular case in a clinic where such matters are dealt with.

After 10 the psychological factors have usually become less important, though at all ages any cause of deep anxiety should be sought out and eliminated.

Any special strain associated with the trouble may be enough to keep it going. Even the popular "star charts" often do more harm than good. Punishment because it is called "just laziness" is quite hopeless, and so is the attitude that the child is doing it as a revenge. Children will often wet their beds after a family row, but it is the anxiety following the incident that causes it, not revenge.

As in all mental matters there are exceptions. There are parents who have "cured" the habit by punishment. There are some few children who do it deliberately. But in these cases skilled advice should be sought because there is something seriously wrong somewhere.

Now let us talk about the commonest form and some of the symptoms that are found frequently to accompany enuresis.

The wetting may happen every night, or only after a long and tiring day, or excitement, but, associated with it is *precipitancy,* which means that when the desire to pass water (or to micturate, in medical language) comes, it is sudden.

Often it is only just possible to get to the lavatory in time. This accentuates the anxiety. It often happens that the sufferer wakens from sleep when he begins to pass water, and can stop before passing much.

Usually it is noted that it does not matter much whether drinks are stopped for a time before going to bed, though drinking a lot of tea or coffee late at night may make wetting more likely.

Besides precipitancy by day there is often frequency. The desire to micturate comes on often, and the tendency is to visit the lavatory on any possible occasion, and to sit through a film or theatre performance is uncomfortable.

The cause behind the trouble, when it has been established for a long time, is that the bladder has become accustomed to hold much less than it normally should.

Every hollow organ in the body has in it a mechanism that makes it tend to empty when it is filled up to a certain extent. The bladder is no exception. Normally it fills up, and when it is getting nearly full, one becomes aware of the fact.

This signal, however, gives considerable latitude. It can fill up a good deal more before it empties automatically, and there is a point beyond which no effort of will can prevent this.

In people who have frequency, however, this emptying reflex happens before the bladder is full, because it has been so constantly emptied before it has fully filled, and, what is more important, before it is full enough to send the message up to the brain to tell of the need to empty. The message that comes then is often not from the bladder but from just beyond it, and is caused by the first drops coming away. This is what wakens the sleeper, or causes slight "leakage" in the daytime.

Enuretics are usually said to be heavy sleepers, and it is easy to see that these weak messages are often not strong enough to wake the sleeper. That is also why drugs which lighten sleep are sometimes helpful, while sedatives can make matters worse.

The first part of treatment must be, therefore, to accustom the bladder to hold more and more, until its content becomes normal. To do this, control must be practiced during the day, gradually teaching it to hold back by not going to the lavatory so often. If this is persevered in, the frequency will decrease.

It is known that bladders that have become accustomed to too frequent emptying get atonic. The muscles are weak; therefore, after seemingly emptying, there will still be a certain amount of fluid left behind.

Therefore, it is very important that at each act of micturition the bladder must be emptied, and when the flow first stops that that must not be taken as indicating that there is no more to come. There we find the second part of the curative "drill."

When a person lies down, the kidneys secrete, so, when we go to bed, a slightly increased production of urine occurs. Therefore, on going to bed, one should go to the lavatory, and pass all the fluid that will pass, and then lie down for half an hour and read, and then go and pass what has since collected.

When a drink is taken, the kidneys become active for a short period, and so the enuretic subject should not drink for at least an hour before going to bed. Fluids, within reason, at any other time do not matter at all.

There is another "drill" that sometimes helps, and that is to increase control by voluntarily starting and stopping the flow say three times in each act of micturition.

In the majority of cases this "five point drill," if really persevered in, will show effects within six weeks, and often the whole trouble will have gone in three or four months.

Sometimes certain drugs help, but they are usually quite useless without the bladder re-education.

Behind all this the importance of anxiety must always be kept in mind. There is nothing that upsets all reflex mechanisms so much as an uneasy mind.

It is therefore very important to concentrate on the removal of anxiety at every stage. Any drill must be carried out with a completely optimistic spirit, and failures must be overlooked and made light of. All the time the child must be kept in a hopeful mood and success continually kept in front of him.

There Seem To Be Several Causes Of Enuresis

Dr. John W. Gerrard, Professor of Pediatrics at the University of Saskatchewan, presents evidence that bedwetting is sometimes the result of an allergy.

Bedwetting

Reporting on his studies in February 13, 1974 *Medical Tribune,* Dr. Gerrard said, "The prime problem is that the bedwetting youngster has a small bladder capacity and that the bladder capacity has shrunk because the detrusor muscle is in spasm, a spasm which is often a manifestation of an allergy." Dr. James B. J. McKendry of the University of Toronto reported at the 1974 meeting of the American Academy of Pediatrics that certain foods such as milk, chocolate and eggs can cause a bladder hypersensitivity which in turn causes bedwetting. Removal of the offending foods results in cessation of wetting. If a child wets only when he is in a certain home, it may be in reaction to a particular food (or brand of food) he eats only at that place.

At the same meeting, Dr. Gerrard described a study comparing the bladder sizes of 223 normal and 75 enuretic children. The bladders of the normal children had about double the capacities of the bladders of enuretics. The children who were wet both day and night had the smallest bladder capacity of all the children tested.

Another speaker at the meeting, Dr. Alan D. Perlmutter, pediatric urologist at Children's Hospital, Detroit, said that of the 15 to 20 percent of children who still wet their beds at age five, only one percent still suffer from this problem at age 15. Either their bladder sizes increase or they learn to awaken at night to urinate.

Dr. McKendry warned that while, "No one ever died of this common complaint, a few patients have died of overdose of drugs used to control it."

This view was supported by an August 17, 1973 article in the *Washington Post* warning against the use of Tofranil for bedwetters. "Many more deaths will occur," claimed the *Post,* from Tofranil overdoses "unless the medical profession is warned of the toxicity of this tiny sugar-coated tablet."

Imipramine is another drug, used for treatment of enuresis, which has caused numerous deaths when misused.

There are many forms of treatment being used successfully for enuresis.

In Toronto in 1974 Dr. Franz Baumann reported successful use of hypnotherapy in treating 14 enuretic boys, ages eight to 11. None of these children had obstruction or neurologic disorders. They did, however, display frequent urinary infections. It was suggested under hypnosis to the patients that they could control their urine flow and that doing so would make them happy. Those boys who were not completely cured were markedly improved.

The use of self-hypnosis was studied by Dr. Karen Olness and reported in the March, 1975 edition of *Clinical Pediatrics.* Dr. Olness observed 20 boys and 20 girls ranging in age from four to 16 years. None of these children had organic problems of the urinary tract and none were severely emotionally disturbed. The subjects were taught a simple form of self-hypnosis. Within one month 28 of the 40 were cured. The study ran 28 months. At the end of this time 31 were cured, six improved greatly and only three showed no change.

Dr. Olness believes "Many parents prolong bedwetting by expecting their children to be dry at night by age three. Their pressure on children who still bedwet after three may prolong the symptom beyond age five, which is a more reasonable time to expect bladder control."

Acupuncture has also been employed as a treatment for enuresis. The July-September, 1973 issue of *American Journal of Acupuncture* carried the report of two Czechoslovakian doctors who used acupuncture in the treatment of 29 children, aged six to 15, who suffered functional enuresis. Doctors K. Tabarka and R. Cupalova used three series of ten daily acupuncture treatments on all but four of the subjects. (These four were cured at the end of the second series.) At the conclusion of the treatments 18 children were significantly cured and the other 11 were only slightly improved or remained unchanged.

The *Journal of the American Medical Association* (April 21, 1975) reported on an anti-bedwetting measure that consists of a battery operated alarm set off by moisture. This device is set up by placing two electrodes, separated by gauze, under the child. It only takes a small amount of urine to close the circuit and activate the alarm. This method works best when the child does not wear pajama bottoms. Of course, the child must understand the reason for the alarm.

It is important that the parents get up with the child in the initial stages of this treatment to make sure he doesn't sleep through the alarm.

This treatment was first used around 1900 and enjoyed a revival in the 1930's. In 1971 S. Dische conducted a study of 84 enuretic children using this treatment. Thirty-three percent of these children were cured in one month, two-thirds after three months and at the end of six months 90 percent of the children were dry. There was, however, a relapse in 30 percent of the cases. Although this problem is generally controllable or curable by the child taking an active role in his own treatment, on occasion surgery or medication is necessary. These should be a last resort.

Section 10
Birth Defects

38. What Are The Major Causes Of Birth Defects?

Birth defects, the leading child health problem in the United States, was once considered primarily a disease of heredity. However, today, heredity alone accounts for only 20 percent of the 200,000 infants born every year with some form of deformity, either mental or physical. These statistics do not indicate a de-emphasis of the role of heredity in the causation of birth defects. Rather they reflect the increasing recognition of the influence of environmental factors. According to the records of the National Foundation—March of Dimes, it is the interaction between the environment and heredity that now accounts for 60 percent of those children born every year with deformities.

Environmental influences include teratogenic (fetus-damaging) drugs, environmental pollutants, poor nutrition and viral, parasitic or bacterial infections. The latter three cause the majority of birth defects by reacting with genetic predispositions which can seriously deform the fetus at any time during the term of pregnancy. However, like heredity, environmental influences alone account for only 20 percent of the total yearly number of babies born with defects.

The correlation between birth defects and poor maternal nutrition is commonly accepted by scientists. Babies who weigh less than five and a half pounds—a generally accepted dividing line between normal and low birthweight—are 17 times more likely to die in infancy than those weighing more. Although low birthweight is not exactly a cause of birth defects, infants who are born too prematurely or too small are likely to suffer from defects, according to the National Foundation—March of Dimes. Researchers at the Foundation also estimate that approximately 245,000 children are born every year under five and a half pounds, of whom 45,000 have birth defects.

All the building material required by the fetus during its life in the womb must be supplied by the mother. Her body processes the food she eats, which is transmitted through the placenta to be assimilated by the fetus. To a large degree, then, her child is what she eats. If, through adulteration or refining or just poor dietary habits, her food intake lacks some nutritional element— vitamin, mineral, or enzyme—the construction of the fetus may be weakened.

Pregnant Women Need Food, Not Weight Control

Every pregnant woman leans heavily on the advice and guidance of her obstetrician. She is, after all, really "eating for two people." But, nine out of ten obstetricians are still recommending a restrictive diet that is not adequate for two, and many a pregnant woman dreads the monthly weighing-in for fear that her increased appetite has caused a weight gain beyond her doctor's orders.

If your obstetrician is still severely restricting your weight gain, then he hasn't been doing his homework. After a thorough study, the National Research Council (NRC) now recommends that a pregnant woman be free to gain weight on good food.

For generations it was believed that an unborn infant holds a privileged place because it can "rob its mother of any nutritional ingredients essential to its own development." But now there is growing evidence that the unborn baby has to compete with its mother's body for the available nutrients. If the mother doesn't eat properly, it is more likely to be the baby who will suffer severe and permanent effects. In other words, when there is a shortage, the baby loses the battle with disastrous results. The mother suffers too. She may suffer the heartache of a stillbirth, a premature infant of low birthweight, a baby with brain damage and impaired intelligence, or a baby who contracts infections easily.

Because of the increasing number of low birthweight babies in this country, not only among poverty-stricken mothers, but at all social levels, the NRC, a part of the National Academy of Sciences, instituted a study to reappraise the whole subject of maternal nutrition. As a result of this study, the Academy struck down the old taboo of limited weight gain for pregnant women stating that *they should be allowed to gain as much as 24 pounds or more.*

While this is a form of emancipation and great news for the pregnant woman who is always fighting a losing battle with the scales in her obstetrician's office, it does not mean that she is free to gorge herself on doughnuts, creampuffs and the like. It is *not* a license to overeat or indulge. There is an important distinction in the kind of weight a woman gains when she is pregnant. When she eats foods of low nutrient and high calorie value, she gains weight. But this weight is nothing but accumulation of fat or fluid. When she eats foods that are high in nutrient value, the weight gain represents an increase in her tissue and in fetal tissue. This is of vital importance, much more serious than most of us, including most obstetricians, realize.

Doctors' Orders Have Caused Complications

Dr. Charles Lowe, former chairman of the American Academy of Pediatrics Nutrition Committee, noted that a poorly nourished mother will give birth to a lower than average weight baby. This infant is in danger of serious malnutrition which, if uncorrected, can lead to growth depression and possibly to mental retardation. "An infant so endowed most likely will become a handicapped adult, if he survives," Dr. Lowe warned (*Chicago Tribune*, Nov. 9, 1971).

Some of the most devastating and heartbreaking effects are caused by malnutrition, according to Dr. Myron Winick, a nutritionist at Cornell University Medical School. "If malnutrition occurs during pregnancy or the first six months of life when brain cells are rapidly dividing, permanent stunting of the brain may occur," he said. "If malnutrition occurs after the first six months, a child's learning ability may be seriously reduced. While the second type can be remedied with proper diet, the first type of damage is uncorrectable."

What you eat when you are pregnant has a far greater impact on the destiny of your child than is generally realized. Dr. Philip Handler, President of the National Academy of Sciences, reported that "There is ample evidence that protein malnutrition in pregnancy leads to a reduced number of brain cells."

In fact, the study conducted by the NRC was instigated by a group of knowledgeable people concerned with the growing problem of mental retardation. And what did this landmark study reveal? That *many problems of premature birth and retardation are probably due to the traditional advice given by doctors to pregnant women cautioning them to keep their weight down.*

Another error committed by many obstetricians is the treatment with diuretics for edema of pregnancy. What they don't realize, says Swiss obstetrician Dr. Frank Hytten, is that the normal pregnant woman often stores far more water in her tissues than had been previously thought (*Die Spatgestosc*, Basel, Switzerland, Schwabe & Company, 1970, p. 150). Dr. Hytten found that the well-nourished, nontoxemic pregnant patient often develops a generalized type of edema contrary to classic teachings. This physiological edema is protective for both mother and fetus and *should not be blindly treated with low-salt diet and salt diuretics*. Obstetricians must learn how to differentiate between benign physiologic edema and pathological edemas.

Why is the obstetrician unaware of these facts? Because most textbooks on the subject, with one notable exception, have generally ignored this point of view. The exception is *Management of High Risk Pregnancy and Intensive Care of the Neonate* by Babson and Benson (C. V. Mosby, Second Edition, 1971). These authors have recognized that inadequate diets during pregnancy lead to both maternal and fetal diseases and deaths. They put emphasis on a "well balanced, high protein, high vitamin, high mineral diet." They also point out the protein-sparing effects of calories from carbohydrates and fats, and decry the use of low-calorie diets and blind weight control which disregards the basic principles of good nutrition. "Patients will fare better if the physician stresses *good diet* rather than total weight gain," the authors emphasize.

39. Good Diet Encourages Healthy Childbirth

A study at Harvard University's School of Public Health showed that among women with good-to-excellent prenatal diets 95 percent of their babies were born without complications and in good-to-excellent condition. Among women with poor-to-very-poor prenatal diets the results were almost exactly the reverse.

Similarly, the introduction of any non-nutrient chemicals—nicotine, alcohol, chemical food additives, drugs, etc.—may affect the fetal enzyme system and interfere with its delicately balanced growth factors, the study reveals.

It was pointed out in the *Medical Tribune* in 1962, that any interference with folic acid metabolism in the fetus will produce deformities. Likewise, a vitamin imbalance, a deficiency of the vitamin B complex, can produce abnormalities, and such antibiotics as streptomycin and tetracycline can cause precisely that deficiency.

According to Dr. W. Coda Martin in his book, *A Matter of Life* (Devin Adair, New York, 1964) an imbalance of the body's stores of B complex "was illustrated by the thalidomide tragedy in which many pregnant women who were taking the tranquilizer produced malformed children. Subsequent research indicated that thalidomide interfered with metabolism of nicotinic acid (a B complex vitamin) in the fetus. This vitamin is essential for normal fetal development during the first and second months of pregnancy. Thus, if the mother transmits too little of it to the unborn child or if some other element she transmits interferes with fetal utilization of it, a birth defect will be a likely result." Not all of the mothers who took thalidomide gave birth to deformed babies. Those who were spared this tragedy may well have been those whose diets included enough of the B vitamins to compensate for what the thalidomide destroyed.

B complex deficiencies have also been associated with birth defects in other well-known studies. "Studies on the Molecular Basis of Congenital Malformations," by Dr. Bruce Mackler and colleagues, which appeared in the June 1969 issue of *Pediatrics*, showed how riboflavin deficiencies in varying degrees affected four separate groups of pregnant laboratory rats. In all the groups, more than 95 percent of the fetuses developed gross malformations.

Most of the defects, reported Dr. Mackler, a researcher at the School of Medicine, University of Washington, Seattle, were skeletal anomalies—abnormal development of the bones. The most common were incomplete development of the bones of the extremities—the baby rats' fore and hind paws—and abnormal smallness of the lower jaw. Dr. Mackler also mentioned cleft palate as an example of "a wide number of other anomalies" that have been produced in rat fetuses of mothers with a riboflavin deficiency.

Can these laboratory findings on experimental animals be translated into human terms? How real is the danger that an expectant mother will have so low a supply of riboflavin that her baby may be deformed? This is a difficult question, since no studies have been made of malformed babies in relation to the mother's riboflavin nutrition. But this much is known: riboflavin deficiency is considered the most common of vitamin deficiencies, and malnutrition in this nutrient is widespread.

Not too long ago, the fact of widespread malnutrition was ridiculed by official government sources and by organized medicine. But now it is openly acknowledged that we face a hidden hunger problem in this richest country of the world.

One especially tragic result of malnutrition in the formative months is the behavior problem child who may well be expressing his mother's poor diet. This youngster, sometimes termed brain-damaged, is not mentally retarded or abnormal in the usual sense, but constantly has trouble at home and at school. He tends to be nervous, irritable, emotionally unstable and uncooperative with his parents and teachers. He is prone to illness and psychological disturbances and cannot seem to concentrate on anything long enough to make passing grades in his studies. Such children are so numerous that they can be classified as a major health and sociological problem. Many schools are now setting up special classes for such children.

Intelligence And Pre-Natal Nutrition

Will my baby be bright? Though few expectant mothers are aware of it, the intelligence of their children is affected by their diet

Birth Defects

during pregnancy. In *Science* (September, 1967, Vol. 157), Marilyn T. Eryckson of the Department of Pediatrics, University of North Carolina says that, "nutrition during pregnancy not only influences the condition of the child but that, when vitamin supplementation was given to pregnant and lactating women with poor nutritional environment, the offspring at four years of age had an average I.Q. score eight points greater than the average score of the children of mothers given a placebo over the same period."

So important is diet in terms of the child's intelligence, that researchers have been able to relate a pregnant woman's change of diet, when her appetite was depressed by the heat of the summer months, to the eventual intelligence of her child. The seat of the baby's mental facilities develops in the eighth to twelfth week of gestation, or the third month. In 1959 Hilda Knoblech, M.D., and Benjamin Pasamanick, M.D., presumed that congenital mental defectiveness would occur in the fetus at this time of pregnancy if it were to happen at all, and conducted an investigation. If a mother's diet is a factor, they reasoned, babies in the third month of gestation during hot weather are more likely to be born mentally disadvantaged than others. *An analysis of birth dates at a home for mentally defective children bore out the theory.*

40. How Radiation Causes Disease And Hereditary Alterations

Drs. John W. Gofman
and Arthur Tamplin

The radiation delivered to humans from beta rays, X-rays, gamma rays, or alpha particles is commonly referred to as *ionizing* radiation. The name is appropriate because the high speed electrons (beta rays) transversing tissue actually rip negatively charged electrons from atoms, leaving positively charged ions. Such electrons in turn ionize other atoms until finally all the initial energy of the high speed electrons is dissipated. X-rays and gamma rays by one or another mechanism set electrons in motion in tissue, and once this is done, all the events which occur are similar to those for an original beta ray. Alpha particles also ionize atoms in their path, again setting electrons in motion, which cause further ionization. This disruptive action, namely, producing electrically charged ions, is a major, but not the only way such radiations injure tissues. Many chemical bonds between atoms are shattered over and above the ionization produced, and this is an important additional damage mechanism.

Such disruptive actions of ionizing radiation can best be regarded simply as a massive, non-specific *disorganization* of biological cells and tissues. Biological cells are remarkably organized accumulations of chemical substances, arranged into myriad types of sub-structural entities within the cells. The beauty of such organization can only be marvelled at when revealed under the high magnifications of such instruments as the electron microscope or the electron scanning microscope. In stark contrast, there is hardly *anything* specific or orderly about the ripping of chemical bonds or of electrons out of atoms as ionizing radiation passes through biological cells. Rather, this represents disorganization and disruption. Perhaps a reasonable analogy would be the effect of passage of jagged pieces of shrapnel through tissues. One hardly expects nature's architecture to be improved by the disruptive action of shrapnel or ionizing radiation. Instead, what we can anticipate are varying degrees of disorganization of the delicate internal cellular architecture. If the disorganization thereby induced is sufficient, the result is death of the cell which has experienced the radiation insult. If the disorganization is of lesser degree, the cell can go on living, though wounded, for long periods of time. Not only can the wounded cells go on living, they can divide and thus reproduce new cells. Unfortunately, such new cells also may carry the injury sustained by the irradiated cell from which they arise.

While not yet proved, the leading concepts suggest that the crucial site of cell injury by ionizing radiation is the *nucleus* of the cell. It appears likely, further, that within the nucleus the critical structures injured are those known as *chromosomes*. In every normal human cell (except for certain stages of sperm and ova cells) there are 46 such chromosomes. These chromosomes are considered by most biologists to carry all, or almost all, the information in the cell. It is such information which provides the cell with the directions for all of its activities, including growth, cell division, production of a host of biologically important chemicals such as proteins, and diverse metabolic activities.

When ionizing radiation interacts with one of the chromosomes, there are two major ways in which the information system of the cell can be permanently altered. The units of information within the chromosome are known as genes, composed largely of the chemical known popularly as DNA (deoxyribonucleic acid). Radiation *can* produce a chemical alteration in a part of a single gene, and the result is that the gene functions abnormally thereafter, providing the cell with false directions. When such cells divide, the altered gene may be reproduced in the descendant cells. If a single gene on a chromosome has been chemically altered to provide new directions, a *point mutation* is said to have occurred.

Radiation can also produce a different type of change in the information system of the cell. This change occurs if the chromosome is physically broken. A human chromosome has two arms and a small region between known as the centromere. When a cell divides, the centromere leads the way for the chromosome to go to the daughter cell. When radiation breaks off a piece from one of the arms of the chromosome, this piece no longer has a centromere. As a result, it gets lost from the cell on the very next cell division. A single chromosome has hundreds or thousands of genes within it. Thus, one piece of chromosome broken off may have tens or even hundreds of genes in it. Such genes are lost to the daughter cells when their chromosome piece is lost. (For a short period of time [measured in hours] a broken piece of chromosome may rejoin its chromosome. Our concern, of course, is with the loss of those pieces which do *not* rejoin their own or some other chromosome in the cell.) Presumably if too many crucial genes are lost thereby, the cell may die. With lesser losses, the information alteration is not sufficiently severe for cell death to occur. Instead, it is possible that the loss of genes so imbalances the cellular information as to lead it ultimately to become a cancer cell. Loss of a piece of a chromosome and the genes within it is also called a mutation. This loss is appropriately designated as a *deletion*, for we have truly thereby deleted a piece of a chromosome and its genes. So radiation can provoke both major types of mutations, *point mutations* and *deletions*.

Hereditary Alterations

Radiation injury to the germinal cells of the testes, ultimately providing spermatozoa, and the germinal cells of the ovary, ultimately providing ova, has even more far-reaching consequences than radiation injury which leads other types of cells to leukemia or cancer. Changes in the chromosomes of sperm or ova precursor cells may be transmitted to all future generations of humans. The heredity of man, his greatest treasure, is thereby at stake. Once irreversibly injured, the chromosomes cannot be repaired by any process known to man.

The sperm precursor cells are called spermatogonia. Ultimately, these spermatogonia cells provide all the sperm in the male. The ova precursor cells are called oocytes, and they ultimately provide the ova. Mature spermatozoa have 23 chromosomes. Mature ova have 23 chromosomes. Upon fertilization of the ovum by sperm, the number is returned to 46 chromosomes, which characterizes all cells from the fertilized ovum through to the entire adult human.

Injury to the sperm or ova chromosomes while in the testis or ovary, either by point mutation or chromosome deletions (see above), can thus have the chance of being carried forward into *every* cell of a new human being. Worse yet, since every cell of a new human can carry such a mutation, the sperm and ova of this human can carry them also, so that the original injury persists through successive generations. We are probably fortunate that some of the mutations have sufficiently severe deleterious effects that the sperm or ova bearing the mutation fail to lead to a fertilized ovum, or if this does occur, the conceptus is lost in utero. Unfortunately, all too many serious mutations do permit the development of humans whose cells bear the mutation, and who suffer serious health consequences as a result.

An Increase In The Mutation Rate Is Undesirable

How serious are the health effects upon new generations of humans carrying mutated genes or altered chromosomes? We are only recently beginning to perceive the full extent of the hazard to health of future generations from such chromosomal or gene alterations—indeed to realize that it may be possible to tolerate only a very small number of additional mutations of genes or chromosomes as a result of technological poisons if humans are to continue to produce new generations of humans. Countless geneticists have repeatedly cautioned society about the danger of allowing *any* increase in the rate at which mutations (of any type, point mutations or chromosome injury) are introduced into the population at large. These geneticists know very well that mutations do occur naturally due to natural sources of radiation and to other causes, many of which are not understood to this date. Some who attempt to make light of the hazards of introducing unnecessary mutations are quick to point out that some mutations are beneficial, and indeed they may be. But prevailing genetic opinion indicates that natural selection most probably has already gone on long enough to maximize the occurrence of favorable mutations. Hence, we cannot hope to improve man by increasing his mutation rate. We can, however, assuredly count upon doing a great deal of harm, measured in untold human suffering from physical and mental deformities, and a higher incidence of many serious diseases if we allow mutation rates to increase.

The Nobel Laureate in Genetics, Professor Joshua Lederberg (Dr. Joshua Lederberg, Professor of Genetics, Stanford University, Palo Alto, California, Affidavit Sept. 8, 1970 [Docket #3445] before Public Service Board of Vermont), indicated his grave concern about the implications of increasing the existing mutation rate of our genes, and stated that present radiation standards allow for a ten percent increase in mutation rates. And he said, "I believe that the present standards for population exposure to radiation should and will (at least de facto) be made more stringent, to about one percent of the spontaneous rate, and that this is also a reasonable standard for the maximum tolerable mutagenic effect of any environmental chemical (better for them in the aggregate)."

Dr. Lederberg is suggesting that *all* forms of influence in our environment which can provoke genetic mutation or chromosome injury be one percent of the spontaneous rate, yet he points out the serious situation that we are currently legally permitting ten percent of the spontaneous rate from radiation alone. Let us quote Professor Lederberg on this: "*A ten percent increase in the existing 'spontaneous' mutation rate is, in effect, the standard that has been adopted as the 'maximum acceptable' level of public exposure to radiation by responsible regulatory bodies.*"

One wonders how it can be that responsible regulatory bodies would allow ten times as much genetic injury to the population from radiation *alone*, when a highly respected geneticist (and others concur) suggests one percent as a maximum for radiation plus chemicals combined.

A multitude of unsatisfactory answers to this question have been provided. One such answer is that we can not afford to impede technological progress by undue restrictions. Thus, it is reasoned, atomic energy programs in various forms such as nuclear electricity generation "must" be beneficial to humans and hence, must be allowed to pollute the environment with radioactive substances that will ultimately produce genetic changes in man. A reasonable view would be to ask why release of radioactivity must occur at such a high level for atomic energy programs to proceed. This is never done, but the answer is, of course, obviously, *economics*. It is cheaper to pollute than to take the necessary steps to prevent pollution. Promoters of all technology realize this intuitively and overtly. Hence, they press for the loosest possible standards of pollution or, better yet, no standards of restriction at all. And the pressure of such promotional interests is staggering. Generally all they need do is to mention the magic word "economics," and everyone falls into line. If it is uneconomic to prevent radioactive pollution, then assuredly we must allow the pollution to occur unimpeded. That we may pay an enormous price in the future through deterioration of our genes and chromosomes and, thereby, cause fantastic human misery and suffering hardly enters this "economic" picture. This is not because the proponents of atomic (or other) technologies are hard-hearted, evil individuals, bent upon injury to humans. Far from it. The *apparent* insensitivity arises from our widespread false definition of the term "economic." We only include short term considerations in our economic calculations—those concerned with days, weeks, months, or a few years. More ultimate costs to be borne by future society, or future generations, are scarcely visible (they almost appear "theoretical") and they routinely are avoided in economic considerations.

Another common, but unsatisfactory, answer is given for why we would legally permit enough radiation (and radioactivity contamination) to cause a ten percent increase in mutation rate. This approach points to the fact that we already are being irradiated from natural sources (cosmic rays, radioactivity of substances in the earth's crust, carbon-14 produced by cosmic rays) in an amount that can also cause about ten percent of the spontaneous mutation rates. As this specious argument goes, "we can't do much harm if we do to humans the equal of what nature is already doing." Fallacious as it is in every respect, this argument seems credible to many in the public, the medical and the scientific communities. They all fail to realize that natural radiation and the genetic and chromosomal mutations caused thereby are doing a very great deal of harm. The genetic disorders and deaths caused by "natural" radiations are no different from those caused by man-made radiation. All we can say is that, at this moment, we know of no way to turn off the various natural sources of radiation and we, therefore, suffer an enormous toll of disease, debility and death as a result of natural radiation. As a minimum element of common sense, we should refrain, except under the most dire circumstances, from adding to this enormous burden of suffering by adding the insult of man-made radiation. The benefits to society should be required to be enormous and obviously so before permitting any amount of increase in radiation mutations due to man-made sources.

When the argument is raised that natural radiation-induced mutations "cannot" be harmful since humans have evolved this far in a "sea of radioactivity," this argument should be countered with several cogent points. First, while we have evolved to our present state in spite of radiation, we do have a limited life span and we do have an enormous toll of suffering, disease, and premature death due to genetic disorders. And natural radiation probably accounts for about five to ten percent of such suffering and disease. We, societally, are at least humane enough to devote a sizeable share of our funds to medical care and medical research in the endeavor to alleviate the suffering and premature deaths caused by genetic mutation-induced disease, five to ten percent of which is due to natural radiation. We must assuredly think very seriously of having to expend ten percent more on medical care and consider having the massive increase in disease (genetic) that would go with man-made radiation starting to exact a toll comparable with or higher than that exacted by natural radiation.

What Kinds Of Genetic Diseases?
In recent years in medicine our horizon has broadened considerably concerning the implications of genetics and mutation for human disease. Whereas in the past, genetic diseases were considered to be a relative rarity among the causes of disability and death, we now realize that this rarity was an illusion, which led to a grave underestimation of the role of genetic mutations in human diseases. Today we recognize that a large proportion of all human afflictions are at least partially determined by heredity, and hence related to genetic mutations. Numerous authorities and authoritative bodies consider that the developing evidence may finally indicate that most, if not all, human disease has a genetic component.

The United Nations Scientific Committee on the Effects of Atomic Radiation states:

"It is generally accepted that there is a genetic component in much, if not all, illness. This component is frequently too small to be detected; in other instances, the evidence for its presence is unequivocal. Nevertheless, the role of genetic factors in the health of human populations has not in the past been considered seriously in vital and health statistics. As a consequence, data on the prevalence of hereditary diseases and defects are now largely restricted to that collected by geneticists for special purposes in limited populations from a small number of countries. An assessment of the hereditary defects and diseases with which a population is afflicted does not necessarily provide a measure of the imposed burden of suffering and hardship on the individual, the family or society" (Report of the United Nations Scientific Committee on the Effects of Atomic Radiation. General Assembly. Official Records: Seventeenth Session. Supplement No. 16

Birth Defects

[A 5216] Chapter IV, "Hereditary Effects," paragraph 56, page 19).

Professor Lederberg ("Government Is Most Dangerous of Genetic Engineers," Joshua Lederberg, *The Washington Post,* Sunday, July 19, 1970) stated the following:

"We can calculate that at least 25 percent of our health burden is of genetic origin. This figure is a very conservative estimate in view of the genetic component of such griefs as schizophrenia, diabetes, atherosclerosis, mental retardation, early senility, and many congenital malformations. In fact, the genetic factor in disease is bound to increase to an even larger proportion, for as we deal with infectious disease and other environmental insults, the genetic legacy of the species will compete only with traumatic accidents as the major factor in health."

Professor Lederberg has stated the problem succinctly and well. In the earlier days of medicine our techniques of sorting out genetically-determined diseases were cruder and tended only to find the diseases that had a simple so-called *Mendelian* form of inheritance. These are diseases which could be referred to as single-gene diseases. The inheritance patterns expected were known, and hence the genetic basis for the diseases relatively easily ascertained by studies of the occurrence of the disease in families and their ancestors. Among the classical cases of such diseases are the well-known phenylketonuria, galactosemia, cystic fibrosis, sickle-cell anemia, hemophilia, and others. However, altogether such diseases, numerous as they are, only accounted for less than one percent of deaths. This is very serious, but still is small compared to the now greatly expanded list of genetically determined diseases, the now well-known multigene diseases.

For many years medical experts realized that a host of the more common and serious diseases of man had a familiar pattern, but not one as readily ascertainable as was the case for the single-gene diseases listed above. Dr. C. O. Carter, in a recent compilation of the evidence ("Multifactorial Genetic Disease" by C. O. Carter, *Hospital Practice*, Vol. 5, pp. 45-59, May 1970. [Dr. Carter is Director, The British Medical Research Council's Clinical Genetics Unit]), has shown that a whole group of important human diseases are indeed genetically determined, but it appears that these diseases are determined by the interaction of more genes than one, and that this is complicated by further interactions with environmental factors. As a result of such work, we now are forced to consider not only the rarities like hemophilia as genetically determined diseases, but also diabetes, mellitus, atherosclerosis (the major form of hardening of the arteries), schizophrenia, and rheumatoid arthritis all as being genetically determined diseases and, hence, all subject to increase in occurrence as a result of increase in genetic mutation rates by radiation or any other mutagenic influences.

How do such diseases, added to the genetic list, lead Professor Lederberg to say a conservative 25 percent of all diseases are genetic, or lead others to say possibly all diseases (aside from trauma) may have a genetic component? Let us focus our attention on the disorder known as atherosclerosis, which, as stated above, is the major form of hardening of the arteries. This disorder underlies most cases of the most serious form of heart disease in the USA, namely, coronary heart disease. It is coronary heart disease that accounts for the great majority of "heart attacks." And coronary heart disease kills Americans prematurely more than twice as often as all forms of cancer plus leukemia combined! What is more, atherosclerosis not only affects the arteries of the heart, but also those of the brain, many internal organs, and the legs. The total disability and death from atherosclerosis is really not fully realized at all, for as a complicating factor in many diseases, its role may as yet have been underestimated—and underestimated seriously. The fact that atherosclerosis and coronary heart disease must now be regarded as genetic in origin really means that at least over 50 percent of all disease is genetic. The implications of genetic mutations are thereby rendered grossly more serious than previously realized, when only single-gene diseases were considered as the genetic disorders of man.

It was stated previously that a ten percent increase in genetic mutation rate would ultimately lead to ten percent more of the biological damage produced per generation by this particular defective gene or chromosome. The cost in health per generation can exceed the ten percent increase in biological damage. Let us consider atherosclerosis. While we know that more atherosclerosis will result in a higher frequency of heart attacks, we do not know the precise relationship between degree of atherosclerosis in the arteries of the heart and the occurrence rate of heart attacks. Indeed, the available evidence on this subject suggests that the risk of a premature heart attack may rise much more steeply than simply in proportion to the degree of atherosclerosis. It may well be that an increase of ten percent in the average degree of coronary artery atherosclerosis of the cerebral arteries will increase strokes by ten percent, twenty percent, or fifty percent.

As a result, while we can anticipate that a ten percent increase in mutation rate will ultimately increase the biological damage resulting in major diseases by ten percent, it is also quite possible that the increased disease incidence may exceed this ten percent increase in damage (already of grave consequence) by quite a lot. The consequences of genetic mutation, as a result of the new medical concepts of the important role of genetic factors in health and disease, are indeed far more serious than were realized ten short years ago. Incidentally, many of the standards for so-called "allowable" doses of radiation to the public for atomic energy programs such as nuclear electricity generation were set before the new implications of human genetic diseases were appreciated! This fact alone requires a total re-evaluation of atomic energy programs, nuclear electricity generation among them.

41. Learn Which Commonly-Used Chemicals Can Deform Your Children

Pollution doesn't simply mean barely tolerable filthy surroundings, stale air and foul-tasting water. Nor are pollutants only the dirt that peppers your freshly washed automobile or even the airborne corrosives that cause your house paint to chip and peel. If pollution meant only annoyances, we could live with it, however miserably. But it also makes people sick, and perhaps sicker than we ever dared guess.

We know that some common chemical agents that we are liable to encounter every day have been found to cause birth defects and mutations in experimental animals. These mutagens, and other pollutants like them, if not removed from and kept out of man's environment, could ultimately mean the end of the human race.

At a January, 1971, Symposium on Environment and Birth Defects in New York City, a herbicide, a gasoline additive and an "antipollutant" substitute for phosphates were fingered as possible threats to unborn human beings, to which was added a plea for stringent testing of any chemical agent to determine its effects on living creatures before it can be released into the natural environment.

In 1960 a drug named thalidomide came before the FDA for approval. The official directly concerned, Dr. Frances O. Kelsey, insisted that the drug had not been safely tested and could not be approved until further testing had proven it harmless. She maintained her position even against the pressure of her own superiors. Thus, the United States was largely spared the worldwide tragedy of thalidomide that surfaced in November of 1961, and which since then has been linked to the birth of at least 7,000 deformed babies missing limbs, parts of limbs and even organs, whose mothers had been given the tranquilizing drug during pregnancy.

When it was revealed how much damage was prevented by the

refusal to approve thalidomide, it was supposed by many that government bureaus generally and the FDA particularly would be far more careful in the future not to allow chemicals into the environment until thoroughly tested and proven harmless. But that still is not the case.

What is particularly frightening is that after a chemical has been marketed, no matter how harmful it might later be proven, it is almost impossible to recall it effectively before serious consequences have taken place.

Common Herbicide Causes Malformations

In 1969, according to *Medical World News*, Dr. Samuel S. Epstein was serving as chairman of the mutagenicity panel of the Mrak Commission, which was formed to study the relationship of pesticides to environmental health, and responsible to the Department of Health, Education and Welfare. At that meeting Dr. Epstein, chief of the carcinogenesis and toxicology laboratories at Children's Cancer Research Foundation, heard that scientists funded by the National Institutes of Health, working at Bionetics Laboratories from 1965 to 1968, had found the herbicide 2,4,5-T, whose safety regarding birth defects had never been questioned by the Department of Agriculture nor the Food and Drug Administration, to have caused congenital malformations in mice and rats. At first he was not even able to secure a copy of the report about this poison which had already been applied to an estimated 30 million acres of American soil, and which had stirred controversy for its role as a defoliant in the then Republic of South Vietnam. By the time that he obtained the report, the herbicide's defenders were claiming that impurities in the samples used, and not the herbicide itself, were responsible for the birth defects.

The government did not halt the distribution of the herbicide until the threat could be pinpointed. Instead, it allowed this agent to be used while new tests were arranged.

Subsequent tests not only confirmed the mutagenic potential of purified 2,4,5-T in experimental animals, but also showed that some forms of its chemical relative, 2,4-D, which is used more extensively on food crops than 2,4,5-T, also cause birth defects. The July-August, 1970 issue of *Environment* magazine, reported that "more than three and one-half years after the initial Bionetics findings, 2,4,5-T and its cousin 2,4-D are still widely used in the environment."

Another mutagen named at the New York Symposium is one that everyone encounters whenever he drives in traffic—a gasoline additive known as TMP, which stands for trimethyl phosphate. In a car, this chemical will keep spark plugs working longer, but in the bodies of test rats it induced defective offspring by breaking the chromosomes that carry the cells' genetic instructions.

Doctor Epstein's concern about the additive is that, "Some unreacted TMP escapes from the exhausts of cars, resulting in the exposure of the general population . . . we have no idea how many people breathe this unreacted TMP." The *Medical World News* also reported that TMP is used as a methylating agent and an ingredient in paints and polymers, adding that "a closely related substance—triethyl phosphate—has recently been proposed as a food additive for keeping beaten egg whites stiff in cooked food."

The third chemical pinpointed as a threat to unborn children, called nitrilotriacetic acid, or NTA, is ironically one which was meant to help save the environment by replacing phosphate detergents. The greatest problem with NTA is its tendency to join with metals into combinations called chelates (KEY-lates), increasing the toxicity of the metals to such an extent that they can damage embryos in pregnant females, as shown by experiments with rats. The evidence was so convincing that then Surgeon General Jesse L. Steinfeld asked detergent manufacturers to remove this chemical from their products.

Dr. James F. Crow, of the University of Wisconsin, said at a Washington conference on human mutations that many genetic changes which may occur naturally in man, to a small degree, are accumulating faster than they can be naturally eliminated, according to a report in the *New York Times* (November 5, 1970). He added that the rapidly growing number of new chemicals must be tested for their mutagenic potential before being released into the environment, for they may be partly responsible for this dangerous trend.

While discouragingly little is known about the environmental causes of birth defects, we can profit from what has already been learned about cancer-causing agents in the environment, many of which are also linked to birth defects. Doctor Wilhelm C. Hueper, former chief of the environmental section of the National Cancer Institute, found that in animal experiments the fetus reacts more to carcinogens than do adult tissues. He believes that because carcinogens are also capable of causing birth defects, all avoidable ones "should be eliminated, and all unavoidable carcinogenic risks should be reduced to a lowest possible minimum."

A carcinogen can also cause birth defects, explains an article in *Medical World News* (February 1, 1971), since "many carcinogens, and a wide variety of other substances, are capable of crossing the placenta and entering into the tissues of the fetus. Known carcinogens enter the mother's body by a variety of routes. She eats them (saccharin), inhales (insecticides), touches (paints), or absorbs them unknowingly (fabric dyes)."

In many ways, suspected congenital threats from environmental pollution resemble what had years ago been thought to be hazards only from radiation. Then, in 1966 a report by the genetic study section of the National Institutes of Health warned, "There is reason to fear that some chemicals may constitute as important a risk as radiation, possibly a far more serious one. Although chemical mutagenesis in man is much less certain than that of radiation, a number of chemicals, some with widespread use, are known to induce genetic damage in some organisms." In the short time span since that report, man has had more reason than ever before to suspect an unknown quantity of chemicals of causing damage to unborn babies.

Accepted Chemicals Should Be Properly Tested

The National Foundation—March of Dimes, the largest and best-known campaigner against birth defects, has said in its "Leaders' Alert" bulletin to volunteers that, "Nothing whatsoever of unknown toxicity should be introduced into the environment, either as a pesticide, herbicide, defoliant, insect repellant, or food additive. The teratogenic effect is the vital key. Any agent found to be toxic or teratogenic in test animals should be excluded from public use." Teratogenic is a term denoting an agent which causes monstrosities at birth.

Vigilance against suspected mutagens and teratogens, said Dr. Epstein, can be strengthened by renewed investigations of chemicals now accepted as safe, but not necessarily tested for their role in inducing birth defects, and by a policy of openness and honesty in revealing test results as soon as possible after experiments are performed. He said that the FDA's *Generally Regarded as Safe* food additives, numbering some 600, would be a good place to start checking for safety against congenital malformations.

"Further legislation concerning access of data is critically needed," he said. "All formal discussions between agencies, industry, and expert committees on all issues relating to human safety and environmental quality, and all data relevant to such discussions must be made public. Records, including clear statements by all concerned of possible conflicts of interest, should be immediately available to the scientific community and to anybody else concerned."

42. Undefined Sexual Development In Newborns

There are solid grounds for believing that maternal lack of vitamin A and/or vitamin B₃ may sometimes bring about the birth of an apparent girl, although the fetus, as conceived, was intended by nature to be a boy.

The whole subject of bisexuals, or hermaphrodites—individuals who seem to be part man and part woman—is one that has long been shrouded in mystery. In times past, the general public had only the haziest notion of what it was all about and referred to suspected bisexuals in whispers and innuendos. Two decades ago, however, the highly publicized surgical conversion of "Christine" Jorgenson opened the subject to public discussion. At the 1972 Olympic Games, which were held in Munich, Germany, the problem of hermaphroditism was dealt with in the most open, public, and matter-of-fact fashion.

For the first time, all female contenders in the Olympic Games submitted to a chromosome test. A hair of the head was examined microscopically to see if its cells carried the male chromosome or the female chromosome. Contenders who showed male chromosomes—or who refused to submit to the test—were disqualified. Their masculine make-up, despite female body form, was considered an unfair advantage in competition with other women.

In an article on the Olympic "hair test," published in *Parade* magazine (April 16, 1972), author Connecticut Walker noted the high proportion of women sports champions who have been found to be hermaphrodites. When sex-testing was introduced at the European track championships in Budapest in 1967, he reported five of eleven women champions proved to have masculine chromosomes. Two famous Russian sisters—Tamara Press, the world's female shot-put champion, and Irina, the Olympic Pentathlon champion—retired from athletic competition when chromosome tests were made a prerequisite. A number of champion women athletes later chose to convert to male status—the most famous being Erika Schinegger, Austrian ski champion, who after four sex-change operations is now Erik and works out with the Austrian men's team.

What biological "mistake" causes these sexual anomalies? And how could simple nutrients, such as vitamin A and vitamin B₃, possibly be the instruments that determine normal sexual development in the fetus?

The XX And XY Chromosomes

Before attempting to answer these questions, let's briefly review what is known about the chromosomal determination of sex. In normal human cells, there are 44 regular chromosomes (all containing the genetic material coded into their DNA strands) plus two sex chromosomes. In females, these are two X chromosomes; in males, there's an X chromosome and a Y chromosome.

If the Y chromosome is present in the hair cells of a would-be female competitor in the Olympics, the individual is identified as a genetic male and ruled out of the contest. Any other cell of the body, of course, would be equally accurate and tell the same story. Hair is used because it can be removed for examination easily, painlessly, and without embarrassment.

The individual's genetic sex is established at the moment of conception. Unlike all other cells in the body, the male and female reproductive cells (sperm and ovum) have only half the normal number of chromosomes—22 regular chromosomes and one sex chromosome—so that when the two cells join in the creation of a new life, their combined chromosomes will add up to the normal number.

Every ovum ready for fertilization has one X chromosome. But the male's sperm carries either an X or a Y. If a Y sperm penetrates the ovum, then the new individual will be a male with an XY pattern. A female, with an XX pattern, develops if the sperm carries an X.

During the early weeks of prenatal growth, however, chromosomes are the *only* distinction between the male and female fetus. As reported by Dr. Ursula Mittwoch in *New Scientist and Science Journal* (July 15, 1971), gonads are first discernible at about five weeks gestation time, but these primitive organs are identical in both sexes. Dr. Mittwoch called them "basically bipotential and composed of the same components, an outer cortex (from which a testis can develop) and an inner medulla (from which an ovary can develop)."

In the normal genetic male, the outer cortex differentiates into

199

testicular tissue while the inner medulla recesses (and vice versa for the genetic female). But except for the gonads there is still no other sex differentiation until the specialized hormone-producing cells of the testis (interstitial cells) develop and start synthesizing male hormones (androgens) in quantity to influence male body development.

Referring to animal experimentation on fetal sex differentiation, Dr. Isobel Jennings explains in *Vitamins In Endocrine Metabolism* (Charles C. Thomas, publishers): "Loss of testicular activity just before gonadal sex differentiation, by castration or by chemical means, inhibits the process, and the animal develops along the female line of differentiation. In such a case, a genetic male acquires the feminine characteristics and is therefore pseudohermaphrodite. The gonadectimized female (one whose ovaries have been removed) suffers no such disability and continues to develop along the female pattern . . . The interstitial cells of the embrionic testis are thus the major factor in deciding somatic (or body) sex differentiation in mammals."

Vitamin Needs Of Male Hormones

Because Dr. Jennings is primarily concerned in her book with the effect of nutrition on endocrine metabolism (or hormone activity), she stresses the vitamin requirements for the synthesis of the steroid hormones, which include the androgens or male sex hormones.

The androgens, which the testis must manufacture in order to develop the male body pattern, need both vitamin A and coenzymes or vitamin B_3 (niacin) for their synthesis, Dr. Jennings says, "and possibly other vitamins" as well. Referring to experiments with rats, she notes that the ability of the fetal testis to manufacture androgens is at its height at exactly the time that bodily sex differentiation is under way. "The vitamin-containing coenzymes necessary for steroid biosynthesis will therefore be required for several days prior to this time," she states.

Or, translated into human terms and getting back to the Olympic Games: vitamin deficiency in the maternal diet may have so deprived the unborn child, at the critical time when he needed male sex hormones, that the boy baby was disguised as a girl, later to become an outstanding "female" athlete—until the new regulations for chromosome-testing ruled her/him out of further competition.

There are, of course, several different types of bisexualism, or intersex as it is often called. In some types, the cause is known.

In others it is a matter of speculation. In an article in the *British Medical Journal* (August 11, 1962), Dr. J. I. Forbes and colleagues categorized the types as (1) *true hermaphrodites* (where there is both ovarian and testicular tissue and the individual may be either genetically male or genetically female); and (2) *pseudohermaphrodites.* While the word hermaphrodite is often used loosely to include all types of intersex—and this is how we've used the term earlier in this article—actually the true hermaphrodite is very rare (only 80 cases have been reported in all medical literature, Dr. Forbes said). Pseudohermaphrodites are far more common.

Female pseudohermaphroditism, a baby conceived as a girl but with masculinized external genitalia, can be caused in uterus by hormone therapy of the mother or by a disruption of the mother's own hormone regulation. Most cases, however, develop from a genetic defect that prevents the fetal adrenal cortex from synthesizing hydrocortisone. This hormone apparently is the decisive "messenger" that tells the pituitary gland not to produce more ACTH—the hormone that stimulates the adrenal cortex to synthesize all of its steroid hormones. Normally, the feed-back communication between hydrocortisone and ACTH keeps steroid output at the normal and desired level. But when hydrocortisone is missing, ACTH continuously stimulates production of the steroids, and among these substances produced in such overabundance is the male hormone, which the adrenal gland as well as the testis can manufacture.

The *male pseudohermaphrodite* is the type of intersex we have been discussing in terms of "female" athletes with male chromosome patterns. Often these apparent women have undescended testes, which are discovered as "hernias." Though their vaginas and exterior genitalia seem female, they lack ovaries and may lack a uterus. In some cases the hidden testis produces estrogens, the female hormones. It is generally agreed that fetal deficiency of the male hormones—whether because of damage to the testes or other cause—is responsible for male pseudohermaphrodites. Dr. Jennings adds the thought that these hormones are vitamin-dependent.

Through surgery and hormone treatment, doctors can help almost all intersex patients to become more pronouncedly male or female, depending on their choice of sex. If discovered at infancy and chromosome tests made, the child can be converted to conform to his genetic sex long before any psychological problems develop.

But prevention, of course, is what is most important. And here the greatest hope would seem to lie in the knowledge that vitamins—specifically vitamin A and niacin—are essential for the synthesis of male hormones. And without these hormones, a normal male baby cannot develop.

Nutrition In Pregnancy

Faulty nutrition of the mother certainly cannot be suggested as the cause of all problems of intersex. But it may be responsible for a portion of them. And, if so, these can be prevented. Supplementary fish liver oil for vitamin A and foods rich in the vitamin B complex, such as whole grains, wheat germ, brewer's yeast, and liver, may well serve as protection for the sexual integrity of the unborn child.

Of wider interest, Dr. Jennings' emphasis on these nutrients as important to normal male fetal development gives us a striking illustration of how devastating even a brief deficiency of a nutrient can be to an unborn child if it happens to come at a critical moment of organ growth. In her chapter entitled "Hormones and Vitamins in Prenatal Life," this British scientist states that "the whole wide range of defects in human morphogenesis (differentiation of cells and tissues during development) can be duplicated in most cases in experimental animals by dietary manipulation."

In other words, birth defects caused by radiation, viruses, hormone therapy, harmful chemicals and drugs, and hereditary or genetic errors can also be induced by depriving the fetus of essential nutrients. Except for genetic defects, the type of abnormality—cleft palate, absence of limbs, heart anomalies, etc.—depends primarily "on the specific period of pregnancy during which the noxious stimulus acts," Dr. Jennings says, rather than on what the teratogenic agent happens to be. And, as animal experimentation has shown, nutritional deficiency must be counted as one of these "noxious stimulants," a teratogen no less effective than the commonly acknowledged inducers of birth defects.

If all future mothers knew about these animal experiments, and knew also that only natural unprocessed organic foods, supplemented by natural vitamins and minerals, can guarantee the full quota of essential nutrients (known and unknown), surely the number of mentally and physically defective babies would shrink to a fraction of the present tragic load.

43. Mongolism

Down's Syndrome, popularly known as mongolism, is an aberration that occurs at the time of conception. As nearly as science can determine—and knowledge of this phenomenon is by no means complete—it is caused by the presence of a single extra chromosome among the 46 that are normally present when a sperm cell and an ovum join together. The general scientific opinion is that the extra chromosome produces extra enzymes that are normal in themselves, but excessive in quantity. The function of these enzymes is to permit the developing cells of the fetus to process, absorb and use nutrients of all types from the mother's bloodstream. It is believed that the excess of these enzymes somehow causes them to interfere with each other, with the result that the developing cells are insufficiently nourished while the bloodstream of the embryo becomes clogged with unused nutrients, hormones and waste products. As a result the organs and tissues grow more slowly, do not mature and develop properly and do not function well.

By birth many of the basic structures of the infant such as the heart, the lungs and brain are malformed and functioning badly. The result is a mongoloid child, a child retarded not only mentally but in nearly every function.

There is no known way to alter the inborn chromosomal pattern of any person. It is conceivable that science may ultimately discover some way to accomplish just this. But even at such a time, it is extremely unlikely that there are many scientists who would even dare attempt to alter a chromosomal pattern of a human being. The consequences would be too unpredictable and the possibility of producing monstrosities too great.

A Treatment For Favorable Change In Mongolism

Dr. Henry Turkel of Detroit, Michigan, and Lugano, Switzerland, has never claimed to cure mongolism. He has never attempted to do so. He is a scientist and does not waste his time attempting to accomplish what is known to be impossible.

But what he does do is impressive. If you were told that there is a treatment for mongoloids that can change their appearance so they look almost normal; that under this treatment they can be taught to read and write, to speak intelligibly and to learn a simple trade that will help them become self-supporting; that some have even progressed to the point where they can marry, cook, clean and run a home and even have "normal" children, you would very likely say, "But, that's ridiculous. Everyone knows that there's no cure for mongoloids. It's a genetic defect—an extra chromosome."

That's exactly what the FDA said about Dr. Turkel's "U Series" treatment which, before they stopped its interstate sale, brought tremendous improvement in the appearance and physical and mental performance to almost 200 mongoloid children.

The treatment helps to correct the damage caused by the extra chromosome that causes mongolism. It consists mainly of vitamins, minerals, enzymes and some drugs—50 different ingredients in amounts which the mongoloid's disturbed metabolism can assimilate.

After hearing more than two hundred case histories, supported by X-rays showing remarkable changes over the course of treatment, supported by the opinions of other doctors and the testimony of parents, schoolteachers and nurses, the FDA banned interstate sale or shipment of the substances used in the treatment.

The "U Series" treatment includes such drugs as pentylenetetrazol and thyroid. The dose of pentylenetetrazol which Dr. Turkel gives to adult mongoloids is only one-sixth the amount in a simple geriatric cerebral oxidant prescribed regularly for symptoms of atherosclerosis. The quantity of thyroid in the formulations is exceeded five times in prescriptions written by doctors to combat overweight and other problems which are relatively simple when compared with mongolism.

Extra Chromosome Causes Nutritional Blockage

The rationale for Dr. Turkel's treatment is impressive in its simplicity. The mongoloid has an extra chromosome in each cell. That extra chromosome triggers a tremendous chain reaction. The chromosome contains genes; the genes produce enzymes; and the enzymes produce metabolites that have nowhere to go. And that's what makes all the trouble. These extra metabolites, mostly calcium, clog up the tissues and blood vessels. Though they accumulate in tiny amounts, so small that they are hardly discernible by the average microscope, they aggregate into larger quantities, causing calcification of the soft tissues which is always a serious problem. They prevent growth, prevent assimilation of nutrients, and prevent proper elimination of waste products.

It is this blockage in the cells and tissues that causes retardation both of the brain and the body, Dr. Turkel says. It also causes water retention. That is why mongoloids usually have enlarged hearts, as well as tongues that seem too large for their mouths and make their speech thick and unintelligible. They have edema of the lungs which makes them prone to bronchial infections. Their sinuses are not developed, which gives them a flat-nosed appearance. Their lacrimal (tear-forming) ducts are blocked; their tears go into their noses. A mongoloid is subject to many ailments, but he is not diseased; he is retarded. His mental and physical growth has been stunted.

The problem then, in Dr. Turkel's opinion, is to eliminate the accumulations of these metabolites which the mongoloid cannot utilize, to clean out the tissues, to provide free passageways, and then to supply the nutrients, vitamins and minerals and hormones which he, for the first time, becomes able to utilize.

The first step was to determine just which elements are in an abnormal state or quantity. Dr. Turkel was eminently equipped for this painstaking task because he himself had invented the special instrument which was indispensable to this investigation. The Turkel biopsy punch is an ingenious device that permits a doctor to take a tissue sample from bone, from a vital organ, or from any tissue of the body, without having to perform surgery and with practically no damage. With this instrument, Dr. Turkel was able to obtain samples of the various tissues of mongoloids.

With high-powered microscopes, chemical analyses and hundreds of X-ray studies, Dr. Turkel determined that the organs and tissues of the mongoloid are indeed clogged with a remarkably complex aggregate of nutritional materials which he is unable to either metabolize or eliminate.

After years of study and experimentation, Dr. Turkel developed a number of separate combinations of drugs, enzymes, hormones, vitamins and minerals, each of which had a specific purpose in relation to what he had discovered about the mongoloid metabolism. Their modus operandi is to clear the blood, the tissues, the system generally of all those unused materials that clog up the works and interfere with the development and functioning of the organs.

Dr. Turkel found at least 50 different substances which the mongoloid is unable to properly metabolize. He found it necessary to include these in his "U Series" medications. A scientist by training and inclination, Dr. Turkel kept a constant check by X-ray and microscopic examination of the blood and tissue specimens of the mongoloid children he was treating.

X-Rays Showed The Improvements Sought

It soon became apparent that he was getting the kind of chemical reaction he was seeking. Great clogging deposits of calcium in the lungs and around the aorta, the artery which conveys blood from the left ventricle of the heart, began clearly to diminish. This was apparent in the step-by-step X-ray studies. Medical examination revealed that his patients were breathing easier and more normally, and that their hearts were taking on a more regular beat. These were the signs of improvement that were apparent to the eye and ear of a trained physician.

Parents were looking for other signs—signs of the child's ability to learn, to take care of himself, to accept toilet training, to talk intelligibly. They had to wait a little longer. It took daily use of his medications over a long period of time to bring about this kind of improvement.

In an attempt to bring the price of the medications down to a level that everyone could afford, Dr. Turkel tried to get a pharmaceutical company to make up his medicines in standard dosages which would then make them available at much lower prices. He approached several major pharmaceutical houses. None were interested. The Turkel formula is compounded of combinations of standard materials, mostly vitamins and minerals, all of which are in the pharmacopeia. Although his concept and combinations are original and specially devised to fit the circumstances of the mongoloid, the formulations cannot be patented. No pharmaceutical company was interested in manufacturing a substance that it could not patent, which would then only result in a loss of money.

Eventually, in order to make it possible for parents to continue their children's medications week after week, Dr. Turkel invested in a small pharmaceutical company, the Ubiotica Corporation, which agreed to manufacture his formulations.

This corporation, though it was fully qualified and licensed to manufacture pharmaceutical products, though it was using only approved drugs listed in the U.S. Pharmacopeia, though it was, in fact, doing no more than any pharmacist in any drugstore in the country does every day, was nevertheless constantly badgered by the FDA until it was forced to close its doors when the FDA finally terminated the interstate sale and shipment of the "U Series" treatment. The FDA considered mongolism an incurable disease since it was caused by a genetic flaw, i.e. the extra chromosome, and, according to dominant medical opinion, there is no treatment that can correct a genetic flaw.

"Granting that there is no cure for mongolism or for the many other inborn errors of metabolism, the goal of medical treatment is not to correct the abnormal chromosomal pattern, but to alter the various inborn abnormalities of body organs and tissues so that they become as near normal in structure and function as is possible within the present limits of medicines," Dr. Turkel replied to the FDA's pronouncement.

While the 200 cases treated by Dr. Turkel are certainly significant, they are too few to represent irrefutable scientific proof of the worth of Dr. Turkel's formulations. It is possible, for instance, that only a small part of the treatment is responsible for its success and that these ingredients in a concentrated form might be even more successful. It is also conceivable, though hardly likely, that coincidence, favorable circumstances and good luck were involved.

Such questions and others of a similar nature regarding the merits of a new treatment would normally be answered in time as many doctors attempted to use the treatment and duplicate the results. In time the body of knowledge would grow much greater and the treatment would be improved and refined.

But this normal scientific evolution has been prevented from developing because the government has made the "U Series" unavailable to doctors anywhere outside the state of Michigan and has prevented its manufacture at a cost that would make the treatment accessible to most families who have a mongoloid.

44. Cystic Fibrosis

Cystic fibrosis is the most prevalent hereditary disease among children today, afflicting an estimated 37,000 children. The life expectancy of cystic fibrosis (CF) victims was once very short. Prior to the mid-1950's most patients died before the age of five. However, new advances in therapy and medication have extended the life expectancy for many into late adolescence. The CF patient has symptoms similar to bronchitis and asthma, with chronic coughing and wheezing a common feature. He also shows a very strong appetite, though his heavy eating results in little weight gain. There are frequent bowel movements throughout the day, all of them bulky and foul. If a couple has a child suffering from CF and they decide to have more children, the chances that the other children will have the disease are very great, and the disease usually occurs with greater severity.

The lubricating mucus secreted inside the body to help carry on the digestive processes, as well as other important body functions, is the source of the problem. Instead of the normal water consistency, the mucus in cystic fibrosis victims is as thick as molasses. It blocks ducts in the pancreas so that essential enzymes cannot be secreted, and, in the case of the lungs, oxygen cannot pass through as it should. The activities thus curtailed are so basic that life without them is exceedingly difficult to sustain.

Where the lungs are affected the problems of pneumonia and lung infection are a constant threat, and CF victims are often kept on daily doses of antibiotics to defend against these complications. The children build natural immunities to these antibiotics, one after the other, and eventually parents are faced with the possibility of exhausting the potency of all known drugs.

Enzymes Shut Off And True Digestion Impossible

Most commonly, cystic fibrosis attacks the pancreas. It is in this organ that the enzymes are made. These juices are secreted into the intestines and they break down the foods we eat into nutritional components the body needs for self repair and normal function. When these enzymes do not appear, the food passes through the body intact, without having had the least bit of nutrition extracted from it. This is the case when CF affects this organ. It becomes coated with a thick layer of mucus which prevents the enzymes from being excreted into the intestines where they are needed. Eventually the victim of such a situation is bound to die of starvation, no matter how much he eats, because his food does him no good whatsoever. Parents and doctors try to forestall this eventual consequence by feeding foods that are very rich in nutrition, hoping that some will remain behind, and by feeding large doses of vitamins to the patient. But neither of these can be effective for very long.

Diagnosis Difficult Until Recent Years

Because of the symptoms presented by cystic fibrosis, it was often confused with other diseases and difficult to diagnose accurately. A great step forward was taken when a simple test was devised to ascertain the presence of CF. It was discovered that CF patients sweat profusely and that their perspiration contains an unusually high percentage of salt. A system was devised for obtaining and analyzing samples of perspiration taken from the hand of the suspected victim.

While there is a great deal known about the nature of CF, little has been discovered up to now about how and why it occurs. For some unknown reason, American blacks rarely contract CF, and it is practically unheard of among Eastern populations. There is no problem of contagion with CF.

Hereditary In Nature

Cystic fibrosis is strictly hereditary, in fact, it is "the most prevalent inherited disease among Caucasions," according to a report by researchers at the University of Texas (*Texas Reports on Biology and Medicine*, Winter 1973). And it is in this area where *prevention* of the crippling respiratory disease can be best implemented by the use of genetic counseling.

According to an article by Victor Cohn in the *Washington Post* (March 15, 1973), there are now blood tests which are capable of detecting an "apparent cystic fibrosis factor" in the blood stream. "The blood tests offer the first possibility of prevention through genetic counseling of potential parents, who might decide not to have children if both show positive results on the tests," reported Cohn.

One out of every 25 people carry the gene that causes the disease. "If two carriers marry," wrote Cohn, "there is one chance in four that each birth will produce a cystic fibrotic child who will often not live past adolescence. The matter becomes urgent, doctors say, for young persons who know that the disease runs in their family and who have had no way except childbearing of learning whether they are carriers." The use of these new blood tests will help to alleviate a good deal of the anxiety which envelops such situations.

News of these tests was reported at a meeting of the Sixth International Cystic Fibrosis Congress in March of 1973 by Dr. Kurt Hirschhorn of Mount Sinai Medical School, New York, and Dr. Barbara Bowman of the University of Texas Medical Branch at Galveston. However, according to Dr. Hirschhorn, widespread use of the tests are hindered because of 1973 cuts in federal health funds which are needed for further development of genetic testing through blood tests.

The Nutritional Aspect Of Cystic Fibrosis

While most researchers concentrate on new ways to treat cystic fibrosis patients with antibiotics to prevent infection, others are pursuing a different angle—nutritional deficiency. It is known that the muscles of cystic fibrosis patients show the same kind of fatty degeneration which is found in the muscles of animals deficient in vitamin E. A certain substance found in the livers of deficient animals is also found in livers of CF patients.

An article in *Pediatrics* (January, 1960) by Dr. Harry Schwachman reported that "most patients with cystic fibrosis have low levels of vitamin E in the blood." He went on to state that adding vitamin supplements to the diet is extremely important for these patients. He gives twice the commonly recommended dose of vitamins. Vitamin K is important, especially for children who have been operated on.

There may also be signs of vitamin A deficiency, reported Dr. Schwachman, although, since water soluble vitamin A has been available, this is less common. He recommended that vitamin E be added to the diet. All of the vitamins so far mentioned are fat-soluble vitamins. It seems reasonable that cystic fibrosis patients would be deficient in these, since one symptom of the disease is a disorder in the way the body handles fat.

Claims of vitamin E deficiency in CF patients were confirmed again when researchers from the National Institutes of Health, meeting in Atlantic City, New Jersey, emphasized the need for vitamin E supplements for people unable to absorb the vitamin naturally, according to a report in the *Medical Tribune* (May, 1974).

In advocating the needs for vitamin E supplements, the researchers told the 58th annual meeting of the Federation of American Societies for Experimental Biology that the study groups used in coming to their conclusion consisted of 50 patients with cystic fibrosis. "Patients with cystic fibrosis were selected for the study because the marked pancreatic insuffiency characteristic of the disease leads to profound vitamin E deficiency," the article reported.

Some Children Very Deficient In Vitamin E

An article was published in the *Canadian Medical Journal* (May 28, 1960) on the subject of the condition of infants and children where vitamin E is concerned. Richard B. Goldbloom, M.D., of Montreal, author of the article, stated that for unknown reasons infants and children are much more susceptible to a lowering of the vitamin E in the blood by a deficiency in diet than are adults. So individuals of the younger age group offer far greater opportunity for the study of possible effects of deficiency in vitamin E.

Interestingly enough, Dr. Goldbloom discovered that the levels of vitamin E are especially low in infants and children who suffer from diseases which cause steatorrhea (an excessive loss of fat in the feces and one of the difficulties in cystic fibrosis) and also that the vitamin E levels are much higher in the case of infants which have been breast-fed. He suggested that we should consider adding vitamin E to the formula of children who are bottle-fed. He said that this is even more important in the case of children who are fed on skimmed milk formulas. Since the fat has been removed from the milk, there is no chance of their getting any vitamin E from it, since the vitamin E is contained in the fat—and precious little of it there is in milk to begin with—a mere "trace."

One More Note On Cystic Fibrosis

Dr. Schwachman, in his article in *Pediatrics*, stressed the importance of a diet high in protein and low in fat. He said that the amount of fat allowed depends on the patient's reaction to it. Most patients can tolerate the amount of fat in homogenized milk, but he advised not giving them butter, ice cream, peanut butter, potato chips, fried potatoes and mayonnaise if these foods produce cramps, discomforts, or bulky or frequent bowel movements. In some patients considerable reduction in fat intake is necessary, he said.

45. Cerebral Palsy

Cerebral palsy is a comprehensive term for a broad category of brain-centered motor disturbances which usually appear at birth or during early childhood. The motor dysfunctions of the cerebral palsied generally manifest themselves as loss of control over voluntary muscles and abrupt, jerking, muscular contractions, and they occur as a result of clogged or hyperactive motor control centers in different locations in the brain.

The conditions which comprise cerebral palsy affect more than 15,000 new babies annually, and though they all share the same distinctive pattern, there is considerable latitude in the intensity and number of symptoms in a single cerebral palsy victim.

There are two basic forms of cerebral palsy: *spastic* and *atheotosic*. The spastic forms show generalized involuntary muscular contractions and paralysis in the lower body; all muscle tone is absent and attempts at voluntary movement of the affected muscles is hopeless. In the atheotosic category there is less paralysis of entire muscle groups; however, there is continual and uncontrollable tremor movement in the limb extremities, as well as involuntary spasms of the neck and facial muscles.

Aside from the varying forms of muscular and neurological dysfunction, ranging from severe paralysis with intermittent and abrupt jerking movements to less severe forms of muscle stiffness, cerebral palsy sufferers may also have other marked symptoms such as problems in maintaining balance, speech difficulties, intellectual and emotional disturbances, epilepsy, and sight, hearing and other sense impairments.

Most people picture the average CP victim as having a staggered gait, shuffling feet, limbs and extremities that flail about awkwardly and a head that hangs loosely with the mouth agape. This may describe the severely afflicted, but there are many cases with other, milder symptoms. These include chronically stiff joints, an abnormally prolonged inability to concentrate and occasional seizures. These less obvious symptoms of cerebral palsy can easily go undiagnosed—and often do. That is why the parents and physician must be particularly alert, since early diagnosis might lead to therapy which will prevent some of the more crippling disorders known to accompany the disease.

What Causes Cerebral Palsy?

The exact cause of the motor impairment in the brain that causes the many symptoms of cerebral palsy is still not known. Heredity, although it may play a part in other birth defects such as mongolism, cystic fibrosis and muscular dystrophy, is not considered as a major cause in cerebral palsy; however, a form of cerebral palsy known as the Lesch-Nyhan syndrome has been identified as congenital. Researchers are currently attempting to develop a test which will detect this particular form of cerebral palsy in the fetus. Such a test would allow doctors to start therapy soon after birth.

The Myth Of Retardation

A common misconception about the cerebral palsied is that they are all mentally retarded. Although cerebral motor dysfunction often impairs intelligence levels, a great many victims possess normal or above normal (including genius) intelligence. Despite the problems involved in testing individuals with severe sensory impairments, more than 55 percent of the cerebral palsied tested have shown normal and above normal intelligence.

The problem is basically one of communication, not native brain power. Seizures, speech difficulties, hearing and sight impairments, the extreme physical discomfort of involuntary muscle contraction or paralysis, and the accompanying emotional stress are almost insurmountable handicaps to the learning process. But with the aid of new innovations in physical therapy techniques, drugs which can control seizures, and surgical advances such as the cerebral "pacemaker" which have alleviated muscle tension and spasms in some cases, breakthroughs in the communication barrier are being achieved.

The treatment of the disease becomes, then, one of "management" rather than "cure." Physical therapy is viewed as a matter of teaching rather than as a matter of medical treatment. A special regimen of teaching, exercise and other orthopedic measures, counseling, plus perseverence on the part of the teacher and the patient, are the requisites of most programs to lessen the disability.

Whatever form the course of the management takes, it is imperative that it begins as soon as possible.

Birth Injury The Leading Cause

Although brain damage at any time during life can cause cerebral palsy, the majority of the cases have occurred at birth or during early infancy. There is a great deal of information which links prenatal injuries of the fetus and injuries caused at birth to a majority of the reported cases of cerebral palsy, according to a comprehensive study begun in 1959, which included the combined efforts of such agencies as the Department of Health, Education and Welfare and the National Institutes of Health.

The researchers stressed the importance of a routine monitoring of a pregnant woman's blood. They discovered that an Rh incompatibility between the blood of the mother and the blood of the fetus can cause brain damage and resulting cerebral palsy. If such an incompatibility is discovered, a total exchange transfusion either at birth or prior to birth will protect the infant from brain damage. Diminished oxygen (anoxia) in the mother's bloodstream can result in brain damage in the fetus and possible subsequent cerebral palsy. The time immediately around or before birth is considered the most critical time for this form of brain injury.

Other external causes of cerebral palsy which could affect a pregnant woman are physical injuries, infectious viruses, such as German measles (rubella) and exposure to X-rays during physical examination. In the case of German measles, the researchers expressed hope that the new nationwide immunization program of all children between the ages of one and puberty would wipe out this threat of cerebral palsy.

Prenatal Nutrition Extremely Critical

The researchers involved in the 1959 comprehensive project also noted a striking correlation between the incidence of premature births and cerebral palsy. There are a number of factors which can lead to premature births: drug abuse; excessive alcohol consumption; age (it appeared that more premature births occurred in pregnant mothers less than 16, or older than 40); and *poor nutrition.*

The evidence of an association between birth defects and poor maternal nutrition has always been far too weighty a correlation to be dismissed. All the building material required by the fetus during its life in the womb must be supplied by the mother. Her body processes the food she eats, which is transmitted through the placenta to be assimilated by the fetus. To a large degree, then, her child is what *she* eats. If, through adulteration or refining or just poor dietary habits, her food intake lacks some nutritional element—vitamin, mineral, or enzyme—the construction of the fetus may be weakened.

This premise was illustrated by the thalidomide tragedy in which many pregnant women who took the tranquilizer produced malformed children. Subsequent research indicated that thalidomide interfered with metabolism of nicotinic acid (a B complex vitamin) in the fetus. This vitamin is essential for normal fetal development during the first and second months of pregnancy.

Not all of the mothers who took thalidomide gave birth to deformed babies. Those who were spared this tragedy may well have been the same women whose diets included enough of the vitamin B's and other nutrients to compensate for what the thalidomide destroyed.

External Causes Of Cerebral Palsy In Early Infancy

Other external conditions which can adversely affect the nervous system during early infancy and cause brain damage—and possible cerebral palsy—include lead paint poisoning, blows to the head and infectious diseases which will cause extremely high fevers and damage the fragile nervous system of infants. One such disease is meningitis, an inflammation of the outer layers of the brain. Even though drugs can cure meningitis quickly, the disease is still responsible for many cases of cerebral palsy. The reason for such disastrous complications is delay in diagnosis and treatment. As in all cases of cerebral palsy, the key words are *early diagnosis* and *prompt therapy.*

Section 11
Bone Disease

46. Why Your Skeleton Might Be Disintegrating

A woman in her late fifties described, in a magazine, a series of experiences involving her diet and her health which shocked her, but also taught her a lesson—the hard way.

For quite a few years, the woman said, she had had rheumatoid arthritis, and had been on cortisone therapy for some years at the direction of a specialist at a well-known hospital. Years later, after bumping her upper arm against a piece of furniture, she realized that her arm was aching long after it should have healed itself. A visit to her family doctor revealed the first shock: her arm wasn't just bruised, it was broken!

The second shock came just seconds later, when her family physician said, "This is one of the results we often see with cortisone treatment." He went on to explain briefly that cortisone interferes with calcium metabolism and people on such therapy frequently develop osteoporosis.

Osteoporosis Eats Away The Bones

Bones that are osteoporotic are like beams in a frame house that have been eaten away for years by termites. But instead of termites, what's eating away the calcium from the bones of an osteoporotic woman is her own blood. That's because every nerve in the body—including those which cause the heart to beat and the brain to function—needs a precise amount of calcium to carry out its job. Our bodies are strictly programmed to keep this calcium at the required level. And if there isn't enough of this mineral coming in from dietary sources, complex metabolic machinery immediately removes the required amount from the legs, hips, spine, ribs and arms.

Ordinarily, this is a slow but relentless undermining process. But with cortisone administration, it is swift and relentless. Just as bad, it usually produces no symptoms—until the patient discovers that a minor bump or fall has broken an arm, a leg, or—worst of all—a hip.

This explanation didn't exactly make the woman happy. Why

hadn't the specialist who put her on cortisone warned her that the drug would cause her to lose calcium? And why didn't her family physician, who had known for several years that she was taking cortisone, warn her?

Fortunately for this woman, about a year before she broke her arm, she had begun taking dolomite tablets which also contained vitamin D. Dolomite is two parts calcium to one part magnesium. All three nutrients, but particularly calcium, help build and maintain strong bones.

The next shock came when she went to visit an orthopedic surgeon, who had just received her X-rays. "So you're the woman whose arm healed so beautifully!" he declared. Showing the woman her X-rays he remarked that her fracture was healing itself at an amazing rate, faster than "what we hope for in the best cases."

Thinking about this, the woman came to the conclusion that although the supplemental calcium and vitamin D she had been taking for a short time was not enough to reverse the effects of years of cortisone treatments, it at least had given her bones the nutrients they needed to heal themselves. Her only regret is that she didn't begin taking the supplements sooner.

Increased Risk Of Fractures

An article on the subject was published in the newsletter (February 1974) of the Jewish Hospital of St. Louis. It begins by pointing out that cortisone and its derivatives are being administered to several million patients in the United States who suffer from a number of chronic disorders, rheumatoid arthritis being just one of them. But it warns that however useful these compounds may be in alleviating these disorders, "They result in a number of potentially serious side effects, including the production of often severe bone loss with an increased risk of bone fractures. It is not unusual for patients to have a loss of 30 to 50 percent of their bone mass after several years of high-dose cortisone treatment."

Dr. Theodore Hahn, a spokesman for a bone research team at the Jewish Hospital, says it appears that cortisone directly blocks the activity of the bone-forming cells and at the same time decreases intestinal absorption of calcium. As if these two effects weren't bad enough, the calcium deficiency in turn can produce "secondary hormonal changes which increase bone breakdown."

But Dr. Hahn and his co-workers have some good news for

people who have been taking cortisone drugs: large, but carefully controlled doses of vitamin D, along with calcium supplements, can reverse this severe degeneration of the skeleton. "Preliminary results from a group of 30 patients treated with this regimen," the article states, "indicate that bone mass can be increased by as much as 25-30 percent over a six-month period, thereby greatly decreasing the risk of bone fracture in cortisone-treated patients."

Doctors Are Warned . . . But Patients?

How many people who are taking cortisone—all those several millions of them—are aware that the drug can cause brittle bones? And how many doctors are going to tell their patients that it is a good idea to get substantially more calcium and vitamin D into their diets *before* they begin splintering their bones?

It does seem that many doctors pay scant attention to the possible side effects of drug therapy, particularly when those side effects are intimately linked to nutrition. This attitude seems to be reflected even in the *Merck Manual*, a standard reference book for physicians. In the section on adrenocortical steroids, which include cortisone and its derivatives, this medical text says under the subheading "Management During Long-Term Treatment":

"If back pain occurs, X-ray of the spine should be made for possible osteoporosis. . . If pathologic fractures occur but the patient's condition warrants continuation of hormonal therapy, additional calcium and protein probably are more effective than the anabolic steroids."

No advice about giving more calcium as a preventive measure is offered. Presumably, the doctor is not expected to do anything until the patient begins complaining of back pain or comes in with a fracture that resulted from a slight bump.

47. Simple Dietary Protection For Your Bones

In a sense, those who have the special kind of osteoporosis produced by chronic administration of cortisone may be luckier than those who have the more common variety of osteoporosis which frequently hits post-menopausal women. This latter form of osteoporosis is not as easily reversed as the former. In talking about post-menopausal osteoporosis, we are talking about a condition which doctors at the Jewish Hospital in St. Louis call "the most disabling, frequently occurring and socially costly metabolic disease in the country."

The significance of this is that those who don't take cortisone have just as much need—if not more!—to try to *prevent* osteoporosis as those who do take the drug. Because once they develop osteoporosis, repairing the damage is no easy matter. While several studies have shown that nutritional supplementation can often stop the osteoporosis and sometimes produce modest degrees of remineralization, the kind of swift and very dramatic bone-rebuilding that can be achieved with cortisone-produced osteoporosis cannot be counted upon.

Few people need to be reminded how fragile is the health of anyone whose bones have become demineralized through osteoporosis. Most of us know at least one mature person whose health may have been otherwise excellent until she or he suffered a fracture, wound up in the hospital, and while trying to recuperate from surgery developed all kinds of serious complications.

How Much Calcium Is Enough?

Here are some findings from a leading nutrition researcher that give us a more accurate guide than we have ever had before of how much calcium most of us really need to keep our bones strong and healthy. Herta Spencer, M.D., of the Veteran's Administration Hospital in Hines, Illinois, summarized her work at the annual meeting of the Federation of American Societies for

Experimental Biology, on April 12, 1974, in Atlantic City, New Jersey.

Dr. Spencer said that she and the other members of her team (Lois Kramer, B.S., Clemontain Norris, R.N., and Dace Osis, senior technician) carried out 80 metabolic studies on 21 hospital patients in order to find out what amount of calcium is most desirable for the general population of adults.

At present, the recommended dietary allowance (R.D.A.) of calcium for adults is 800 milligrams a day, and—theoretically—this amount is supposed to provide a margin of safety in the event that a few people have extra calcium needs. There are even some medical and nutritional people who have expressed the opinion that most adults don't really need 800 milligrams of calcium, because they have stopped growing.

What Dr. Spencer found was that "although a daily intake of 800 milligrams of calcium was sufficient for most people studied, some patients receiving that level had a negative calcium balance—that is, they excreted more calcium in the urine and in the feces than they were consuming."

The Road To Osteoporosis

When you are in negative calcium balance, you are on the road to osteoporosis, because, as Dr. Spencer puts it, "When the body receives too little calcium, the element will be removed from its storage depots in the bones to meet calcium needs in blood. Years of chronic calcium depletion may lead to osteoporosis, a painful, disabling bone condition in which the long bones become porous and fragile. The condition is quite common, especially in women after menopause."

Dr. Spencer has stated that when the patients were given 1,200 milligrams of calcium a day, an amount which is 50 percent higher than the RDA, all of them achieved positive calcium balance—even those who had osteoporosis.

When calcium intakes were raised higher than 1,200 milligrams a day, there didn't seem to be any additional benefits for any of the 21 people tested. This, of course, does not rule out the possibility that some people require even more than 1,200 milligrams of calcium a day, but it does at least establish the fact that, as Dr. Spencer stated, "It is more desirable for adults to consume 1,200 milligrams of calcium daily than 800 milligrams."

Dr. Spencer believes that her findings should be translated

into action, "because it is not yet possible to predict the development of osteoporosis, and because of the difficulty in diagnosing and treating this painful and disabling condition."

The fact is that osteoporosis usually cannot be diagnosed radiographically until at least 30 percent of the bone mass is lost. Early detection, except through actual biopsy of bone tissue, is just not possible.

For this reason, every adult—especially every woman—is wise to check her diet carefully to see how much calcium she is getting. Dr. Spencer says that in order to get 1,200 milligrams of calcium a day, you must eat a balanced diet and also drink at least two to three glasses of milk every day.

Few adults regularly drink three glasses of milk a day. Many don't even get a "balanced" diet. But for those who like to drink milk and whose digestion isn't bothered by it, milk is certainly one good way of getting calcium into the system. It's also an excellent source of protein.

Bone Meal—A Natural Calcium Source

There are several supplemental forms of calcium for people who aren't big milk drinkers or cheese eaters. The most natural source of calcium is bone meal, tableted, or preferably powdered. Bone meal is derived from the long bones of young cattle, and contains all the minerals and trace elements—in the right proportions—which we humans need to build our own bones. It is well absorbed and utilized by most people, except those who have a deficiency of hydrochloric acid in their stomachs. These people may have difficulty with bone meal, and can turn to calcium gluconate, a naturally derived form of calcium which is easier for them to absorb.

Dolomite is usually valued more as a magnesium supplement than a calcium supplement, but it contains very useful amounts of calcium. Many people prefer to divide their calcium intake between bone meal and dolomite, thereby getting calcium, phosphorus, magnesium, and all the trace elements they need to keep their bones healthy.

Minerals are deposited in the bone on a matrix of protein, and as the *Merck Manual* pointed out, people taking cortisone may have difficulty synthesizing this protein. Anyone taking cortisone would be well advised to take extra protein in his daily diet.

Bone Disease

Vitamin D, of course, is another necessity for healthy bones. Those who live in the South and spend a good deal of time outdoors in the sun need minimal dietary vitamin D. But those who live where sunny days are rare would be well advised to take daily vitamin D orally, from a natural source such as fish liver oil.

48. A Closer Look At Osteoporosis

To many people it will come as a shock to learn that it is possible for bones to lose minerals. What? Those hard, solid, supporting structures? Their minerals can be dissolved away and washed out into the bloodstream?

But the fact is that bones are not stable but physiologically dynamic. They *normally* lose minerals all the time, and just as normally take up new minerals. It's only when the mineral loss is greater than the mineral gain that the health and integrity of the bone is in danger.

There are reasons, as you might suppose, why this active metabolism of the skeleton is beneficial. In the first place, the skeleton can be (and is) constantly and subtly remodeled to accommodate to changes in the individual's weight distribution and changed conditions of stress. Secondly, and of crucial importance every minute of life, the bones serve as a reservoir of calcium for replenishing the bloodstream when serum-calcium levels drop. Adequate calcium in the blood, instantly available to nerve cells, is essential for the functioning of the nervous system. Several hormones, plus vitamin D, help both store this mineral in bone deposits and release it as needed to maintain constant serum-calcium values.

Once we understand this turnover of bone calcium, the importance of adequate intake of dietary calcium becomes very apparent. Hormone-triggered mechanisms will readily sacrifice your bones on the altar of a dropping serum-calcium level, minute by minute. It's much more vital to your life and health to insure that your nerve cells continue to be bathed in circulating calcium than it is to protect the hardness of your skeletal structure. Fragile bones are less threatening than an impaired nervous system. You can't move a muscle, entertain a thought, or even take a breath if the proper nerve cells aren't working.

The trick, then, is to make sure your bloodstream is so supplied with dietary calcium that your bones needn't be robbed in order to make up for faulty eating habits.

Bone Disease

Forearm And Hip Fractures Most Common

"The principal clinical manifestation of osteoporosis is fracture," Dr. B.E.C. Nordin, professor of mineral metabolism at the University of Leeds, points out, "and three osteoporotic fracture syndromes can be defined: the lower forearm fracture, which predominantly affects women between the ages of 50 and 65; the fracture of the proximal femur (the hip), which affects both sexes over the age of 70; and the relatively rare vertebral crush fracture syndrome, which may be present at any age but is most common in elderly women" (*British Medical Journal*, March 13, 1971).

So you see that osteoporosis cannot be taken lightly, and it most certainly must be dealt with, for every one of us who approaches the half-century mark in age is likely to encounter it unless we do something about it preferably well in advance of that time.

Osteoporosis characteristically occurs in women after menopause and is presumably related to low estrogen output—the female hormone that dwindles when ovulation and the monthly periods cease. In men, fragile porous bones typically develop considerably later in life and the disorder is less severe. But though the disease is associated with late middle age and old age, the process probably begins many decades earlier.

"I would advise women to start calcium and vitamin D supplements at age 30, or perhaps 25," says Dr. Jennifer Jowsey of the Mayo Clinic. With the average American diet, there's apparently a long-term gradual loss of bone mineral exceeding the rate of mineral uptake and bone formation. In later years, when hormonal changes increase the susceptibility to osteoporosis, the skeleton has already lost a good deal of its substance. By then, because of previous loss, the rate of bone formation must not only equal the rate of bone demineralization (the normal condition) but must *exceed* it if bone strength is to be restored.

It's far more difficult, Dr. Jowsey warns, to induce new, compensatory bone formation than it is simply to slow down bone demineralization. Adequate calcium and vitamin D in the diet will go far to accomplish the latter. But preliminary findings, the Mayo scientist says, indicate that lost bone tissue will not automatically be restored by such dietary correction.

Osteoporosis, Puff By Puff

We can believe from what Dr. Jowsey says that long-term marginal deficiency in calcium and vitamin D is the principal villain in the tragedy of osteoporosis. However, other factors, too, influence bone health. We now know, for example, that cigarettes contribute to bone demineralization and that we should swear off smoking, supposing we're still hooked on this altogether harmful habit.

In a letter appearing in the *Journal of the American Medical Association* (July 31, 1972), Dr. Harry W. Daniell reports his findings that heavy cigarette smoking appears to be a prominent factor in inducing osteoporosis. Dr. Daniell, who practices in Redding, California, was prompted to undertake his study when he realized that most of his under-65 patients suffering from osteoporosis were habitual heavy smokers. (When it occurs before 65, osteoporosis is considered "premature.") The West Coast physician and his associates then studied records from the three small hospitals in the area, coming up with the cases of 17 women who had had at least one characteristic osteoporotic bone fracture prior to age 65. Follow-up interviews with the patients or surviving relatives revealed that, of the 17, only one was a non-smoker; one smoked less than 20 cigarettes a day; and 15 of the 17 had smoked 20 or more cigarettes daily for many years. An 88 percent correlation between heavy smoking and early incidence of osteoporosis is "statistically significant!"

As to how cigarette smoking could so affect the bones, Dr. Daniell points out that bone minerals (mostly calcium and phosphorus, responsible for the bone's hardness) are "known to be strikingly more soluble in acid solutions," and cigarette smoking is known to increase the acidity of bone tissue. Thus the bone minerals could be expected to dissolve and be absorbed into the bloodstream at a much faster rate when smoking provides the acid environment.

Studies have shown, Dr. Daniell says, that three consecutive cigarettes cause a prompt transient hypercalcemia—or high content of calcium in the blood. This finding, he explains, suggests that the act of smoking is associated with rapid calcium loss from bone structures.

Parathormone And Bone Resorption

Still other factors can influence the onset of osteoporosis. Writing in the *British Medical Journal* (June 2, 1973), Dr. P. E. Belchetz and colleagues suggest that taking your daily calcium supplement just before going to bed might make a difference in preventing excess bone mineral loss.

Here's the rationale: regular meals during the day constantly provide at least *some* calcium to the bloodstream. But calcium absorption from the gut continues only three to five hours after eating, and therefore from about midnight on, the lack of incoming calcium from the intestinal tract triggers the action of the parathyroid hormone (parathormone), which stimulates bone demineralization or "resorption." The female hormone, estrogen, the authors note, to some extent desensitizes bones to the action of parathormone. But in postmenopausal women this protection has been reduced.

Initial clinical studies by the investigators tend to confirm their hypothesis. So take your bone meal or dolomite or glass of milk just before retiring and you may counteract those bad night hours when your bones are most likely to dribble away their substance.

Another factor that triggers the action of parathormone, according to Dr. Jowsey and her associates at the Mayo Clinic, is a mineral imbalance, with phosphorus intake grossly exceeding calcium intake (*Postgraduate Medicine*, October, 1972). Heavy meat-eaters are at risk of this condition because meat, while very poor in calcium, has a high phosphorus content. It's meat-eaters' unbalanced high phosphorus intake, in Dr. Jowsey's opinion, that accounts for the now established fact that longtime vegetarians are less susceptible to osteoporosis than are omnivores.

How Magnesium Helps

Finally, let's get back to magnesium, which is contained in the supplement dolomite and is believed to contribute to bone strength. This mineral has been used to treat a number of brittle bone disorders and the related problem of resistance to vitamin D—that is, failure of the body to utilize vitamin D properly. Drs. Ariel Rosler and David Rabinowitz, writing in *The Lancet* (April 14, 1973), suggest that magnesium may be necessary for the conversion of vitamin D to its active forms. As scientists have learned in recent years, the vitamin D we ingest or synthesize from sunshine is itself biologically inert until it has been converted by the liver and the kidneys into active derivatives.

If this conversion is magnesium-dependent, as *The Lancet* authors propose, then even a large supplement of vitamin D would be of little use to an individual who was magnesium-deficient. The recommended daily allowance for magnesium is a sizable 300 milligrams for women, 350 milligrams for men. Yet not many foods provide significant amounts of this mineral. Egg yolks and brain have exceptionally high values, and other good sources are kidney, liver, almonds, cashews, peanuts, black-eyed peas, blackstrap molasses, curry, and mustard powder.

But we haven't really faced, yet, the question of how to *reverse* the disease process once it's begun nor to restore the bone tissue that has been lost. Are any measures available?

Dr. Jowsey and her colleagues review some of the medical measures that have been tested. At one time it was widely believed that the hormone, estrogen, given to postmenopausal women, would stimulate normal bone formation and thus contribute to the build-up of denser, stronger bones. It is now known, Dr. Jowsey says, that estrogen temporarily slows down bone loss but doesn't do a thing for bone build-up. Other hormones have also been tried with no success.

Fluoride Affects Bone Density

The one substance, according to Dr. Jowsey, which is known to actually contribute to bone build-up is fluoride. You will probably read a lot about fluoride as the "solution" to osteoporosis, since public health authorities of this country have latched on to the partial evidence to boost their arguments for mandatory fluoridation of public drinking water. An example is an article in *Medical World News* (January 18, 1974), reporting on research at the University of Tennessee; here investigators found that bone density measurably increased in a group of older women following a regimen of fluoride treatment.

But the question to ask is: What *kind* of density? For when fluoride is given in sufficient quantity to increase bone density, the results are likely to be the same as in regions of endemic fluorosis—communities where the natural water supply contains too much fluoride, and abnormal bone density and bone deformities are prevalent.

As Dr. Jowsey explains it, the new bone formed following fluoride treatment is not normal healthy bone but "poorly mineralized." Furthermore, the parathyroid hormone is actually stimulated so that the rate of bone loss as well as bone gain is stepped up.

The Mayo researchers, however, do believe that fluoride can be helpful if used always and *only* in conjunction with heavy supplements of calcium and very large doses of vitamin D. Their clinical studies indicate that under this regimen, normal bone formation will be simulated and normal bone strength restored in about five years. Even under their cautious guidance, however, the researchers found that one patient developed a bony spur, or spine-like outgrowth, characteristic of fluoride poisoning.

But if we stop looking around for another "substance" and search for a life-style factor instead of a pill, then we find that the medical world long ago discovered something that actually does promote normal uptake of mineral by the bones: exercise.

49. You Can Strengthen Your Bones With Exercise

Many things can be done to build the strength of the bones and ward off chronic bone weakness. Most important is to realize that exercise or stress builds bone just as it builds muscle. Professional athletes not only have bigger and stronger muscles than non-athletes, but they have thicker and stronger bones as well. The pull and tug of muscle against bone that occurs when you exercise stimulates the vital life processes which go on in healthy bones, and causes them to grow in size.

The opposite is true when a person does not exercise. Bones become weaker. That has been proven beyond doubt by several experiments with healthy young people who volunteered to lie in bed with their bodies encased in plaster casts. Within a few days they began to excrete much larger than normal amounts of calcium in their urine, proving that the stores of calcium in their bones were being depleted by lack of exercise. If bed rest or sedentary habits are continued for long periods, bones can become seriously weakened.

Bones Need Some Stress And Strain

In the June, 1969, issue of *Geriatrics*, Dr. Charles D. Bonner writes: "Although there are many causes for the clinical syndrome of osteoporosis, the one most commonly seen in patients admitted to a chronic disease hospital or rehabilitation center is that caused by lack of physical activity and muscular contraction."

Dr. Bonner explains that decalcification can take place in isolated bones that are immobilized for fracture. However, when inactivity is generalized, as in the case of some older people, the osteoporosis is also generalized. All the bones are affected. The rehabilitation specialist urges careful mobilization and gradual increase in activity to reverse the disease process. Even more important, he emphasizes the need for day-to-day activity as a preventive—one that provides the bones with the stresses and strains they require to stay strong.

How does exercise produce such beneficial effects? Part of the credit goes to an unusual phenomenon called the piezo-electric effect.

When certain types of crystalline structures—and bones contain these—are subjected to pressure, a weak electric current is generated. Somehow, and researchers have been looking into the hows and whys for several years, this electric current seems to draw calcium and other minerals out of the blood and into the bone, which is rebuilt and strengthened.

When a person jumps, for example, this creates pressure and a small amount of electricity is generated in the bone. When the bone is jarred from the bottom, such as would be the case with walking, hiking or skipping rope, the piezo-electric effect eventually causes the bones to become more dense. And increased density means stronger bones, something which the elderly would be happy to have.

Activity Fortifies The Bones
In 1970, at the annual meeting of the Swedish Medical Society held in Stockholm, Drs. Nils Westlin and Bo Nilsson of Malmo, Sweden, reported that when they measured bone densities in young men they found that 64 athletes had significantly higher bone density than 39 non-athletes of the same age. Density was found to increase with increases in physical activity (*Medical Tribune*, February 6, 1970).

Highest densities were observed among weight lifters. Next came discus throwers and shot putters. They were followed by runners and then soccer players. Swimmers (whose exercise does not involve impact on the bones) were found to have densities not significantly different from controls. The investigators also noted that the non-athletes who jogged and skied had significantly denser leg bones than non-exercisers.

Dr. Carlton Fredericks has said that women with bones weakened by osteoporosis should, if they are capable of doing it, skip rope as a means of therapeutic exercise. The impact on the spine, vertically exerted, generates the electrical forces that drive calcium to the bone areas requiring reinforcement (*The Carlton Fredericks Newsletter of Nutrition*, July 1, 1972).

Obviously, an elderly man or woman isn't suddenly going to take up jumping rope after not having exercised for several years. But much the same effect could be gained from walking. A brisk walk at least, for those unable to perform more vigorous exercise, is essential if bones are to stay healthy.

If the small amount of electricity generated by the piezo-electric effect helps in the construction of stronger bone, it seems obvious that electricity would be valuable in healing bones as well. The medical profession has already taken this next step and has found this to be true.

Bone Healing Aided By Electricity

Two surgeons at the University of Pennsylvania, Dr. Carl T. Brighton and Dr. Zachary B. Friedenberg, reported that electricity healed the broken ankle of a 51-year-old woman who had suffered for almost two years (*New York Times,* October 30, 1971).

The woman broke her ankle in 1969. The ankle was in a cast for 13 weeks. Then she walked unaided for a year. But the ankle never healed properly, and she returned to the hospital in February, 1971.

This time the surgeons connected wires to the fracture. A cast was put on, the wires were run through the cast, and a source of power attached. Ten micro-amperes of current were applied for nine weeks, causing the bone to grow together. The patient used crutches for two weeks, and then walked unaided without any further problems.

According to Drs. Brighton and Friedenberg, the point where new bone normally grows, (the end) is electronegative. The rest of the bone is less electronegative unless there is a fracture. When there is a break, the entire bone surface develops a negative charge, strongest at the fracture site. They also found that electrical activity in the bone returns to normal only as healing is completed. Further research found that application of electricity produced bone growth at the negative pole, until current was increased beyond 20 micro-amperes. At that point there was bone destruction.

In another case, a 14-year-old Brooklyn, New York, boy, who was born with a rare defect in his leg bone, was cured by the application of electricity (*Science,* March, 1972). Dr. Leroy S. Lavine, an orthopedic surgeon at the State University of New York's Downstate Medical Center, directed the effort which cured the boy of pseudoarthrosis of the tibia.

In the main bone of the boy's lower leg, part of the structure that should have been strong bone had developed as wobbly, cartilage-like tissue instead. As a result, the halves of the tibia on either side of the defective area would slip apart if he tried to stand on the leg. In addition, the leg failed to grow properly.

Bone Disease

A bone graft when he was four had temporarily repaired the defect, but seven years later he injured the leg and broke through the old defective area. Subsequent bone grafts, immobilization with a metal rod and other treatments failed to heal the defect. So Dr. Lavine decided to try electricity. It worked, and within four months the bone was completely healed.

50. Osteomalacia, Rickets And Vitamin D

For many years, it has been generally assumed that "typical" hip fractures of elderly men and women are invariably caused by the pathological loss of bone density known as osteoporosis. But, as new research in Great Britain reveals, in actuality a significant proportion of hip fractures in the elderly may not be due to this gradually-developing and difficult-to-cure disorder. Rather, they can be the result of a *temporary* condition—deficiency in vitamin D. The patient may be suffering not from osteoporosis but from frank vitamin D deficiency disease, which is called rickets in children and osteomalacia in adults.

Essentially, rickets affects bone growth in the very young. It throws their bone-growth metabolism off, resulting in malformation. Manifestations of rickets include fragile bones and soft teeth, extremely susceptible to decay. The outward signs of rickets include bowed legs and bent backs. In adults, vitamin D deficiency can bring osteomalacia, a condition marked by the softening of the bones along with accompanying pain, tenderness, muscular weakness, anorexia (lack of appetite) and loss of weight. In either case, the cure is simplicity itself: vitamin D supplements.

The very real danger of vitamin D deficiency in adults—particularly older people—was pointed up in a British study conducted at the General Infirmary at Leeds. Here doctors made microscopic examinations of bone samples from 125 elderly patients who were hospitalized following a common form of hip fracture (fracture at the neck or top of the femur, which is the long bone of the thigh).

As Dr. J. E. Aaron and colleagues reported in *The Lancet* (February 16, 1974), nearly a fourth of the patients (21 percent) were unequivocally diagnosed as suffering from the vitamin D deficiency disease, osteomalacia. If patients who revealed one (rather than two) characteristics of this bone disorder were included in the calculations, then osteomalacia could be diagnosed for more than a third (37 percent) of all patients studied.

Bone Disease

"We have so far treated eight of our osteomalacia cases with vitamin D," the authors wrote, "and obtained histological evidence (evidence from microscopic studies of bone structure) of cure of the osteomalacia in every case."

The Two "Osteo's"

Let's take a closer look at the two bone diseases—osteoporosis and osteomalacia—in order to get a better understanding of exactly what the Leeds doctors discovered.

In osteoporosis, the bone has lost minerals, and its density or volume has so diminished that it crumbles easily. In the center of the bone, normally tiny spaces have enlarged at the expense of the solid portion, so that thin spikes of bone are unsupported by surrounding bone tissue.

You can see why osteoporosis is not as easy to prevent or cure as the frank vitamin D deficiency diseases, rickets and osteomalacia. What happens in those disorders is that soft matrices in the bone (osteoid), which the bone-building cells have prepared for calcification, remain uncalcified because deficiency in vitamin D has reduced absorption of dietary calcium. Both rickets and osteomalacia are characterized by an abnormally high proportion of uncalcified osteoid. This is where new bone formation *should* have taken place, but the calcification never occurred. Also, "calcification fronts"—that is, the beginnings of new calcification—cover an abnormally low proportion of all osteoid tissue in individuals with vitamin D deficiency diseases.

These two characteristics are the criteria the Leeds investigators used in determining whether or not their fracture patients suffered from osteomalacia. For determining osteoporosis, bone density or volume was the determining factor.

Of the 125 patients (23 men and 102 women), 26 could be positively diagnosed as suffering from osteomalacia, while 20 had only one of the two characteristics of this deficiency disease and were classified as "probable osteomalacia." Of the osteomalacia cases, 10 also had osteoporosis.

Normally, we are protected against osteomalacia in a wonderfully simple way. When natural sunlight strikes the bare skin, the ultraviolet portion acts on a lipid substance, 7-dehydrocholesterol, just below the surface to form cholecalciferol (vitamin D_3). It has always seemed plausible to suspect, however, that those of us who live in temperate zones far north of the Equator might risk vitamin D depletion in late winter when sunshine wanes.

Winter—A Bad Season For The Bones

The existence of just such a seasonal variation in bone health has been conclusively demonstrated by Dr. Aaron and his associates. Examining biopsy samples over a five-year period, they discovered that disease symptoms were heavily clustered in those patients whose fractures occurred in February through June (*The Lancet,* July 13, 1974).

"As would be expected if this seasonal variation was attributable to variation in the supply of vitamin D dependent on sunlight," they reported, "the proportion of cases with osteomalacia is highest in the spring and lowest in the autumn."

The two- to six-month lag between the days of absolute least sunlight (the third week of December) and the highest incidence of osteomalacia is explained when we remember that vitamin D is fat-soluble, and thus easily stored in the body. All summer while the sun shines brightly you are stockpiling this vitamin for the cold dark days ahead. Reserves are most likely to run out at the very tail end of winter or even early spring.

This was confirmed by Professor W. Farnsworth Loomis, a biochemist at Brandeis University, who reported in *Scientific American* (December, 1970) that "rickets occurs most severely and most frequently at the end of winter" in children. The painfully crippling and deforming bone disease strikes its young victims then, he said, because the "winter sun, hanging low in the sky, is almost without potency in effecting the crucial conversion of 7-dehydrocholesterol into calciferol."

Why Mature People Are More Vulnerable

Each winter brings a new and serious challenge to your bones. As you grow older, that challenge becomes more severe with each passing year. After the age of 30 to 35, the total amount of bone in an individual actually shrinks "about 10 percent per decade in women and five percent per decade in men," explained mineral metabolism expert Dr. Louis V. Avioli in an interview with *Medical World News* (October 19, 1973). That's probably why seasonal bone loss may cause no aches or pain in a woman of 25, but real suffering in a woman of 55.

Whether or not you can ignore diet and depend on sunlight for your vitamin D depends on where—and how—you live. "In many populations exposed to adequate sunshine, the dietary intake of vitamin D is probably irrelevant," said Dr. J. Chalmers, a physician at Princess Margaret Rose Orthopedic Hospital in Edinburgh, Scotland, in a letter to *The Lancet* (June 7, 1969). "In

Hong Kong, for example, the average Chinese diet contains less than 70 I.U. per day, and yet osteomalacia is excessively rare, owing to the generous exposure to sunshine enjoyed in that part of the world."

But he cautioned that the disease is on the rise in temperate climates: "Since we have become aware of this situation in recent years, nearly 150 cases of osteomalacia have now been recognized in this area alone, and I have little doubt that these represent only the tip of the iceberg."

Subsequent reports confirm Dr. Chalmers' prediction. Dr. Aaron and colleagues at Leeds have concluded that "it seems reasonable to suggest that for every case of proven osteomalacia, representing severe vitamin D depletion, there must be others with minor degrees of vitamin D deficiency. In view of the dominant role played by vitamin D in calcium absorption, possibly malabsorption of calcium in elderly people may be a manifestation of a degree of vitamin D deficiency falling short of osteomalacia, and this must at least contribute to senile bone loss."

The best way to avoid those kinds of problems is to take a daily supplement of vitamin D, naturally derived from fish liver oils. For just as the diet can't be counted on to meet your vitamin D needs (unless you're an Eskimo eating oily fish for breakfast, lunch and dinner), we have seen that even sunshine, the very best and most natural source, fails us in the winter.

Rickets: The Earliest Air Pollution Disease

One important reason why wintry skies just can't deliver the sunshine vitamin in amounts we need is the staggering concentration of dirt and grime that modern man has added to the atmosphere. Soot and other particles do a very effective job of filtering out the sun's vital ultraviolet rays. In fact, the first widespread epidemics of rickets occurred in Europe in the 18th century, when the air had become fouled with a pall of smoke from the increasing use of soft coal.

Professor Loomis at Brandeis called rickets "the earliest air-pollution disease." He said that it took years for researchers to realize that people who suffered rickets were simply not manufacturing vitamin D in their bodies. They were thrown off the track for a while by the fact that rickets was not rampant in other Northern European countries where sunlight also was scarce, but where the population ate a lot of fish. Only later did they discover that fish are able to manufacture vitamin D without the aid of ultraviolet rays from the sun, and that these people who ate the fish acquired the vitamin in their diets. Later studies showed that certain fish liver oils were rich in the anti-rachitic ingredient, and that cod-liver oil, for example, taken over the sunless winter months, offered effective protection from rickets.

Then in 1927 two scientists found a way to add ergocalciferol, a form of vitamin D, to milk. Ultraviolet irradiating activated the vitamin and made it readily available to children who shunned the taste of cod-liver oil. Irradiated milk for children was believed to have closed the book on rickets.

Why is it, then, that today, more than half a century after the cause and cure of rickets were discovered, cases of vitamin D deficiency are still being found across this country and in other nations? The blame must be put at the doorstep of nutritionists who were so certain that rickets had to be eradicated by the addition to bottled milk of 400 units of vitamin D per quart, that they never bothered to check.

Proof That Rickets Still Occurs

The main reason that you don't hear much about rickets and osteomalacia today is that they are rarely recognized by doctors as such, and so, in turn, are rarely reported. Physicians have been taught that there is no longer a vitamin D deficiency in this country, so they look for other causes. But rickets does exist, and evidence of this was reported in the November, 1967, *American Journal of Clinical Nutrition* by Sister Mary Theodora Weick of the Nutrition Department of Mercy Hospital, Buffalo, N.Y. She found, in studying official records from 1910 through 1961, that 13,807 deaths were caused by rickets, and that from 1956 to 1960, 843 new cases of rickets were reported. She doubts that *all* cases of rickets are reported, and states that rickets "is still noticeably prevalent, and only constant, continual efforts will bring about its complete elimination."

So 200 years after the Industrial Revolution, people who live in industrialized, urban areas are still succumbing to what Professor Loomis called "the earliest air pollution disease." The number of elderly people dying after bone-breaking falls in Britain over a 35-year period was closely related to the amount of coal smoke in the air, Dr. T. P. Eddy of the London School of Hygiene and Tropical Medicine reported in *Nature* (September 13, 1974). Bone fragility caused by lack of sunshine is the suspected cause.

Bone Disease

"When smoke pollution was at its height in 1937-39," Dr. Eddy noted, "it was estimated that in Leicester (latitude 53 degrees north) at least 30 percent more ultraviolet daylight would have reached the center of the city in winter if all the smoke in the atmosphere had been eliminated, and occasionally the loss was more than half." He concluded that "The steep rise in femoral fractures with advancing age in Britain may be attributable to an absolute or relative deficiency of vitamin D."

But even if air pollution could be eliminated tomorrow, winter would still play havoc with our bones. From November through March, the sun rises so late and sets so early that those of us who work in offices or factories often go from weekend to weekend without spending any time in bright sunshine. And what little time we do manage to spend out-of-doors is virtually useless for vitamin D accumulation, because we are heavily wrapped in coats, scarves and gloves.

In fact, the farther north you live, the more futile it becomes trying to obtain your sunshine vitamin D out-of-doors. You can, however, be certain of getting all the vitamin D your bones will need for the long winter by supplementing your diet with natural vitamin D derived from fish liver oil.

Section 12
Bronchitis

51. The Battle For Breath

51. The Battle For Breath

Every winter, many millions of people on both sides of the Atlantic suffer from bronchitis. They have spasms of coughing that leave them weak and breathless, with aching chests. Breathing is wheezy, indicating that there are large amounts of phlegm in the respiratory tract. Many doctors who once prescribed antibiotics for this drawn-out chest disease, now have learned that the antibiotics don't work. But they don't know what else to do about the ailment. Some recommend that patients stop smoking, and they may prescribe a medicine to help bring up some of the phlegm. But no cure is known for bronchitis. Of the millions who contract it, many will die.

Bronchitis is often coupled with emphysema in medical statistics and investigations, since both are part of the same syndrome. Chronic bronchitis, if it does not become acute and kill immediately, leads to the chronic condition known as emphysema—inability of the lungs to extract enough oxygen from the air to enable the body to carry on such rudimentary tasks as walking, dressing or even eating. The emphysema section of this book discusses that dread disease in more detail. It is a terrible end-stage of the progressive deterioration of the respiratory tract.

Emphysema-bronchitis deaths have increased so alarmingly in the past 25 years that these chronic respiratory diseases are referred to as the "fastest growing cause of death in the United States" and "a health menace of major magnitude." And in England and Wales, the rate of deaths from these diseases is between four and five times as great as it is in the U.S.

Most Bronchitis Sufferers Are Smokers

Cigarette smoking is considered to be the chief cause of bronchitis. In a very thorough statistical study comparing the prevalence of bronchitis in the British Isles and America, made by an international team of experts and published in the *British Medical Journal* (December 12, 1964), it was established that in the

242

U.S. only nine percent of those suffering from bronchitis were non-smokers. The comparable figure for Britain was 16 percent. There could hardly be a clearer demonstration that, while cigarette smoking is not the only cause, it is of enormous importance in the development of this disabling and deadly disease.

The cigarette hazard even extends to non-smokers living in the same house. An infant in the first year of life is twice as likely to get bronchitis if both parents smoke, British researchers report in the November 2, 1974, issue of *The Lancet*. If only one parent smokes, the risk of serious chest illness drops, but it is still greater than for children of non-smokers, according to Dr. J. R. T. Colley, of the London School of Hygiene and Tropical Medicine, and two associates.

It would seem, then, that the first and most important measure for anyone who wishes to avoid bronchitis in himself or loved ones is to stop smoking, or better yet, never start.

Even if you are a smoker, however, there is evidence that the possibility of your contracting bronchitis or other diseases of the respiratory tract is much less if you are getting generous amounts of vitamin C in your diet.

Vitamin C Lessens Effects Of Bronchitis

This good news comes from Dr. E. G. Knox of the University of Birmingham in Great Britain (*Lancet,* June 30, 1973). Dr. Knox, availing himself of a tremendous amount of health statistics, set up a table which correlates increasing amounts of intake of various nutrients with increasing incidence of various fatal diseases. A correlation of zero, in this table, means that there is no correlation at all between how much of a certain nutrient a person consumes and his statistical chances of dying from a certain disease. A correlation of +.20 means there is some correlation between the nutrient and the disease, but it is not all that significant. Correlation of +.30, +.40, and up indicate that the statistical link is probably quite significant.

For example, the correlation between consumption of fat and the incidence of death from high blood pressure is +.38.

One of the causes of death on Dr. Knox's chart is bronchitis. The correlation between vitamin C intake and bronchitis as a cause of death is *minus* .52. In other words, the more vitamin C a person consumes, the less his chances of succumbing to bronchitis.

Air Pollution, A Factor In Respiratory Ills

If cigarette smoking is the leading cause of bronchitis, there is little doubt that polluted air is also involved. Fertilizer factories, canneries, paint factories, rubber plants, metal fabricating industries, and automobiles, all contribute to the haze of toxic filth that lies over our metropolitan areas. In the *Archives of Environmental Health* (January, 1963), Dr. Richard W. Stone, Medical Director of the New York Telephone Company blamed this increasing level of pollution for the high incidence of chronic respiratory disease. The Metropolitan Life Insurance Company has found that chronic respiratory ailments such as bronchitis are 33 percent more common among holders of its industrial policies, who breathe polluted factory air on a daily basis.

For those of us compelled to earn our livings in areas of heavy air pollution, there is no way we can avoid breathing chemical toxins, notably sulfur dioxide. But we can give ourselves a significant measure of protection with vitamin C, and also vitamin A.

A London physician, Dr. Max Odens, conducted a long term clinical study, based on the knowledge that vitamin A is involved in the maintenance of a healthy mucous membrane lining of the respiratory tract. As reported in the German medical publication, *Vitalstoffe* (December, 1967), Dr. Odens gave 17 people suffering from chronic bronchitis daily doses of vitamin A (in addition to traditional therapy) over a 15-year period. All showed improvement. There were no mortalities, although the patients' ages ranged from 48 to 67, and the period took in one of London's most severe and fogbound winters when thousands of elderly people died of chronic bronchitis.

Two Common Foods That Can Trigger Bronchitis Symptoms

Food allergies are commonly overlooked as a factor in some stubborn bronchitis cases. Strangely enough, there is good reason to suppose that one of the guilty substances is bread. Irvin G. Spiesman, M.D., and Lloyd Arnold, M.D., described in the *American Journal of Digestive Diseases and Nutrition* (September, 1937) a sensational investigation they had conducted. They investigated cold susceptibility in 63 patients at their clinic who were under observation for three years. The patients were divided into three groups: those who seldom had colds, those who were frequent cold sufferers, and those whose colds appeared to be related to allergies and extreme sensitivity, rather than germs.

Specifically forbidden to those who participated in the study were all products made from wheat flour. Spiesman and Arnold credited the absence of wheat as a major factor in the success they experienced in reducing colds in all of the participating patients.

The scientific team remarked that others have related high carbohydrate ingestion to catarrhal illnesses. If we remember that bronchitis frequently starts as a common cold, or occurs in the individual who is particularly susceptible to colds, it can be seen that there is a strong possibility that simply eliminating bread, macaroni and other wheat products from the diet could have an enormously beneficial effect in the prevention of bronchitis.

Other physicians have obtained seemingly miraculous results by eliminating milk from their patients' diets. "One of the common problems facing both pediatricians and family physicians," reported Dr. John Gerrard, a pediatrician at the University of Saskatchewan, "is the child who seems to have one cold after another, each cold being followed by an attack of bronchitis or bronchial pneumonia, often necessitating admission to the hospital. The fundamental cause of the child's repeated respiratory tract infections frequently remains obscure . . . We have recently encountered four children with predisposition to respiratory tract infection which was relieved by the simple expedient of excluding cow's milk and dairy products from their diets . . ."

One of the cases Dr. Gerrard described in the November, 1966 issue of the *AMA Journal* was that of a baby boy who caught a cold at two months and had to be hospitalized with serious bronchitis. In the hospital he got worse in spite of oxygen and antibiotics. His lungs became increasingly congested. He ran a constant fever, and was periodically unconscious.

At last, he was put on a milk-free diet, and he recovered quickly. The symptoms returned only when he drank ordinary cow's milk. From then on, he was on a beef-base formula with vitamin supplements. But even a year later he suffered with nasal congestion and wheezing whenever he was given milk.

Aside from dramatic cases like this where an underlying

Bronchitis

allergy is discovered, medical science does not offer any cure for bronchitis, although your doctor can do much to bring you temporary relief. Give up tobacco, fortify yourself with a highly nutritious diet every single day and see whether that better opportunity doesn't enable nature to help.

Section 13
Cancer

52. The Cancer Problem And How To Cope With It

R. A. Holman, M.D.
Honorary Consultant Bacteriologist
United Cardiff Hospitals

The very mention of the word cancer to the ordinary layman strikes a note of fear, because he knows only too well that, despite the tremendous advances in medical science, there seems to be no solution to the problem which this very grave disease presents. Cancer is, of course, a condition which has been recognized in man for thousands of years; and generation after generation of deep-thinking workers have attempted to explain the cause of the development of the malignant tumors, and have tried their hand at discovering a cure. Although a vast amount of work has been done and recorded in the literature, the progress is disappointing.

During the past 100 years our knowledge of disease in general has advanced rapidly, and as a result there have been revolutionary changes in the understanding of both human and animal medical problems. The greater part of this advance was due to the pioneers of medical laboratory work, namely the bacteriologists. Enormous strides were made during the latter half of the 19th century by such famous workers as Pasteur, Koch, Hansen, Ogston, Neisser, Klebs, Salmon, Bruce, Gaertner, Kitasato, Shiga, and others, who firmly established the bacterial origin of a large number of common diseases from tuberculosis down to simple lesions like the boil. Following this terrific period of discovery and the development of better microscopes, numerous workers attempted to show that malignant tumors were caused by bacteria or larger cells like the protozoa. At the turn of the century, eminent men put forward strong evidence in support of a causative factor of this nature, but we know, and have known now for many years, that there is no real scientific support for this. We do know that one or two specific tumors in experimental animals are caused by certain smaller particles which we call viruses, but in the cancer field as a whole there is still no good evidence that all tumors are derived from normal cells by such viral action.

Compounding A Problem

Apart from the intense work on the bacterial, protozoal and viral origins of cancer, there have been a great number of suggestions, from vague generalizations such as chronic irritation and chronic irreversible injury of cell respiration to specific theories of embryonic rests and so on. None of these theories is adequate or specific enough to explain the greatest problem which faces medicine today. When no obvious cause of a disease is to be found, one always finds a great deal of speculation based on such diverse factors as climate, soil, food, radiation, cigarette smoke, diesel fumes, etc.; and whenever such a multiplicity of agents is implicated, then the problem appears to be extremely complex.

A Civilized Disease

Barker, as long ago as 1928, wrote: "Cancer is a disease of over-civilization or faulty civilization, and is caused by chronic poisoning in almost any form, and it cannot be doubted that much disease is caused by our being bombarded with chemicals and poisons in minute quantities at all meals." Four years later Cope wrote: "One in nine die of cancer in this country, and the time is fast approaching when we may expect one in four or five will die from this disease; but long before that the encroachment of this dreaded enemy may suddenly awaken the nation from its apathy and arouse such a panic of terror as may compel attention to the causes of this scourge." We now know that in the civilized populations this forecast is coming true; but there is no panic of terror—at least not on the surface. Now, almost thirty years after Barker's book (*Cancer, the Surgeon and the Researcher*), we find Berglas, in his book, *Cancer, Nature, Cause and Cure*, pointing out that current figures show that one out of every four persons in the U.S.A. will contract cancer during their lifetime. These, he says, are the figures to be anticipated which in reality may be still higher, and, in his opinion, before very long everybody will be threatened with death through cancer. The ominous rise in the incidence of the disease he blames on the increasing toxicity of our environment. He rightly points out that the food we eat has, in a few decades, been so altered and contaminated that every mouthful we consume contains some trace of harmful substances, and that, on top of that, the human organism in the course of present-day therapies is subjected to still more chemicals, with little thought given to any long-term effects.

Cancer's Common Cause

In recent decades we have become aware that there is an ever-increasing number of physical and chemical agents which can cause cancer in laboratory animals and in man, e.g., X-rays, U/V light, radium, certain dyestuffs, soot, tar, etc. J. W. Cook is of the opinion that the study of cancer-inducing substances is likely to prove one of the most profitable forms of cancer research, but it is quite obvious to well informed opinion that as we have a host of quite unrelated agents capable of producing the malignant change, then it is wiser to concentrate our attention on the processes occurring in the reacting cells. In my opinion, the only common denominator is the cell upon which these agents act. As O. H. Warburg recently wrote, in his *New Methods of Cell Physiology*: "Just as there are many remote causes of plague—heat, insects, rats—but only one common cause, the plague bacillus, there are a great many remote causes of cancer, but there is only one common cause into which all the other causes of cancer merge—the irreversible injury of respiration."

One of the few well-established facts about cancer is that the important enzyme catalase (so called by O. Loew when carrying out experiments on the curing of tobacco leaves) is progressively diminished in the host as well as the tumor. Catalase inhibition is known to be associated with mutagenic processes and the development of viruses, and it is also known that some of the proven carcinogenic agents can inhibit this enzyme. In fact, catalase inhibition in red blood corpuscles, which results in the formation of Heinz bodies, has been suggested as a rapid method of screening agents for carcinogenic activity.

It is now realized that the wide-spread distribution of catalase in living cells is essential for their ability to live in the presence of oxygen. Catalase is intimately concerned in the control of the effects of hydrogen peroxide. It is generally agreed that hydrogen peroxide is a substance normally produced, used or destroyed by a wide variety of living cells. Just as with bacteria, it is very probable that there is a specific catalase-peroxide balance for each type of animal cell; and if this is interfered with for a long enough time, the abnormal biochemistry occurs which could lead to the development of cancer cells. Numerous workers are coming to the conclusion that the key to the cause, treatment and prevention of cancer lies in this altered fundamental biological mechanism.

Environmental Causes

In order to understand the problem of cancer it is essential to realize that man is a complex organism composed of physical, chemical and parasitic structures, surviving in a more complex environment of similar agents. A few of the well-known cancer producing materials have been part of man's environment throughout the ages, and this probably accounts for the fact that the existence of cancer has been noticed for thousands of years. Solar radiation is known to increase the incidence of skin cancer in certain occupational groups, e.g. sailors and agricultural workers in dry and sunny climates. Water, air and certain foodstuffs have been found in certain regions to be contaminated with radioactive materials, or chemicals such as arsenic, which results in local increase in the incidence of certain cancers. Soot, a substance known to cause cancer, and primarily produced by man, has become increasingly released into the environment as carboniferous fuels gained in popularity for heating, cooking, lighting and smoking. Much has been written in the past 100 years about the pollution of air in this respect, but little has been done to control this obvious source of carcinogens.

The Chemical Life

Probably of much greater import is the fact that during the past seventy years, as a result of the rapid technological advances, large numbers of physical and chemical agents have been placed or released into man's external and internal environment with little thought about the possible long-term effect of these on his own cells. Civilized man today, living in overcrowded cities, is being exposed day and night, in some cases for the whole of life, to agents which were not available a century ago, or were found in such minute amounts as to have a negligible effect on living cells. These agents may affect our own cells through diverse routes, i.e., by inhalation, ingestion, injection, irradiation, or by absorption through the skin. On top of these, the body may manufacture certain cancer-producing chemicals as a result of other stimuli. Not all the agents recently introduced are carcinogenic, but the fact is that many have not been tested, and the tests on some already examined have not been very comprehensive. Even if many substances prove to be negative with the methods at present available, it is a fact that there are large numbers of these being placed on, around and in us which together provide a considerable insult to the cells so exposed.

Most Cancer Environmental

W. C. Hueper, who retired in 1965 as head of the Environmental Cancer Section, National Cancer Institute, stated: "The evidence on hand, when critically and competently evaluated, in fact strongly suggests that the majority of cancers affecting the following organs are attributable to exposures to environmental carcinogens: skin, mouth, paranasal sinuses, larnyx, lung, esophagus, stomach, intestine, liver, blood-forming organs, bone, bladder, kidney and thyroid. The probable existence of similar casual relations can be suspected, moreover, for at least a part of the cancers affecting the brain, breast and uterus."

If the catalase-peroxide balance is interfered with for a long enough time by physical and chemical agents present in our environment, whether in food, drink, drugs, or in the air we breathe, then we shall see in races so exposed a progressive increase in the incidence of cancer. By contrast, in those primitive communities where such agents are not used or encouraged the incidence will remain at a very low level. A. Berglas regards the notion that we could control these environmental agents as utopian, and, therefore demands an all-out attack on finding a cure for cancer—a truly defeatist attitude.

The Cure Of Cancer

Like Berglas, the majority of people interested in cancer during the past 200 years have searched and searched for the cure which they unwisely think would be the greatest blessing to mankind. It is altogether humane and desirable that we should attempt to develop means of curing cancer victims, but it must be realized—and this point cannot be stressed too much—that no effective cure can ever reduce the high incidence of this disease in the civilized races. It is far more important that the main attack on the cancer problem should be focused on the preventive aspect.

The real attack on the treatment of malignant growths must come from intelligent interference with the catalase-peroxide mechanism. As the enzyme is progressively depleted in the tumors and in the cancer patient as a whole, it is highly probable that any physical or chemical method of either depressing the catalase content further, or increasing the concentration of peroxides will have a detrimental effect upon the tumor. This is the probable explanation of the action of ionizing radiations, and may also explain the temporary regression which follows the removal or destruction of certain endocrine glands. Almost thirty years ago, Maisin succeeded in controlling certain animal tumors with dihydoxymethyl peroxide. Motawei, in Cairo, reported significant results in animals and humans with hydrogen peroxide alone or combined with X-rays. Certain American workers, who have been recently working on the same lines with H_2O_2, have caused rapid destruction of tumors in man in periods as short as seven days.

To develop a far more effective cure it is essential that the catalase-peroxide mechanism be exploited in order to determine the most efficient way of over-oxidizing the catalase-deficient cells. A perfect method of doing this is going to be very difficult to produce because, in certain sites, e.g. the liver, where the catalase concentration of the normal cells is high, it will be extremely unlikely that the cancer cells growing there can always be affected when so well buffered by the surrounding catalase.

The Prevention Of Cancer

Louis Pasteur emphasized that it is far more important to prevent a disease than to treat it. It is eminently obvious to all that the majority of those diseased processes which have been almost abolished from the civilized races, e.g. plague, typhoid, cholera, have been controlled by preventive means and not by cure. The direct treatment of such diseases by chemotherapeutic and antibiotic agents has not been, and never will be, responsible for their elimination. So it is with cancer. We have a terrible disease which is one of our worst killers; and to stop this we must prevent the tumors from starting. It is the only sure way.

During the past thirty years, famous men like the Nobel Prize winners Alexis Carrel and Szent Gyorgyi, and others have emphasized that until we intelligently reform some of our habits of civilization there will be no measurable reduction in the incidence of this disease. How is this to be done? Many cancer research workers believe that this is just a question of screening thousands of chemicals for their ability to produce tumors, and then attempting to eliminate the positive ones from our environment. This method of attack becomes valueless when we realize that relatively common everyday substances such as salt and sugar are proven tumor-producing agents. Furthermore, as J. Holtfreter points out, practically any kind of continuous maltreatment can provide a potential cancer-inducing stimulus.

It is no use requesting the public to cease smoking tobacco or to cease ingesting food containing carcinogenic dyes in order to significantly reduce the incidence of lung and stomach cancer respectively, when at the same time large numbers of other noxious agents are being deliberately placed on, around, and in us, and no one takes heed of their long-term effects. As Berglas points out, modern civilization has become toxic in every sense of the word.

Threefold Plan

Since many physical and chemical agents can alter the catalase-peroxide balance, and some of these are cumulative, then the prevention of cancer, which must be our ultimate goal, can be realized if we see to it that our cells have a high concentration of catalase, and that this is not depleted over the years by exogenous and endogenous factors.

The plan for the prevention of cancer should be threefold:

(1) *To increase our intake of catalase.*

Man, having discovered fire, has, over the centuries, progressively utilized heat for the preparation of his food. Catalase, as well as many other enzymes, are destroyed by heat. Civilized man now lives primarily out of the can, the bottle and the package. Most of the foodstuffs in these are practically sterile. The fear of the microbes has gone too far, and it is now high time that, while being on our guard for certain pathogens, we should view the majority of organisms in a different light. The agents used to destroy the bacteria invariably destroy the catalase in the food. Cancer of the stomach is one of our common tumors; and yet we continue to ingest very hot materials coupled with catalase-deficient food and catalase-destroying chemicals. No other species of animal has such a diet. It would be to everyone's advantage if the consumption of fresh fruit and vegetables were to be markedly increased, thus ensuring a far greater intake of catalase and peroxidase. There are numerous references in the literature to the fact that garlic-eating people have an increased resistance to cancer. This is not surprising when one realizes that garlic is very rich in the catalytic systems containing catalase and peroxidase.

(2) *To increase the manufacture of catalase by our own cells.*

It was shown many years ago that if a normally active creature is forcibly imprisoned in a cage so as to limit its normal muscular activity, after some weeks the catalase content of the body decreases. Conversely, normally inactive creatures can be made to develop more catalase if forcibly exercised. It is very probable, therefore, that the chronic habit of limiting the muscular activity of man, by encouraging him to imprison himself in cars, trains and other forms of mechanical locomotion, which has developed on a world-wide scale during the past 40-50 years, is doing much to diminish his normal catalase level. Many other habits adopted by civilization decrease the ability of our cells to respond to those normal stimuli which reflexly induce the synthesis of catalase. Puig has already shown that, according to our daily habits the body catalase level varies; and it is, therefore, of the utmost importance that our normal animal physiology must be considered when designing our civilized way of living. In general, a high concentration of catalase implies an increased consumption of oxygen, which provides a catalytic system of prime importance in the detoxification of our bodies.

(3) *To curtail the intake of agents which destroy or inhibit the action of our cell catalase.*

This is probably the most important mode of attack. As others have pointed out, civilization is becoming toxic in every sense of the word; and, as man reproduces his species relatively slowly, it will take many thousands of years for him to adapt—if this is ever possible. It is important, therefore, that we should recognize the pollutants in our environment and set about removing them or controlling their distribution.

The toxic agents can be considered according to the mode of entry into the body. The main pathways are (*a*) Ingestion; (*b*) Inhalation; (*c*) Injection; (*d*) Irradiation.

(*a*) *Ingestion.*

During the past fifty years many diverse alien chemical agents have been added to food and drink in order (i) to kill bacteria resulting in a longer shelf-life; (ii) to color the products, resulting in increased sales; (iii) to act as sweeteners, flavoring agents, antistaling agents, etc.; (iv) to accelerate the growth of chickens, bullocks, fish, etc.; (v) to have some effect on man's own cells, e.g., iodine, fluoride.

Synthetic Poisoning

Hueper observed that trout reared in hatcheries in the United States suffer from an epidemic of liver cancer which in some instances affects practically 100 percent of the trout population over three years of age. The bulk of available evidence incriminates some constituent in the feed as a nutritive factor, or chemical additive or a medicinal agent. As Hueper writes: "The occurrence of this epidemic amongst edible fish subject to an artificial nutritive regimen provides a serious warning of the possible future production of a similar cancer epidemic in the human population through an increasing contamination of the human environment."

Destroyers Of Catalase

It has been estimated that there are more than 1,000 additives to our food and drink. Many of these interfere with the catalase-peroxide balance, e.g., sulphur dioxide, sodium nitrate, sodium fluoride, certain hormones, insecticides, fungicides and dyes. One of the main arguments in favor of adding chemicals is that this prevents much bacterial food-poisoning in the consumers. This attitude is overstressed. It is not only the catalase of the bacteria which is destroyed, but also that of the food. This enzyme is all important in the prevention of cancer. The majority of the chemicals added to food and drink for preservation, coloring or sophistication could and should be abolished. Most of the additives are not essential, and many are harmful. The obvious way to preserve food is to make use of the energy provided by atomic power for deep-freeze transportation and storage. This would ensure a non-toxic food supply with many vital enzyme systems intact, assuming, of course, that the foodstuffs are not covered or impregnated with toxic chemicals as a result of spraying, etc.

Fluoridation

The deliberate addition of that poisonous substance sodium fluoride to public water supplies, with the intent of delaying the onset of dental caries, is a most unscientific and unethical measure. Sodium fluoride is a potent catalase poison and is cumulative. Its use is not backed up by sound medical facts, and in any case it does not deal with the prime cause of dental decay, which is generally recognized as being due to a sophisticated and chemically adulterated food supply.

Insecticide—Homicide

The uses of multitudinous agents, e.g., insecticides, fungicides, weed killers, antibiotics, etc., for the killing of multicellular or unicellular forms of life can and does result in some temporary amelioration of the problem of pest control. But in the long run such methods are doomed to failure for the very simple reason that even the most delicate single cells can, under certain conditions, adapt and produce descendents which will ultimately resist the agent which is trying to kill them. This problem has been known and recognized for many years by bacteriologists, with the result that most of the serious pests which affect man have been controlled by preventive means and not by direct treatment with drugs. The control of the various pests in agricultural practice can be affected by the encouragement of methods which result in the production of animals and plants with much enhanced immunity. This would ensure a food supply free from the toxic residues of the numerous lethal sprays now in common use.

The indiscriminate consumption of catalase-destroying drugs by the civilized races is a matter of serious import. The control of these very important preparations is a matter for the serious consideration of the medical profession.

(b) *Inhalation*.

The majority of the poisonous chemicals which pollute the oxygen so vital for our health have been placed there by man. Vast amounts of sulphur dioxide and sulphuretted hydrogen—two very potent catalase poisons—are released daily into our environment as a result of the burning of fuels of various kinds. Many other toxic chemicals are ejected in the effluents from furnaces, fires, rail, road, air and sea transports, as well as from tobacco smoking.

The indiscriminate use of aerosols containing insecticides, fungicides, antibiotics, etc., on farms, in hospitals and in domestic institutions is a matter of deep concern to us all. The inhalation of small amounts of these agents is not necessarily harmful, but the continual use of such agents over a period of years, particularly if they contain cell poisons, as many of them do, will have an adverse effect upon our cells, particularly those lining the respiratory tract.

It is obvious that the control of air pollution demands our most urgent attention.

Diminished Oxygen

A good oxygen intake is essential for good health. Some workers go so far as to explain the high incidence of cancer in the human race on the basis of poor or diminished oxygen consumption, and in a sense they are right. Oxygen is essential for the removal and destruction of many toxic agents present on or in our cells, and it is, therefore, quite obvious that the more actively oxygenated our bodies the better we shall be able to combat the toxic agents which help to influence adversely our normal cells.

(c) *Injection.*

Modern therapy of disease processes relies to a large extent on the injection of drugs. The sulphomanides, which have been known for a long time to inhibit catalase *in vivo* and some of which are proven carcinogens, have been widely used for almost thirty years. Who can tell what part these have played in increasing the incidence of leukemia in children or cancer in adults?

Many drugs now used can interfere with cell respiration, and there is an urgent need for work to be done in this field before we can assess the long-term risk.

(d) *Irradiation.*

For more than sixty years we have increasingly exposed ourselves to man-made radiation. X-rays and other forms of irradiation are known to inhibit catalase. These rays have helped enormously in elucidating certain aspects of disease; but, like most other key discoveries in nature, these have been widely applied for decades without the mechanism of action being understood. At last we are beginning to realize that we do not know where the threshold lies below which these rays cease to be harmful, with the result that in various civilized countries mass X-ray programs are advisedly being curtailed, and individual dosage limited. The indiscriminate use of such rays should be more effectively controlled. There are many other forms of radiation being placed around and in modern man, but no one is able to predict what the effect of these will have on the incidence of cancer twenty years hence. It is already too late to reverse some of this activity, but the civilized world has been repeatedly warned of the very real and serious dangers of allowing this problem to get out of hand.

Chemical Filth

The once dominant problems of bacterially-contaminated air, water and food have now been replaced in considerable degree by chemical pollution. Chemical filth is the major public health hazard of our time, and it is important that all levels of society should appreciate this fact and see to it that measures are urgently introduced through education, controls, etc., to deal with this rapidly deteriorating situation.

Cancer prevention, the only effective scientific method of controlling the disease, can show results if we pull together and reform some of the bad habits so prevalent in our civilized way of living.

Exercise And Cancer: Another View

One of the best preventive measures against cancer may be exercise. It may sound too simple for such a complex disease, but the work of Drs. R. A. Holman and Warburg certainly suggest that impaired utilization of oxygen by the body's cells may be responsible for the beginnings of many cancerous growths, and the hearty breathing resulting from good exercise is one of the best ways to insure that you are providing your entire body with enough oxygen.

The importance of the oxygenation process and cancer prevention appears to have been borne out in a study conducted in Germany in 1971 when a doctor evaluated the medical histories of runners belonging to a long-distance running club.

German Dr. Ernst van Aaken kept close tabs on a group of 454 members of a club for older long-distance runners. He found that in the six-year period of his study, only four of the runners got cancer, and all recovered and are now running again. He also kept records of a parallel group of 454 normal men who didn't run, and found 29 cases of cancer during the same period. And 17 of the non-runners died of the disease.

The fascinating results of Dr. van Aaken's study were reported in a January 15, 1971, article in the Cologne *Stadt-Anzeiger*. The report emphasized that the low-cancer group formed no human elite, but was simply a bunch of older men who liked to run three to five miles a day. There is plenty of reason to believe that *anybody* in reasonable health can get the same results—if they can motivate themselves to get out and run every day. Other "huff-and-puff" exercises like cycling, climbing, long-distance swimming and cross-country skiing would be just as good.

The reason the runners didn't get cancer is that they were constantly providing their bodies with more oxygen than they needed, says Dr. van Aaken.

53. Artificial Lighting Could Be A Factor In Cancer

Dr. John Ott speculates that cancer may be causally related to our artificial lighting environment—our closed-in way of living behind walls and window panes and under man-made light—and he suggests that outdoor light therapy (or its equivalent) might be a way to prevent or even treat cancer.

Dr. Ott's theories are as unconventional as they are controversial, but his warnings that cancer may be influenced by "malillumination" or "polluted light"—that is, a lighting environment markedly different from the natural outdoor spectrum under which all life on earth evolved—appear credible enough to some of the most august bodies of medical learning, such as the prestigious Wills Eye Hospital in Philadelphia, to grant him a forum for his theories.

John Ott is founder and head of the Environmental Health and Light Research Institute, Sarasota, Fla. He is not an M.D.; his doctorate is an honorary one from Loyola College in Chicago. But he is a self-educated investigator "uncluttered by scientific training," (as he was introduced when he lectured at Philadelphia's famous Wills Eye Hospital) whose inquiring mind and experimental work have contributed notably to the growing body of literature on light's influence on biological activity.

No one else, it is safe to say, is as committed a crusader against light pollution as John Ott. No one else is so keen an advocate of putting our knowledge of light to work in the study and practice of medicine. But it should be stressed that his basic theory—that light received through the eye influences bodily functions—is a scientific fact accepted by researchers in the field at university centers throughout the world.

With the aid of Dr. Ott's Institute, researchers have learned that when normal natural light is distorted, animals respond abnormally and pathologically. His experiments on the effect of lighting on mouse tumor development have been tested in various versions at Wills Eye Hospital and the opthalmology department of Temple Medical School, Philadelphia, Pa. The results of Dr. Ott's experiments were as follows: In mice inbred for cancer, those in daylight cages develop malignant tumors on an average of two months later than mice kept under white artificial light and three months later than those under pink lights (*Annals of the New York Academy of Sciences*, Vol. 117, pp. 624-635, Sept. 10, 1964).

So far, we've been talking about animal experimentation. But what about people? Would natural light, for example, be beneficial to cancer patients? Have controlled clinical tests been made?

No, not yet, though Dr. Ott in his missionary role is working hard to persuade medical investigators to institute such programs. But, though scientific experimentation is missing, Dr. Ott does have suggestive evidence that human cancer can be beneficially influenced by exposure to natural light.

During the summer months some years ago, fifteen terminal cancer patients attending the outpatient department at New York's Bellevue Medical Center agreed to follow Dr. Ott's suggestions for prolonged hours outdoors minus eyeglasses. At the end of that summer, the hospital staff reported to Dr. Ott that, while it was difficult to make an evaluation, fourteen of the fifteen patients showed no further advancement in tumor development and several showed possible improvement. Most significantly, Dr. Ott later discovered that the one patient whose condition deteriorated had misunderstood the instructions; while she stopped wearing sunglasses, her regular glasses always covered her eyes.

Ott's Own Recommendations

Dr. Ott proposes a method, which he follows himself, to counter light pollution: 1) stay outdoors as many hours a day as you can (without your glasses), since completely unhindered natural light is the best preventive; 2) substitute ultraviolet-transmitting plastic for glass (which screens out ultraviolet) in your windows and in your eyeglasses; 3) for indoor lighting, use a new type of full spectrum fluorescent bulb specially designed to mimic natural light both in invisible ultraviolet emission and in the distribution of color bands of the visible spectrum.

If you want to go all the way with Dr. Ott, you'll consider ultraviolet transmitting plastic for your windows. Hardware stores sell this type of plastic that looks like glass. However, you will have to check carefully that it has not been treated to do precisely what you don't want—i.e. to screen out these invisible rays that are of such importance to health.

Ultraviolet rays have gotten a "bad name," as Dr. Ott says, because in large overdoses they cause cell damage, and they have been linked to skin cancer in people overexposed to direct sunshine over long periods of time. But the ultraviolet band, Dr. Ott stresses, is similar in nature to the visible rays. In fact, ultraviolet *is* visible to some species, for example bees; thus it is just as similar to light (as opposed to mysterious "rays") as tonal pitches we cannot hear (but dogs can) are similar to sound.

Striking the skin, ultraviolet light is essential for the synthesis of vitamin D, as we have known for a long time. Now we know, from experiments by Dr. Ott and others, that it is also essential for other physiological functions which it stimulates when it strikes the eye's retina.

Man needs full spectrum natural light, Dr. Ott says, just as he needs full nourishment. He can no more safely skip particular ingredients of natural light than he can go without essential vitamins. Nor is it necessary, to receive the benefits of ultraviolet light, to bake in direct sunlight and risk devastating effects on your skin.

Far safer, and all that one requires, is to spend several hours a day outdoors in the shade, leaving the eyes unshielded and exposed to natural daylight. It is a gentle, natural way to avoid the possible ill effects of *malillumination,* a general condition today that may be found to be as devastating to health as *malnutrition.*

54. Asbestos And Talc— Surprising Carcinogens

The air of city streets is loaded with asbestos. The average vehicle wears out three or four sets of asbestos brake linings and one or two asbestos clutch facings in its lifetime. This is probably a major cause of asbestos dust in our environment. In addition to brake linings and clutch facings, there are floor tiles, building materials which include shingles for roofing and sidings, sheets for exterior and interior walls, insulation board, clapboard, casings for electric motors, pipes to carry water, sewage and gas. Asbestos textiles are used in fireproofing theater curtains, in conveyor-belting and safety clothing, in potholders, ironing-board covers, draperies, rugs, motion picture screens, as filters in gas masks, in the processing of fruit juice, acids, beer and medicines, in mail bags, airplane fittings, stove and lamp wicks, sparkplugs and fire hoses. Virtually thousands of products are made with asbestos. Are you using a torn ironing-board cover, or a torn potholder, unsuspectingly being exposed to dangerous asbestos particles you may be inhaling?

By virtue of being almost immune to the force of corrosion and decay under almost every condition of temperature and moisture, asbestos particles are resistant to the action of most acids, alkalies and other chemicals, and are practically indestructible.

Back in the first century, the adverse biological effects of asbestos were observed by the Greek geographer and historian, Strabo, and by the Roman naturalist, Pliny the Elder. Both of these men mentioned the "sickness of the lungs" in slaves whose occupation was to weave asbestos into cloth. Early history records these two great men calling attention to the disease that would one day be known as asbestosis, a form of pneumoconiosis (the term for all dust diseases of the lungs caused by inhalation of fine fibers and particles of minerals).

Asbestos, once inhaled, continues to react within the lungs for a lifetime. Many doctors believe that there is a definite relationship between asbestos exposure and lung cancer.

There are case histories of children who lived and played near asbestos mines, who died of cancer due to asbestosis. In South Africa, small barefooted Bantu children were forced to trample down fluffy amosite asbestos as it came cascading over their heads into bags. These children developed asbestosis with corpulmonale (right sided heart failure) before the age of twelve. None of them lived long enough to develop either lung cancer or mesothelioma.

Cigarette Effect Is Reinforced

Dr. Irving J. Selikoff and others, surveying people with bronchogenic carcinoma, stated that people who smoke cigarettes are 90 times more likely to die of lung cancer than men who neither work with asbestos nor smoke, and that a definite co-carcinogenic effect exists between asbestos exposure and cigarette smoking.

Asbestos fibers, which are highly absorbent as well as virtually indestructible, may retain the substance known as benzopyrene from cigarette smoke for long periods of time in lung tissue, thus tending to produce lung cancer by combining the worst effects of both. One out of every five asbestos insulation workers who die in the New York-New Jersey area, dies of lung cancer.

The asbestos insulation workers are not the only group that risks lung cancer. They share their exposure with more than three and one half million other construction workers, steam fitters, electricians, welders, carpenters, ironworkers, plumbers, masons and tile setters who are inhaling the same dusts.

All over every city, millions of sub-microscopic and highly respirable particles are sprayed on buildings every time they are made fireproof. That snowy white material you see fluttering down to earth when they are building the skyscraper, is a combination of amorphous glass fibers (rock wool) and amosite asbestos. Whenever you see belts of yellow canvas girdling a skyscraper under construction, it means that asbestos is being sprayed somewhere inside, and the contractors are making an effort to prevent billions of asbestos fibers from being blown all over the city.

Talc Related To Asbestos

In the March, 1971 *Journal of Obstetrics and Gynecology* (British) there is a paper on "Talc and Carcinoma of the Ovary and the Cervix" prepared by Dr. Keith Griffiths, Director of

Cancer Research in Cardiff, Wales. "Researchers found particles of talc in approximately 75 percent of the ovarian tumors and 50 percent of the cervical tumors examined. The implications were obvious. Talc, the principal 'active ingredient' in talcum and baby powders and in a wide variety of other cosmetic preparations, including some of the so-called feminine hygiene sprays, may cause cancer." Most talcs contain some asbestos contaminant, so the real villain may prove to be the asbestos in talcum powder.

Talc, both chemically and geologically, is closely related to three of the five types of asbestos. The two families of minerals are so intimately linked in nature that it is difficult, if not impossible, to separate them. A well known brand of talcum powder was quietly removed from the market in England when it was discovered to be laced with asbestos.

It is known that older talc workers die of lung cancer at a rate four times higher than would be expected. Talc workers are also subject to talcosis, a disease which scars the lungs.

Doctors Abandon Talc—Quietly

It was common practice for some doctors to use talcum powder to preserve rubber gloves they wear during surgery and pelvic examinations. For the same reason some women dust their birth control diaphragms with talcum. Most doctors stopped using talc because they found they were developing granulomas, a type of skin lesion on their fingers. In its place they substituted cornstarch, a substance cheaper and by no means considered a carcinogen. However, the use of talc on diaphragms continues, in spite of the talc particles found inside cancerous tumors of the ovary and cervix.

Dr. Pierre Biscaye (Mineralogist at the Lamont-Doherty Geological Observatory of Columbia University) decided to find out what the label wasn't telling. He analyzed one of the feminine-hygiene deodorants by X-ray diffraction, and found it was composed almost entirely of talc. The X-ray diffractogram also revealed minor amounts of some other substance which he was not able to identify. Dr. Biscaye stated that, "In this type of analysis, minerals such as asbestos could be present up to several percent and not be detected."

Dr. Langer, a mineralogist with New York Mount Sinai Hospital, believes that the real villain in this controversy may prove to be asbestos in talcum powder and not the talc. His staff has prepared a report on the confirmation study it did on one of the ovarian cancer slides used by Dr. Griffiths as the basis for the paper on talc and carcinoma. Mount Sinai found the talc, but also found something the British missed. It is difficult to imagine how asbestos fibers could find their way into the female reproductive system, if they weren't introduced there along with talcum powder . . . unless, he stated: "One could speculate they arrived via the bloodstream, after having been absorbed through the walls of the digestive tract."

H. Cunningham and R. Pontrefact (*Nature* Magazine, July 30, 1971), reported finding asbestos fibers in the tap water of Toronto, Montreal and Ottawa. Ranging from 2.0 to 4.4 million fibers per liter in filtered water systems; unfiltered water from a lake in the asbestos mining region of Quebec showed an asbestos content of 172.7 million fibers per liter. Water from Ottawa River showed 9.5 million fibers per liter. Even melted snow which feeds lakes, rivers and streams was discovered to have 33.5 million asbestos fibers per liter. Asbestos fibers have been found in U.S. and Canadian beers (some breweries use asbestos filtering pads), in soft drinks, sherry, port and vermouth. The magnitude of the problem begins to be apparent.

The asbestos industry maintains that the case against asbestos or talc in our food and drinking water has not been proven. But as far as the tobacco industry is concerned, the case against cigarette smoking has never been proven either. There is an important difference between these two health problems. Smoking is a voluntary act. If you want to live longer you will stop smoking, but people who do not want asbestos in the air they breathe and the water they drink have no choice.

Asbestos In Children's Cosmetics

According to Dr. Langer: "Big companies like Johnson & Johnson are not as likely to have an asbestos problem since they have the resources to select only high-grade talc and free it of any remaining impurities, but there are many types of talc used by the cosmetic industry in this country and abroad. There are French talcs, Italian talcs and talcs that are not really talc at all, such as tremolite asbestos. Cheap cosmetic products of all kinds, including children's play-lipstick, powder and rouge have been found to contain asbestos. There is some evidence that the fibrous varieties of talc may be more hazardous than others. Unfortunately these talcs are favored by manufacturers of certain lines of cosmetics because they adhere to the skin more readily . . . ."

Clark Whelton (*The Village Voice*) writes: ". . . garment workers in New York manufactured 100,000 coats from Italian cloth, that was, unknown to them, eight percent asbestos. How much fiber was released into the air by the cutting and stitching of that cloth is not known . . . neither is the effect these coats will have on the people who bought them."

There are many hidden hazards revealed daily: hidden dangers in foods; in highly toxic pesticides and fungicides; carcinogenic drugs in animal feeds; dangerous chemical preservatives, sweeteners, flavorings, coal tar colors, etc., etc. The public relies on U.S. regulatory agencies for *responsible* protection and assurance. *How much real protection do these agencies give us?*

55. Can Your Emotions Lead You Into Cancer?

"Let me speak to you regarding the things of which you must most beware. To get angry and shout at times pleases me, for this will keep up your natural heat; but what displeases me is your being grieved and taking all matters to heart. For it is this, as the whole of physic teaches, which destroys our body more than any other cause."

The physician who wrote this to his patient was Maestro Loranze Sassoli, and he inscribed this letter in the year 1402. He was revealing a common medical notion of the times that cancer, specifically, was related to one's temperament. Galen, the father of modern medicine, who lived in the second century A.D., believed that melancholic women were more prone to cancer than those whom we today would call happy-go-lucky.

By the eighteenth century, European physicians were noting in their medical articles that a severe emotional shock (usually the death of a loved one) contributed to a large extent to the onset and development of cancer. Physicians of that time had available none of the tests which modern researchers use to discover facts about personality and personality difficulties. So they could do nothing but record their observations about personality and cancer. Here are some of the notes they made:

1822—Nunn described a woman who died of breast cancer shortly after the death of her husband.

1846—Walshe wrote in part as follows: "Much has been written on the influence of mental misery and habitual gloominess of temper on the deposition of carcinomatous (cancerous) matter. If systematic writers can be credited, these constitute the most powerful cause of the disease; and Lobstein, assuming the fact as established, exercised his ingenuity in tracing the connexion of cause and effect: moral emotions produce defective innervation, this perversion of nutrition which in turn caused the formation of carcinoma (cancer) . . . I have myself met with cases in which this connexion appeared so clear that I decided questioning its reality would have seemed a struggle against reason."

On the basis of this conviction Walshe advised patients with a family background of cancer to select their professions with great care. Avoid those which entail constant care and anxiety, he cautioned. Clearly, he believed that an inherited tendency to cancer plus a long-term period of psychological stress might result in cancer.

1885—Willard Parker, an American, studied 97 cases of breast cancer and reported that grief is undoubtedly associated with the disease. Cancer patients are not people who have been noted for cheerfulness before the disease struck them. Another physician, Cutter, remarked that mental depression is too common an element in cancer to be overlooked. He believed, furthermore, that the disease could be cured by diet combined with stimulating the patient's will to live.

An English physician reported, "Great mental stress has been assigned as influential in hastening the development of cancer." Another said that cancer of the breast and uterus follow immediately upon depressing emotion too often to be mere chance.

By 1921 Willy Meyer, who introduced radium therapy for cancer into America, had stated his belief that cancer is often the result of social and emotional stress because of changes in the body produced by such stress—in other words, changes in the actual chemistry of the body necessitated by its reaction to severe stress.

Distinct Personality Types Related To Cancer

Frederick L. Hoffman, LL.D., wrote in 1915, "From dietary disorders to nervous disorders is but a step. The two are frequently interrelated and cause and effect are often hopelessly confused . . . This naturally brings me to the question of the interrelationship of cancer and worry, or the mental attitude of the patient toward the development, spread and curability of the disease." Another researcher, Foque, in 1931 spoke of the "role of sad emotions as activating and secondary causes in the activation of human cancers." His theory, important and well-conceived, was that the stress or emotion affects the nervous system which in turn affects the body's metabolism which acts on the glands in such a way as to make individual cells susceptible to the effects of a cancer-causing substance. He spoke of his patients thus, "... you can see in the patients prolonged and silent sorrow without the release of sobs and tears."

In this book *Happy People Rarely Get Cancer*, J. I. Rodale summed up observations he had made over the years which led him to conclude that certain people are more prone to develop cancer than others because of their predisposition to depression, melancholy and general despondency. He deduced that cancer occurs in definable and distinct types of personality and in response to specific psychological problems.

Mr. Rodale compared the recorded studies on the Hunzas and the Nagyri people, who are both neighbors and relatives to each other. There is a great deal that is strikingly similar about their diet and environment, yet the physiques of the Nagyri, he reports, are vastly inferior to those of the Hunzas, and the Nagyri are more prone to disease. After mentioning several medical studies, including his own personal study of the Hunzas, he suggests that the difference in their health patterns is simply due to the fact that the Hunzas are happier people.

The medical profession is beginning to recognize the relationship between cancer and personality. They call it the "cancer syndrome." According to Dr. Philip Rubin in an article entitled "The Cancer Syndrome" (*Journal of the American Medical Association*, Sept. 16, 1974), "... seemingly remote pathophysiological occurrences may offer a clue about the pathogenesis of the neoplastic state. The increasing awareness of syndromes in cancer has allowed for new diagnostic and investigative pathways. The debilitation of a cancer patient may not be related to the invasion of normal and vital organs by the neoplasm, but to the tumor's capability to create or be causally related to certain distant functional aberrations."

Medical authorities are now beginning to suspect that latent cancers may cause some change in the person's psychological makeup. Distress, anxiety and despondency can be looked upon as suggestive of an incipient case of cancer. Or could it be, as J. I. Rodale reported, that the constellations of fears and anxieties that cause depression may in and of itself cause cancer?

Mr. Rodale reported on studies showing that some forms of cancer, such as Hodgkin's Disease (a disease of the lymph glands, including the spleen), tend to occur in people who have a unique personality pattern. He cited the work of Dr. Lawrence LeShan, of the Institute of Applied Biology in New York, a pioneer and authority in the investigation of the possible relationship between the personality and development of cancer. Using a control group of patients admitted to the Institute, Dr. LeShan noted, "This investigation into the life history pattern of patients with Hodgkin's Disease revealed a sequence of events which appears more consistently in these patients than in our control groups. This sequence appears to antedate the first noticed symptoms of the disease by many years, and may have important implications for the pathogenesis and etiology of this process."

Dr. LeShan found that all the patients had childhoods in which unhappiness, alienation, repression and a general feeling of unworthiness were the dominating moods, but he found that later in life all the patients seemed to have gravitated towards an outgoing mode of living, rejoicing in the aspects of acceptance and devoting themselves entirely to the welfare of a social group.

In *A Psychological Study of Cancer* (Dodd, Mead and Company), Dr. Elida Evans, an analyst, compiled her studies, done over a 15 year period, which identify a certain type of personality that seems more prone to develop cancer than others. "I began to find a similarity in their psychological histories until the cancer patients took the form of a distinct type." Dr. Evans stressed the need for people to be happy in their work and other life pursuits.

The role that emotions play in the development of physical ailments has been recognized by even the most orthodox members of the medical establishment under the name of psychosomatic illness. However, the role that emotions may play as a causal effect in the development of cancer is just beginning to awaken concern in some medical authorities. J. I. Rodale's uncanny blending of intuition and research more than a generation ago paved the way for contemporary investigation of this relationship. He wrote: "In considering the relationship between cancer and the emotions, it is certainly appropriate to ask whether it is possible to influence the kind of patterns into which our personalities fall. We have already seen that the characteristics of the cancer-prone personality, such as alienation, hostility, hopelessness, and lack of focus or objective, are psychiatric classifications that a strictly medical man might well translate into the single word—depression. And considering the problem as simply one of depression might be a very helpful thing to do."

56. The Unsuspected Threat Of Fluoride Pollution

Researchers looking at the total fluoride picture now recognize that, aside from food and water, the very air we breathe may be loaded with fluoride compounds that are quickly absorbed by plants and animals (including man). Fluoride is a trace mineral with a relatively narrow margin of safety. Our bodies can only tolerate so much before there are serious toxic effects. And one of these toxic effects may be cancer.

In a Japanese study by two faculty members of the Agricultural School of Meijo University, the effects of the heavy use of fluoride-containing phosphate fertilizer on the fluoride content of "favorite foods" was measured. Total fluorine ingestion (consisting of a large number of specific flouride compounds) from the same diet tripled over a seven-year period from 1958 to 1965. And a strong geographic correlation was found between "a very high fluorine content of common foods and increase in the incidence of gastric cancer" (*Japanese Journal of Public Health,* Vol. 4, 1969).

Experiments have also shown that fluoride compounds injected into chicken eggs caused malformations in the embryo. Hydrogen fluoride air pollution caused mutations in fruit flies. The addition of sodium fluoride to the diet of fruit flies caused a high frequency of melanomas (tumors).

When we understand that the genetic material of life (DNA) occurs in all living things, apparently operating precisely the same in all species, we can more easily understand why scientists are concerned when they find that an environmental pollutant changes the DNA of a fruit fly, a chick embryo, or a tomato plant. For we know that the resulting deformed insect, chick, or plant is not just a scientific curiosity, but may have serious implications for us and our children.

Joshua Lederberg, Nobel Prize winner and professor of genetics at Stanford University, has written that studies on the immunobiological system "indicates it (DNA) may play a part in protecting the body against cancer as well as infectious diseases, and that a weakening of this system might allow a potential cancer to grow."

The implications of a possible mutagenic (and carcinogenic) capability of fluoride compounds in human populations make discussions of toxicity and tolerances dwindle almost to the level of nitpicking by comparison. Nevertheless, while the scientists are investigating, the least that can be done is to try to reduce human fluoride exposure to the lowest possible minimum.

While more comprehensive research is needed into the toxic effects of fluoride on man and environment, it is already apparent that fluoride pollution is becoming a critical problem in this country. One measure which may help to resist fluoride-induced injury is to make sure you get enough calcium, magnesium, vitamin C and protein in your diet. Research shows that an individual's nutritional status can help him withstand the toxic effects of fluoride.

57. Bladder Cancer Rise Traced To Popular Eating Habits

Between 1971 and 1974, the estimated yearly number of newly detected cases of bladder cancer more than doubled, while the number of estimated deaths per year increased by approximately 74 percent, according to American Cancer Society figures.

But does this dramatic increase come as such a surprise considering the trend in American dietary habits towards more processed and chemicalized foods? After all, it's the bladder that eventually becomes the last repository for most of the body's fluid wastes before excretion via the urethra. And these fluid wastes contain many of the known and suspected carcinogens that were part of the commercial foods and beverages we ingested.

Few of us think of the bladder as a vital body organ. All the bladder appears to do is provide a convenient collection point for the urine excreted by the kidneys. But the importance of that function must not be underestimated.

The bladder is a muscular reservoir lined with a mucous cell coating. When not overdistended, the bladder's capacity is one pint. The number of times a human urinates is an individual matter and depends on such variables as solid or liquid intake, physical well being, climate, etc. But the bladder, by its very nature as a transient pool for the body's liquid and minute undiluted waste by-products, makes a likely environment for carcinogens to take a parting shot at its delicate lining before excretion.

For about 43,000 people in 1974, recognition of the bladder's susceptibility to cancer came too late. In May of 1972, the Labor Department's Occupational Safety and Health Administration (OSHA) said it had proof directly linking benzidine and its salt (chemicals used in the manufacture of aniline dyes) with cases of human bladder cancer. According to OSHA reports, benzidine tumors do not appear until at least ten years after exposure to the chemical. The agency reports that any exposure at all to benzidine presents a "grave danger" to workers. Along with benzidine, OSHA indicted and subsequently banned thirteen other industrial chemicals linked to human cancer. Among these were BCME, used widely in the permanent press industry, and MOCA, widely used in the manufacture of natural and synthetic rubber products.

All of the chemicals banned had been known to cause cancerous tumors in test animals, but it was not until they were directly linked to human cancer cases that government officials deigned to consider them hazardous to the public. In fact, it was this information that led to giving bladder cancer a category listing all its own in statistical surveys. Before that, bladder cancer figures were simply combined with kidney cancer statistics.

The Saccharin Controversy

Urine is comprised of approximately 96 percent water, with the remainder made up of minute metabolic wastes such as urea, uric acids, creatinine and ammonia salts. Along with these waste products of the body's protein metabolism are such water soluble substances absorbed by the body but not utilized, such as saccharin.

Cyclamate, an artificial sweetener like saccharin, was banned from use and sale by the Food and Drug Administration after it was found to induce cancerous tumors in the bladders of rats and mice. Yet saccharin, which can produce the same results in test animals, is still very much on the market.

In 1972 the Food and Drug Administration officially proclaimed that saccharin was not 100 percent safe. Dr. George T. Bryan, the University of Wisconsin researcher whose tests had led to the ban on cyclamates, performed tests on mice with saccharin implants showing cancer rates of 47 and 52 percent on the test animals. Largely as a result of the latter tests, the FDA proposed removing saccharin from the Generally Recognized as Safe (GRAS) list. Yet, unlike cyclamates, it was not removed from the market; FDA officials were merely content to order that foods and beverages containing saccharin bear complete label descriptions. And the public was warned not to take more than a gram a day of the substance.

Attempts to ban the use of saccharin go back to the beginning of the century. Harvey W. Wiley, the author of the nation's first Pure Food and Drug Act of 1906, tried desperately to have it banned. But his arguments were shattered when President Theodore Roosevelt, a diabetic who used saccharin liberally, bellowed, "Anyone who says saccharin is injurious to health is an idiot!" Teddy Roosevelt's reasoning must still live on in the halls of the FDA because, despite Bryan's tests, no real restriction on its use as an additive has been effected, nor even proposed.

Dr. Bryan feels that the tests he performed indicated that saccharin is every bit as dangerous as cyclamates. He said he had removed all saccharin products from his household and advised others to do likewise.

Vitamin C And Bladder Cancer

The incidence of bladder cancer in smokers is approximately twice that found in nonsmokers (J. M. Price, *Benign and Malignant Tumours of the Urinary Bladder,* New York, 1971). L. Holsti and P.Ermala both reported in *Cancer* (October, 1965) that when they applied tobacco tar to the mouths of mice, instead of developing buccal (cheek) or lung cancer, 75 percent of the animals developed tumors of the bladder. Whatever chemical inherent in cigarette smoking that causes these tumors also lowers the levels of vitamin C.

Dr. Gordon U. Schlegel, head of the Department of Urology at the Tulane University School of Medicine, New Orleans, La., suggests large amounts of vitamin C as a protective against cancer of the bladder. In May of 1968, Schlegel told the American Association of Genito-Urinary Surgeons that vitamin C appears to destroy certain cancer producing substances commonly known to chemistry as "aromatic amines," produced by smoking. In a test, the amount of the suspected carcinogen was greater in the urine samples of cigarette smokers than in samples of nonsmokers. When those tested were given large amounts of ascorbic acid for a number of days, their urine was free of the substance. Theoretically, the vitamin C prevented the accumulation of the cancer-producing material in the bladder fluid of the smokers.

But "if you have had bladder cancer, take lots of vitamin C and chances are the trouble will never come back," advises Schlegel. By "lots of vitamin C," Schlegel means 20 times the 75 mg. recommended for the maintenance of good health by the National Research Council's Food and Nutrition Board.

The aim, according to Dr. Schlegel, is to exceed the body's requirements so that the excess of ascorbic acid will spill over into the urine. Dr. Schlegel has studied the effect of massive doses of vitamin C for five years and he, along with Tulane biologist George E. Pipkin, has been able to demonstrate that in the presence of ascorbic acid carcinogenic metabolites will not develop in the urine.

Drs. Schlegel and Pipkin told the American Association of the Genito-Urinary Surgeons that they were able to gauge the carcinogenic potential of urine by chemiluminescence, which is the amount of light generated by high energy electronic excitation. They found it was considerably higher in the urine of nine smokers and 18 patients with a history of bladder tumors than in the urine of 17 normal nonsmokers. But after the subjects took ascorbic acid for several days, chemiluminescence decreased significantly in all three groups.

Coffee And Bladder Cancer

In an article in *Lancet* (June 26, 1971), Philip Cole of the Harvard University School of Public Health reported that there appeared to be a relationship between coffee drinking and cancer of the lower urinary tract, more specifically the bladder. Cole based his conclusions on a case-control study involving subjects from the Boston area. The participants in the study were carefully matched for age and sex, with necessary consideration for cigarette smoking and occupation.

From this study, Cole hypothesized that one-quarter of the bladder cancer cases reported among men could be "due to coffee drinking." And the results on women in the test, according to Cole, indicated "that about half of their disease experience might be so caused." From the conclusions he reached, Cole asserted that "the relationship between coffee drinking and bladder cancer warrants investigation."

Cole's theory was followed up by officials at the Roswell Park Memorial Institute (RPMI), Buffalo, New York. The RPMI study, which was supported by a grant from the Public Health Service, supported Cole's findings. However, the RPMI study, which took into account data on patients admitted to the Institute between the years 1957 and 1966, found the relative risk factor of coffee for men but not for women.

The RPMI study, which was reported in the second quarterly issue of *Preventive Medicine* (1973), did not rule out "the possibility of a causal relationship" between coffee and bladder cancer.

Alcohol And Cola

Canadian Drs. Meera Jain and Robert W. Morgan, members of a Toronto medical team, proclaim that they have established the first definite link between the two beverages, alcohol and cola, and bladder cancer (*Medical-World News*, Sept. 13, 1973). In a controlled study of 233 bladder cancer patients against a matched number of cancer free controls, they found alcohol and cola consumption to be strong relative risk factors.

58. How To Protect Yourself Against Bone Cancer

Radioactive Strontium And Bone Cancer

Soviet academician, A. V. Topchiev, declares in his book, *Nuclear Explosions, A World-Wide Hazard,* that we already have dangerous amounts of radioactive strontium in our bones. The "we" means everyone in the world. This has come about only through nuclear bombs let loose in the world and nuclear testing of all kinds. Dr. Topchiev has further declared that within the next decade radiostrontium poisoning will reach such serious levels that sarcoma of the bone and leukemia cases will become epidemic. Within the foreseeable future, he predicts we will have upwards of 200,000 cases of leukemia from worldwide fallout alone.

Strontium 90 is the radioactive form of strontium. Although strontium is found naturally in the earth, strontium 90 is man-made through nuclear fission. It is a chemical cousin of calcium, which makes it a great danger to us all—it acts like calcium, has characteristics similar to calcium—but is a *killer.* Strontium 90 is often absorbed by plants and animals when there is not enough calcium around.

Since all living things need calcium, strontium 90 contamination besets the whole world. It is now found in every corner of the earth, in every continent and is especially prevalent in milk and cereals. With each new nuclear test, the strontium 90 increases everywhere in the world.

Strontium 90 and its lesser radioactive elements like cesium 137 (a chemical cousin of potassium, and also a product of fallout) stay in your body throughout your lifetime, emitting radioactive rays (like X-rays). They produce bone cancer, anemia and leukemia (cancer of the blood).

To quote two noted research scientists of McGill University, Montreal, Canada, Yukio Tanaka and Stanley C. Skoryna, "Ingested radioactive strontium as a bone-seeking element would be absorbed through the intestinal wall and then deposited in the bone. When a sufficient amount of long-life strontium 90, a fall-out product, is accumulated in the bone, bone tumors and other malignant changes occur." That quotation is from the book *Intestinal Absorption of Metal Ions, Trace Elements and Radionuclides* (Pergamon Press, New York, 1970).

Bone cancer appears to selectively strike the young in most cases. There is one good reason why it should, since radiostrontium as an environmental pollutant falls from the air onto vegetable matter and is most fully absorbed by the plants with a naturally high content of calcium. The most receptive of such plants is grass. The grass is eaten by dairy cows and the radiostrontium gets into the milk, and of course children drink much larger quantities of milk than adults.

"Safe" Levels Not So Safe

And how does the radiostrontium get into the air, now that above-ground tests of nuclear bombs have long been discontinued?

It has been shown by Professor Ernest J. Sternglass of the Department of Radiology of the University of Pittsburgh, in his book *Low-Level Radiation* (Ballantine Books, New York, 1972), that particularly the installations that process nuclear fuel for power plants, and the power plants themselves, release radioactive gases into the atmosphere and thus increase fallout around each plant. Furthermore, as each plant gets older, the quantity of radioactive pollutants it releases increases year by year. In calculating the damage, Professor Sternglass focuses on leukemia, another type of radiation-induced cancer that he demonstrates has been increasing in the vicinities of nuclear establishments. Presumably it takes longer for the same radioactive insults to cause bone cancer than it does for them to cause leukemia. Infants and children develop leukemia. Older children and young adults develop bone cancer. Thus, in his studies, Professor Sternglass did not develop any figures for bone cancer which has begun to show an increase only within recent years. But the cases are so similar in nature that Professor Sternglass' indictment obviously holds just as true in terms of bone cancer.

In the town of Aliquippa, Pennsylvania, nine miles away from the Shippingport Nuclear Generating Plant, the mortality rate for infants is more than double that for the rest of the state. There is more than twice as much leukemia as the state average and infant diseases of all kinds amount to 165 percent of the state average.

Leukemia and infant mortality have been declining throughout Pennsylvania—but not in Aliquippa.

The figures were uncovered by Professor Sternglass when he was asked by the owner of the plant, Duquesne Light Co.— perhaps preening itself on the Atomic Energy Commission's evaluation of Shippingport as one of the safest of all nuclear power plants—to make such a survey.

Naturally, when the facts emerged, Duquesne Light attacked them. But the only defense it could muster was a claim that the black population of Aliquippa has increased, weighting the health statistics. A quick check of U.S. Census figures showed that the black population has actually decreased. A further claim that the high rate of sickness and death are due to non-radioactive air pollution was taken seriously by no one, since that type of pollution is the same in Aliquippa as everywhere in western Pennsylvania.

Duquesne Light, in self defense, contracted for another study by National Utilities Service Corp. Analysis of the statistics of the study was assigned to Professor Morris DeGroot, head of the Department of Statistics at Carnegie-Mellon University.

DeGroot's studies confirmed those of Sternglass.

It was shown that in 1970, the year of highest infant mortality in Aliquippa, the level of strontium 90 in milk at the six local dairies also reached an all-time high. It was actually 75 percent higher than the average concentration for the region.

Unwilling to believe their results, the National Utilities Service technicians repeated their measurements three times. After that there was no longer any room for doubt.

Even from what is considered one of the safest of atomic power plants, there is a discharge of radioactive gases. Kept within the limits that the Atomic Energy Commission considers permissible, as the discharges are at Shippingport, the gases do contain radioactive strontium which falls to the ground. Possessing a chemical affinity for calcium, the radioactive strontium gets into the grass and other high-calcium cattle feed. Through the feed it gets into the milk, and from the milk into the children.

It should also be remembered that while small children are the first to show the physiological effects of fallout, and probably accumulate more because they are heavy milk drinkers, the effects are by no means limited to children. Radioactive minerals will be found in all food and adults accumulate them, too. Deposited in the bone, they can cause bone cancer. They can also damage chromosomes and result in defective or dead babies. And there is some reason to believe they can also simply shorten life, by affecting the nucleic acids, without causing any specific disease at all.

Yet not everybody will succumb to what the Atomic Energy Commission likes to call "negligible" amounts of radioactive matter added to the atmosphere. The difference between those who become ill and those who stay healthy, those who die before their time and those who live out their natural lives, may well lie in the difference in their diets. And one of the important dietary differences may lie in our ability to obtain and make use of algin, a compound found in seaweed, in our daily diets.

Intensive studies and laboratory tests at the McGill Gastrointestinal Research Laboratories in Canada found that sodium alignate (the trade name is algin) is the "most effective preventive therapeutic measure against radiostrontium poisoning." Algin can be purchased in convenient quantities in health food stores throughout the country.

Since radiostrontium poisoning is the only known cause of bone cancer (other than metastases from an already existing malignancy), there is reason to believe that thousands of young people every year could be spared the miserable and untimely end that bone cancer brings if their mothers would just include a gram or two of algin in their daily diets.

It is obviously going to take more than algin to protect us from fire and explosion. But so effective is this kelp derived food product, that in the aftermath of such a blow-up when food and air can be expected to be heavily contaminated with radioactive strontium, it is algin that the medical profession would use in such an emergency and which probably will keep many people alive and unpoisoned.

How Algin Works

The original experimental studies conducted at the Gastrointestinal Research Laboratory of McGill University were supported by a grant from the Bureau of Radiological Health of the United States Public Health Service, particularly because it was important to find a protective material that could be used in a radiation crisis. What the Gastrointestinal Research Laboratory sought, naturally enough, was a material that would protect people against contaminated food. So when they reached conclusions about ingested radioactive strontium, they were considering enormous quantities such as we are unlikely to encounter in any situation short of a blow-up of a nuclear power plant. And even against such an exaggerated level of pollution, algin was found protective. Let us return for a moment to the quotation that was originally cited to make it clear that eating radioactive strontium can cause bone cancer.

"Ingested radioactive strontium as a bone-seeking element would be absorbed through the intestinal wall and then deposited in the bone. When a sufficient amount of long-life strontium 90, a fallout product, is accumulated in the bone, bone tumors and other malignant changes occur." The quotation goes on, however, to point out that: "If alginate is given with a diet contaminated with the radioisotope, however, an ion-exchange reaction . . . takes place in the gastrointestinal tract, forming an insoluble strontium alginate gel which is eventually excreted without causing significant pathological or physiological damage to the body.

"This was quickly confirmed by other investigators using different animal species as well as human subjects. Stara recently demonstrated that the skeletal accumulation of radioactive strontium, even in chronically labeled cats, can be reduced by keeping them on an alginate diet. Thus, alginate became the most effective preventive and therapeutic measure against radiostrontium poisoning."

It should be noted in the above that what actually takes place in the gastrointestinal tract is an ion exchange reaction. It is very similar to what happens in the water softener. In the softener, calcium, iron and other minerals are removed from the water by an electrical reaction that exchanges those minerals for sodium. In the gut, using sodium alginate as the exchange medium, the sodium is exchanged for strontium, and the strontium is incorporated into a gel formed by the alginate and the intestinal fluids it absorbs. Once formed, the gel will not dissolve nor can it be absorbed into the system. It is simply excreted, carrying along with it the strontium it has removed from the food.

It should be easy to understand then how it is that algin, simply by binding the radioactive strontium in food, prevents the deadly material from being absorbed and carries it out of the body. But even better, the algin will also remove from the body a large proportion of the radioactive strontium that enters by being breathed into the lungs. This is shown in a 1973 paper entitled *Prevention of Gastrointestinal Absorption of Excessive Trace*

Elements Intake, which was presented at a symposium on trace substances in environmental health held at the University of Missouri. The paper was presented as a joint study from the Division of Environmental Toxicology of the U.S. Environmental Protection Agency and the McGill Gastrointestinal Research Laboratory. In this paper it is pointed out that the intestines are not a one way track, but that in fact there is a constant exchange between the contents of the digestive tract and those of the blood. Also, it is pointed out, from 25 percent to 75 percent of inhaled pollutants are carried up out of the lungs by the activity of the cilia and are actually incorporated into the saliva, to be swallowed into the digestive tract.

Thus, by one route or the other, nearly all of the pollutants entering the lungs are carried to the digestive tract and, even from the bloodstream, sodium alginate will neatly extract radioactive strontium by the ion exchange method, actually purifying the blood as it flows through the digestive tract that contains algin.

This information is very hopeful. An easily obtained material, algin can be added to the diet simply by using it as a thickening agent in cooking, and will actually protect the body against radioactive strontium.

The November 17, 1973 issue of the *Chicago Tribune* reported that at some of the best medical centers specializing in cancer therapy, the five year survival rate for bone cancer has been pushed up to 30 percent. As described by Ronald Kotulak, Science Editor of the *Tribune,* "The new therapy consists of surgery to remove the affected limb if the cancer is localized in one area. Then powerful anti-cancer drugs are administered to the patient in an effort to destroy any cancer cells that may have escaped into the bloodstream."

No complaints. It's better than dying. But as they write about these great new techniques that are going to rescue children from bone cancer with only the loss of a limb and a great deal of sickness, does nobody give a thought to prevention? Algin is not exactly unknown. It is well known to the Environmental Protection Agency. It is well known at McGill University, the most prestigious university in Canada.

Maybe it's just that prevention of disease isn't very dramatic compared to miracles of surgery. Maybe we need more emphasis on the miracle that is embodied in a healthy, vital child.

59. The High Fiber Diet Fights Bowel Cancer

Diet has long been suspected as playing a significant role in the development of cancer in the digestive tract. In parts of Africa, liver cancer is a thousand times more common than in much of the Western world. In Britain, cancer of the large bowel is ten times as common as in rural Africa.

The implications are clear. Differences in the environment, in diet, surroundings, personal habits, must be responsible for much human cancer. The epidemiologists calculate that 80 percent of all human cancer is probably caused by environmental factors and should therefore be preventable in the fairly near future—if we heed the warnings of environmentalists!

Cancer of the large bowel is, after cancer of the lung, the malignancy that claims the most victims in Great Britain; 12 percent of all cancer deaths. In North America its toll is similar. The American Cancer Society predicts that, excluding skin cancer, cancer of the colon and the rectum will account for the greatest number of newly detected cancer cases in 1975.

Dr. Denis Burkitt, a noted British physician who first identified and described a certain malignancy found in African children, now known as *Burkitt's lymphoma,* states that excessive carbohydrates change the content of human wastes in the intestines. Dr. Burkitt says studies show that persons who eat a lot of carbohydrates have an altered bacterial content which encourages the breakdown of natural bowel substances such as bile salts. In this chemical reaction, he contended, cancer-causing agents are produced.

Besides, Dr. Burkitt remarked, since refined carbohydrates contain little roughage, carcinogenic wastes remain in the bowel and colon for a longer-than-normal time, keeping contact with the intestinal linings and further increasing the likelihood that cancer will take hold. In his studies, Dr. Burkitt found that the "transit time" for an American or European is considerably longer than for an African living in a rural village.

Among rural Africans, colon disease is almost unknown, Burkitt discovered. The cause, he says, is the kinds of foods that are eaten. Africans eat large amounts of unrefined cereals, and very little sugar or other processed foods. Westerners, on the other hand, eat a highly refined diet that gives the gut less work to do, so the passage of food is much slower.

From studies he conducted, Dr. Burkitt found that food eaten by the average Englishman takes 77 hours to pass through the gut. Tests on English vegetarians showed that they passed their food in 49 hours. Yet the average "gastrointestinal transit time" for a rural African is a remarkably short 35 hours. And it is interesting to note that one British woman who was moving her bowels every day did not pass a marker pellet until a week after she swallowed it. So even though a person may be "regular" on a daily basis, food passing through the intestines can still be moving very slowly.

There is also a big difference in the weight of stools between Africans and Westerners. The average for Africans, in Dr. Burkitt's tests, was 470 grams. Two groups eating a combined kind of diet had an average of only 200 grams per bowel movement. But the average Englishman, says Dr. Burkitt, gives forth with "a miserable 108 grams" per stool. "The average stool in England is what I would call just a caricature of a stool," he says.

It's also interesting to note that many rural Africans, especially those on a diet of corn meal and beans, produce such a large weight of stool that they move their bowels twice a day. In fact, they become quite concerned if they don't have a second bowel movement each day.

The fact that cancer of the large bowel is common while cancer of the small intestine is very rare indeed supports the idea that transit time and the gut bacteria are important. Food is held up for quite long periods in the large bowel, and it has a large bacterial population, but food passes rapidly through the small intestine and it is almost free of bacteria.

Dr. Burkitt also reports that where there is a high incidence of bowel cancer there is also a comparable incidence of diverticulitis, which, according to Dr. Burkitt, is caused by the same highly refined carbohydrate diet which he believes is the cause of colonic cancer.

In fact, Dr. Burkitt believes diverticulitis may be a forerunner of cancer of the bowel. Diverticulitis is a disease in which tiny herniations develop in the lower intestine causing the formation of small pouches (diverticula) which ring the inside border of the colon. These pouches become filled with waste matter, which often leads to infection and inflammation.

It is Dr. Burkitt's opinion that the waste matter that is collected and trapped in the diverticula may have as equally a carcinogenic effect within the walls of the intestine as those carcinogenic substances which are broken down in the large intestine and passed along ever so slowly. In both instances, Dr. Burkitt sees precautionary dietary measures as preventive against cancer of the bowel and colon.

Some Useful Ideas From Dr. Burkitt

Using Dr. Burkitt's ideas is not really complicated, but it does call for motivating people to change their food habits. It is simply a matter of reordering the priorities in our diet; placing our attention on the positive, on the things that we should eat to get the food moving faster through our intestines, providing insurance against bowel disease.

Dr. Burkitt puts great emphasis on bran, the outer part of the wheat that is removed during milling. In his household an eight gram spoonful of bran is added to each person's food every day. (Bran can be purchased in many health food stores, and perhaps even in special health food departments in supermarkets.) The Burkitts also eat real whole grain bread, the kind that they make themselves from whole wheat flour. It's important to realize that much of the sliced, plastic-wrapped bread that is labelled as whole wheat is in fact not. It has some whole grain flour in it, usually, but is dyed dark with caramel to give it a brown color. That kind of bread will be of little or no use for the purpose we are recommending.

Eating bran regularly may take some getting used to. The taste is not at all offensive, but your innards could well take a few weeks to adjust to the extra work. That is perfectly normal and is to be expected, and will pass in a short time. And while you're starting on the bran regime, start cutting down on your sugar intake, because sugar is one of the refined foods that has a detrimental effect on the gut, in Dr. Burkitt's opinion.

Corn meal is an important food to include in your diet for bowel health. Rural Africans eat a good deal of corn meal mush and other foods made from unrefined corn. That has been pointed out both by Dr. Burkitt and others working on the same problem. The ability of corn to promote larger stools and more rapid transit of food through the gut is not due to bran (which acts by absorbing moisture) but results from the incomplete digestion of the starch of maize in the human gut. Therefore, corn meal is not reduced in size to one of those "caricatures of a stool" that Dr. Burkitt refers to, but retains a good deal of bulk.

One of the most convenient and tastiest ways to eat corn regularly is in the form of home-made corn pones. They taste much better than bread, and their value is their bowel-bulking action. Here is the recipe:

Heat several cups of water to boiling. While it is heating, put three cups of *white* corn meal and a half-teaspoon of salt in a mixing bowl. If you can get raw peanut flour, add about one-half cup of that, and you can also add some sesame seeds and/or caraway seeds.

Slowly pour the boiling water and one-third cup of corn oil into the meal at the same time. Stir thoroughly. Use only enough of the water to make a firm dough, not too wet.

After the mixture cools, form into about 15 cakes with the hands. Let the imprints of your fingers remain to save time. Bake on a greased pan for 35 to 40 minutes in a 375 degree oven. They are done when the edges get well-browned.

There is more to good diet than vitamins, minerals, fats, carbohydrates and other essential nutrients. We know now that we must also eat to provide the proper physical environment in the gut, if we are to avoid many painful and expensive diseases of civilization.

Getting this information into common use, and overcoming the resistance to change that is built into our highly commercialized and profit-motivated society, is going to be a tremendous task, and will only happen if you—the enlightened health-minded person—accept the challenge of becoming a new kind of missionary of health. So practice overcoming the false dictates of "good taste" and start talking to your friends about their bowel habits.

60. Breast Cancer

Most women when they inquire about breast cancer are governed as much by fear as by curiosity. Although the disease rate for cancer of the breast has been climbing at a slow and steady pace over the past 40 years, breast cancer can hardly be called a *common* disease among women.

The publicity surrounding the 1974 operations of Betty Ford and Happy Rockefeller, both occurring within a month's time, created a climate of hypochondria among American women. The only thing common about breast cancer is the massive wave of anxiety that accompanies the very thought of it.

According to the American Cancer Society, the chances *against* the average woman developing breast cancer are 15 to one, with a survival rate for those detecting a malignant lump at an early stage better than 60 percent (two out of three cases are cured, according to the American Cancer Society statistics).

It is not uncommon for a woman to develop a lump or small hardness in the breast; oftentimes it is accompanied by pain or a discharge. These lumps are known by many names, such as papilloma, fibroadenoma and fibroscsystic disease. None of them is cancerous. But the fear that such a lump may be malignant often leads women to delay seeing a doctor.

According to Dr. Henry P. Leis, Jr., a clinical professor and chief of the breast service department at the New York Medical College, literally hundreds of thousands of women each year undergo surgery for the removal of a suspicious lump in the breast, but less than one out of three of these is cancerous.

But for that one, time is all too crucial. Unfortunately, it takes something like the Ford or Rockefeller operations to get women concerned enough to employ the best and most basic means of self-defense—breast self-examination (BSE).

A Gallop Poll in November of 1973 documented the attitudes of American women on breast cancer, including their views on breast self-examination. At the outset of the interviews, "before any mention had been made of breasts and breast cancer," women were asked, "What are the two or three most serious medical problems facing women? Forty-three percent named cancer first, another thirteen percent referred specifically to breast cancer and six percent to uterine or cervical cancer. No other health problem was named first by comparable percentages . . ."

And according to Dr. Irving Crespi, vice-president of the Gallop organization, some other highlights were as follows:

—Breast removal arouses (quite incorrectly!) deep seated fear of being less a woman. "This attitude is most common," read the report, "among single women (61 percent) and those 18 to 34 years of age (66 percent). In terms of personality, the type of woman who is most likely to feel that breast removal impairs her sense of womanhood is relatively likely to be a highly sociable, tense person who tends to seek out new acquaintances and to be somewhat more concerned than the average person about her physical appearance . . ."

—Despite the high degree of concern, few women have their breasts examined on a regular basis by their physicians or engage in monthly self-examinations, though they are aware that early detection improves the chance of a cure. Forty-six percent of all women felt that having monthly breast examinations would make them worry unnecessarily.

—Most women know about self-examination but few have specific knowledge of how to practice it.

—Physicians and mass-media are the prime sources of initial information about breast self-examination, but most doctors do not instruct patients on how to perform breast self-examination.

Crespi found in addition to the exaggerated idea of the prevalence of breast cancer there is a widespread belief that most lumps in the breast are cancerous. Actually, biopsies reveal that between 65 percent and 80 percent of such lumps are not malignant, according to Dr. Arthur Holleb, chief medical officer of the American Cancer Society.

Another major finding of the poll: "A realization of the extent to which early detection increases the survival rates could also reduce the inhibiting effect of worry upon the desire for frequent breast examinations."

Breast Cancer And Men

Breast cancer is not exclusive to women; men also suffer from it. In fact, one out of every 100 cases detected is a male. A common ignorance about male susceptibility to breast cancer accounts for the disease's high fatality rate among men. When men detect a lump or hardness in their breast, they tend to ignore it, completely unaware that it could be breast cancer. The resulting delay in seeing a doctor often results in needless tragedy. All men should check their breasts regularly for any lumps or abnormal hardenings.

Diet And Breast Cancer

Although there is no conclusive evidence to prove that diet is a specific cause of breast cancer, many authorities believe that increasing chances of developing breast cancer go hand in hand with a large intake of the type of saturated fats found in dairy and beef products.

Scandinavian countries, where consumption of fatty foods is the highest in the world, have the highest rates of breast cancer occurrence. Japan, which is well known for its traditional diet low in saturated fats, has one of the lowest incidence rates of breast cancer in the entire world.

In fact, when Japanese women develop breast cancer they have generally better prognoses after treatment than do American women. This finding was based on studies observed by Dr. E. L. Wynder and others when they made a comparison study of breast cancer patients treated at Japan Cancer Institute and Memorial Hospital in New York City.

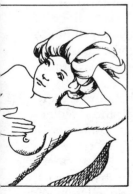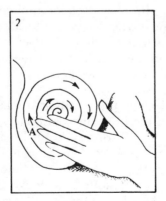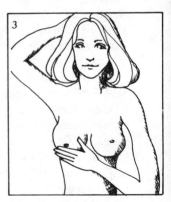

A breast self-check has three steps: 1. Lie down. Place one hand behind the head. With fingers flat, use other hand to gently touch the breast, pressing lightly; 2. Beginning with the area at letter A, follow arrow directions, checking for a lump or thickening. Cover entire breast; 3. After checking both breasts, repeat the same procedure sitting up, one hand behind the head. (This is the procedure recommended by the American Cancer Society.)

A massive study undertaken by the Harvard School of Public Health reported that an increased consumption of saturated fats, along with the concomitant increase in cholesterol, causes increased stimulation of the breast tissue. The report suggested that increased amounts of cholesterol in a diet high in saturated fats can increase the supply of female hormone compounds to above normal levels which may have cancer inducing effects on breast tissue.

The study showed that Japanese women who had immigrated to the United States had increased their risk of developing breast cancer. Although the risk factor does not come anywhere near that of native American women, the risk factor of Japanese women in America does increase with succeeding generations. Experts believe that this is due to the fact that as succeeding generations of Japanese abandon the culture of their homeland they also abandon their low cholesterol diet.

Dr. Philip Cole, who participated in the Harvard Study, noted that daughters of Japanese immigrants residing in Hawaii had hormone levels close to those of the Caucasian residents of Hawaii. Their hormone levels were well above the levels of their contemporaries who were still residents of Japan.

Iodine Deficiency And Breast Cancer

Dr. Bernard A. Eskin, director of endocrinology in the Department of Obstetrics and Gynecology at the Medical College of Pennsylvania, believes that iodine deficiency may contribute to the development of breast cancer. His conclusion is based on extensive tests of laboratory animals and the beginning of clinical studies with humans.

Most convincing of all is the fact that his laboratory experiments, showing the effect of iodine deficiency in the development of tumors and other disorders in rat breasts, concur with known facts about the incidence of human breast cancer in regions of the world that are iodine-deficient. Now, these iodine-poor areas are well plotted in every country—in fact, probably the occurrence of no other single nutrient has been pin-pointed around the globe as comprehensively as this one. This is because lack of iodine causes the extremely visible deficiency disease of goiter. Iodine is needed by the thyroid gland, located in the throat, to manufacture the hormone thyroxin. In the absence of iodine, the thyroid swells to gross proportions (goiter).

Regions of endemic goiter—that is, areas where goiter is prevalent because iodine is lacking in the soil and food—have been identified for many, many years. And now, comparing these regions with areas high in breast cancer deaths, it turns out that the two coincide to a remarkable degree.

Japan and Iceland, for example, have few instances of goiter and few instances of breast cancer. (Japan, where iodine-rich seaweed is a favorite food, has a death rate from breast cancer five times lower than that of the U.S.)

On the other hand, in Mexico and Thailand both goiter and breast cancer are common. Since these are both countries where babies are commonly breast fed, this information tends to contradict the belief that nursing improves resistance to this form of cancer, while it reinforces the idea that iodine in the diet is a determining factor.

Breast cancer death rates are high specifically in endemic goiter areas in Poland, Switzerland, Australia, the Soviet Union, and the United States. In the U.S., the highest death rate from breast cancer anywhere in the country is found in what is known as the "goiter belt" in the Great Lakes region.

"The similarity of high mortality regions to endemic goiter areas is striking," Dr. Eskin told the National Medical Association at its 1971 convention in Philadelphia. A lengthy summary of his work was published earlier in *Transactions of the New York Academy of Sciences* (December, 1970).

Tumor Growth Studied

Dr. Eskin's laboratory studies of the effect of iodine levels on tumor development cover a long series of tests done with thousands of laboratory animals. Perhaps the most striking of these is one in which a cancer-causing agent—DMBA—was injected into 200 rats. Some of the experimental animals had been fed an adequate diet, sufficient in iodine. Others had been made iodine-deficient. While all the animals eventually developed breast tumors from this powerful carcinogen, those that were unprotected by iodine did so measurably sooner. In fact, the process of cancer development was speeded up 25 percent in the animals on the iodine-deficient diet.

The Pill And Breast Cancer

Linked to strokes, diabetes, mental depression, gall-bladder diseases and a wide spectrum of other metabolic and physiologic changes, the oral contraceptive has also been linked to cancer.

Cancer

"Women who use the Pill are sustaining irreversible and permanent breast changes. The cancer risk factor in women taking the Pill is 2.8 times greater the world around, than in women who do not use the Pill," said Dr. Otto Sartorius, director of the Cancer Control Clinic at Santa Barbara General Hospital in California.

Dr. Sartorius noted a correlation between the increasing number of women contracting breast cancer today and the formation of abnormal nodules in the breasts of women who are taking the Pill or who have been on the Pill at one time or another.

After examining 3,000 patients over a period of three years, Dr. Sartorius found that regardless of whether a woman had just started to use the Pill or whether she had been off it for two or three years, her breasts were *harder and more nodular* than those women who had never been on the Pill.

Concerned with these findings, Dr. Sartorius undertook a controlled study of 200 women, only half of whom were on the Pill. With the necessary data collected by his technicians in preliminary studies, Dr. Sartorius examined the breasts of each patient not knowing to which group she belonged. His findings were then compared with the records of his technicians. By palpation (the manual examination of the breasts), Dr. Sartorius achieved 92 percent accuracy in determining which of the women were on the Pill. His results indicate how widespread and profound are changes in the breasts of those using the Pill.

Today's Pill, which comes in sundry dosages and is marketed under approximately 30 brand names, is made of either of two estrogens (female hormones) combined with one of six different progestogens. The progestogens are the sex hormones that can also be used alone as contraceptives.

The sex hormones occur naturally in the body to make fertilization and pregnancy possible, but the Pill upsets this natural balance by increasing the amounts of estrogen in the female body on a frequent and fixed schedule; consequently, the lining of the uterus is changed so that the egg cannot affix itself to the wall of the womb. Scientists admit that they do not know exactly what the Pill does to stop pregnancy.

But the high estrogen level of the Pill is of concern to Dr. Otto Sartorius. "Estrogen is the fodder on which carcinoma grows," he says. "To produce cancer in lower animals, you first introduce an estrogen base."

There is controversy, however, about whether estrogen affects humans in the same way. Physicians who advocate estrogen replacement therapy (estrogen is widely prescribed for women at menopause and in the postmenopausal years), for example, point to the curious fact that women are *most* susceptible to breast cancer at the time when their own bodies are producing the *least* estrogen—that is, breast cancer risk rises with age, and estrogen production declines with age. Time will doubtless solve this medical argument, since so many women serve as "guinea pigs" on the Pill. But, if the estrogen advocates are proven wrong, it will surely be a tragedy of immense proportions.

Canadian physician and researcher Evan Shute, M.D., long known for his pioneering studies with vitamin E, believes estrogen production does not necessarily diminish as the ovaries become inactive. The hormone is produced by other glands, and, in some cases, its production can actually increase with age.

Be that as it may, there is little argument that the condition known as breast dysplasia (abnormal changes in the tissues, nodules, benign tumors, cysts) is stimulated by taking the hormone.

"If I were a girl," Dr. Sartorius said, "I would not be on the Pill. The Pill is producing abnormal changes in the breasts and I know I wouldn't want them in my breasts. What will happen to millions of women with these breast changes? I worry about this."

But what about prevention. Can the woman who has been on the Pill take any measures which might help her to avoid these ominous changes in the breasts?

Supplemental Iodine For Women Taking Estrogen

The protective role of iodine seems to be related in a curious way with the carcinogenic properties of the female sex hormone, estrogen. Dr. Eskin, who was discussed in the previous section, explores this relationship in much of his work.

Through his animal experiments, Dr. Eskin has definitely established that iodine deficiency induces dysplasia. Furthermore, the effect of the deficiency on breast dysplasia is greatly augmented by administering estrogen at the same time. The combination of the two causes far more damage than either one by itself.

Definitely encouraging, on the other hand, is the fact that dysplasia yields to iodine therapy. The condition gradually

297

improves and reverses when the animal is given a high iodine diet.

Iodine is active in the breast tissue itself, as you might surmise. Through quantitative measurement, Dr. Eskin has shown that the amount of iodine in the breast is inversely related to the extent of dysplasia. Rats that measured lowest in breast-iodine content were those that showed dysplasia in the severest form.

In Dr. Eskin's work with humans, the lessons of the laboratory seem to apply. He writes of ten dysplasia cases—five of whom had their first discomfort after starting on estrogen. All ten women were tested objectively for breast lesions with both mammography (X-ray) and thermography (an extremely sensitive measure of heat, an indication of abnormal tissue growth). Thyroid activity was also tested as an indication of iodine status.

After adequate iodine therapy, Dr. Eskin recounts, the objective tests were given again. In all cases the condition had decreased or disappeared. "The treatment," he states, "seemed to be effective and at least temporarily improved the breast condition. There is need for further basic information on these therapeutic regimes and longer periods of follow-up on these patients."

Patient's Deficiency Should Be Checked

In light of his studies, Dr. Eskin is particularly concerned that doctors commonly prescribe estrogen without any investigation of the patient's iodine sufficiency. As he points out, he is suggesting that iodine inadequacy is a cause in progressive breast disease and induced carcinoma. Sex hormones have a profound effect on the mammary gland, he says, and "estrogen is increasingly used for contraception and postmenopausal medical maintenance. Since no evaluation of iodine status is usually made before this therapy is given, sensitive women could be exposed to a greater risk of dysplasia or neoplasm."

He recommends that iodine tests be given by all practitioners before prescribing estrogen. And this is certainly sound advice. Even more to the point, if in spite of all you know about estrogen's bad side effects you still insist it's worth the risk, at least you should protect yourself as much as possible by taking supplemental iodine.

The really exciting thing about Dr. Eskin's discoveries, however, is not just this warning about the Pill and "estrogen maintenance" therapy. Rather, it's the whole preventive opportunity he opens up for all women.

It is not safe to count on unsupplemented diet alone for your iodine requirements. Vegetables will give you this trace mineral only if they happen to have been grown in iodine-rich soil. Water supply is equally chancy. And milk supplies iodine only if the cow has been eating grain that was grown in an iodine-rich area.

Seafood is a particularly good source of iodine—but, of course, many fish and shellfish have been found to be contaminated by industrial pollutants and bacteria of the coastal waters. Commercially iodized salt will supply enough iodine if you shake the salter generously—but salt is harmful to health.

Undoubtedly, the safest and best source for iodine in your diet is the seaweed product, kelp. Unlike fish, seaweed is at the bottom of the food chain and does not accumulate pollutants as do the higher forms of life. You can get kelp in tablets or powder. Many people use it regularly as a salt substitute.

It is known that a deficiency in vitamin B_6 hinders the uptake of iodine by the thyroid gland (*Vitamins in Endocrine Metabolism* by Isobel W. Jennings, published by Charles C. Thomas, 1970). Would such a deficiency also hinder iodine uptake by breast tissue? Nobody knows, but it would seem a sensible precaution against breast disorders to insure this vitamin, as well as iodine, in your daily diet.

61. The Prime Suspect In Cervical Cancer—DES

Cancer of the uterine cervix (that is, the opening of the uterus), at one time the second most prevalent type of cancer among women in America and Europe, is on a steady decline. Cervical cancer now accounts for one-third the number of deaths attributed to it 35 years ago.

According to the American Cancer Society (ACS), the decline in the national toll of victims (11,000 estimated for 1975, 1,700 less than 1971) is in large measure due to better understanding of health hygiene by more women and the widespread use of the Pap test. Profiles drawn up by the ACS indicate that those most susceptible to cervical cancer come from a low income background, have never had regular medical examinations or Pap tests, have borne children and have a history of early sexual intercourse with multiple partners.

Caesarian births and miscarriages do not seem to have any bearing on the incidence of the disease. But it does seem to occur more widely among populations where early marriages and large families are the rule. The risk is twice as great among women who have had five or more children as among those who have had one to three children. The actual physiological changes that a woman experiences during pregnancy and childbirth seem to retard the development of cervical cancer in some respects while they are known to favor it in others. It is very much more likely, experts tell us, that frequent lacerations of the cervix during labor and consequent inflammatory processes play a predominant role.

Of all the suspected causes of cervical cancer, no carcinogen is more clearly indicted than *diethylstilbestrol* (DES), a synthetic sex hormone.

The first report came in the spring of 1971 from gynecologist Dr. Arthur L. Herbst and his associates at Harvard Medical School (*The New England Journal of Medicine*, April 22, 1971). Investigating the unusual clustering of seven cases of adenocarcinoma of the vagina in seven New England girls between 1966 and 1969, they discovered that diethylstilbestrol (DES)—a synthetic sex hormone still being used to fatten beef cattle and other food animals—had been administered to the mothers of all seven during the first three months of pregnancy to guard against miscarriage. Because DES was prescribed often back in the early 1950's to treat pregnant women with a history of miscarriage, Dr. Herbst noted ominously that, "It is likely that more patients with this tumor will appear as girls who were exposed *in utero* come to maturity."

Prior to the cases reported in 1971, the occurrence of adenocarcinoma of the vagina in young women was extremely rare; in fact, the number of cases in the entire world literature for such tumors in girls born before 1945 could be counted on the fingers of one hand.

"Although we do not know how frequently these compounds were used," the article noted, "obstetricians in several upstate New York cities believe that stilbestrol for threatened abortion was used fairly widely and in large doses during the early 1950's. (Such doses) were recommended by two major pharmaceutical companies in the 1950 *Physicians' Desk Reference....* This raises concern about the future. It is not known how many more vaginal carcinomas will be developing ... or whether a longer induction period may be present for those who received a smaller dose. There can no longer be doubt that synthetic estrogens are absolutely contraindicated in pregnancy."

Other Avenues Of Risk

But almost every expectant mother is still eating meat from animals treated with stilbestrol. As Dr. Judah Folkman cautioned in an editorial appearing in the same issue of *The New England Journal of Medicine*, "By avoidance of the prescription of stilbestrol to pregnant women, this unusual cancer may be prevented in the future. But more worrisome is stilbestrol residue in meat. Of 40,000,000 cattle slaughtered in this country each year, 30,000,000 have been fed stilbestrol that remains undetected by the current government assay method."

Pregnant women and young children and all of us are ingesting this carcinogenic hormone unless we use meat from animals that are organically raised or practice vegetarianism.

Stilbestrol is so potent that as little as 2ppb (parts per billion) are toxic in the diets of experimental mice. Cancers in these test animals have been induced by daily doses as low as .07 millionths of a gram.

No Detectable Residues—But Effects Are Apparent

How much of this hormone do you get in the meat you are eating? Enough to make British school girls mature at least three years earlier than in the past, it was reported in the *Medical Officer*, an English journal for government health officers.

More important and perhaps more dangerous than an occasional large dose of stilbestrol, as was taken by the women cited by Dr. Herbst in the original Massachusetts study, is the hazard of repeated small amounts, it was pointed out by Knight, Martin, Iglesias and Smith in a symposium on medicated feeds reported in the *Medical Encyclopedia*, 1956. When you stop to consider that you are ingesting small amounts repeatedly every time you eat a hamburger or steak or any other kind of stilbestrol-treated meat through the years, this becomes a factor of great concern.

62. Leukemia—What Is It? How Does It Occur?

Leukemia, cancer of the blood, is characterized by the uncontrolled proliferation and accumulation of leukocytes (white blood cells). Just as there are many different types of leukocytes, there are many different types of leukemia, but the four most important forms are derived from only two types of cells.

Acute and chronic lymphocytic leukemias (also known as lymphoblastic leukemias) are malignancies of lymphocytes, cells produced in the lymphoid organs (the spleen, lymph nodes, and thymus) and in the bone marrow.

Acute and chronic myelocytic leukemias (also known as granulocytic or myelogenous leukemias) are disorders of granulocytes. Granulocytes, produced by bone marrow, engulf and digest bacteria and other small particles.

Most leukemia cells never mature into functioning leukocytes. That means the body is deprived of vital components of its immune system. Also, the cells accumulate in the blood and in certain organs, forcing out healthy cells and interfering with the function of that organ.

Acute leukemias generally appear suddenly, with symptoms like those of a cold, and progress rapidly. The lymph nodes, spleen, and liver may become infiltrated with leukocytes and enlarged; there is often bone pain, paleness, a tendency to bleed easily, and a high susceptibility to infections. The most common causes of death, which occurs, on the average within three months without treatment, are hemorrhaging and uncontrolled infections. The chronic leukemias take a much slower course; many cases are discovered during routine blood examinations, and several years may pass before significant symptoms appear. The symptoms are similar to those of the acute leukemias, but the life expectancy without treatment is about three years after onset.

Acute lymphocytic leukemia is the most common cancer of childhood (about 3,000 cases per year), but it is even more common in adults. Acute myelocytic leukemia occurs much less frequently in children, and the chronic forms occur almost exclusively in adults. Leukemias strike about 19,000 individuals in the United States each year and take the lives of approximately 14,000.

Chemotherapy For Leukemia Victims

Twenty years ago the life expectancy for a leukemic child was three months after diagnosis of his disease. Today, it is two to three years, and some survive five years or longer.

A remission is a temporary arrest of the leukemic process. When remission occurs, there is often a complete return to the normal state: the symptoms disappear, the physical findings become normal, and the abnormal cells are no longer found in the bone marrow and peripheral blood. Sometimes the remission is only partial, and one or more signs of leukemia may not completely disappear. The increases in remission are credited to more sophisticated chemotherapy, or drug treatment. Unfortunately, most remissions are only temporary and there are some patients who never achieve one.

The drugs used to treat leukemia are members of several different families of anti-cancer drugs: antimetabolites, alkylating agents, hormones, antibiotics, and enzymes. Scientists have found that the interaction of two or more of these drugs produces a combination with greater ability to induce remissions than any one individual drug. Combination therapy has increased the likelihood of response in adult acute leukemia to approximately 50 percent or more in some studies.

There are, however, side effects from these drugs which can threaten the patient's life. Some of the drugs eat away at the stomach lining. Both the drugs and leukemia damage the bone marrow. This impairs the patient's ability to produce platelets, tiny disc-shaped particles that prevent hemorrhage, and white blood cells that help control bacterial and fungal infections. Tranfusions of blood platelets have been effective in stopping hemorrhaging, but the donor platelets must be carefully matched with the patient's platelets, or the patient may develop a resistance to the donor platelets. Powerful antibiotics must be used to curb infections, and they can destroy the patient's natural bacterial defenses.

Radiation Linked To Leukemia

Medical researchers do not know what causes leukemia, but they do know that certain substances can help produce it. The most damning factor involved in the onset of leukemia, the factor now believed responsible for most leukemias, is radiation. According to the National Cancer Institute's booklet, *Progress Against Leukemia* (1973), "an unusual incidence of leukemia has been recorded among persons exposed to radiation: survivors of the atomic bomb explosions in Japan; persons who received large amounts of radiation for treatment of conditions other than leukemia; and radiologists (in early years of the specialty)." A report appearing in *Science* (July 5, 1975) indicated that the unusually high rate of leukemia among radiologists has declined since the routine use of protective precautions.

Research at the Atomic Bomb Casualty Commission revealed that the frequency of leukemia increases proportionately to doses of radiation above 35 rads. Further studies indicated that there may be a latent period of up to 20 years before leukemia develops. In recent years the rate of chronic myelocytic leukemia in the atomic bomb survivors has returned to normal, but the excess of acute leukemia has persisted.

The greatest present danger of radiation comes from the excessive use of medical X-rays. While it is true that everyone is exposed to a certain amount of radiation from the sun, the amount is one ten-thousandth of a roentgen per day. In contrast, a full chest X-ray gives off one-half of a roentgen, and a single tooth X-ray can run from four to 14 roentgens (*Radiation*, Schubert and Lopp, Viking Press). A G.I. series (gastrointestinal X-rays) will give a patient 15 roentgens; a barium enema with two films, five roentgens; and a full "preventive" checkup can run up to 40 roentgens (*Radiology*, vol. 61, W. E. Nolan and H. W. Patterson).

While no threshold has been set below which radiation can be said to be safe, Dr. Shields Warren, professor of pathology, Harvard Medical School, believes that the human body can handle up to 50 roentgens without detrimental effects. He set down a rule of thumb that between 50 and 100 roentgens can bring on leukemia.

The real danger of X-rays is that the radiation received is cumulative; two separate X-rays of five roentgens have the same effect as one X-ray of 10 roentgens. The National Cancer Institute warns that "the leukemogenic effects of small doses, such as those used in diagnosis, cannot be discounted" (*Progress Against Leukemia*, U.S. Department of Health, Education, and Welfare, 1973). Dr. Herman E. Hilleboe, of the Columbia University School of Public Health and Administrative Medicine, stressed that the practice of modern medicine would be impossible without X-rays, but he warned that unnecessary exposure should be prevented and all X-rays kept to a minimum.

Susceptibility Linked To Genetic Factors

Even among persons who received the largest radiation doses from the atomic explosions in Japan, only one in every 100 has developed leukemia. Thus, it is possible that factors other than more exposure to radiation are involved in the susceptibility to radiation-induced leukemia. Just such a possibility was convincingly demonstrated in a study reported in *Preventive Medicine* (vol. 3, 1974, 361-369). Reporting the results of their study, Drs. Irwin D. J. Bross and Nachimuthu Natarajan, of the Department of Biostatistics, Roswell Park Memorial Institute, Buffalo, New York, stated: "Further statistical analysis has clarified the hypothesis that there exists a susceptible subgroup of children who are prone to develop leukemia after exposure to low doses of diagnostic radiation which have no effect on normal insusceptible children. The susceptible group does not show marked increase in relative risk when there is no report of exposure. The risk of developing leukemia among the susceptible children with any of the three types of radiation exposure (preconception, *in utero* and postnatal radiation) is markedly increased in the appropriate age groups."

This varying susceptibility is, according to some researchers, an indication that leukemia may have, in part, a genetic basis. This is also suggested by the frequency with which childhood leukemia occurs in identical twins, who have the same genetic makeup. If one identical twin develops leukemia before the age of five or six, the other has about one chance in five of developing the disease within a short time. This is not true of fraternal twins, who are no more similar in genetic makeup than any other brothers or sisters.

It has recently been found that leukemia occurs together with certain congenital defects more often than can be attributed to chance. Some of these diseases are characterized by abnormal numbers or shapes of the chromosomes, the structures that pass hereditary information from one generation of cells to the next. For example, children with Down's syndrome (mongolism), a congenital disease, characterized by an extra chromosome, have a risk of developing leukemia that is about 15 times greater than that for the general population.

Chromosomal abnormalities have been found in the bone marrow cells of a high percentage of patients with acute leukemia who show no congenital defects. The abnormalities disappear during remission—periods when signs and symptoms of the disease are temporarily in abatement.

The only consistent chromosomal abnormality ever found in studies of cancer cells is one present in the majority of patients with chronic myelocytic leukemia. This abnormality, known as the Philadelphia (Ph¹) chromosome, has been found in most patients with this type of leukemia; it has been observed in all phases of the disease and is unaffected by treatment. It has also been seen in acute myelocytic leukemia and other allied diseases, but rarely.

In animals, chromosomal abnormalities are known to occur after exposure to radiation, chemical carcinogens, and certain viruses. According to the National Cancer Institute, some scientists feel that chromosomal abnormalities, whether inherited or acquired, may be a common factor in the origin of leukemia but that the disease may be triggered by a combination of environmental carcinogens, of which radiation is a leading suspect.

Is There A Leukemia Virus?

Recent medical research has focused a great deal of attention on the possibility that leukemia is caused by a virus. A worldwide research effort conducted by the National Cancer Institute's Special Virus Cancer Program has as its primary objectives: (1) to determine whether viruses comparable to those known to induce cancers in laboratory and domestic animals are causative agents of human cancer, and (2) to develop therapeutic and preventive measures for control of human cancers when such causative agents are found. Certainly, the discovery of a virus that causes leukemia in humans would be a great step toward controlling the disease with a vaccine, much as polio is controlled today.

In 1973, researchers for the National Cancer Institute discovered a virus known to cause leukemia in the gibbon ape. This virus is called a "Type C" virus. Since then, several viruses distinct from, but related to, the "Type C" virus have been isolated from leukemia patients, but according to the National Cancer Institute, "there is no evidence that they are causally related to the disease" (*Progress Against Leukemia*, U.S. Department of Health, Education, and Welfare, 1973). Furthermore,

Cancer

Dr. Robert C. Gallo, of the National Cancer Institute's laboratory of tumor cell biology, reported that these viruses in no way indicate that leukemia can be passed from person to person as in an infectious disease. Dr. Gallo believes that these viruses interact with heredity and environmental influences in the onset of leukemia (*Medical Tribune*, vol. 16, no. 11, March 19, 1975). While the research concerning viruses is still inconclusive, it is known that radiation can activate latent viruses. Also, according to Dr. Robert Miller, of the National Cancer Institute, chromosomal breakage makes cells more susceptible to viral infection or to expression of latent viruses (*Science*, July 5, 1974, p. 50). This chromosomal breakage can result from radiation or genetic factors, or a combination of the two.

63. A Healthy Liver Is An Anti-Cancer Agent

The liver is our largest and most versatile organ, having approximately 500 known functions. It filters out dangerous substances, controls metabolism, manufactures essential chemicals, stores nutrients and sends them through the bloodstream on demand. Several doctors have suggested studying closer the linkage between liver and cancer. One of them, Dr. Martin Protzel, chief of oral pathology at City Hospital, Newark, has shown evidence that the liver may be degenerated by heavy smoking, heavy drinking and nutritional deficiency. When the organ which the body depends upon to neutralize and eliminate its poisons becomes impaired, cancer may be the result, in his opinion.

Dr. Protzel induced liver degeneration in rats by injecting the animals with an olive oil-carbon tetrachloride solution and allowing them free access to drinks containing ethyl alcohol. When a known cancer-causing agent, 3-4 benzopyrene (found in auto exhaust) was painted on the insides of their mouths, tumors developed in 43 percent of the animals.

In a similar group of mice whose livers were not tampered with, the 3-4 benzopyrene caused only 16 percent to develop tumors. And of this group only those mice whose livers had somehow been damaged developed advanced cancers.

Dr. Protzel's studies indicate that the great majority of humans with mouth cancer have a history of heavy smoking, drinking and poor nutrition. However, even feeble agents for cancer can be damaging to tissues "rendered more susceptible to tumor genesis by some unknown mechanisms, possibly liver imbalance," according to Dr. Protzel.

A wide-range exploration of this liver-cancer combination was made by Kasper Blond, M.D., in his book, *The Liver and Cancer*, published in 1960. Dr. Blond suggests that modern medicine pays too much attention to the alarming multiplication of cancer cells and fails to consider the possibility that some metabolic disorder outside the affected cells or organs might be causing the unregulated growth. This influence could be common to all malignancies. The liver, he believes, is that universally affecting center.

Because cancer is a growth, it must be involved with growth metabolism. Normal metabolism would hardly produce pathological changes, Dr. Blond reasons, so only a disordered metabolism could be responsible for cancer. The liver is the central controlling organ for metabolism.

For Blond it follows logically, then, that the liver functioning properly and healthfully can prevent cancer, and that a diseased liver, incapable of exercising full control over metabolism can be the basic cause of cancer. Blond reinforces this conclusion with the fact that about 90 percent of all cancers in the adult population originate in what he classes as metabolic organs.

To make sure your liver keeps regulating your metabolism in a healthy way, make sure your liver gets a steady supply of vitamin C to fight toxic substances. Get it from fresh fruits and vegetables, plus insurance by way of a supplement. Include a mineral supplement (bone meal) for zinc and selenium. And obtain the vitamin E you need for a healthy liver from wheat germ oil and either alpha or mixed tocopherols. Avoid the thieves of the essential B vitamins—alcohol, drugs and smoking—and air pollutants, including sprays and insecticides that are hard on the liver, too.

64. Lung Cancer From The Air We Breathe

Open Door To Cancer

Lung cancer among males has gone up nearly 2,000% since 1914. Dr. Eugene Houdry, who invented the high cracking of petroleum and who has spent his life studying petroleum chemistry, reported that this increase corresponds exactly with the increase of gasoline consumption. He also noted that lung cancer declined 35% during the war years 1941-1945 when gas consumption was reduced because of rationing. It is not difficult to understand this in light of the fact that 600,000 tons of pollutants are poured into our atmosphere daily. Besides the known poisonous gases such as carbon monoxide, sulphur dioxide, nitrogen dioxide and nitrogen oxide, there are also particles of lead and a number of hydrocarbons which are carcinogenic. They make up a large percentage of the pollutants and are highly virulent.

Premium gas is especially cancer-dangerous. W. A. Cruse, an expert in the field of motor fuel, described premium gas in his book, *Motor Fuels, Performance and Testing*. He said that premium gas consists mostly of high boiling fractions over 700 degrees. (In the fracturing of raw petroleum all fractions coming off above the 700 degree boiling have been proven to be highly carcinogenic.) The chemists and engineers of Standard Oil and Esso concurred with this.

Regular gas normally contains less carcinogenic fractions, but the car engine acts as a cracking plant heating the gas from 700 to 1,000 degrees, so that the unburnt gas emerging from the exhaust is also highly carcinogenic. The truck diesel engine is even worse, for besides giving off formaldehyde and acrolein (this one is the main ingredient in tear gas), the engine temperature runs even higher than an ordinary car (3,500 degrees). What comes out of that exhaust is not perfume.

These high boiling aromatic hydrocarbons were thoroughly examined by Dr. Cornelius Rhoades of Memorial Hospital for

Treatment of Cancer and Allied Disease in New York at the instigation of Standard Oil and Esso. The conclusion of these studies upon test animals showed that any component of petroleum boiling over 700 degrees was highly cancerous to mice, rabbits and monkeys.

Jet airliners have engines that reach temperatures of 6,000 degrees. The emission of smoke is a sign that all the fuel is not being burned. The takeoff of one commercial jetliner emits pollutants equivalent to 10,000 cars. About one jet a minute takes off or lands at an airport the size of Kennedy.

The stationary emitters, factories, plants, etc., contribute to our carcinogenic air by converting coal into benzopyrene—a well known carcinogenic agent, also found in cigarette smoke. This gas has been found in skies above every American city.

Here are some mortality figures from the American Cancer Society. In 1930, 3,000 deaths from lung cancer: 1947—17,000; 1963—25,000; 1974—75,000! Cigarette smoking is no doubt a large factor, but Professor A. Haddow, Director of the Chester Beatty Cancer Research Institute of London stated in 1966 that as much as 80 percent of lung cancer may be due to environmental causes.

Vitamin A Protects Against Cancer

What may turn out to be one of the most important pieces of research in the history of modern medicine was unveiled at the Ninth International Cancer Congress. Dr. Umberto Saffiotti, then a pathologist at the Chicago Medical School, reported that he had virtually 100 percent success in giving lung cancer to laboratory animals by exactly the same means that the disease is supposed to be caused in humans. In identical animals, however, he was able to reverse the process and render the animals immune to cancer-causing chemicals he used on them, by giving them vitamin A as well.

Dr. Saffiotti himself, in the manner typical of scientists, warned that his findings were not yet conclusive, and while he felt that they might "possibly lead to results of practical significance for the prevention of lung cancer," he also felt that such results had not yet been achieved.

Top Expert

There is little possibility that Dr. Saffiotti could be mistaken about whether he was truly dealing with cancer. A pathologist's specialty is the examination of diseased tissue and the precise determination of what disease if any is present. We can assume that the Doctor knows what he is talking about when he says that he had practically 100 percent success in giving lung cancer to hamsters. Why hamsters? Because these animals never contract lung cancer by natural means. If the hamsters got lung cancer at all, it could only be because of what Dr. Saffiotti was doing to them.

What he did was to subject their lungs to benzopyrene, the hydrocarbon that is believed to be the chief cancer-causing chemical in cigarette smoke as well as in automobile exhausts, and smoke from the coal and oil fires of home and factory. This material was permitted to fasten itself to inert particles of dust, in exactly the same way it does in the atmosphere. The dust was then placed in the windpipes of hamsters.

The particles were found to lodge in the lower portion of the lungs. Cell fluid in the lungs washed the dust particles, separating out the benzopyrene and dispersing the cancer-causing material throughout the lung tissue. When the benzopyrene reached the cells lining the bronchi—the tubular passages through which air is channeled into the lungs—the cells began to grow and divide in a rapid, irregular manner. It was soon evident that the animals that were, in effect, subjected to the same air pollutants as a smoker and city dweller, had developed lung cancer.

Vitamin A Protects

It is well known that vitamin A is intimately connected with the health and functioning of the lining of the bronchi. Dr. Saffiotti experimented with giving large doses of vitamin A to his laboratory hamsters to see if that would have any effect on the rate or manner of development of the lung tumors.

And what an effect it had! ". . . when he also feeds them vitamin A, very few come down with lung tumors," according to the Associated Press report of his paper.

Dr. Saffiotti was careful to warn that he did not intend his report to be taken as advice for smokers to start dosing themselves with massive amounts of vitamin A. He also warned that excess vitamin A can be harmful. Vitamin A, as is true of all the oil-soluble vitamins whose surpluses are stored in the liver rather than being excreted, cannot be taken without limit. What your personal limit is depends very much on how you react to the vitamin.

65. How Oral Cancer Can Be Controlled

Cancer of the mouth is easily detectable and, in most instances, treatment immediately after detection and prior to metastasis (spreading) is successful; yet the number of deaths resulting from this type of cancer is increasing every year. The estimated number of newly detected cases of oral cancer has nearly doubled over the past five years. Despite new and better methods of treatment, deaths due to oral cancer increased by about 1300 from 1974 to 1975.

In a five year study, reported by Dr. Daniel M. Laskin, editor of the *Journal of Oral Surgery,* the survival rates for oral cancer patients jumped a dramatic 45 percent when the cancer was detected prior to metastasis.

In analyzing cancer statistics over a period of time, Dr. Laskin, an oral surgeon, observed that fewer patients survive oral cancers than other cancers much more difficult to diagnose, such as cancer of the bladder, colon and breast.

Commenting on the need for a re-educational program for dentists which would familiarize them with the obvious symptoms of oral cancer, Dr. Laskin said it "is particularly distressing when one realizes that 85 percent of oral cancers are either visible directly or indirectly with a mirror, and 11 percent of those not visible are palpable on careful clinical examination."

Because dental disease usually does not keep people from the performance of their routine duties, the dentist sees far more well persons in a medical environment than does any other person in the health field. Many times the dentist is the first person in a position to see certain pathologic changes. The fact that people visit dentists on a regular basis makes it possible for him to observe changes in the tongue, lips, teeth, gums and adjoining bone structure which would not necessarily be observed by the family physician. The dentist is in a position to note the changes which lead to disease, to alert the patient to see his physician, or change his habits and thus avert a head-on collision with a debilitating condition.

Other Causes

A relatively high incidence of oral cancer has long been associated with heavy smokers. But according to Dr. Morris E. Chafetz, director of the National Institute of Alcohol Abuse, "When heavy drinking and heavy smoking are combined, the risk factor jumps enormously . . . Those who do both are fifteen times as susceptible as people who neither drink nor smoke." Dr. Chafetz made his remarks in August of 1974 at a White House Health Seminar under the auspices of the Department of Health, Education and Welfare.

If you take your whiskey "neat," that is, undiluted by anything else, the risk of mouth cancer is greater for you than if you smoked cigars or a pipe, in the opinion of Professor Jens J. Pindborg of Denmark's Royal Medical College. In a refresher course given for dentists at the University of California Medical School, Dr. Pindborg said: "Not all cancers of the mouth are due to tobacco. Smoking a pipe or cigars increases the risk, but not as much as hard liquor." Six shots of straight whiskey a day boost the chances of mouth cancer to ten times the normal rate. About five percent of all cancers in the Western world—and 20 to 40 percent of cancers in Southeast Asia where chewing tobacco and betel nut are common—are mouth cancers, concluded Dr. Pindborg in *MD* (October, 1966).

Cancer From Ill-Fitting Dentures

Nearly half of the cases of oral cancer (the cause of 7,000 deaths annually) occur in toothless patients over fifty who wear badly-fitted dentures. Researchers say this statistic could be reversed if more dentists would perform complete oral examinations and educate their patients to know when dentures need adjusting. *The Cancer Bulletin* (September-October, 1968) warns that regular check-ups for proper fit are important. Too often, patients wearing false teeth accept discomfort as inevitable, putting up with years of irritation before complaining to a dentist. By that time it is likely to be too late.

66. Skin Cancer— The Sunbathers' Disease

The rays of the sun embrace you with a seductive warmth. It is so tempting to surrender to them. But try to remember that, "Sunlight ranks as the major cause of skin cancer, which is one of the most common forms of malignancy," according to Dr. John N. Knox, of the Baylor University College of Medicine (*Roche Report*, September 6, 1963). In fact, skin cancer has sometimes been called the farmers' disease and the sailors' disease. It is more common among men than women, simply because men work and take their recreation out-of-doors to a much greater extent than women.

Today, skin cancer could also be known as the sunbathers' disease. An occasional sunbath probably won't hurt you—except perhaps to give you a bad case of sunburn if you aren't careful. But constant exposure to sunlight can be dangerous—especially if you are a blue-eyed blonde. Fair people are much more susceptible to skin cancer than others. Those who tan easily and black or copper-skinned people have plenty of pigment cells which seem to form a protective barrier against the damaging ultraviolet rays of sunlight. But if exposure is long and frequent, brunettes, too, can push their luck too far and lose the skin game.

Too many of us tend to relax our vigilance against the danger sheathed in the rays of the sun because we have heard that skin cancer has a low mortality rate and can often be cured. This is perfectly true, but it doesn't mean that sunlight-induced skin cancer isn't dangerous. Indeed, according to American Cancer Society figures, over 95 percent of the over 300,000 estimated cases of skin cancer reported in 1974 were treated successfully. But deaths do occur: an estimated 5,000 will occur in 1975, the same number as those deaths estimated from bone, connective tissue and thyroid cancers *combined.*

Protect Yourself

There are several steps that can be taken to safeguard against the sun's rays if you spend a lot of time out-of-doors during hot summer days. If you intend to enjoy yourself this summer by sailing, water skiing, swimming, golfing, playing tennis, fishing or gardening, is there anything you can do to protect yourself from the cancer-causing rays of the sun without wearing so much protective clothing that your movement is restricted and you begin to drown in your own perspiration?

Yes, there is. The two antioxidants, vitamins C and E, show promise that they can help prevent sun-induced skin cancer, according to recent findings of Dr. Homer S. Black and Dr. Wan-Bang Lo, dermatology researchers associated with the Baylor College of Medicine, Houston, Texas (*Nature*, December 21-28, 1973).

Two Vitamins Help Prevent Dangerous Oxidation

The Texas researchers studied the mechanism by which sunlight triggers skin cancer and discovered a very interesting phenomenon. After human or animal skin is exposed to ultraviolet light, cholesterol in the skin oxidizes and forms by-products (*Nature*, December 3, 1971). One of the by-products of this oxidation process is a substance called cholesterol alpha-oxide, a known cancer-causing chemical.

Since vitamins C and E are known to reduce the oxidation of fats, Drs. Black and Lo wondered if adding extra antioxidants to the diet might block the formation of the cancer-causing cholesterol oxide in the skin.

The first step was to determine if antioxidants taken orally would affect the concentration of antioxidants in the skin. To find out, they fed one group of mice an ordinary diet and another group the same diet supplemented with vitamins C, E, and other antioxidants of a chemical nature.

Skin was obtained from animals sacrificed at intervals of two weeks, and irradiated for 30 minutes to simulate the effect of several hours of ultraviolet light.

The researchers discovered that those animals which had received a supplemented diet had 64 percent more antioxidants in their skin after two weeks than the other animals. The level decreased somewhat after this, but was maintained at about 18 percent above the control level for the next 24 weeks.

The really important finding, though, was that as the antioxidant content of the skin increased, the formation of cholesterol alpha-oxide decreased. In fact, complete protection against formation of this carcinogen was observed in those animals which had received the vitamin supplements during the first two weeks of the study, when the maximum increase of antioxidant content of the skin occurred. Approximately 50 percent protection against formation of cholesterol alpha-oxide was afforded those animals fed the supplemental diet for four to 24 weeks, at which time the experiment ended.

This study shows that when supplemental antioxidants are consumed, they *do* get to the skin, and they *do* act as a deterrent to the formation of a carcinogenic substance induced by ultraviolet light. The fact that the greatest amount of inhibition occurred after two weeks, and fell somewhat later, is an interesting phenomenon.

Whatever the cause of this drop in antioxidant concentration in the skin and the subsequent lowered protection, the implications are clear. Your need for vitamins C and E tends to increase with time, and as you are repeatedly exposed to sunlight. They won't give you complete protection, but there's every reason to believe that they will help significantly.

Even if you do increase your intake of vitamins C and E throughout the long hot summer, it would not be wise to throw precaution and your sunbonnet to the wind.

Many of us look upon extensive sunbathing as a natural and healthful activity. But even aside from the possibility of developing skin cancer, this is not exactly true. In fact, our contemporary adulation of a deep bronze tan is really a fad. Throughout most of history, men and women alike have usually taken careful precautions against excessive exposure, and for good reasons, science tells us.

Dr. Knox of Baylor, whom we mentioned earlier, says that "Unlike areas covered by clothing, exposed skin tends over the years to become dry and wrinkled, with a coarse, leathery look and changes in pigmentation. This aging of exposed areas is the first degenerative change. The next stage, for susceptible skin, may be development of actinic keratoses. Such growths are pre-malignant."

The process by which you become tanned is the result of a traumatic disturbance that occurs under the skin. The elastic fibers of the skin become heated and their shapes become distorted. The melanin pigment, found in the deepest layers of the epidermis, begins to migrate upward towards the surface. Repeated and prolonged exposure of the skin results in a chemical breakdown of the cells in the dermis, causing chronic irreversible changes, especially in the elastic fibers. These fibers may multiply in number and become extremely disorganized in their arrangement. The results are wrinkling, sagging and drying of the skin, as well as localized areas of thickening.

The worst damage occurs when the ultraviolet radiation from the sun reaches its greatest intensity between the hours of 10 a.m. and 2 p.m. If you're on a boat, or on the beach, you will not only be burned by the rays of the sun, but by reflected rays from the sand and water. Significantly, grass reflects only about one-seventh as much light as sand. So you might plan on spending a little more time in the garden and forego a few days at the beach.

But in all honesty, we expect that very few people who love the beach and other summer activities are going to give them up for any reason. Which brings up the subject of suntan lotions.

The Best Suntan Lotion Of Them All

There are many suntan lotions on the market, and many of them are helpful to some extent. Some work by reflecting the sun's rays away from the skin, while others absorb the rays before they hit the skin. Still others allow only certain rays, which cause tanning but not burning, to penetrate.

You may be surprised to learn that the most effective suntan lotion you could use consists solely of a B vitamin in solution with ethyl alcohol. The vitamin is para-aminobenzoic acid, or PABA. German researchers showed over 40 years ago that PABA is effective as a sunscreen agent, but recent research has found that when five percent PABA is mixed in solution with 70 to 95 percent ethyl alcohol, the result is a suntan lotion which is far and away the most effective protection against sunburn available.

This discovery was made by a team consisting of Drs. Pathak, Fitzpatrick and Frenk from the Department of Dermatology at Harvard Medical School, who reported their research in the *New England Journal of Medicine* (June 26, 1969).

The Harvard scientists tested a large number of suntan lotions in the Arizona desert and high in the Swiss Alps. They found that the PABA solutions "after a single application, can protect fair-skinned persons undergoing long exposure (over four hours) under natural sunlight, and *are more effective than 24 of the commercially available products tested.*"

Two things ought to be emphasized about this excellent lotion.

First, although PABA by itself is partially effective as a sunscreening agent, its vast superiority over all other products only emerges when it is mixed with the proper amount of ethyl alcohol. If a pharmacist has some PABA and some ethyl alcohol on hand, he can easily prepare the solution. Second, although this lotion offers excellent protection against sunburn, it does allow tanning. Therefore, it will probably permit a certain amount of the damage associated with long exposure to the sun.

Another Way To Protect Against Harmful Sun Rays

There is yet another way in which nutrients can help protect against the sun. Anthony C. Turner and co-workers of the British Air Corporation's Joint Medical Services reported in *The Practitioner* (206:662, 1971) that a preparation containing 25,000 I.U. of vitamin A and 120 mg. of calcium carbonate in tablet form, taken orally, is very useful in preventing painful sunburn. They gave the combination of vitamin A and calcium to 3,000 people, 163 of whom had previously reported severe or uncomfortable sunburn at some time in the past. During the period of the test, only 15 people suffered severe sunburn, while the others had either complete protection, or suffered only very mild symptoms.

If you're wondering exactly what calcium carbonate is, this is the form of calcium which is found, along with phosphorus, in bone meal supplements.

One last word of caution. There are many drugs and chemicals in the environment today which can increase your sensitivity to the sun to the point where exposure that would normally cause only the slightest redness will produce a fiery agony. These various chemicals are known as photosensitizing agents, and there is no shortage of them. The article, "Problems of Sunlight Sensitivity" by Dr. John H. Epstein (*Medical Digest*, August, 1970), tells us that among the agents which can produce this abnormal sensitivity to sunlight are antihistamines, barbiturates, tranquilizers, antibiotics, diuretics, and antidiabetic drugs. If you are taking any of these drugs, it is best to stay out of the direct sun completely. At the very least, you should be extremely cautious, and get inside at the first sign of discomfort.

In addition, photosensitization can be produced by antibacterial soaps, and a number of cosmetics and lotions—even some suntan lotions! Only a small number of people suffer photosensitization after contact with these substances, but it is wise to be aware of the potential danger.

Another Way To Protect Against Harmful Sun Rays

If medicinal drugs of nearly every variety can turn the rays of the sun into a potentiator of disease, is it possible that some of the other innumerable chemicals which pollute our bodies can have a similar effect? This question has been raised by some fascinating experiments carried out by Yoho, Weaver, and Butler, three entomologists at West Virginia University. In a series of studies, the latest of which was published in *Environmental Entomology* (December, 1973), the researchers demonstrated that a variety of fluorescent dyes can react with sunlight in entirely unexpected ways. Working with common house flies, the entomologists discovered that when the insects were fed the dyes, and kept in darkness, very few deaths resulted. But when they were put into either artificial or natural light, they died . . . well, like flies. With three of the dyes, the mortality was very close to 100 percent.

As entomologists working in the Division of Plant Sciences of West Virginia University, the researchers are primarily concerned about the possibility of using these dyes as potent insecticides. But they note that, "at the same time, this work has revealed the possible dangers of photo-dynamic effects occurring in our environment." In other words, the food additives, dyes and other chemicals which we eat, drink, breathe, and rub against every day, may appear to be safe when they are given to animals kept under laboratory lighting conditions. But what happens when these chemicals get into our systems or on our skins and we are then exposed to bright sunlight? Do they become subtly toxic, perhaps allergenic, or even carcinogenic? These are questions that must be answered, and until they are, give us yet another reason to reduce our internal and environmental pollution to the absolute minimum. If there's a choice between chemicals and sunlight, we'll take the sunlight any day.

So go ahead and get all the exercise, fresh air, and just plain fun that you can this summer. With a few simple precautions, you will have little or nothing to fear from the sinister side of our good friend, the sun.

67. Common Causes
Of Stomach Cancer

Smoked Meats

Smoking has been documented as the leading cause of lung cancer. But there's another kind of smoking that's almost equally dangerous, it seems. It's the kind that is used to process meat.

During exposure of meat to smoke to preserve it, millions of tiny carbon particles are lodged in the meat—carbon particles that resemble lamp black, and like it have been seriously implicated as a cause of stomach cancer.

Although stomach cancer is on the decline in America, it is still a prevalent health problem, and is very often fatal because of the difficulty of detecting it in its early stages. The decline in incidence of this killer may very well be related, in part at least, to a decline in the consumption of smoked foods.

Years ago smoking meat was commonplace. There were no refrigerators, ice boxes were costly, and ice was hard to find around the summertime farm. Smoking, the biggest development in embalming since the Egyptians, was used to preserve meat.

Today, however, freezing techniques allow a far safer form of meat preservation, and refrigerated transportation speeds fresh meat to us daily. Thus, smoked meat declined in use in the United States. Perhaps this is a reason why stomach cancer is declining in most areas where smoked meat is not a staple item of the diet.

But smoked sausage, fish, hams, bacon, and other products are still in widespread use in this country.

What happens to the population of an area that subsists mainly on smoked meat or fish? The stomach cancer rates rise. This fact was borne out in a study conducted by Dr. Niels Dungal of Reykjavik, Iceland, and reported in the *Journal of the American Medical Association*. Dr. Dungal became interested in the problem of stomach cancer in his own country because the disease accounts for up to 45 percent of all cancers in males there.

The link between smoked meat and cancer of the stomach was further strengthened by the report of Dr. Charles C. Stock, biochemist in charge of experimental cancer chemotherapy at the famed Sloan-Kettering Institute, delivered before the Montreal Medico-chirurgical Society in Montreal, Canada. He said the incidence of stomach cancer is extremely high in regions where meat and fish are smoked before consumption.

"Statistics show that in Japan alone 50 percent of cancer histories are stomach cases, whereas in the central United States, where fresh meat is plentiful, the number of stomach cancers is very low.

"In Iceland the number of stomach cancer cases is also very high," he said. "There is a very strong suspicion that this is in some way related to the large amount of smoked fish the natives eat."

He fed smoked fish—a favorite food of the Icelanders—to laboratory rats, and one-third developed malignant tumors. Further, he found a higher rate of stomach cancer in areas where people fish for their food.

"Smoked fish," Dr. Dungal reported, "contains large quantities of polycyclic hydrocarbons, known cancer-causing agents."

Nitrites

It would be a simple matter of willpower if the only carcinogenic (cancer-causing) effects of commercial meat products were confined to smoked meat products. We would simply have to choose between eating them or not eating them. But the cancer threat in commercial meats does not stop there: As long as nitrates are used to color and preserve meats, as well as being lacquered onto our croplands every year as fertilizers, our stomachs will be exposed to carcinogens—specifically, nitrites.

Usually, nitrite starts out as nitrate, a relatively harmless compound. Nitrates, which as the name implies, are nitrogen compounds, are essential to plant life. The bacteria in soil, by metabolizing organic nitrogen compounds, release nitrates, in which form the nitrogen can be readily absorbed and utilized by plants for growth. Some plants, especially greens such as spinach, accumulate relatively large but highly variable amounts of nitrate. Ordinarily, we wouldn't be eating enough of this natural nitrate to pose any problems. But there is nothing ordinary—or natural—about the food and water most of us eat in this super-technological age.

In the natural state—and in organic farming—plants get their nitrogen slowly as organic matter in the soil slowly decays. But today, to spur the maximum amount of growth from overworked soil, nearly all farmers use tremendous amounts of chemical fertilizer, in which all the nitrogen is already in the inorganic or nitrate form in which it can be immediately used by the plant. The more of this fertilizer which is used, especially as the crop is ripening, the more nitrate winds up in our food and in our drinking water (Wolff and Wasserman, *Science*, July 7, 1972). When vegetables are grown under shade, as they sometimes are in very hot areas, the nitrate count rises still higher, while the vitamin C content diminishes! (*Miss. Farm Research*, July, 1962)

And don't forget human sewage, millions of tons of which winds up in rivers every day, further adding to the nitrate burden of drinking and irrigation water.

But there is yet another way in which added, unnatural amounts of nitrate enter our food. Fully eight billion pounds of beef and pork, mostly in the form of hot dogs, luncheon meats and canned hams, are impregnated with nitrates and/or nitrites and eaten by Americans every year, according to Robert Rust of Iowa State University (*National Hog Farmer*, July 22, 1972). The major function of this nitrate is to give aging and decomposing meat a healthy-looking pink or reddish color and perk up the flavor. The dire need for such a lift in hot dogs, for example, becomes all too plain when you realize that most hot dogs contain liberal amounts of added fat, cereal, water, and goat or old chicken meat. Nitrate allows this garbage to be kept in storage for weeks before the unsuspecting consumer buys it and feeds it to her children.

Some processors claim that it also retards bacterial growth and even inhibits growth of the spores that cause botulism. Other processors cite tests which show that this is unlikely, and point out that some nations have banned the use of nitrate without triggering an epidemic of food poisoning. These foreign processors often use natural preservatives or boil foods for longer periods of time prior to processing. In fact, one of the best safe preservatives is ascorbic acid or vitamin C, the very factor which protects against nitrite by destroying it.

Meat processors depend upon this fact to keep their products looking fresh. That's because it really isn't the nitrate, they discovered, that keeps the color in meat. What happens, tests showed, is that the bacteria normally found in meat work on the nitrate and reduce it to nitrite. And it's the nitrite that does the cosmetic and preservative work. Entirely disregarding the fact that nitrite is far more toxic than nitrate, many processors simply quit using nitrate and replaced it with nitrite, or used some nitrate along with it as a sort of nitrite time-release capsule. The label on the lunch meat may say "sodium nitrate added" but you can be sure that by the time you eat it, much or all of the nitrate has been transformed into nitrite.

Nitrosation: The Cancer Risk

For many years, it was thought that this transformation could only take place in the stomach of an infant less than five months or so old. But recently, evidence has been published that this is not the case. Dr. Johannes Sander of West Germany, according to an editorial in the *Journal of the American Medical Association* (May 17, 1971), has shown experimentally that adult stomachs can also reduce nitrate to nitrite if acidity is low, as it is in many people most of the time, and in most people toward the end of a meal. The sheer size of adults, however, precludes that kind of acute reaction that can swiftly kill infants.

Now that we understand how nitrite reaches our stomachs, we must be perfectly honest and state that nitrite as such isn't what cancer and public health specialists are worrying about—except for contamination of well water and the subsequent deadly threat to babies. True, some adults have been fatally poisoned by eating foods containing excessive amounts of nitrite (*Eleven Blue Men*, B. Roueche, 1954), but there is another danger involving nitrite in our stomachs which is of far greater concern to these scientists—and should be to you, too.

That fear is that nitrite, once in the stomach, combines with substances called *secondary amines* to form compounds known as *nitrosamines*. Nitrosamines are known to cause cancer.

All that is necessary for this reaction to take place is for nitrite and a secondary amine to be present together in the stomach. A process called *nitrosation* takes place, and the results of this process are the cancer-causing nitrosamines.

Lijinsky and Epstein (*Nature*, Jan. 3, 1970) cite literature showing that various nitrosamines fed to animals produce cancer of the esophagus, stomach and lungs. The *Journal of the National Cancer Institute* (48; 1972) abstracted the most recent test results reported by S. S. Mirvish and others at the Eppley Institute which demonstrate, quite plainly, that nitrite and amines fed to a mouse at the same time also result in lung tumors (as many as ten times more than control animals), and overwhelm the liver with toxins.

These animal studies, along with test tube procedures, and a knowledge of human stomach chemistry have convinced most researchers that there is no known reason why this same process of nitrosation does not take place in a human stomach when nitrites and secondary amines come together.

By now we know where nitrites come from, but what about the secondary amines? According to Lijinsky and Epstein, you are eating large amounts of these amines when you eat any kind of fish, especially salt water fish. Do you have cereal for breakfast? You are eating secondary amines. Do you enjoy a cup of tea? You are enjoying secondary amines. Have you ever sat next to a person who was smoking? You were inhaling his secondary amines along with his smoke. And if you have ever taken any one of a rather large number of drugs, you were also taking secondary amines.

Dr. Moizo Ishidate, director of the Tokyo Biochemical Research Institute, was quoted in *Medical Tribune* (March 22, 1972) as singling out powdered milk and sausage as foods especially high in nitrosatable amines. He also points out that cooked or processed foods tend to be higher in secondary amines than raw foods. Other researchers have named various grains, as well as alcoholic beverages made from these grains as sources of amines.

Clearly, it would be just as difficult to design a diet free of secondary amines as it would be to choose one free of all nitrates. It would be almost as difficult never to eat the two together in an attempt to block nitrosation. You would never be able to eat vegetables with any kind of bread, grain or fish; never drink tea at the end of a meal, and never so much as sip a glass of wine if anyone at the table was smoking a cigarette.

You are probably thinking, in that case, why doesn't everyone have cancer?

Well, that is the very question which many researchers in various parts of the world are asking themselves. They are probing their statistics, examining small differences in regional diets. Dr. Sander, whom we previously mentioned, says there is a link between weak stomach acidity and cancer of the stomach. The weak acidity could permit a much higher production of nitrites, as occurs in babies. Any one or many of an infinite number of metabolic differences could also enter the picture.

We must also keep in mind that when cancer develops in a human being, it doesn't happen in a matter of months, as it does in a laboratory mouse. Typically, carcinogenesis in a human being takes 20, 25, or 30 or more years. It is not the kind of process that can be followed closely in a laboratory. At this point, there has never really been established a thoroughly scientific cause-and-effect relationship between cancer and cigarette smoking, so it should not be surprising that there is no definitive link between nitrosamines and stomach cancer in humans.

The official position of the Food and Drug Administration is that you shouldn't start to worry about excess nitrates and nitrites until it has been proven beyond doubt that cancer-causing compounds are being churned out in your belly. That is why so many people worry about the FDA. (The FDA for years actually defended the use of nitrites in fish, loaded with secondary amines, and even in foods for babies, so vulnerable to nitrite-induced methemoglobinemia.)

But until now, whatever your attitude toward the danger of nitrites was, there wasn't too much you could do about it, except avoid foods to which nitrate had been artificially added, eat organically grown food, and keep the detoxifying enzymes of the liver in full potency by a good diet rich in the B-complex vitamins. But this would only reduce the potential danger, not eliminate it.

Dr. S. S. Mirvish and others at the Eppley Institute for Research in Cancer combined nitrite with various secondary amines under varying conditions of acidity which had already been shown to produce nitrosamines. But when they added vitamin C to the brew, and analyzed the contents, they discovered that, on the average, the process of nitrosation had been blocked about 97 to 99 percent!

In one case, though, there was more nitrosation, but only under conditions of extreme acidity. In all likelihood, the nitrite in the food would be destroyed before the food reached that point of acidity.

Dr. Mirvish and his colleagues mention eight drugs as being among those known to contain secondary amines. If they were taken just before some nitrited fish, or hot dogs or luncheon meat or even spinach, eggplant or other nitrite-loaded vegetable, the stage would be set for nitrosation and the production of nitrosamines. Therefore, they urge the medical-scientific community, doesn't it make sense to prescribe a small amount of vitamin C to be taken with every pill? They also suggest that vitamin C be added to any food product which contains nitrates or nitrites, as a preventive measure. Why gamble with cancer when prevention is so simple and so inexpensive?

68. Cancer Of The Thymus—A Consequence Of Radiation Therapy

Radiation therapy, sometimes valuable in the treatment of cancer, at other times has been found more damaging than helpful. Even though it is chancy, its use for cancer can probably be justified. However, the evidence is overwhelming that when used indiscriminately to "treat" a variety of malignant and benign ailments, radiation techniques do more harm to the human body than good.

Two New England physicians demonstrated that irradiation of the thymus gland during childhood—once a routine procedure if the gland was considered "enlarged"—increases the risk of thyroid cancer in later years. Dr. Murray L. Janower of the Department of Radiology, Massachusetts General Hospital and Harvard University, and Dr. Olli S. Miettinen of the Department of Epidemiology, Harvard School of Public Health, studied the long-term effects of X-ray therapy on 466 patients. Their findings were published in the *Journal of the American Medical Association* (February 1, 1971).

The pair didn't have far to look for the ideal study situation: From 1924 to 1946, prophylactic irradiation of enlarged thymus glands in infants was standard policy at the Massachusetts Eye and Ear Infirmary in Boston. Usually a cumulative radioactive dosage of 400 roentgens was administered—four treatments of 100 roentgens each at 10-day intervals spread over 30 days.

Of the 1,131 children exposed to such treatment over the 22-year period, Janower and Miettinen were able to obtain complete follow-up information in 466 cases. These irradiated patients were designated Group 1. A control group, involving 506 unirradiated subjects treated at the same hospital, became Group 2. Brothers and sisters of these first two groups provided additional controls; 993 in Group 3 and 1,105 in Group 4.

The investigators discovered a significantly higher tumor incidence among the irradiated subjects. Two malignant and 9 benign thyroid tumors were reported and verified in Group 1. But there were *no* malignant tumors in the other groups, and fewer benign tumors: two in Group 2, two in Group 3 and six in Group 4. In addition, three cases of breast cancer were reported in Group 1.

From this data, Janower and Miettinen concluded that irradiation, erroneously being administered for the benefit of patients, is actually causing cancer. "In our group of irradiated patients," they wrote, "the finding of two malignant and nine benign thyroid neoplasms (tumors) suggests an increased risk which is, very roughly, 30-fold for malignant and five-fold for benign tumors."

As alarming as their conclusion was, the two doctors hastened to add that the effects could have been much worse if the X-ray beam had not been properly focused. "It should be noted . . . that the positioning of the beam in the cases in our series probably resulted in relatively minimal exposure of the thyroid gland to the primary radiation beam," they said.

The conclusions of Drs. Miettinen and Janower were confirmed by those of Dr. Leslie DeGroot and Dr. Edward Paloyan, of the University of Chicago, who found that among 50 patients with thyroid cancers seen over four years, 20 had received prior X-ray treatment. These patients, the two researchers said, developed tumors an average of 20 years after X-ray exposure, and were nearly all under 35 years of age.

The doctors reported in the *Journal of the American Medical Association* (July 30, 1973), that a majority of all patients with thyroid tumors had a history of prior radiation to the neck, typically 300 to 600 rads delivered sometime during the first five years of life. This compares to between eight to ten rads the average adult receives by the time he reaches 30, said Dr. DeGroot.

Why did these future cancer victims receive radiation treatment? For cancer? No. For the most part, the researchers point out, they were given X-rays during their youth for tonsilitis or acne! At that time, radiation was in vogue for these and other conditions among doctors who simply didn't know any better.

69. Vitamin A: Cancer Inhibitor

Vitamin A And Lung Cancer

Vitamin A seems to prevent cancer of the lung. A report by Dr. Max Odens of London to this effect came quietly in the German medical publication *Vitalstoffe* of December, 1967, without any ballyhoo or screaming headlines. Yet, in its implications, the report is of far-reaching significance.

For while the American Cancer Society recommends such methods as chemotherapy, radiation and surgery as cancer treatments, the dietary pathway to prevention and cure of this dread disease has been largely ignored by orthodox medicine.

Yet recent research on the effect of vitamin A on cancer and precancerous conditions should most certainly give this vitamin top priority in the arsenal of weapons effective in the prevention of malignancies.

Dr. Odens bases his conclusions on both his own research over a period of 15 years on the effect of vitamin A on bronchitis, and the report on vitamin A's ability to prevent cancer by Dr. Umberto Saffiotti presented at the Ninth International Cancer Congress in Tokyo in October, 1966. Dr. Saffiotti, now a research pathologist affiliated with the National Cancer Institute, was, at the time of his report, affiliated with the Institute for Medical Research at the Chicago Medical School.

Vitamin A is necessary, according to Dr. Odens, to the maintenance of all surface tissues: the skin, the mucous membrane lining the mouth, the throat, the eyelids and outer coat of the eyes, and the mucous membrane lining the respiratory tract. It was the fact that vitamin A is involved in the maintenance of the mucous membrane lining of the respiratory tract that gave him the idea to start a clinical trial and to treat patients suffering from chronic bronchitis with daily doses of vitamin A in addition to conservative methods. He treated 17 patients, aged 48 to 67, and followed their state of health for 15 years. All 17 patients showed considerable improvement in spite of the unfavorable English climate.

Dr. Odens explains how vitamin A acts to protect the lungs

from bronchitis, lung cancer, and other respiratory diseases. He maintains that if lysosomes—the minute bodies inside cells containing protein-splitting enzymes—are damaged and, if the enzymes leak to the cell substances, chromosomal material could be damaged and could lead to malignant changes. In other words, the vitamin A helps the lysosomes to withstand the effects of carcinogens so that they do not leak into and damage the cell substance. It is as if the vitamin A provided an armor around the lysosome which the carcinogen cannot penetrate.

Safeguard Against Pollution

Also known for its ability to enable your body to ward off communicable infectious diseases, vitamin A can also help you to stave off the ill effects of environmental carcinogens. Much of this effectiveness is concerned with the cilia, the microscopic hair-like projections of the cells lining the lung's air passages. These cilia perform the necessary functions of trapping and removing from the lung the inhaled foreign substances including dirt, irritants and potential carcinogens. Without vitamin A, the cilia dry up and lose their function. Vitamin A owes much of its effectiveness to the fact that it can restore the cilia to functioning status.

In 1966 Dr. Saffiotti reported laboratory results which implied that the cilia could trap and reject foreign substances, including carcinogens. It is well known that the inhalation of the carcinogen benzopyrene (found in smoke) produces lung cancer. In tests, Dr. Saffiotti gave benzopyrene alone to 57 hamsters. Fifty-nine hamsters were given benzopyrene plus 5 mg. (5,000 International Units) of vitamin A palmitate twice weekly in oral doses. Of the 57 animals receiving only the carcinogen, 30, or more than one-half, developed 42 squamous tumors in the bronchi and 27 developed 51 papillomas (tiny precancerous growths) of the forestomach. Of the 59 animals receiving the carcinogen plus vitamin A, only 13, or less than one-fourth, developed 25 papillomas of the forestomach.

What was particularly notable about Dr. Saffiotti's experiments was that of 17 animals that received the carcinogen plus the vitamin A, 10 exhibited squamous metaplasia (abnormal changes in the cells) *with no tumors*. But all the animals who got the carcinogen without the vitamin A had tumors along with squamous metaplasia. Dr. Saffiotti explained that the vitamin A prevented the squamous metaplasia initiated by the carcinogen from becoming squamous cell carcinoma.

This is information of the utmost importance to all of us whether we are smokers or not, for all of us are subject to the pollutants in the air. If we must inhale these cancer-causing benzopyrenes why not include the protective action of the vitamin A? Further experiments performed in 1968 by Dr. Saffiotti showed that vitamin A also inhibited cancer development in the upper stomach, the gastrointestinal tract and the uterine cervix of laboratory animals.

Much the same conclusion was reached by Raymond J. Shamberger, Ph.D., a Cleveland biochemist who published his findings in the *Journal of the National Cancer Institute* in May, 1971. Dr. Shamberger found that locally applied vitamin A had a powerful inhibitory effect on the development of cancer of the cervix, vagina, and lungs of hamsters which had been treated with a powerful chemical, DMBA, known to cause cancer.

Vitamin A Fights Cancer Virus

In tests with laboratory animals, vitamin A has shown promise as a health protector against a cancer-causing virus, specifically a virus known to cause cancer of the thymus in mice.

The new tests were carried out at the well-known Albert Einstein College of Medicine in New York City, supported by a grant from the National Institute of Health. Drs. Martin Zisblatt, Mark Hardy, Giuseppe Rettura and Eli Seifter published an abstract of their work in the *American Journal of Clinical Nutrition* (July, 1973) and reported on it at the First Joint Fall Meeting of the American Institute of Nutrition and the American Society for Clinical Nutrition at Cornell University, held August 14-17, 1973.

In the discussion of their experiments they point out that the thymus gland, located in the human being in the middle of the upper chest, plays a crucial role in the body's immunity system. Both in animals and in human beings, they say, if this gland is either surgically removed or has dwindled in size, the entire body becomes less able to carry out immune reactions. In the laboratory mouse, the gland will shrink when the animal is subjected to unusual stress. This particular kind of shrinking, the researchers previously demonstrated, can be partially prevented by feeding the animals a vitamin A supplement. However, the involution or shrinking of the thymus also occurs when the animals are inoculated with a cancer-causing virus known as murine sarcoma virus (MSV).

The researchers wanted to see what would happen to the

thymus if vitamin A were given to mice infected with the cancer virus. And their work showed that vitamin A does, in fact, delay the degeneration of the thymus when it must cope with the invasion of cancer virus. The mice were divided into a number of groups, receiving varying amounts of viral tumor extract, with each group further divided into those animals which did not get supplemental vitamin A and those that did.

Vitamin A dramatically reduced the incidence of tumors which developed in the infected animals, at least when they were infected with large amounts of the virus. In one group, 20 out of 20 control mice infected with the virus developed tumors, while only 13 of those who got the vitamin A developed tumors. In another group, 19 out of 20 unsupplemented animals developed tumors while only 11 of the supplemented animals did so. When a relatively weak concentration of the tumor virus was given to the animals, supplementation seemed to make no difference: the tumor rate was four out of ten in both groups.

The animals who developed tumors despite their vitamin A supplements did not develop the growths as quickly as the others. And once they appeared, *they regressed twice as fast* as the tumors in the other groups. In all animals that developed a tumor, the thymus gland decreased in weight, DNA, RNA and protein. This weakening of the thymus was delayed in those animals that received vitamin A. Likewise, the thymus gland recovered its normal weight faster in the supplemented animals.

From everything that they learned, the researchers tentatively concluded that "vitamin A appears not to be working directly as a selectively anti-tumor compound, but rather, it appears to affect the process of rejection of the tumor." They said that this ability to help the body reject the abnormal growth may be related to the antagonism of vitamin A to substances called glucocorticoids, which the body produces in response to stress associated with the invasion of the virus.

No one, it must be stressed, has proven clinically that vitamin A can prevent or cure human cancer. At the same time, a number of researchers have shown over and over again that vitamin A has a remarkable protective effect on laboratory animals that are exposed to irritating chemicals and even cultures of cancer cells. It would be remarkable indeed if this effect occurred only in test animals and not in human beings—even if it occurs in a slightly different way. Obviously, this thought is what is motivating the many researchers testing vitamin A and the officials of the National Institutes of Health and other major research organizations who are · funding continuing research into vitamin A's ability to fight cancer.

70. Vitamin B Deficiency, An Open Door For Cancer

One of the world's foremost authorities on the physiological development and effects of cancer was the late Professor Otto Warburg, two-time Nobel Prize winner and director of the renowned Max-Planck Institute for Cell Physiology in Berlin, Germany. At an assemblage of Nobel Prize recipients meeting in Lindau, Germany, in July of 1966, he declared that the three B vitamins, riboflavin (B_2), niacin (B_3) and pantothenic acid, together form a powerful team to fight off cancer. These are prominent constituents of brewer's yeast and desiccated liver.

Dr. Warburg's address, entitled "Concerning the Ultimate Cause and Contributing Causes of Cancer," explained that, in the final analysis, the thousands of secondary causes that stimulate and induce cancer are all reduced to a primary cause: oxygen starvation.

As little as a 35 percent reduction in the oxygen available to the cell, according to Dr. Warburg, causes the cell in its efforts to stay alive to make a fundamental metabolic switch. It gives up attempting to derive its energy from the oxidation (or burning) of food and instead turns to securing energy by fermenting sugar, a process that requires no oxygen. And it is this fermentation process which provides impetus for the growth of cancer cells.

Where do the B vitamins come in? The three named by Dr. Warburg—riboflavin, niacin and pantothenic acid—all act within our bodies as co-enzymes that are essential to the production and the full activity of the respiratory enzymes within the individual cells. In other words, according to this scientist, a basic reason for the formation of a cancerous tumor may well be that the particular tissues where the tumor forms lack one or another of these B vitamins and thus are unable to breathe properly.

B_3: Cancer Inhibitor
Before 1971, researchers were unable to isolate a specific member of the B complex family which had a distinct cancer

inhibiting effect. Researchers such as Dr. Kanematsu Sugiura of the Sloan-Kettering Institute had shown that desiccated liver and brewer's yeast, which both have a full complement of B vitamins, have an anti-cancer effect on test animals. Then a six-member West Coast research team identified nicotinamide, or vitamin B_3, as a cancer inhibitor. The team, under the direction of Dr. Loraine Bush, found nicotinamide to be consistently lacking in cancer cells and consistently present in normal cells. And it's nicotinamide that, when added to cancer cell cultures, has been shown to inhibit the cells' characteristic abnormal protein synthesis. In other words, vitamin B_3 may turn out to be the crucial ingredient that prevents a cell from proliferating and thus guards against the killer disease, cancer. The research team reported its findings in the February 1, 1972, issue of *Biochemistry* (journal of the American Chemical Society).

One of the differences between a normal cell and a cancer cell is that the normal cell contains an inhibitor of a certain enzyme involved in protein synthesis and cell reproduction, while the cancer cell does not. The enzyme, and therefore protein synthesis, is controlled by the inhibitor in normal cells. In cancer cells it is uncontrolled; cell proliferation goes wild.

Characteristically in cancer development, something goes wrong with a single cell, which multiplies to tumor size. It is only after the tumor is well developed that cancer spreads to distant sites—a process known as metastasis. And even when cancer has spread extensively and the patient is near death, most of his millions of cells remain normal; in light of the new research we can say that most of his cells continue to receive and contain enough vitamin B_3 to inhibit the activity of the enzyme in question—transfer RNA methylase, or tRNA methylase.

Why is the cancer cell lacking B_3 when it is nourished by the self-same bloodstream that provides the normal cells with adequate amounts? Perhaps, as Dr. Bush and colleagues speculate, cancer cells metabolize or degrade B_3 more rapidly and thus become depleted of the nutrient. Or perhaps there is something about the cancer cell that makes B_3 uptake difficult. Whatever the reason, it is clear that here we're dealing not with a simple deficiency but rather an unexplained abnormality of the cell in its relation to vitamin B_3 uptake or vitamin B_3 metabolism.

Nevertheless, the work of the West Coast researchers offers much hope in the fight against cancer. The discovery that abnormal enzyme activity can be inhibited in cancer cell cultures by the addition of nicotinamide suggests the possibility that here may be a new and better weapon for cancer treatment—an injectable anti-cancer agent that for once would not be a poison, a destroyer of normal cells along with cancer cells, but rather a nutrient that the entire body uses and needs.

71. Vitamin C Defends Tissue Against Cancer

The possibility that vitamin C deficiency may be causally related to cancer was a conclusion reached after years of study by the late Canadian physician Dr. W. J. McCormick. It is possible, he said, that "all physical and chemical carcinogens may act indirectly by bringing about or exaggerating a latent deficiency in vitamin C."

Dr. McCormick believed that an injury (whether it is an actual physical injury or a chemical injury) could lead to cancer if the body tissues affected were not cared for properly.

Dr. McCormick warned that the injury that leads to cancer produces a certain condition resulting in the formation of what some researchers call "pseudoelastic tissue." He quoted Dr. T. Gillman and colleagues, writing in the *British Journal of Cancer* (Vol. 9, pp. 272-283, 1955), as saying that such tissue is regularly encountered in sites of chronic injury to connective tissue in the skin as well as in other parts of the body—arteries and gallbladder, for example.

This tissue, which is preceded by and associated with an invasion of dermal cells by epidermal cells, can consistently be produced in human beings who have injuries. Dr. McCormick quoted the British researchers as stating, "It is shown that similar elastotic degeneration of collagen (tissue) is invariably present in the dermis in many degenerative skin conditions which may and frequently do become precancerous." They contended that such a degeneration of this layer of cells may play an important part in causing cancer.

Dr. McCormick often referred to a researcher who wrote in 1908 (long before vitamin C was discovered) that precancerous tissues always show a loss of connective tissue: the edges of the cells in the epithelium (the lining of all parts of the body) are frayed; yellow elastic tissue disappears; *and it is in this de-elasticized area where connective tissue has disappeared that the first beginnings of cancer occur.*

How Vitamin C Protects Intercellular Cement

We know that the cement holding cells together can be manufactured only if vitamin C is present in ample quantity. This cement becomes watery in an individual suffering from scurvy, the disease of vitamin C deficiency. The protein contained normally in this cement disappears into the blood. In cancer patients, tests have shown that there is an increase of this particular protein in the blood. When vitamin C is given, almost immediately the intercellular cement begins to reform in its normal consistency.

Several researchers have found that there is a pronounced deficiency of vitamin C in the blood of cancer patients, compared to that of healthy persons. It has been found that guinea pigs suffering from scurvy and given just enough vitamin C to be kept alive are far more susceptible to cancer and get it sooner than healthy guinea pigs.

Dr. McCormick believed that all this evidence shows definitely that the degree of malignancy of an illness is determined inversely by the degree of connective tissue resistance. And this, in turn, is dependent on the adequacy of vitamin C intake. In other words, the less resistant the connective tissue is, the more serious the trouble is likely to be. And lack of vitamin C is perhaps the basic cause of lack of resistance.

Hard Cancer Spreads Slowly

To illustrate this point, Dr. McCormick said that the scirrhus or hard cancer of the breast is slow to metastasize or spread throughout the body. It may remain just as it is, completely inactive for years. On the other hand, soft cancer of the breast is "extremely invasive." That is, it spreads rapidly to other parts of the body. In the former there is plenty of connective tissue which binds the cells together more effectively. In the second kind of cancer there are mostly only cells and the connective tissue is lacking.

It may be, said Dr. McCormick, that cancer cells, which are known to move around in the body, may do so because of an inherent propensity which becomes manifest solely because they have lost their connective tissue anchorage as a direct result of vitamin C deficiency.

So cancer may not be a "malignant" disease, striking its victims like a bolt of lightning out of the blue, but rather, said Dr. McCormick, it may be an ailment that we cultivate all during our lifetime by our habits.

Preventing Cancer Is The Important Thing

We should, then, direct our attention to preventing the cause of cellular disarrangement—that is, the breakdown of connective tissue. What about sores or fissures that fail to heal? What about unusual and easily produced hemorrhages—not necessarily with visible blood as in a nosebleed, but the bruises so many of us take for granted?

Dr. McCormick found that fully 90 percent of our adult female population show bruises or "black and blue marks," yet little or nothing is ever done about it. No one should ever show bruises unless he is in an extremely serious accident. The bumps and knocks we get in everyday living should never produce bruises. They are as easy to prevent as the nearest vitamin C tablet and a glass of water.

Easy bruising is one of the earliest—hence one of the most important—symptoms of vitamin C deficiency. And, make no mistake about it, bruising is a serious symptom. As Dr. McCormick suggested, it may be your first and most valuable warning of a predisposition to cancer.

Dr. McCormick believed that one reason we moderns are likely to be deficient in vitamin C is the almost universal habit of smoking. Smoking destroys or neutralizes to a large extent what little vitamin C is taken in food. The smoking of one cigarette, as ordinarily inhaled, tends to neutralize in the body about 25 milligrams of vitamin C, or the vitamin C content of an average orange. This fact alone would do much to explain the terrible increase in lung cancer in recent years.

But poisons other than nicotine are counteracted by vitamin C in the body. And the vitamin C is used up in the process. We know of many. Could it be that all physical and chemical carcinogens (causes of cancer) may act by using up the body's supply of vitamin C, thereby destroying the connective tissue and leading the way to cancer that spreads rapidly through the body?

Vitamin Status Study Advised For Middle-Aged

Dr. McCormick suggested that all persons of middle age or over should have a study made of their vitamin C status. Your doctor should be able to do it.

Or, as a general overall test, ask yourself these questions: Do your gums bleed or do you have some loose teeth? Do you bruise easily? Do you get colds easily? Do open sores heal slowly? Are you exposed to tobacco regularly, or smoke, or fumes of some materials like solvents, fresh paint, etc.? If you answer yes to any of these questions, better get concerned about your vitamin C status. Now, before there is any possible chance of a serious deficiency that might mean a predisposition to cancer.

A vitamin C supplement is your best assurance that you won't be short. In addition, concentrate on getting as many fresh raw foods as possible in your diet every day.

72. Folic Acid Acts As A Buffer In Cancer Treatment

After cancer surgery, powerful and potentially lethal medication is sometimes given to kill off any possible stray cancer cells that might have wandered to other parts of the body. A simple nutrient, folinic acid, the "active" form of the familiar B vitamin, folic acid, is used to protect other tissues against this poison.

Nutritionally minded people, of course, have long been familiar with the human need for folic acid. This B vitamin is one of a triad of nutrients (folic acid, vitamin B_{12}, and iron) essential for healthy red blood cells and for protection against anemia. We're beginning to realize that folic acid deficiency, brought on by a variety of factors—faulty diet, alcoholism and many commonly prescribed drugs—is probably a threat to a large portion of the American population.

Dr. Emil Frei III, of Harvard Medical School and the Children's Cancer Research Foundation in Boston, told about the treatment given to children suffering from bone cancer in an arm or leg at a St. Augustine, Florida seminar for science writers sponsored by the American Cancer Society.

Dr. Frei explained that after the patient's primary tumor is removed (usually by amputation), the great danger is that secondary cancer cells (metastases) will later show up elsewhere in the body, the lungs being particularly vulnerable. This spread of malignancy, according to Dr. Frei, occurred in 80 percent of the cases he had studied prior to the development of the new technique—a technique which involves a dangerous overdose of the anti-cancer drug, methotrexate, followed by a "rescuing" dose of folinic acid. Of the patients treated by the new method, he added, none has died over the observed period of 21 months and the spread of cancer cells has occurred in only one of the 17 cases.

Methotrexate inhibits cancer growth and is highly toxic to the rest of the body for one simple reason: it blocks the normal action of the nutrient, folic acid. The blocking action takes place at an early stage of folic acid metabolism in the body. The drug prevents the conversion of the nutrient to folinic acid. Since folinic acid is essential for the growth or multiplication of cells (because it is needed for the synthesis of the nucleic acids, DNA and RNA), this blocking action inhibits the multiplication of cancer cells. The catch is that it also hinders the renewal of billions of healthy body cells, including the red blood cells and the antibody-producing white blood cells, whose rapid multiplication is the body's normal immune response to threatened infection.

"Brinkmanship": A Vitamin Vs. Death

Dr. Frei practices what has been called "sophisticated brinkmanship" to obtain the anti-cancer benefits of methotrexate while minimizing its dangerous consequences. As he explained to the science writers' seminar, the drug in "potentially lethal doses" of about 200 times the conventional "safe" amount, is given to patients intravenously for about six hours; then, two hours later, folinic acid (also called "citrovorum") is injected. Folic acid itself, of course, would be useless in this treatment, since the methotrexate in the body would prevent the nutrient's conversion into its active coenzyme form. By injecting the preformed folinic acid, the physicians bypass the step where the drug plays its anti-folic acid role.

This whole procedure is repeated at intervals over a period of months. With the "rescuing" doses of folinic acid to save the patient's health and life, it is hoped that the massive drug therapy will "eradicate the cancer cells and not merely suppress their growth," Dr. Frei told the science writers.

The same technique has also been used in treating other forms of cancer, including cancer of the pancreas, colon, lung, breast, and liver, it was reported at the seminar by Dr. Isaac Djerassi of Mercy Catholic Medical Center, Darby, Pa.

This treatment is a very striking example of the grave consequences from a lack of functioning folic acid in the body. Recall that methotrexate's one property as a drug is to inhibit the action of folic acid, and this drug is known to bring death if given in large enough quantities to massively curtail folic acid's activity.

We can thankfully say that most of us will never come near the anti-folic acid drug, methotrexate. But can we be equally thankful that we *do* have our full complement of active folic acid helping to keep us healthy day after day?

73. Magnesium, Unheralded Cancer Preventive

In 1974 physicians were again noting patterns of correlation between magnesium deficiency and a higher incidence of cancer. The late J. I. Rodale discovered and interpreted reliable research materials on magnesium that had been overlooked for several years by most American medical authorities. In *Cancer: Can It Be Prevented?*, summing up earlier articles he had first written in 1950, he wrote: "We will talk about the researches of Professor P. Schrumpf-Pierron (a professor of medicine at The Sorbonne in Paris) whose work is written up in the *Bulletin de-l'Institute d'Egypte* (volume 14, February 15, 1932, and others). He talks about the rarity of cancer in Egypt where malignant cases are only about one-tenth that of Europe. What is the cause? After exhaustive studies in research, the professor came to the conclusion that it was due to too much potassium and too little magnesium in the food of the Europeans. On the other hand, in the soils of Egypt the conditions are reversed; that is, more magnesium in relation to potassium.

"There seems to be a definite relationship between magnesium and potash wherever it is found, whether in the soils, rocks, or other places. Where there is an oversupply of the potash there is always an undersupply of magnesium and vice versa. Schrumpf-Pierron studied the cancer statistics of France in relation to the rock structure underlying its soils. It worked most uncannily. Wherever he found an excess of potash, there he discovered less magnesium and more cancer cases. Wherever he observed a minimum of potash, he found a maximum of magnesium and fewer cancer cases. This means that people who eat food raised in certain soils obtain a nutrient from the rocks which underlie them, get certain elements into their food because of this . . . ."

But Mr. Rodale noted that the mineral value of potash should not be misinterpreted: "In connection with this information, let me stress that potassium is not a factor in cancer. On the contrary, potash compounds have been given as a medication in cancer. But evidently the reason Schrumpf-Pierron found more cancer in regions where the soils abounded in potassium was because of the low magnesium in such soils."

Mr. Rodale also drew from other works frequently overlooked by medical scholars, such as the work of F. L. Hoffman of the Biochemical Research Foundation of the Franklin Institute, Philadelphia, Pa., who, in 1937, also noted a correlation between cancer and areas of magnesium deficient soil. He included Hoffman's comments on the treatment of cancer patients with magnesium chloride. In all the cases observed, according to Hoffman's records, the cancer was "retarded considerably as the result of magnesium treatment."

From these studies Mr. Rodale formed his own theories as to the importance and interrelation of magnesium with other minerals and its effect on cancerous growth.

"Potash is as useful and indispensable to the plant as to man, but only when it is associated in a favorable ratio to magnesium and calcium. Magnesium acts as a 'brake for Cancer' (Pierre Delbert, *The Prevention of Cancer*), as much as an antitoxic potash. That is why 'the predisposition to cancer accompanied the deficit of magnesium reserve' (Dunbar and Voisnet). The older the individual is, the easier the intoxication by potash, because the organism grows older and becomes poorer in magnesium than the young organism; because this loss in magnesium decreases vitality, resistance, the power of regeneration of cells (Delbert) provoking a sort of cellular anarchy which favors the evolution of cancerous processes," concluded Mr. Rodale.

Recent Studies Support Mr. Rodale

These early writings of Mr. Rodale's have been supported in recent years by several medical tests and findings. Dr. P. Bois, M.D., Ph.D., chairman of the Department of Anatomy at the University of Montreal in Canada, startled members of the Federation of American Societies for Experimental Biology meeting in Atlantic City, New Jersey, in 1968 when he reported that he had performed a series of tests which demonstrated that merely by eliminating magnesium from the diet of rats, tumor growth could be triggered within a matter of 64 days. (Ordinarily, rats rarely develop cancer spontaneously. Scientists even have trouble causing tumors artificially in the laboratory.) Even more astounding, the site of the tumors developed in magnesium deficient rats was predictable: the thymus gland. And if the deficiency was not corrected, cancer developed in other parts of the body; eventually lymphoid leukemia followed.

"Magnesium is essential for numerous enzymic processes in the cell as well as for the integrity of the structure of the chromosomes and nucleic acids," Dr. Bois stressed. "Withdrawing magnesium may lead to mutation of those chromosomes, and the mutation may lead to tumor growth." Dr. Bois went on to explain that low magnesium levels produce high calcium levels and a loss of phosphate; hence, it may not be the lack of magnesium itself, but the result of other changes brought on by a lack of magnesium that is directly related to tumor growth.

Dr. Bois also explained that "there is a lot of magnesium in humans, in bone and urine. All foods have magnesium in them. But if your diet is too high in fats or lipids, you may need more than ordinary amounts of magnesium because you lose too much of the mineral in those substances."

Studies completed in 1974 by the Department of Pediatrics at the Fitzsimmons Army Medical Center, Denver, Colorado, appeared to bear out Dr. Bois's earlier reports when the Colorado tests indicated that magnesium deficient rats had impaired cellular immunity (*Lancet*, Sept. 7, 1974). "Because immunological surveillance including cellular immunity plays an important role in preventing carcinogenesis," read the report, "impaired lymphocytic function may explain the increased incidence of certain malignancies in magnesium deficient rats." The conclusions of these findings appear very much in line with J. I. Rodale's interpretation of Pierre Delbert's findings 24 years earlier.

Earlier in 1974 Herbert I. Sauer, of the Extension Environmental Health Surveillance Center at the University of Missouri, Columbia, told members at the annual meeting of the Water Quality Research Council that death rates attributable to cardiovascular-renal diseases, heart diseases and cancer in white, middle-aged people tends to rise as the amount of dissolved solids such as magnesium in their drinking water drops.

"Calcium and magnesium, which are the major constituents of hard drinking water," according to the report in *Family Practice News* (June 15, 1974), "have consistently negative correlations with cardiovascular-renal diseases and cancer."

Most food buyers in the United States don't know when they are buying foods grown in magnesium deficient areas. As J. I.

Rodale noted in his book, *The Prostate* (Rodale Books, Inc., 1967), "there is widespread magnesium deficiency in the states of New Jersey, Maryland, Virginia, both Carolinas, Georgia and Florida, and there is some lack in Illinois, Michigan, New York and the New England states. With our nationwide distribution of food, we can never tell when we might be getting what we eat from one of these low magnesium regions."

In May, 1968, Dr. Lewis B. Barnett, a retired orthopedic bone surgeon from Center, Colorado, reported on tests he conducted involving 5,000 people in which 60 percent of the subjects proved to be deficient in magnesium. On the basis of his findings, Dr. Barnett recommended 600 milligrams of magnesium a day. How can you be sure of getting that much? Make sure your diet is rich in green leafy vegetables (uncooked), in raw nuts and seeds and, to be on the safe side of the mineral balance, take a dolomite supplement. Dolomitic limestone supplies a good balance, not only of calcium and magnesium, but also of many trace minerals which in minute quantities play an important and often overlooked role in human nutrition.

74. Nitrilosides: A Natural Cancer Fighter In Search Of Recognition

The existence of cancer-causing factors in processed foods is a fact with which most of us are well acquainted. Certain coal tar dyes used to artificially color a wide variety of foodstuffs, the synthetic hormones and chemical additives fed to livestock and sometimes found as a residue in their meat, cyclamates once used as artificial sweeteners—these are just a few examples of the substances which have produced cancer in test animals and are therefore presumed dangerous for people to eat.

But few of us have even considered the possibility that certain *natural* food substances may have just the opposite effect— hindering or halting the growth of cancer within the body.

This idea is not quite as whimsical as it may sound. Scurvy, after all, once killed thousands of sea-going men before it was discovered that citrus juices contain a natural substance (later dubbed vitamin C) which prevents its outbreak. The idea that food could prevent this horrible disease seemed so strange at the time it was first published that many decades passed (many sailors, too) before all ships began to stock fruit. Today we know that pellagra, beriberi and rickets are also diseases brought on by a deficiency of naturally-occurring beneficial food substances.

And we are only just beginning to find out that natural food substances do more than prevent deficiency diseases. There is accumulating evidence that they play a vital role in protecting the body from disease and healing damaged tissue. Dr. Gordon W. Schlegel at Tulane University, for example, has shown that vitamin C blocks the invasion of bladder cancer in mice. Dr. Daniel Menzel of Battelle-Northwest Institute has demonstrated that vitamin E can protect mice against the deadly effects of air pollution. Umberto Saffiotti of the National Cancer Institute blocked lung cancer in mice with vitamin A. We now know that the trace element zinc plays a vital role in healing burns and speeding the mending of fractured bones in animals. Ample niacin and pantothenic acid have now been proven necessary for the production of infection-fighting antibodies, and so it goes, as researchers begin to understand the multiple protective roles of each and every dietary element for health.

Vitamin B$_{17}$

Some researchers who have spent a quarter of a century or more studying the question are convinced that there is one class of natural food substances which have a specific anticancer effect. These substances are known variously as nitrilosides, amygdalin, or vitamin B$_{17}$, and are found in the seeds of fruits and grains. The theory that nitrilosides actually prevent or retard the growth of cancer cells is based on two lines of evidence. One is that doctors who have used nitrilosides on thousands of cancer patients are enthusiastic about the results. They don't say it cures cancer, only that in many instances it halts the deadly progress of the disease. Dr. Ernst T. Krebs, Jr., a biochemist and co-discoverer of Laetrile, a controversial cancer treatment (Laetrile is the proprietary name for one nitriloside), says nitrilosides are nontoxic, water-soluble accessory food factors found in abundance in the seeds of almost all fruits.

The other line of evidence is of a purely deductive nature. And that is that so-called primitive peoples, among whom most forms of cancer are extremely rare, eat a diet very high in nitrilosides. Conversely, in nations where cancer is near the top of the killer list, the diet contains very little or no nitrilosides.

Cancer is a rare occurrence among the Taos (New Mexico) Pueblo Indians and the residents of a place called Hunza, a tiny country hidden in the mountain passes of northwest Pakistan. Both groups are known to have diets rich in foods containing nitrilosides. The traditional beverage of the Taos Pueblo Indians is made from the ground kernels of cherries, peaches and apricots. Robert G. Houston, who has written several articles on the New Mexican Indians, said that he enjoyed this beverage when he was in New Mexico gathering material for a book dealing with cancer prevention.

When he came home, Houston began to make blender shakes based on an Indian recipe. Into a glass of milk or juice he mixed a tablespoon of honey with freshly ground apricot kernels (1/4 of an ounce or two dozen kernels) which had been roasted for 10 minutes at 300°. It is vitally important to roast the kernels first, Houston said, "in order to insure safety when you are using the pits in such quantities." Roasting destroys enzymes which could upset your stomach if you eat too many at one time. In any event the drink was so delicious that Houston kept having it daily. On the third day of drinking this concoction, Houston said that a funny thing happened. Two little benign skin growths on his arm, which formerly were pink, had turned brown. The next day, he noticed that the growths were black and shriveled. On the seventh morning, the smaller more recent growths had vanished completely and the larger one, about the size of a grain of rice, had simply fallen off. Houston says that two of his friends have since tried the apricot shakes and report similar elimination of benign skin growths in one or two weeks.

How Nitrilosides Fight Cancer

It is illegal for a doctor in the United States to prescribe nitrilosides. Although they are included in the diets of millions of healthy people, the Food and Drug Administration believes that because nitrilosides contain cyanide, they are potentially hazardous. People who have studied the nitrilosides chemically and clinically agree that the cyanide in them is indeed a killer—but only, they claim, the cancer cells.

Here is the explanation of this strange phenomenon given by Emory W. Thurston, Ph.D., Sc.D., executive secretary of the Institute of Nutritional Research in Los Angeles: "The cyanide contained in amygdalin can be split off only by a special kind of enzyme. Fortunately, cancerous growths possess such an enzyme, thus making cancer cells vulnerable to the poisonous cyanide. Furthermore, cancer tissue does not possess a certain protective enzyme which is found in normal, non-cancerous tissue. This enzyme transforms cyanide into a relatively harmless substance.

"Although cyanide is very poisonous, it is not destructive to noncancerous tissue in small doses as it is converted by the body's protective enzyme into a substance which is harmless to man. Therefore the cancer cell is poisoned by even small amounts of cyanide, while the healthy tissues are unharmed. Circulating through the body is this enzyme. It must have sulphur present in a form the body can use. Where the body is deficient in sulphur, it can be supplied by taking a very small amount of sodium thiosulphate. So little of the protective enzyme is present at any time that cyanide compounds still remain a dangerous poison unless administered very slowly. Cancer tissue, fortunately, having none of this protective enzyme is very vulnerable and the cyanide is extremely poisonous to cancer tissue, even in small amounts, no matter how slowly the cancer is exposed to the cyanide."

Dr. Dean Burke, chief cytologist at the National Cancer Institute, calls Laetrile "remarkably nontoxic . . . compared with virtually all cancer chemotherapeutic agents currently studied."

Where To Look For Nitrilosides

Ernst T. Krebs, Jr., a prominent biochemist from San Francisco, California, is perhaps the one man best qualified to speak on the subject of nitrilosides. He says: "Nitrilosides are non-toxic, water-soluble, sugary-looking accessory food factors, found in abundance in the seeds of almost all fruits and over 1,200 other plants. Wherever primitive peoples have been found to have exceptional health, with a marked absence of malignant and degenerative disease, their diet has been shown to be high in the naturally occurring nitrilosides. These substances, which are accessory food factors and as such might be classified as vitamins, are widely distributed in nature. They're in the arctic tundra, with its mosses and lichens, cloud-berry and salmon berry. They're found in the grassy plains, with their mountain blueberries and common pasture grass. And they're found in the tropics, with its profusion of delicious fruits."

In a lecture before the New England States Natural Food Associates Convention in Manchester, Vermont, Dr. Krebs emphasized the wide availability of nitrilosides in several rich sources common to Vermont. The wild crabapple, the market cranberry, the smaller cranberry found growing in moist places, all contain from one-half to one percent nitrilosides, or B_{17}. Also on the list of plants named are the scarlet strawberry and the hawthorne apple. Among the wild grasses mentioned were the common vetch, white clover and lupine.

Other familiar foods, wild and cultivated, and occurring in many states, include the quinces, peaches, plums, apricots, cherries and apples, *when eaten whole including the kernel or seeds;* red and black raspberries, blackberries, huckleberries and gooseberries. All contain the nitrilosides in great quantity when made into fresh raw juice, stewed fruit, or jams and jellies in which the pits or seeds are utilized.

Now we know why our grandmothers, in their primitive wisdom, cracked the apricot or peach kernels and included them in stewed fruits or canned fruits for winter. In fact, in the less affluent societies, the kernel of such fruits was always used as part of the diet.

From the legume family many varieties were mentioned by Dr. Krebs; Mung beans and lentils (especially high in nitrilosides when sprouted), shell beans, lima beans (a particularly rich source), garbanzos or chick peas, fava beans and some varieties of garden peas. Grains high in nitrilosides are millet, buckwheat and the flax family. All species of the passionflower fruit, and cassava, the bread of the tropics, are rich sources of B_{17}.

Dr. Krebs reminded his listeners that bears and other animals always eat the whole fruit. They eat first the sweet flesh, then hoard and eat the pits. "If we were cast upon a desert island," said Dr. Krebs, "we might see many fruit trees. At first we would likely eat only the sweet watery fruit. If we continued to do so, we would become very sick and die within three months. We would lack proteins, fats, and vitamins. But if we ate the whole fruit, including the seed or pit, the proteins, fats and vitamins contained in this vital natural food would allow us to live in health to a ripe old age."

We may ask ourselves, if such an abundance of nitriloside-bearing foods are all about us, why is it that so little finds its way into our daily diet? One answer is that we have selectively bred out of our plants and taken out of our diet these highly protective food factors. At first this was accidental as men bred wild peaches, plums, apricots and the like, for sweeter, more abundant fleshy fruit in place of the somewhat bitter flesh of the wild varieties. This bitterness, of course, was due to the nitrilosides in the flesh of the fruit. The soft edible seeds of any of the common fruits are still a very rich source of this protective vitamin.

In addition to accidental elimination of the nitrilosides, man-made changes in seed-bearing plants to obtain higher yields or longer shelf life have depleted food plants even further. Before its hybridization corn carried B_{17} in large quantities. A few open-pollinated strains are left today and they are still rich in this nutrient as well as higher in other vitamins and minerals. Navy beans, broad beans, garden peas and most other legumes were rich in nitrilosides in their native state. Those grown today in Burma may run over 1,500 parts per million.

Another important reason for the acute deficiency of the nitrilosides is that in the last 50 years people in this country have begun to eat great quantities of poor quality carbohydrate foods.

Prepared cereals, syrups, candies, white sugar and white flour, bakery products, macaroni, white rice, pastries, sugary jams and jellies are being consumed in ever increasing amounts. These foods are being used to replace many of the vital protective foods, the fresh fruits and vegetables, whole grains and high grade proteins that formerly made up a large portion of our diets. This severely limits the amount of nitriloside-bearing foods we eat, as well as other important nutrients.

When cattle are fed on the quick growing green grasses, such as alfalfa, Johnson grass, clover, vetch and Sudan grass, their milk and the cheese made from it are high in B_{17}. Today, most milk and cheese no longer contain these protective elements.

Sorghum cane is high in nitrilosides; sugar cane and the sugar made from it have none. Most people in our country today do not use sorghum from the whole sorghum grass, but instead use white sugar made from only part of the sugar cane. Molasses has value as a source of minerals, but it contains no B_{17}.

No area of the earth that supports vegetation lacks nitriloside-bearing plants; all life on earth participates directly or indirectly in the chain of nitriloside metabolism, yet we are living in the face of a great deficiency. Dr. Krebs and others claim this is evidenced by the shattering fact that one out of every three of us is dying of cancer.

75. Predictive Medicine Can Anticipate Cancer

Predictive medicine is a discipline Dr. Emanuel Cheraskin, M.D., D.M.D., Department of Oral Medicine, University of Alabama Medical Center, and a small group of doctors have been advocating for more than 15 years. Unlike traditional medicine, predictive medicine helps to intercept disease rather than wait for disease to develop and then try to cure it.

"With illness rampant nationally," Dr. Cheraskin wrote, ". . . the cost in time, money, grief, productivity, makes it imperative to exploit immediately all avenues leading to the *anticipation* or primary prevention of disease. For too long, attention has been simply directed to the *identification* and treatment of long-standing common killing and crippling disorders. Hence, there is a real and long overdue need for a fresh approach to health. The singular features of *predictive medicine* provide the possible solution. . . .

"For practical purposes and as an immediate working hypothesis, *predictive medicine* may be defined as the clinical discipline designed to *anticipate* disease. The intent, by such an approach, is to foretell illness before it erupts and thus institute *primary* prevention (prevention of occurrence). This philosophy immediately sets *predictive medicine* apart from conventional medicine where the cardinal theme is the *identification* of disease with subsequent treatment and, at best, *secondary* prevention (prevention of recurrence)" (*Journal of the Southern California Dental Association*, Vol. 37, No. 7, July, 1969).

Sugar And Cancer

For instance, Dr. Cheraskin and his associates have discovered that a study of carbohydrate metabolism—fundamentally of the way your system reacts to an overload of glucose—can give significant indications of whether or not you will develop cancer in the future.

What Professor Cheraskin and his associates did was to take advantage of the annual diabetes detection drive in Birmingham,

Alabama, as well as the availability of dental patients at the Department of Oral Medicine at the University of Alabama. They gathered what most doctors would consider unrelated statistics to see if a correlation could be established between them. They studied two groups of dental patients, one comprising 120 and the other 170 persons, all of them well by normal medical criteria. Three hundred and sixty-two more people were examined in the course of the diabetes detection drive for 1964. Values were obtained from all persons for fast blood glucose. These were then compared to figures revealing the incidence of tumors in these persons.

They found here a predictive tool of tremendous importance. There was a definite correlation between the incidence of tumors and a high blood glucose level. Even small variations in blood glucose provided some measure of predictiveness, Dr. Cheraskin told an American Medical Association convention in June, 1966. There is then a strong indication that anyone whose metabolism is unable to rapidly clear the blood of an excess of sugar is more likely to develop tumors in later age than one whose blood clearing mechanism is more efficient.

How much better to have a test that will show you when you are 20 how you can avoid tumors that might devastate you at age 40 than a "smear" technique that tells you when you're 39 you've already got it, you need surgery, or else.

This is the big difference between Cheraskin's predictive medicine and what the medical profession hails as the great advances in preventive medicine. Make no mistake, preventive medicine has its place and it is, of course, much better to remove a carcinoma before it metastasizes. But, how much better never to get a tumor at all!

76. A Survey Of Unorthodox Cancer Treatments

Everyone has his own idea of just what a "quack" can be. To most of us it means a crackpot who peddles useless products at exhorbitant prices. In recent years the term has been widened to include anyone who promotes a treatment which is not in complete accord with the policies or attitudes of organized medicine. People who are against fluoridation, no matter what their background, are classified by some as quacks; those who are convinced of the power of vitamin E are called quacks; an advocate of natural food in the diet is labeled a quack, etc. But the term, in its most damning sense, is reserved for those who would presume to treat cancer by means of anything but surgery or radiation. It might be an untrained country boy who has treated his local neighbors with a homemade remedy, or a bona fide researcher who has tested his treatment in a hundred scientific ways. If the medical fraternity frowns on the treatment, the treatment is finished. The developer and his associates are branded as quacks. Your doctor will be told it is a worthless treatment. He might run into serious professional trouble if he uses it.

Actually how good is the treatment? Medical authorities say it is no good. The researchers says it is beneficial. He has lists of patients who are willing to testify that they were helped, even completely cured, by the treatment. But once that first verdict has been handed down, nobody of any influence or authority will listen, or look at the evidence.

If the medical profession wants to find a cancer cure, why is it not willing to look for it wherever it might be? Are we to miss it because it originates in a small laboratory in the Southwest instead of the stainless steel and stone skyscraper of a multimillion-dollar research center? It is as though we had refused to use electricity because it was discovered by a publisher instead of a scientist, or refused to enjoy the Mona Lisa because it was painted by an inventor, instead of a fulltime artist.

Laetrile

Laetrile is a controversial anti-cancer agent made from apricot pits. Though it has been in and out of the headlines, hailed as nature's answer to cancer and condemned as a worthless sugar molecule, actually the average doctor knows no more about it today than he did 40 years ago.

Thus, in spite of the fact that the federal government and most politicians are now firmly committed to the establishment of a "Conquest of Cancer" agency—funded with hundreds of millions of dollars—not one dollar will be used to conduct Laetrile tests on humans, even though advocates of Laetrile include a number of outstanding doctors and scientists around the world—in Germany, Italy, the Philippines, Canada, Mexico, Belgium and a few in the United States.

To explain their rejection, the cancer specialists said that Laetrile might be poisonous and had no effect whatsoever on the regression of tumors in test animals. This is directly contrary to the results of extensive tests made by Dr. Dean Burk, chief cytologist of the National Cancer Institute, who has reported that Laetrile is "remarkably non-toxic . . . compared with virtually all cancer chemotherapeutic agents currently studied." It is also not much of an explanation in view of the fact that every substance used in the accepted treatment of cancer, drugs and radioactive materials alike, is definitely and beyond doubt poisonous. Furthermore, in answer to claims by the National Cancer Institute (NCI) and the federal government's Food and Drug Administration (FDA) that there is no proof substantiating the claim that Laetrile has any inhibiting effects on tumor growth, Dr. Burk states that tests have been performed which prove that the product has an effect on tumor regression in test animals. Dr. Burk calls the claims by the NCI and FDA "deceptive," asserting that the anti-cancer activity of Laetrile has been shown in "at least five independent institutions in three widely-separated countries of the world, with a wide variety of animal cancer."

Laetrile is a natural substance, discovered by Dr. Ernst Krebs, Sr., of San Francisco, California, who was always careful to explain that he did not develop Laetrile—nature did that. He considered it a vitamin, which he called B_{17}, maintaining that Laetrile is to cancer what vitamin C is to scurvy; what vitamin B complex is to pellagra; what B_{12} is to pernicious anemia. His son Dr. Ernst Krebs, Jr., says in a paper, *The Laetriles–Nitrilosides in the Prevention and Control of Cancer*, (published by The

McNaughton Foundation), "Cancer is a chronic disease and no chronic disease has yet found therapeutic or prophylactic resolution except by accessory food factors (vitamins) which are normal to the normal diet; one of the truly fixed laws of physiology, without exception. Night blindness, once considered incurable, found resolution in vitamin A; beriberi through vitamin B_1; rickets through vitamin D. Even mental illness is now known to be due to the deficiency of micronutrients normally present in the brain."

The McNaughton Foundation, a nonprofit organization formed originally in Canada, has significantly funded research into the value of Laetrile as a cancer fighter over the years. Other sizable donations have come from the government of the province of Quebec, Timex Corporation and several other large industrial organizations in the United States, Canada and Europe, as well as public-spirited individuals in other countries.

Serving with Andrew McNaughton, president of the McNaughton Foundation (whose late father was General A. G. L. McNaughton, commander of the Canadian Armed Forces in Wolrd War II and president of the Security Council of the United Nations and of the National Research Council of Canada), are three directors and thirteen advisory board members, all with distinguished credentials in the sciences or in the business community.

The purpose of Laetrile, according to Andrew McNaughton, is that in advanced cases of cancer it has a palliative effect, reducing the need for narcotics, improving the subjective condition of the patient—he feels better and doesn't have pain. Objectively, his blood pressure picture improves and he gains weight and frequently goes back to work until eventually he dies of cancer because he's an advanced case. But he dies without the pain and the total dependence on narcotics, generally because the damage to vital organs has eliminated his ability to sustain life.

"We claim it on the basis of thousands of cases observed. In earlier cases where there's not been damage to vital organs beyond the point where there's inadequate capacity for the organ to sustain life, in those cases patients frequently live to die of other causes.

"The real quacks are those who pretend to knowledge they don't have about Laetrile, and condemn it without knowledge. We have many patients," McNaughton said, "who say Laetrile has cured their cancer. We don't agree—we never say it cures. At best, we say it will eliminate a tumor. To remove the tumor, however, is only attacking symptoms. The disease is an underlying deficiency of nitrilosides (B_{17}), inadequate pancreatic function, the presence of trophoblasts at a site of estrogen production."

Some of the controversy surrounding the manufacture of Laetrile is due to the fact that when the apricot pits are crushed a certain amount of cyanide is secreted, but, according to McNaughton and the developers of Laetrile, cyanide naturally occurring in food is not dangerous. Primitive people who eat only whole natural organic and unfractionated foods, they say, regularly ingest from 250 to 500 milligrams of organic cyanide each day. This natural cyanide is locked in a sugar molecule. It is normal to our metabolism and is found in over 1200 known unrefined foods and grasses. When it is eaten and taken into normal cells, the enzyme rhodanese detoxifies the cyanide and releases it into the urine.

But,—and this is the rationale of Laetrile treatment—cancer cells are completely deficient in rhodanese, and are surrounded instead by another enzyme called beta-glucosidase. This enzyme, they claim, which is secreted by the cancer cell, in turn releases the bound cyanide from the amygdalin (another name for Laetrile) at the site of malignancy, and the released cyanide destroys the cancer cells. Thus, in the belief of its advocates, organic cyanide is a highly selective substance which shoots at the enemy only. It is toxic to cancer cells—and completely nontoxic to normal cells.

Dr. Ernst T. Krebs, Sr., of San Francisco was the first in this country to experiment with its therapeutic properties. He worked with it from the 1920's until his death in 1969. Another pioneer in its use is Charles Gurchot, Ph. D., former biochemistry instructor at Cornell University Medical School, author of *Biology–Key to the Riddle Cancer,* former assistant professor of pharmacology at the University of California Medical School, San Francisco, and for more than a decade, research consultant to the McNaughton Foundation.

So ingrained is the concept of surgery/irradiation as the sole hope for whipping cancer that a Laetrile patient often has trouble convincing family and friends that the drug has saved his life. But whether others believe it or not, the patient whose life is at stake usually gives credit to the drug and diet and other elements of the treatment, as well as to the doctors.

The Gerson Treatment

Max Gerson, M.D., who died in 1958, was a German-born doctor who discovered a dietary treatment for a type of skin tuberculosis in 1929. Arriving in America in 1936, he brought with him another dietary "cure"—this time for cancer. His clinic in Nanuet, New York, claimed considerable success in curing without surgery or radiation, cancers of the skin, esophagus, liver, bone, lung, breast, stomach and brain in terminal cases given up by doctors.

It was Dr. Gerson's theory that cancer results from faulty metabolism, aggravated by long-term exposure to the irritating agents of civilization—pesticides, chemical fertilizers, and pollution of water and air. He believed in restoring proper body chemistry by enabling the most vital organ—the liver—to rid the system of accumulated poisons resulting from the inability of a damaged digestive tract to cope with these irritants in the body. The medication and diet he developed for promoting such liver function relied upon the juices of many kinds of fruits and vegetables, iodine solutions, vitamins, and liver extracts to restore proper enzyme performance and metabolic function—and as many as six enemas a day to prevent the re-absorption of toxic elements through the intestinal walls. Foods rich in potassium, needed for muscular and kidney function, must saturate the cells in order to drive out sodium, the surplus of which hampers recovery of organs.

The treatment prohibited bottled, canned, frozen, refined, preserved, and flavored foods in addition to coffee, sugar, chocolate, alcohol, salt, tobacco, berry fruits, mushrooms, nuts, pickles, water (since stomach capacity was needed for the great quantity of juices), and the use of hair dyes, aluminum utensils, pressure cookers, fluorides, mouthwash and plastic bags. Animal protein is omitted for the first six weeks. Oatmeal, apples, potatoes, and fresh greens were highly recommended.

Dr. Gerson believed that the chemical and artificial treatment of the soil was depriving us of greatly needed natural elements. For this reason, the dietary treatment consisted of organic foods to fortify the liver, which would then be better able to combat the unnatural condition of cancerous cells. In his book, *A Cancer Therapy: Results of Fifty Cases* (1958), Dr. Gerson wrote: "For the benefit of coming generations, I think it is high time we change our agriculture and food preservation methods. . . . The coming years will make it more and more imperative that organically grown fruits and vegetables will be, and must be, used for protection against degenerative diseases, the prevention of cancer, and more so in the treatment of cancer."

The writings of Dr. Gerson always emphasized that this drastic treatment was designed specifically for cancerous conditions, and was by no means to be used as preventive therapy by a healthy person. Dr. Gerson believed that a patient cannot treat himself at home alone since medication and diet must be adapted to individual needs. In addition, another person must be available to administer enemas and to provide a constant supply of nourishment from a busy kitchen. Yet, even the expectation of some physical discomfort and exertion did not discourage a large number of patients from besieging the already filled-to-capacity clinic.

Dr. Gerson was highly esteemed by such honored men as the late Dr. Albert Schweitzer. Although his clinic claimed to have cured patients of cancer, the extent of such claims remains unconfirmed because no one was willing to investigate.

Insulin—The Beale Treatment

Dr. Samuel Beale, of Sandwich, Massachusetts, used insulin to treat cases ranging from minor skin cancer to cancers of the eye and the breast. Records and pictorial slides show the progress they made. The need for surgery, he said, was eliminated in many of the cases and tumors unaccountably regressed and disappeared. "I have never claimed insulin as a cure for anything, but as an adjunct to accepted methods. This statement applies particularly to cancer, although sometimes insulin alone is all that is required."

Dr. Beale discovered insulin's regenerative action on abnormal tissue totally independent of any other research. In treating a near-gangrenous infection of the toe in a 63-year-old patient, he found the patient slightly diabetic and began insulin injections. A remarkable improvement in the toe as well as the diabetes followed. The diabetes was soon controllable with diet alone. But when the insulin was stopped the toe changed for the worse. Dr. Beale suspected that the insulin had exerted a healing influence on the degenerating tissue of the toe. He began using small doses of insulin for healing and continued using it on ulcers and other serious skin breaks from that time, with no dangerous side effects.

Dr. Beale did not realize then that the rationale for using insulin to treat cancer was gaining support. Scientists knew then that each cell contains a minute amount of insulin. Was this factor missing from malignant cells? Dr. Beale believed it was, and it was this lack that caused the cell to go haywire.

The reaction encouraged by insulin in the cells is oxidation, the burning of oxygen. This gives the cell its energy and promotes its proper function, according to Dr. Beale. No other substance but insulin can do this job as nature intended, and that is why all normal cells are equipped with it, said Dr. Beale. He suggested that malignant cells short on insulin, or without it entirely, use sugar erratically, through undisciplined fermentation. He believed that insulin, restored to the cells through injections of small doses (two to three units) encouraged malignant cells to revert to a normally regulated energy supply.

Critics have raised the question that if an insulin shortage of the cells is related to the development of cancer, all diabetics should be likely candidates for this disease (there is no proof that this group is any more susceptible than others), and diabetics who have cancer should be relieved of the cancer when insulin is used. Dr. Beale answered that the exact cause of diabetes is not yet understood by medical men. Diabetes itself may be caused by the body's inability to use insulin properly, rather than an actual shortage of this hormone. Also, the effect of the minute doses of insulin Dr. Beale prescribes was entirely different from that of the large doses used in treating diabetes.

While Dr. Beale may have been the American physician most experienced in using insulin to treat cancer, he was not the only one using it. Serge A. Koroljow, M.D., a New Jersey physician, reported on insulin for cancer in *Psychiatric Quarterly*, April, 1963. He was convinced too, that somehow insulin can help to control the spread of cancer in some (not all) cases. Koroljow said the insulin somehow interferes with the capacity of cancer cells to reproduce, or it might act to strengthen the normal cells which border the cancer so that they can resist invasion.

Dr. Koroljow reported that in Germany insulin is used routinely in the treatment of cancer. In Russia results have been demonstrated that make the outcome of accepted cancer treatments in the United States appear very pale indeed. One Russian report describes sixteen cancer patients treated with insulin.

Four of the patients recovered completely, ten had temporary remission of three to six months, and two showed no change. In Italy and Spain, as well as in South America, insulin is an orthodox part of cancer therapy, according to Koroljow. In the United States, it is barely known.

Krebiozen

The drug Krebiozen has had a well-publicized and stormy history. It was first introduced into this country in 1949 by Dr. Stevan Durovic, a former assistant professor at the University of Belgrade, Yugoslavia. He came to the United States after several years of experimentation in South America with a drug which he had discovered and which he believed to be a cure for cancer. Dr. Durovic developed the substance when he injected horses in Argentina with a sterile fungus. The horses' systems produced a natural substance which fought the infection. It was this substance, essentially a fat molecule in combination with six natural sugars, that later became known as Krebiozen. Once in the United States, Dr. Durovic met Dr. Andrew C. Ivy, at that time vice president of the University of Illinois and head of its huge Medical School, who became interested in the theory and possibilities of Krebiozen.

The drug has been the source of both legal and emotional controversy between the FDA and the NCI, who claim that the drug has absolutely no therapeutic anti-cancer value, and Dr. Ivy and other doctors and patients, who claim documented proof that Krebiozen does have a nontoxic, anti-cancer effect on certain types of cancer. The furor over Krebiozen reached a peak in November of 1964 when Dr. Ivy and Dr. Durovic, doing business as Promak Laboratories, his brother, Marko Durovic, a lawyer, the Krebiozen Research Foundation, and Dr. William F. P. Phillips, a Chicago physician who prescribed the drug to several patients, were indicted on 49 counts for violations of the Food, Drug and Cosmetic Act, mail fraud, making false statements to the government, mislabeling and conspiracy. It took nine months for the case to be heard, with 121 government witnesses and 57 defense witnesses taking the stand. The 700 exhibits could literally be weighed by the ton, and court reporters estimated the transcript as running to 20,000 pages of testimony.

Early in the trial, both defense and government attorneys said they would confine the case to an examination of whether the four defendants had violated FDA regulations in shipping the drug out of Illinois. However, this point was never seriously contested by the defense, and the emphasis shifted to the question of fraud: Did the defendants knowingly promote a "worthless drug"? The jury then became involved in determining the efficacy of a drug and a mode of cancer therapy, which Dr. Ivy had earlier said "would be most undesirable." On January 30, 1966, Drs. Ivy and Phillips and Mr. Marko Durovic were acquitted. On the following day, January 31, the jury found Dr. Stevan Durovic and the Krebiozen Foundation innocent of all charges. Several jurors said they had not been convinced that Krebiozen was worthless. "I felt it never did get a fair test," said one (Joseph Bukowski). "Everyone felt that way. We thought the evidence against them was not good enough." The jury foreman, Adolph Beranek, said, "I feel Krebiozen does have merit as a treatment for cancer. It should not be eliminated completely." Despite the verdict, federal law prohibited the shipment of Krebiozen across state lines in late 1966. Several patients who were residents of other states have since moved to Illinois where the dispensing of the drug was still allowed.

Dr. Ivy has carried on his studies on Krebiozen alone since 1967 because Dr. Durovic left the country shortly after the trial. In an interview with CBS News in February of 1967, Dr. Ivy said that he had a new name for his anti-cancer substance; he no longer called it Krebiozen but Carcalon. In an interview in the April 2, 1967 edition of *Chicago's American,* Dr. Ivy said: "I've manufactured some of the drug myself. I call it Carcalon, not Krebiozen. Krebiozen is a commercial name; Carcalon is its biomedical name. But it's the same thing." Dr. Ivy, no longer associated with the Krebiozen Research Foundation, is now Research Director of the Ivy Cancer Research Foundation, where he treats patients with Carcalon, which he derives from cow and horse plasma.

Drosnes-Lazenby Treatment

The Drosnes-Lazenby treatment was developed by two lay people, Philip Drosnes and Lillian Lazenby, who had worked for years in their Pittsburgh, Pennsylvania laboratory conducting experiments with a mold substance they grew. Excited about the possibilities of using the mold for cancer treatment, they went to the Director of the National Cancer Institute who listened to them carefully and encouraged them to go ahead. Six years of hard work went by—years in which Philip Drosnes and Lillian Lazenby spent their own time and money buying laboratory equipment and working almost around the clock on experiments to prove cancer tissue could be broken down and destroyed by the substrate of their mold. (A substrate is the liquid that drips from the mold—the extract of the mold.)

They had gotten something started that they couldn't stop. What if this were the long-sought key to the problem of cancer? Or what if it might throw some light—even if ever so little—on the problem? This was the thought that kept them going through one discouragement after another. Finally they were convinced that they had found an organism under their microscope which existed in cancerous tissue and also existed in the mold they had grown. By injecting the substrate from their mold they could stop cancerous growth in their laboratory animals. And the organism no longer appeared in the formerly cancerous tissues.

Analysis of the mold product made by the National Institute of Health showed that it contained two substances called Rhizopus and Mucor as well as various strains of penicillium. The name of the substance—Mucorhicin—is derived from the names of these various elements. Sending a report of this to Mrs. Lazenby, the National Institute suggested that she interest some local physician in giving the antibiotic (as it could now be called) to cancer patients and make careful studies of results over a long period of time. Paul A. Murray, M.D., of Pittsburgh, who was already using the antibiotic, proceeded enthusiastically to give it to cancer patients and to work closely with the discoverers to keep records of his patients.

At the Drosnes-Lazenby Clinic a rule was made to take only "terminal" cases of cancer, that is, patients whose cases had been declared hopeless by their physicians and who had been sent home to die. They must present at the clinic a statement from their physician or hospital giving the diagnosis of cancer.

But the Drosnes-Lazenby Clinic did not claim to have a cancer cure. They believed wholeheartedly that they had discovered something of great value to humanity and they wanted the chance to try it out on people already given up for dead. But it was not as simple as it sounds. Mr. Drosnes and Mrs. Lazenby were eventually arrested on the grounds of practicing medicine without a license.

If you inquire, you will probably be told that the Drosnes-Lazenby treatment for cancer was thoroughly investigated and found to be worthless. Actually, no bona fide investigation was ever done. No official representative of the Cancer Society, the Public Health Service, the Medical Association, or any other professional group, ever went over the case histories, interviewed patients or studied the formula and processing of Mucorhicin, the mold substance which was used at the Drosnes-Lazenby Clinic.

The Koch Treatment

Dr. William F. Koch used Glyoxylide, a substance designed by Koch to convert the poisons which he believed cause cancer into antitoxins which, by chain reaction, would eliminate the cancerous condition. He used this substance in connection with a rigid diet. Dr. Koch insisted that both must be used, since neither diet nor Glyoxylide would be effective separately.

Dr. Koch was outspoken in his criticism of surgery as a treatment for cancer, and was equally critical of those who promoted surgery in such cases. Due to public pressure, the Wayne County Medical Society of Detroit, Michigan, was forced to initiate an investigation of the Koch treatment. The procedure devised was completely fair and thoroughly practical. The only trouble was that the agreed-upon procedure was ignored by the investigators leaving the initial hearing totally inconclusive.

A second hearing was arranged with much difficulty, and in spite of opposition by the AMA, Dr. Koch presented a number of patients who had been diagnosed as hopeless and whom he said he had cured. The committee simply denied both the diagnoses and the cures. In one case a husband testified that his wife had been cured of Paget's disease after she had refused an operation to remove the cancer that had spread from her breast, because it might have meant the loss of her arm. Her surgeon who examined her during the course of her recovery acknowledged in the presence of her husband that she had been cured of cancer. When he was called before the committee, the surgeon testified that his original diagnosis had been falsified and that the woman's condition had really been a simple ulceration, and not cancer at all. He did not say why he had been willing to operate so radically on such a mild condition.

A campaign against Koch and his formula followed the hearings. Even those who employed Glyoxylide were in danger of losing their professional standing. Meanwhile, still another cancer investigation was set up, this time in Ontario, Canada.

Cancer

Cancer Incidence by Site and Sex*

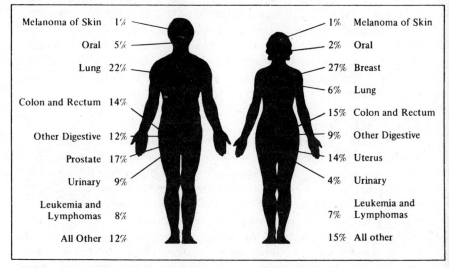

Melanoma of Skin	1%			1%	Melanoma of Skin
Oral	5%			2%	Oral
Lung	22%			27%	Breast
				6%	Lung
Colon and Rectum	14%			15%	Colon and Rectum
Other Digestive	12%			9%	Other Digestive
Prostate	17%			14%	Uterus
Urinary	9%			4%	Urinary
Leukemia and Lymphomas	8%			7%	Leukemia and Lymphomas
All Other	12%			15%	All other

*Excluding non-melanoma skin cancer and carcinoma in situ of uterine cervix.

Cancer Deaths by Site and Sex

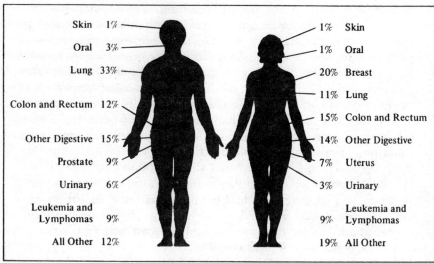

Skin	1%			1%	Skin
Oral	3%			1%	Oral
Lung	33%			20%	Breast
				11%	Lung
Colon and Rectum	12%			15%	Colon and Rectum
Other Digestive	15%			14%	Other Digestive
Prostate	9%			7%	Uterus
Urinary	6%			3%	Urinary
Leukemia and Lymphomas	9%			9%	Leukemia and Lymphomas
All Other	12%			19%	All Other

Credit for illustrations and charts: *Courtesy of the American Cancer Society, Inc.*

Reference Chart: Leading Cancer Sites, 1975

SITE	ESTIMATED NEW CASES 1975	ESTIMATED DEATHS 1975	WARNING SIGNAL IF YOU HAVE ONE, SEE YOUR DOCTOR	SAFEGUARDS	COMMENT
BREAST	89,000	33,000	LUMP OR THICKENING IN THE BREAST.	ANNUAL CHECKUP. MONTHLY BREAST SELF EXAM.	THE LEADING CAUSE OF CANCER DEATH IN WOMEN.
COLON AND RECTUM	99,000	49,000	CHANGE IN BOWEL HABITS; BLEEDING.	ANNUAL CHECKUP INCLUD-ING PROCTOSCOPY, ESPECIAL-LY FOR THOSE OVER 40.	CONSIDERED A HIGHLY CURABLE DISEASE WHEN DIGITAL AND PROCTOSCOPIC EXAMINATIONS ARE INCLUDED IN ROUTINE CHECKUPS.
LUNG	91,000	81,000	PERSISTENT COUGH, OR LINGERING RESPIRATORY AILMENT.	PREVENTION: HEED FACTS ABOUT SMOKING. ANNUAL CHECKUP. CHEST X-RAY	THE LEADING CAUSE OF CANCER DEATH AMONG MEN, THIS FORM OF CANCER IS LARGELY PREVENTABLE.
ORAL (INCLUDING PHARYNX)	24,000	8,000	SORE THAT DOES NOT HEAL. DIFFICULTY IN SWALLOWING.	ANNUAL CHECKUP.	MANY MORE LIVES SHOULD BE SAVED BECAUSE THE MOUTH IS EASILY ACCESSIBLE TO VISUAL EXAMINATION BY PHYSICIANS AND DENTISTS.
SKIN	9,000***	5,000	SORE THAT DOES NOT HEAL OR CHANGE IN WART OR MOLE.	ANNUAL CHECKUP. AVOIDANCE OF OVEREXPOSURE TO SUN.	SKIN CANCER IS READILY DETECTED BY OBSER-VATION, AND DIAGNOSED BY SIMPLE BIOPSY.
UTERUS	46,000**	11,000	UNUSUAL BLEEDING OR DISCHARGE.	ANNUAL CHECKUP, INCLUD-ING PELVIC EXAMINATION WITH PAP TEST.	UTERINE CANCER MORTALITY HAS DECLINED 65% DURING THE LAST 35 YEARS, WITH WIDER APPLI-CATION OF THE PAP TEST. MANY MORE LIVES CAN BE SAVED, ESPECIALLY FROM CERVICAL CANCER.
KIDNEY AND BLADDER	43,000	17,000	URINARY DIFFICULTY. BLEEDING—IN WHICH CASE CONSULT DOCTOR AT ONCE.	ANNUAL CHECKUP WITH URINALYSIS.	PROTECTIVE MEASURES FOR WORKERS IN HIGH-RISK INDUSTRIES ARE HELPING TO ELIMINATE ONE OF THE IMPORTANT CAUSES OF THESE CANCERS.
LARYNX	9,000	3,000	HOARSENESS—DIFFICULTY IN SWALLOWING.	ANNUAL CHECKUP, INCLUD-ING MIRROR LARYNGOSCOPY.	READILY CURABLE IF CAUGHT EARLY.
PROSTATE	56,000	19,000	URINARY DIFFICULTY.	ANNUAL CHECKUP, INCLUDING PALPATION.	OCCURS MAINLY IN MEN OVER 60, THE DIS-EASE CAN BE DETECTED BY PALPATION AND URINALYSIS AT ANNUAL CHECKUP.
STOMACH	23,000	14,000	INDIGESTION.	ANNUAL CHECKUP.	A 40% DECLINE IN MORTALITY IN 20 YEARS, FOR REASONS YET UNKNOWN.
LEUKEMIA	21,000	15,000	LEUKEMIA IS A CANCER OF BLOOD-FORMING TISSUES AND IS CHARACTERIZED BY THE ABNORMAL PRODUCTION OF IMMATURE WHITE BLOOD CELLS. ACUTE LEUKEMIA STRIKES MAINLY CHILDREN AND IS TREATED BY DRUGS WHICH HAVE EXTENDED LIFE FROM A FEW MONTHS TO AS MUCH AS TEN YEARS. CHRONIC LEUKEMIA STRIKES USUALLY AFTER AGE 25 AND PROGRESSES LESS RAPIDLY.		IF DRUGS OR VACCINES ARE FOUND WHICH CAN CURE OR PREVENT ANY CANCERS THEY PROBABLY WILL BE SUCCESSFUL FIRST FOR LEUKEMIA AND THE LYMPHOMAS.
LYMPHOMAS	29,000	19,000	THESE DISEASES ARISE IN THE LYMPH SYSTEM AND INCLUDE HODGKIN'S AND LYMPHOSARCOMA. SOME PATIENTS WITH LYMPHATIC CANCERS CAN LEAD NORMAL LIVES FOR MANY YEARS.		

*All figures rounded to nearest 1,000.
**If carcinoma-in-situ is included, cases total over 86,000.
***Estimates vary widely, from 300,000 to 600,000 or more, for superficial skin cancer.
INCIDENCE ESTIMATES ARE BASED ON RATES FROM N.C.I. THIRD NATIONAL CANCER SURVEY

Chart courtesy of the American Cancer Society, Inc.

Cancer

The proceedings were conducted in a dignified and impartial manner. One witness, Dr. J. W. Kannel of Fort Wayne, Indiana, told of treating 72 patients in 14 years with Glyoxylide, due to their own pleadings, though he considered many of these too hopeless to treat in any way. He reported that 21 of these were still alive and four others had died of other causes. Dr. Kannel said that Glyoxylide was the only remedy that had offered him hope in treating cancer, in contrast to his poor results after 24 years of experience with X-ray or radium treatment and surgery. In spite of such evidence, no formal report of this hearing was ever published. Dr. Koch was prosecuted in two more FDA trials concerning Glyoxylide which ended in a permanent injunction against Koch Laboratories. Dr. Koch finally assigned the manufacturing process of Glyoxylide to a Detroit religious organization where the preparation was incompetently processed and was no longer effective.

Section 14
Celiac Disease

77. The Devastating Gluten Allergy

77. The Devastating Gluten Allergy

Idiopathic celiac disease is a common wasting disease of infants. Children who suffer with it are small and emaciated. The abdomen is swollen and muscles are underdeveloped. The liver is abnormally small, growth is retarded, and there is marked emaciation of the trunk, arms and legs. By impairing the absorption of vitamins, this disease will lead to various deficiency diseases such as anemia, rickets, osteoporosis, and scurvy.

According to three Dutch doctors, Weijers, Vanderkamer, and Dicke, writing in *Advances in Pediatrics* (9: 277-318, 1957), "There are no known specific agents for the treatment of celiac disease . . ." In other words, there are no drugs, no medicines, not even a vitamin that will bring about improvement in this disease, although various nutrients have improved the general condition of patients by counteracting deficiencies caused by the disease. There is only one treatment known for celiac disease. It is to eliminate all gluten from the diet. "The harmful effects of wheat and rye, in contrast to the harmlessness of their starch, have been demonstrated," state the Dutch doctors, and "In a series of investigations, we proved that gluten, the protein of wheat flour, and especially its gliadin fraction, was responsible for the noxious effect."

The authors point out that, while in the past doctors had treated celiac disease by ordering all starch-containing foods removed from the diet, this was not at all necessary and was in fact a shot-gun treatment. The authors demonstrated in controlled hospital experiments that all that was needed was to banish gluten from the diet. "When wheat was banished from the diet and rice or buckwheat flour, cornstarch and peeled boiled potatoes were substituted for wheat in the diet of celiac patients, the anorexia, vomiting, and abdominal pain vanished. There were no more attacks of acute diarrhea, the feces became darker, the patients gained weight and resumed normal growth and height or even more than normal."

One of the nutrients gluten malabsorption causes to be carried out of the system instead of being utilized is dietary iron. Theoretically, simple iron deficiency anemia is an easy disease to treat and cure. Sometimes, however, the disease proves intractable—administration of iron and B vitamins just has no effect on the anemia. In such a case, it is pointed out by doctors Zachary Kilpatrick and Julian Katz in the *AMA Journal* (May 12, 1969), the physician would do well to investigate the possible presence of celiac disease.

Adults who attempt to lose weight by going on excessively rigid diets, may be courting celiac disease. Dr. F. E. Pittman, reporting in *Gut* (April, 1966), found that only a gluten-free diet brings a normal response in such people.

Doctor Pittman believes that the protein deficiency that can occur in extreme reducing diets, or the heavy use of laxatives, sometimes produces alterations in the gastrointestinal tract which make it especially vulnerable to the admitted toxic effects of wheat gluten.

Celiac disease may be a factor in schizophrenia, too. It was Dr. F. Curtis Dohan, M.D., who first noticed that the mental symptoms caused by celiac disease very closely resemble those of the schizophrenic.

Specifically, Dr. Dohan and his associates at the William Pepper Laboratory of Clinical Medicine began suspecting the gluten-like proteins in cereals when they learned that patients suffering from the non-tropical sprue ailment known as celiac disease also demonstrated marked mood and behavioral changes. Dr. Dohan also found that when victims of celiac disease were placed on diets completely free of wheat, rye, barely and oat-meals, their mental conditions improved markedly, followed closely by improvements in their physical symptoms.

Section 15 Childhood Diseases

78. Good Diet Essential For Children Taking Vaccines

Before the various vaccines and antibiotics were discovered, children's diseases were far more prevalent and much more serious than they are today. Smallpox, a dreadful disease which claimed many lives, has practically been eliminated in this country. Polio is no longer a threat. Diphtheria shots, routinely given to infants, have virtually eradicated that disease. There are also vaccines to combat measles, mumps and whooping cough, and if a child does get one of these diseases, it need not prove dangerous if the child is properly cared for.

But the effects of these vaccines are not all positive. Although they perform an invaluable health service they can also heavily tax the resources of a child's body.

Even in the presence of an adequate diet, the strain placed on the body by these medicines threatens protective stores of vitamin C, the B vitamins and intestinal flora. Any child who is receiving treatment to either cure or prevent these childhood diseases should also be getting supplementary vitamins B and C, either in tablet form, or in foods such as wheat germ, brewer's yeast and fresh fruits and vegetables. He should also have a regular intake of foods such as yogurt and buttermilk that encourage the growth of intestinal flora.

79. Crib Death

During the chilly months of winter, thousands of chubby, apparently healthy babies are put to sleep by their mothers and never awaken. In the morning, they are found dead. The parents are dumbfounded, heartbroken; their pediatrician puzzled. In some cases the doctor had examined the infant only a day or two before and pronounced him to be the very picture of health, growing rapidly. And then, from the pathologist who performs the autopsy comes the report: crib death.

And what does "crib death" mean? Only that the baby is dead and all the resources of modern medicine cannot figure out why.

Crib death, also known as SIDS for Sudden Infant Death Syndrome, and in Britain as S.U.D. for Sudden Unexpected Death in Infancy, is the worst killer of children between the ages of one week and one year, far ahead of cancer. It takes the lives of more children under 15 than any other cause except accidents. Its tide of death reaches the flood during winter, but no one knows why. One in every 350 children will die from crib death, and there is evidence that the rate is rising.

The parents of crib death children often spend years dwelling on the circumstances of their children's deaths, possessed by the question: *why*? And although the amount of research money channeled into investigation of crib death is much smaller than its seriousness warrants, there are many medical researchers equally possessed by this question. Drawing on evidence amassed in the last few decades, various doctors have theorized that the deaths are caused by milk allergy, viral infection, bacterial infection, stress, a deficiency of immunoglobulin, or some other cause. But other investigators have shown that all these theories have significant weaknesses, and none of them are completely satisfactory. Crib death remains a terrible but fascinating mystery which continues to attract the attention of many brilliant scientists, who are attempting to put together the diverse pieces of evidence into a meaningful pattern, much as a homicide detective attempts to solve a single baffling murder. And still, the culprit remains unidentified.

One of the most scientifically creative attempts to solve this mystery has been made by Dr. Joan L. Caddell, a pediatric cardiologist affiliated with the St. Louis University School of Medicine. Published in the *Lancet* (August 5, 1972), the distinguished British medical journal, her theory is that the real killer in crib death is a critical deficiency of the mineral magnesium.

Asked how she came to suspect a deficiency of magnesium as the possible cause of crib death, Dr. Caddell explained that in 1962, the Rockefeller Foundation sent her to Uganda to establish a heart clinic for children. "Many of the children were suffering from severe malnutrition, but after treating them, we discovered that the health of their hearts as revealed in the electrocardiogram was getting worse, not better. We then learned that some of the symptoms we were seeing in these children were the same as those produced experimentally in dogs which have been deprived of magnesium.When we added magnesium to our regimen, the children improved dramatically." (Previously, it had been thought that generous amounts of protein, calcium, vitamins and all the other "major" nutrients were sufficient to restore health to the malnourished child. Dr. Caddell's discovery showed dramatically that magnesium in more than merely trace amounts is vital to a child's health.)

First Clues To The Killer

But is it really possible to compare the nutritional status of severely deprived children to that of well-fed American babies? Significantly, at about the same time that Dr. Caddell published her findings in the scientific literature, another major study of magnesium metabolism was published in the *American Journal of Clinical Nutrition* (June, 1964) by Mildred S. Seelig, M.D. Dr. Seelig's own exhaustive studies and her review of previous research showed quite conclusively that most Americans are in fact deficient in magnesium. In most cases, this is a borderline deficiency.

The link between Dr. Caddell's work and Dr. Seelig's work is in the fact that the kind of sub-clinical deficiency described by Dr. Seelig, which does not produce obvious symptoms in the mother, can nevertheless expose that mother's infant, under certain circumstances, to a truly critical deficiency of magnesium.

After her experiences in Africa, Dr. Caddell continued to pursue the relationship between magnesium levels and the health of children. After studying several hundred case histories of crib death, and reviewing a vast body of medical literature, she framed a hypothesis stating that the difference between the 349 children who do not die of crib death and the one child who does is a slight but critical difference in magnesium stores, primarily as a result of insufficient magnesium in the mother during gestation, and secondarily as a result of the infant's own diet.

Growth Taxes Baby's Magnesium

The great preponderance of crib death, or S.U.D., as Dr. Caddell calls it, occurs between the second and fourth months of life, peaking at about two months. This coincides with the infant's most rapid period of growth. And curiously enough, most S.U.D. victims have gained weight well and may in fact be overweight for their ages. At this period of life, children typically exist on a diet exclusively of milk, usually cow's milk or formula, or on milk plus enriched baby cereals. These facts alone made Dr. Caddell suspect magnesium deficiency, because as protein is synthesized in the rapidly growing babies, magnesium stores are swiftly exhausted. The faster the rate of growth, the faster the depletion of magnesium.

Formula or cow's milk is not only rich in protein, but also in calcium and phosphorus. Both of these minerals, necessary as they are, sharply reduce the amount of magnesium the infant can utilize by competing for absorption in the intestines and then for reabsorption in the urinary tract. Milk is a poor source of magnesium to begin with, so the competition is fierce. Because calcium is absorbed preferentially, magnesium always comes in a poor second.

Enriched baby cereals only aggravate the situation, because they are heavily fortified with both calcium and phosphorus but not magnesium. In addition, all cereals contain phytic acid, which interferes with absorption of all minerals from the intestine. There is so much calcium and phosphorus added to this cereal that the interference is insignificant. But for magnesium, it is a loss the infant cannot afford.

Advantages Of Breast Milk

What about breast milk? At one time, crib deaths were associated with nursing mothers, because only the poorest women nursed. Many of these women had grossly inadequate diets and so it is logical to assume that they were unable to provide their babies with sufficient magnesium either before birth or while nursing. But this is no longer the case. Today, most women who nurse their babies are relatively well-educated and sophisticated. More important, they tend to be very knowledgeable and conscientious about dietary matters. Many take vitamin supplements. There is another factor, too. Although breast milk actually contains less magnesium than cow's milk, the amount of calcium, and especially phosphorus, is so much greater in cow's milk that the net effect, according to Dr. Caddell, is that the bottle-fed baby probably receives less usable magnesium than the breast fed baby. Perhaps it is because of this that crib death is very rare among breast-fed babies today.

About one-third of all crib deaths involve babies who are born prematurely. Yet, when they die, they have been gaining weight very rapidly and show no particular signs of weakness. This fits in with the notion that magnesium deficiency is involved, because prematurely born infants are very low in magnesium. (The magnesium level rises sharply during the last period of gestation.) And their subsequent rapid growth may exhaust what small stores of magnesium they have, as the mineral is pressed into service to build protein.

Many crib death babies die very suddenly—usually in their sleep—but some deaths have been observed and the signs and symptoms duly noted. A very common sign is blueness of the skin, along with cold hands and feet, resulting from a lack of oxygen, and difficulty in breathing. About half the infants show relatively mild symptoms during the last day or so of life, including coughing, wheezing, loss of appetite, vomiting or diarrhea. They may be pale, limp, and listless, or they may be restless, irritable, or even convulsing. From a doctor's point of view, findings inside the baby are equally important. Chief among these in the crib death infant are swelling and inflammation of the lungs and respiratory tract, water and blood in the lungs, and marked spasticity of the small tubes connecting the lungs to the bloodstream. The curious thing about all these symptoms is that when you add them up, they create a picture which is identical to fatal anaphylactic shock in adults. Dr. Caddell cites three studies which corroborate this.

But what is anaphylactic shock? Basically, it is an extremely rapid and catastrophic reaction of the circulatory system to some foreign protein or substance. Such shock may occur in a person with a very high degree of allergic sensitivity who is stung by a bee. Within a few moments, the victim's circulatory system is in a virtual state of collapse, his throat may be swollen as to completely block the intake of air, and he may be hemorrhaging severely internally.

But of course, the crib death baby has not been stung by any insect nor even taken any new food or drug which might cause this fatal reaction. What then could bring on all these symptoms? The answer, Dr. Caddell theorizes, might well be magnesium deficiency.

Low Magnesium Can Trigger Histamine Shock

How so? First of all, *magnesium deficiency triggers the liberation of histamine without need of any external irritant.* Histamine is the substance responsible for the swelling and irritation of delicate membranes of the respiratory tract in people suffering from hay fever and other allergies. Some people, of course, are extremely susceptible to histamine-induced pathology. It is a fact that newborn babies can release a far greater relative amount of histamine than adults, or even children past the neonatal period. The flood of histamine released from certain cells causes exaggerated dilation of blood vessels and vastly increased permeability of capillaries, so that the blood with all its vital nutrients, including oxygen, leaks uselessly out of its prescribed course and collects in sites such as the lungs. Histamine can also cause release of heparin from the liver, which decreases the coagulability of the blood and aggravates this condition.

There is a great concentration of crib deaths during the winter, and also between midnight and 6 a.m. This ties in with two other factors which are known to favor histamine release: low temperature and low blood sugar.

Dr. Caddell found another clue in a medical report which suggested that when magnesium levels are low and calcium levels normal, there can be increased acetylcholine at motor-nerve endings, with the result that relaxation of the nerves would be difficult. And this fact, Dr. Caddell suggests, could well account for the nervous irritability, including tetany and convulsions, which are often seen in both crib death infants and older youngsters known to be suffering from magnesium deficiency.

Mother's Diet Is Crucial

One point that we should emphasize about Dr. Caddell's theory is that *this chain of events resulting in death could not begin in the first place unless the mother was deficient in magnesium.* In fact, animal studies show that when maternal magnesium stores are borderline, the mother will retain what she needs and short-change the embryo.

How much magnesium does a woman actually need? The absolute *minimum* amount, according to Dr. Seelig, is about 6 milligrams a day for every kilogram of body weight. This means that a woman weighing 120 lbs. should have a magnesium intake of 330 milligrams a day—at the very least. Chemical surveys have shown that this is just slightly more than the amount that most women actually get from magnesium-rich foods such as beet greens, cucumbers, cauliflower, almonds, and cashews. But many get *much* less. Dr. Seelig says that a safer level would be 10 milligrams of magnesium a day per kilogram of weight, or 550 milligrams of magnesium for a 120 lb. woman. And when a woman is pregnant or lactating, this higher amount should certainly be her minimum intake.

Fortunately, there *is* a way to be totally assured that your magnesium intake is adequate, regardless of your taste buds or dietary habits. And that is to take your magnesium daily in the form of a naturally-occurring mineral substance known as dolomite. Dolomite, or dolomitic limestone, is an edible form of magnesium mixed with calcium which is extracted from deep mines. Its magnesium and calcium occur in the highly desirable ratio of one to two. It is tasteless, prepared both as pills and chewable tablets, and is perfectly safe and non-upsetting to the system. The expectant mother could hardly ask for a more convenient or less expensive form of insurance against magnesium deficiency.

If Dr. Caddell's theory about the cause of crib death turns out to be correct, we should all rejoice, because prevention will be so easy. But even if it should prove no more reliable than the other theories which have been put forward over the years, we should still be thankful to this very talented and dedicated pediatrician for alerting all of us to the crucial role which magnesium plays in maintaining the health of the newborn child.

80. Measles (Morbilli)

In North America and Europe measles is a rare cause of death compared with the high mortality rate (15 percent or more) in primitive countries. According to *Nutrition Reviews* (August, 1968) this difference may be due to differences in the nutrition of the host rather than the virulence of the virus.

A survey of 426 measles cases in Senegal shows that measles frequently precedes severe malnutrition. "In measles cases from six villages there was a higher mortality in those children who were underweight and this was irrespective of the pulmonary complications." The largest number of those who died fell into the age bracket of two to three years. It is possible that protection was provided by better nutritional status in the young, breastfed children. Children one to three are more likely to be malnourished as they go off the breast.

In the opinion of *Nutrition Reviews*, "It seems that a child's nutritional state helps determine the severity of, and the chances of survival from, an attack of measles," and "measles can then seriously impair the surviving child's nutritional status. . . "

The measles vaccines which have been widely used in the United States since 1966 have further reduced our incidence of measles. The vaccine shouldn't, however, be used without regard for the possible consequences. Children who get the wrong kind of measles vaccine are in for quite a time, if they are among the unlucky ones who get a reaction. The *American Academy of Pediatricians Newsletter* (November 16, 1967) said that the reactions include "an atypical rash that begins on the feet and spreads upward, high fever, edema and pneumonia." Children who have been inoculated with an inactivated or killed measles vaccine are especially susceptible. The Academy recommended that these children be given attenuated (weakened) live vaccine as soon as possible. But at the same time it warned that some children might develop a similar reaction from the live vaccine.

The measles virus is a dangerous one, whose effects can lead to encephalitis or retardation. Within one or two weeks of coming in contact with the disease, a bumpy, pinkish rash appears on the neck and face and within a few days spreads over the entire body. Measles is contagious for about nine days. Unfortunately, this period includes four days before the rash has manifested itself and so children are frequently exposed to the virus unknowingly.

Fever, cold, cough and koplik spots inside the throat and mouth precede this rash. When the rash is full-blown, fever dissipates and other symptoms gradually disappear.

Measles is sometimes treated with antibiotics. However, if the exposure is known prior to the time the symptoms show up, an injection of gamma globulin can be given to insure a light case. After symptoms have appeared gamma globulin is not effective. A bout of measles generally insures life-time immunity.

Live measles virus vaccine can be used to produce an immunity that is thought to be good for life. But it may result in fever about a week after the injection.

Killed measles virus provides immunity which only lasts a few years.

81. German Measles (Rubella)

This virus caused disease starts with a slight fever accompanied by a swelling of glands on the back of the head and neck, and a pimply rash starting on the face and working its way downward. This rash covers the entire body within 24 hours. Headaches and red eyes are not uncommon. These symptoms appear about two to three weeks after exposure. This disease is spread through contact with an infected person over the period from the beginning of the symptoms until three or four days after the onset of the rash.

German measles are not usually serious in childhood but they pose the threat of retardation or heart problems to the unborn fetus carried by a pregnant woman who contracts the disease. This is especially true if the woman is in her first trimester of pregnancy.

There is a live German measles vaccine which is administered to children. The specific length of immunization provided by this vaccine is not known but it is presumed to be lengthy.

82. Mumps (Parotitis)

Mumps may begin with fever and vomiting or there may be no noticeable symptoms until the swelling starts in the parotid gland on the jaw line just below the ears. Often one side will swell before the other and sometimes only one side will swell at all.

A severe case may result in swollen salivary glands and swelling of the pancreas, as well as the ovaries in females and the testes in males.

Incubation period for this infectious disease is from two to three weeks from time of exposure. Contagion continues as long as the swelling lasts.

Bed rest is the recommended treatment.

One bout of mumps generally insures a lifetime immunity. It is believed that live mumps virus vaccination also confers lifetime immunity.

The vaccine is usually administered to children and pre-adolescents. It is considered especially important that boys be immunized as a severe case of mumps in a male past puberty may cause infertility.

There is another vaccine which may be given immediately after exposure, but this hyperimmune mumps globulin only protects for a few weeks.

Before being immunized with either of these vaccines, it would be wise to submit to a skin test for mumps immunity. This simple test using mumps antigen, has shown that a vast number of people who have never had mumps are nonetheless immune to the disease.

83. Scarlet Fever (Scarlatina)

A streptococcal infection which starts with fever, vomiting, sore throat and general irritability, scarlet fever is closely related to strep throat. These symptoms appear abruptly and are followed within a few days by a bright-red rash on the back, chest and neck. The rash may cover the entire body, but for some reason it does not affect the face and scalp.

The rash lasts about six to eight days, at which time it fades and the skin commences to peel in tiny pieces.

There is no preventive for scarlet fever, but it is usually treated with antibiotics to control the infection. Bedrest is also prescribed by most doctors.

On rare occasions, scarlet fever leads to rheumatic fever. Earaches and swollen glands are signs that the disease is more severe than usual. The attending physician should be notified at once if these symptoms occur.

84. Whooping Cough (Pertussis)

This acute inflammation of the air passages is characterized by paroxysms of coughing which terminate with a whooping sound. Whooping cough is a pertussis bacterial infection and is transmitted by direct contact with discharges from the mouth of an infected person.

It starts with a dry cough that usually develops from about a week to three weeks after exposure. It is at this time that the disease is more contagious, although some degree of contagion continues for the entire period of the cough, which often lasts a full six weeks. From the third to the fifth week the cough may become very severe. In fact, it is sometimes so difficult for the child to catch his breath that he turns blue.

Either tetracycline or chloramphenisol are used to treat whooping cough.

Three injections of pertussis vaccine administered at once a month intervals are now generally started when an infant is two months old. This only provides partial immunity, however. If a child is exposed to whooping cough he is given a booster shot.

Pertussin immune anti-serum or hyperimmune pertussis gamma globulin provide about four to six weeks immunity. These are often given to those who have been exposed to whooping cough but have never been immunized with the pertussis vaccine series.

85. Diphtheria

Diphtheria is spread through contact with secretions from the nose and throat of an infected person. The disease presents itself within a week of this contact. It is manifest by a high fever, extremely sore throat with a pus-like substance, headache, cough and a nasal discharge often containing blood.

Penicillin injections are usually begun by the doctor as soon as exposure is known, and penicillin is generally continued orally for about ten days. Diphtheria antitoxin and erythromycin are also commonly used in treating diphtheria.

Since the discovery and general use of diphtheria toxoid this disease is no longer the health hazard it once was. These inoculations, which are given during infancy, do not provide lifetime immunity, however, and booster shots are given at ten year intervals.

Section 16 Circulation

86. Thick Blood Imperils Your Health: Vitamin E Thins It Safely And Naturally

If your blood is too thick, it will slow down your circulation. This slowed circulation can be the cause of many life-threatening complications. It is a condition so serious that doctors frequently treat it with special drugs to thin the blood, even though they know it is risking internal hemorrhage.

Even the obsolete practice of blood-letting is being reconsidered to lower the hematocrit (the measurement of blood thickness or viscosity). It was found in a Georgia study (*New York Times*, February 14, 1972) that those men who donated blood every two and one-half months were able to maintain their hematocrit at a normal 42 percent. Acting on such information, Dr. Leonard J. Stutman at St. Vincent's Hospital in New York conducted a blood donation program for 2,500 male volunteers, to see if it would reduce the incidence of coronaries and strokes. The existence of too-thick blood implies an error in the machinery or the metabolism which may temporarily benefit from blood-letting or blood thinning, but will benefit much more from a change in some habits.

To find out if your river of life has become sluggish, try this simple test. Press your fingertips hard against a table top, desk, windowsill, or whatever. Did your nails become red or a deep pink? If so, congratulations. Your blood is doing its job—carrying micronutrients to your extremities. You can probably assume that your blood is fulfilling its primary mechanical function as a conveyor system. It is conveying oxygen from your lungs to your cells; carbon dioxide from your tissues back to your lungs to be expelled with every exhalation; nutrients from your stomach and intestines through your liver to your tissues; waste products from your tissues to your excretory organs; and hormones, enzymes and other chemical compounds between all parts of the body.

If your nails remained pale when you pressed your fingers down, it might be that your circulation has slowed down and nutrients are not being delivered where they are urgently needed. Your blood, because it is not flowing freely, may have a tendency to form clots, and you could be headed for trouble.

The viscosity of your bloodstream is a vital index to your well-being. The delivery of nutrients and adequate oxygen to the many cells of the body is in itself a massive logistics problem which cannot be performed perfectly when the blood is hampered by a sluggish flow. The consequences of failure to deliver nutrients or even of just a poor job are not only cell starvation, but serious damage from inadequately removed waste products. This can lead to many degenerative conditions—kidney problems, faulty memory, as well as heart and blood pressure diseases and strokes.

There is a delicate balance in red blood cell physiology, however, which must be observed. While too many red blood cells impair the circulation, a shortage of red blood cells is anemia. This shortage would, of course, lead to a lower hematocrit and a lower viscosity, but the advantage of a lower viscosity in this instance is outweighed by the insufficiency of delivered oxygen, which of course leads to other serious consequences.

While lots of red blood cells are usually equated with rosy cheeks and robust health, there's trouble ahead if the hematocrit is more than 50 percent, according to Leo Vroman, Ph.D., a physiologist on the staff of Veterans' Administration Hospital, Brooklyn, New York. In his book titled, *Blood* (Doubleday, New York, 1971) Dr. Vroman points out that the increase in viscosity is such that the heart has problems pushing the blood through the vessels. This of course leads to slowed circulation and all the problems that go with it. It defeats the reason for an increase in red cells. The precious oxygen is there, with good transportation that can't get through the traffic jam.

Oxygen Supply And Hematocrit

What is it that thickens your blood in the first place? What causes increased viscosity? The main cause, it would appear, is simply an insufficient oxygen supply to the cells. According to Dr. Vroman, when the kidneys, for instance, are short of oxygen, they put out a hormone-like substance called erythropoietin which signals the bone marrow to produce more red cells. Some experiments have shown that the brain, too, can influence red cell production. The spleen and bone marrow have a reserve of red cells which they release on demand. It seems that anything which tends to create a shortage of oxygen over a period of time will stimulate red cell over-production.

A number of different circumstances are capable of creating this shortage. One of them is high altitudes. People living at an altitude of around 17,000 feet above sea level, where less oxygen is available, have a percentage of red cells near 60, as compared with 46 percent at sea level. Other circumstances which trigger a call for more red blood cell production are, according to Dr. Vroman, hard physical labor, a decreased output by the heart as in heart failure, phagocytosis or destruction of foreign substances and microbes in the blood by white blood cells, as in the case of infectious disease. All these conditions increase the need for oxygen.

Perhaps the most compelling of all the circumstances which trigger the need for more oxygen is premature and undesirable oxidation or rancidity of fatty acids in the blood. According to Dr. Wilfrid Shute, because of this process of spoilage of fatty acids, we waste and lose oxygen (*Vitamin E for Ailing and Healthy Hearts*, Pyramid House, 1969). When we can prevent this wanton waste of oxygen, we increase the amount of oxygen available to all body tissues and thus avoid signaling for erythropoietin and a subsequent higher hematocrit. It is the most effective way to have the use of more oxygen without cluttering the blood with an excessively heavy load of red corpuscles.

Since vitamin E prevents the oxidation of fatty acids in the blood, it increases the oxygen available to all the body tissues. To this extent, vitamin E can be the safest ticket to an adequate oxygen supply without an overproduction of red blood cells. According to Dr. Shute, the decrease in oxygen need affected by regular high intake of vitamin E is as much as 50 percent and in some cases has gone as high as 250 percent.

87. Impaired Leg Circulation

Vitamin E is probably the single most important factor in the battle against circulatory ailments. With extra vitamin E in the muscles, walking can become a pleasure again for those with obstructed leg arteries. The following selection is one doctor's view of the miracle of vitamin E.

Vitamin E And The Circulation:
A Surgeon's Success Story
by Knut Haeger, M.D.

Knut Haeger, M.D., was Chief Surgeon in the Department of Vascular Surgery of Malmo General Hospital in Sweden until 1973, when he accepted the position of Assistant Medical Research Director of the Schering Corp. (Scandinavia). He has published some 200 articles in medical journals on physiology, gynecology, general and vascular surgery.

The story of vitamin E began in the early 20's, when Herbert M. Evans and colleagues found that an unknown substance in wheat germ oil appeared to be necessary for normal reproduction in rats. Some ten years later, the chemical properties of this factor were revealed by Dr. and Mrs. O. H. Emerson. The substance was called tocopherol on the suggestion of a professor of Greek at Berkeley—from *tokos* (childbirth) and *phero* (bring about). There are several varieties of this compound in natural sources, the most potent being alpha-tocopherol.

Good research on the benefits of vitamin E has been scarce. Leg ulcers are a good example. Although there are many reports in the literature of the beneficial effect of vitamin E, the scientific validity of these studies has been challenged for lack of proper controls. For example, the beneficial effects reported for vitamin E on leg ulcers cannot be separated from the effect of bed rest with elevation of the leg. Much the same is true for the work done by the Shutes of Canada, using vitamin E for a variety of circulatory problems. Their findings have never been generally accepted by the medical profession because they neglected to conduct controlled series—giving vitamin E to some patients while denying it to another group of patients with very similar health problems.

Altogether, the results of vitamin E treatment were so vague and partly contradictory that an editor of the *Journal of the American Medical Association* in July, 1967, summed up the status of alpha-tocopherol by dubbing it a "vitamin in search of a disease."

I believe that work done in the Malmo General Hospital in Sweden has shown that vitamin E *can* be therapeutically useful, and for a disease for which there is no other treatment known to be really effective. That is the condition as intermittent claudication. Claudication means limping. In the typical case, the patient, who usually is an elderly male, feels pain and cramp in the calf after walking a certain distance. The pain increases so that the patient starts to limp, and finally is compelled to stop.

It is generally supposed that the pain is a result of the production of abnormal metabolites in a muscle deprived of its normal oxygen supply. The pain is of the same type as if one puts a rubber band tightly around the finger: the arterial blood is prevented from reaching its destination. The pain comes much faster if the finger is moved.

Actually, intermittent claudication is not a disease *per se*. It is, however, a most important and painful symptom of peripheral obliterative arterial disease of the legs. In 99 cases out of 100, the disease is atherosclerosis—degenerative changes in the arterial wall. It starts with deposition of abnormal fats and loss of elasticity in the artery. This is followed by calcification, or hardening, and the clogging up of the blood vessel.

Vitamin E was used as early as 1948 for this kind of obstructive arterial disease by Vogelsang and Shute. Their results were encouraging, and during the following decade a great number of papers were published on the use of alpha-tocopherol in intermittent claudication. But once again, the results were challenged because of the manner in which these tests were conducted.

It wasn't until fully 15 years later that Dr. A. M. Boyd and Dr. J. Marks of Britain proved vitamin E was extremely helpful in treating poor leg circulation. Compared to patients who received identical placebo capsules, they found, patients who took about 400 units of vitamin E a day were able to walk significantly greater distances in carefully observed tests. In fact, those who did not get the vitamin actually deteriorated.

A somewhat unexpected finding also showed up: keeping

track of some 1,476 patients who received vitamin E for a prolonged period, the doctors discovered that they survived longer than any other group of claudication patients which had ever been studied.

Williams and colleagues in Edmondton, Canada, studied a group of patients with femoro-popliteal occlusion (blockage of the major artery nourishing the leg). In the placebo group, consisting of 17 patients, only one patient was able to increase his walking distance. But of 16 patients who were given vitamin E, nine were able to walk a greater distance. Their investigation was later enlarged, and in a report in 1971 they stated that two-thirds of patients with femoro-popliteal occlusion and poor lower leg arteries seem to derive a worthwhile improvement.

My own interest in vitamin E for peripheral arterial disease was aroused by a distinguished member of the Faculty of Medicine at the University of Malmo. He suffered from diabetes mellitus and had considerable claudication due to arterial occlusion in both legs.

The medical literature at that time was not particularly encouraging. At the urgent request of my elderly friend we started, however, a very limited open clinical trial at the Department of Vascular Diseases as a pilot study. When five out of six gentlemen with rather severe claudication reported marked subjective improvement, we decided to go on.

We wanted to have a reliable control series, and also a sufficiently long period of observation. Since the symptoms of occlusive arterial disease of the leg have a tendency to come and go, and also are clearly dependent on the time of the year, it is imperative that the period of observation must be at least two years, preferably longer.

In our first clinical study, we compared the effect of alpha-tocopherol with that of vasodilator agents, anticoagulant therapy, and vitamin tablets without vitamin E. Vasodilating agents are drugs which tend to dilate blood vessels, permitting more blood to flow through them. Anticoagulant agents fight the tendency of the blood to form abnormal clots and are often given to patients with obstructed blood circulation and the tendency to form clots or thrombosis.

We further divided the patients in each therapeutic group into two subgroups, one subgroup being instructed to exercise regularly and the other group not told to exercise.

We found that the patients who received vitamin E were able

to increase their walking distance much more than any other group of patients. Fully 38 percent of patients receiving tocopherol were able to double the distance they could walk before having to halt in pain. In contrast, only 3.5 percent of the other patients showed an increase. In the vitamin E group, 36.7 percent increased their walking distance between 50 and 100 percent; in the other group, only 16.5 percent showed such an increase. We should add that those patients who took vitamin E and also exercised by walking regularly improved most of all.

There was no significant difference in degree of improvement between those who took the various drugs or the vitamins without the vitamin E; whether or not they exercised also made no difference.

We then asked the patients to rate their own improvement in terms of how far they could walk, how much their legs bothered them and to what extent they were troubled with coldness and numbness of the feet, both of which are symptoms of impaired peripheral circulation. Once again, the patients who took the vitamin E scored much higher, particularly those who also exercised. In the other groups, regardless of whether they exercised or not, there was very little difference between the groups using the various regimens.

During the years in which we conducted this study, it was necessary to amputate 12 legs because of intractable pain and/or gangrene. This was, of course, done as a last resort, only after more conservative treatment and operative techniques had failed. In the group of patients who were taking vitamin E, there was only one amputation case out of 95 surviving patients. But of 104 patients who did not receive vitamin E, there were 11 amputations. This difference is very significant.

During the course of this work, we also learned that the clinical effect of vitamin E therapy does not appear until after three to four months of administration. It seemed to us that this is the amount of time needed to load depleted muscles with tocopherol, and this observation has been corroborated by several other Swedish physicians. Nowadays, we always warn the patient not to expect any relief within the first three months on alpha-tocopherol.

In a following investigation, in collaboration with the biochemist Hans Larsson, we discovered that older men with peripheral arterial disease have a lower content of alpha-tocopherol in their skeletal muscles than healthy men. We also observed that the increase of alpha-tocopherol in the muscles after supplementation was proportional to the clinical improvement—another definite sign that vitamin E was really working. In fact, the highest percentage of increase in walking distance occurred in those patients who were capable of storing the most alpha-tocopherol, and vice versa. In a way, this may be regarded as a correlated drug-response curve—if the dose is taken as the amount of the given drug which really reaches the reacting organ.

 ´ So far, we had reasonable proof that vitamin E was helpful in intermittent claudication, and also some theoretical evidence to support this claim. Furthermore, our results corroborated those of the British and Canadian investigators. However, we felt that one important link was missing. We wanted to know if the significantly increased walking distance in claudicators on vitamin E also corresponded to an increase of the arterial flow in the muscles of the calf.

At that time, the best amd most reproducible method of measuring blood flow was venous occlusion plethysmography. Using this technique, we followed 47 patients (mean average age, 67 years) with intermittent claudication for from two to five years. Their disease was rather severe. All patients had been proven by X-ray to have total occlusion or blockage of a major artery. The arterial flow in all patients was lower than 14 ml/100 grams of tissue per minute, while the normal range is from 22 to 30 ml.

Thirty-three patients received d-alpha-tocopherol acetate, and 14 served as controls. The patients took three tablets of vitamin E a day, each tablet containing 100 mg. of a highly purified natural vitamin E with a higher biological activity than synthetic alpha-tocopherol. It was equal to 400 to 500 mg. daily of older preparations which contained synthetic d-alpha-tocopherol acetate.

As expected from our earlier experience, the walking distance improvement caused by alpha-tocopherol was again much better than that in the control group. Our tests stopped at walking for 1,000 meters (about .6 of a mile), but many patients were able to walk much longer without pain or stopping.

Altogether, 29 out of 33 patients who took vitamin E experienced an improvement of blood flow. Only three patients of 14 in the control group improved.

Another finding was that the improvement in blood flow did

not come at the same time as the improvement of walking distance. In fact, the effect on blood flow was delayed for 12 to 18 months after the beginning of the treatment.

The truth is that we do not know exactly how vitamin E works. Its action is probably associated with the known fact that it is intimately concerned in the metabolic cycle.

Folic Acid Effective For Leg Ulcers

While vitamin E is the answer for many circulatory problems, leg ulcers seem to respond well to folic acid. Geriatric specialists say these chronic leg ulcers in older people are among the most severe and disabling conditions of the lower extremities. And more than that, their stubborn resistance to treatment is legendary.

To Tibor L. Kopjas, M.D., these sores are the consequence of poor blood supply. If, as we know, all the nutritive elements, the oxygen supply, immunizing substances and defensive cells are carried by the blood, patients with constricted blood passages are being deprived of the very healing power leg ulcers must have. He reasoned that widening the blood vessels would speed the healing of the leg ulcers. It was as simple as that. And Dr. Kopjas decided to try the simplest and safest of vasodilating agents, the B vitamin, folic acid.

The average age of the three men and seven women selected for a test was 61. Four of them had moderate to advanced hardening of the arteries with resultant leg ulcers. And one of these had had a leg amputated above the knee because of advanced hardening of the arteries and gangrene with ulcers of the leg. Although the usual pharmaceutical vasodilators were used continuously on this patient, the stump had responded very slowly. Another of the patients had vascular surgery for vein grafts because of severe arterial changes in the legs, but only two months after the operation a dime-sized ulcer developed on one of the legs. The other two patients suffering from advanced arteriosclerosis had small ulcers on each toe; the legs were cold, the pulse in the legs was slow and skin color was bad. The six remaining patients had poor circulation in their legs with chronic ulcers of varying sizes.

Dr. Kopjas prescribed five milligrams of folic acid three times a day for three months. Four of the most seriously affected patients received, in addition to the regular dosage of folic acid, 20 milligrams of folic acid twice weekly by injection. All of the patients but two dressed their ulcers every day with plain sterile gauze pads. The two exceptions suffered with infection and edema, so antibiotics and diuretics were prescribed until these conditions improved. Five of the patients continued with a previously prescribed maintenance dose of digitalis. Aside from this, no other medication was used during the three-month study period.

The results of this experiment, reported in the *Journal of the American Geriatrics Society* (March, 1968) speak for themselves. In six to eight weeks complete repair was achieved in the patients with the smaller ulcers (one to three centimeters in diameter). For patients with larger sores, healing took 12 weeks. After only two months of folic acid therapy, satisfactory repair of the ulcer was observed even in the stump of the amputee who previously had healing difficulties. His other leg also showed definite improvement in the skin color and temperature. For the patient who had earlier vascular surgery, the ulcer that appeared near the graft was completely healed in six weeks; both legs became noticeably warmer and walking improved, says Dr. Kopjas. Only one out of the ten cases did not show complete healing of the ulcer in the 12 weeks, although even that ulcer was reduced to about half size. The researcher believes that in this case, chronic atrophy in the toe, plus poor foot hygiene was responsible.

For the many who have tried vasodilating drugs and the popular anticoagulant drugs, it is of special interest that there were no side-effects with this therapy.

X-rays published with the article show how folic acid works, apparently creating auxiliary routes for blood transmission when the major arteries are clogged. Dr. Kopjas explains that "In older patients with generalized vascular disease, the poor blood supply does not provide enough hydro-dynamic pressure to dilate the small arteries and develop collaterals. . . ." That's where folic acid's effective vasodilation of the smaller blood vessels comes in.

Equally important as a clear highway for the blood to travel, is having worthwhile elements for it to carry. "The state of nutrition is important for the efficiency of the healing process," says Dr. Kopjas. "For instance, the protein depletion in malnourishment, chronic wasting disease or avitaminosis C has a profound effect upon wound healing. Collagen formation is depressed, the integrity of the capillary wall is altered, and capillary rupture and hemorrhage hinder the healing process." So good diet counts heavily in speeding recovery.

88. Pulmonary Embolism: Is It Due To Vitamin E Deficiency?

On May 22-23, 1964, in Boston, a conclave of medical experts discussed a major cause of death, pulmonary embolism. Their special concern was that this condition is incorrectly diagnosed so frequently as pneumonia, heart attack, or heart failure. Actually this type of embolism—blood clot—lodges in the lung, causing a pulmonary insufficiency and death.

If properly diagnosed, a pulmonary embolism will respond to medical treatment and almost invariably the patient's life can be saved. However, Dr. Sasahara, chief of the cardio-pulmonary laboratory at the West Roxbury Veterans Administration Hospital told the symposium, with regard to diagnosis, that "our batting average is miserably low. We're only hitting about 30 percent, which is terrible." The Boston conference was called because these diagnostic failures are permitting thousands of people to die unnecessarily.

Why Does It Happen?

The truly dismal failure is that these pulmonary embolisms are ever permitted to happen, when they should be so easy to prevent.

Dr. Sasahara explained the mechanism by which a pulmonary embolism forms. The condition, he said, is brought on by a blood clot which generally forms in a leg vein and moves through the blood stream up to the heart. It is able to pass through the relatively large valves of the heart but when it reaches the lung, it is trapped in one of the tiny blood vessels that carry blood to that vital organ. Blockage and failure of the blood supply results in suffocation combined with acute heart failure, leading to death.

So the real physiological villain is the formation of blood clots in the veins. We know how such clots form. Because of our upright posture, it takes terrific pressure to return blood from our feet and legs to the heart. Any type of unusual abdominal pressure such as may be caused by pregnancy or even constipa-

402

tion, or a job that requires standing for long periods of time without the compensation of vigorous exercise, can slow down the blood in the leg veins to a point that permits clot formation.

Vitamin E

In the *American Journal of Physiology* (Vol. 153, p. 127, 1948) K. L. Zierler, D. Grob and J. L. Lilienthal described experiments in which vitamin E showed a profound effect on the blood's clotting qualities. They found a strong anti-clotting effect both in laboratory experiments and in the veins and arteries of human beings. Dr. Evan Shute, a recognized authority on vitamin E, is convinced that vitamin E not only inhibits the formation of blood clots, but also expands the blood vessels so that any clots that might exist can pass through them more freely.

This trouble with blood clots which can lead to a killing pulmonary embolism might never occur if people ate enough vitamin E in their daily diet. How much is enough? The absolute minimum has been estimated by such authorities as Horwitt and Shute at 50 to 60 milligrams per day of alpha tocopherol alone. In the mixed tocopherols, as vitamin E generally occurs in food, one would have to ingest at least 100 milligrams a day in order to obtain 50 to 60 milligrams of the biologically active alpha tocopherol. Most Americans consume only six to twelve milligrams of mixed tocopherols daily.

Section 17
Colds

89. Common Sense On The Common Cold

It would be hard to guess how many millions of man hours and billions of dollars have been devoted to the attempt to find a drug that will cure the common cold. Every pharmaceutical company has developed at least one product worth millions of dollars in yearly sales that will alleviate some of the symptoms of a cold. Although such so-called "remedies" account for sales of more than a billion dollars a year, none has actually been proved effective in preventing colds or shortening the duration of existing colds.

The medical wiseacres used to put it this way: "We'll land on the moon before we learn how to get rid of the common cold."

That once extravagant prediction has, of course, come true. We have sent men strolling across the lunar plains in a miracle of scientific and engineering precision. But still millions of people back on earth snort, sniffle, and cough their way through the miseries of the common cold, with no medical cure in sight. Science is helpless.

Vaccines Hold Little Promise

The antibiotics and sulfa drugs are useless against the cold virus. Furthermore, the development of a vaccine to immunize us against colds has turned out to be an impossible task—and small wonder! To prepare a vaccine, you must first isolate the infecting agent. But, in the case of the common cold, more than 100 viruses are known to cause the typical symptoms. Still others have yet to be identified, and mutations are believed to be constantly creating virus offspring with changed characteristics. So, no matter what vaccine is made, there will always be resistant viruses on hand to keep humanity sniffling.

It is abundantly clear that anti-cold measures designed to build up the body's own defense mechanisms are the only answer—not just the *best* answer but the *only* answer. Every aspect of healthy living counts on your ability to throw off a cold or not catch one: adequate rest, regular exercise and, above all, a nutritious diet.

An authoritative volume published by the World Health Organization, *Interactions of Nutrition and Infection* (1968), presented evidence from all over the world, collected over the preceding 50 years and more, showing an intimate connection between resistance to infection and adequate intake of protein, trace minerals and every vitamin known to man. None of the essential nutrients can be neglected if we want to avoid colds.

Two of these nutrients—vitamins A and C—play especially vital roles. In subsequent chapters, we will examine their protective properties in considerable detail.

What To Do If A Cold Strikes

Even the best preventive measures, however, cannot guarantee complete freedom from colds. If you should catch a cold, be sure to take common sense measures that will speed it on its way.

1. Maintain an adequate diet. Eat lightly if you must, but eat.

2. Stay home and rest. This doesn't mean you have to "take to the sick bed." But take it easy. Lie down if you feel tired. Stay warm. Don't expose yourself to sudden changes of temperature.

3. If possible, keep your distance from other members of the family so you won't spread the infection. Keep your own towels separate and away from others. Don't leave your glass or dishes where someone else might eat or drink out of them.

4. Blow your nose gently, with both nostrils open. A puddle of warm water held in the palm of the hand and sniffed in gently will flush out excess mucus without irritating tender nasal membranes.

5. A moist atmosphere is particularly important when you are fighting a cold. You want to give the defense mechanisms of your respiratory system every help. A small vaporizer that can be purchased at the drugstore does a good "spot" job by the bedside or chair.

6. Avoid over-the-counter remedies. They won't cure you and they may very well do harm.

90. Vitamin A, First Line Of Defense

Research has shown certain nutrients to be particularly useful in maintaining resistance to upper respiratory infections. Vitamin A is one of these.

Add some potent vitamin A to a culture of cold viruses under laboratory conditions and the viruses roll merrily along, thriving, multiplying and growing more virulent right under the nose of vitamin A. But expose a person who maintains a high level of vitamin A in his system throughout the year, to those same cold viruses, and the march of the infection is halted. Statistically speaking, those with high vitamin A intake get fewer colds, and the ones they do get are less severe.

Colds Unexpectedly Blocked

Spontaneous evidence of vitamin A's power to build resistance to colds came to light in the British Isles during World War II, when the government distributed cod liver oil supplements (rich in vitamin A) to children. Parents and doctors alike were amazed to find almost complete disappearance of the perpetually runny noses so characteristic of children growing up in the damp, chilled British climate. Medical men called it an unexpected dividend of the supplement.

To understand how vitamin A was able to achieve this effect, we need to examine the body's first line of defense when a harmful substance enters the nasal passage.

The mucous membrane, lining the nose, the mouth and all the cavities and passages of the respiratory tract, contains protective devices that guard against invading substances, whether they be chemical pollutants, bacteria or the common cold virus. Attached to the mucous membrane in fantastic numbers are tiny cells, each containing about eight microscopic hairlike structures known as cilia. In each nostril alone there are literally millions of cilia. The mucous glands secrete a moist film of mucus which is kept in constant motion by the cilia, whipping back and forth about 250 times a minute in such a sequence that they form waves.

The motion of the cilia sweeps unwanted substances (including viruses and bacteria) back from the nose into the mouth, where they are expectorated or swallowed. (The gastrointestinal system has its own protective devices to deal with invaders that are sent on to the stomach in this fashion.) Cilia elsewhere in the respiratory system perform similar work where viruses or other intruders get past the first defense, which is the nose.

The secretions of the mucous glands work with the cilia to physically remove foreign objects. They also contain an enzyme, lysozyme, which was discovered and found to be a microbe destroyer by Alexander Fleming (the discoverer of penicillin) in 1922. Since then, lysozyme has been shown to be active against viruses as well.

You can see that the common cold virus has to get past some formidable barriers before it can get a toehold in your system and cause sniffles, sore throat and other familiar symptoms. The barriers we have described, however, depend on the health and efficient functioning of the mucous membrane. And this lining of the respiratory tract—like the eyes, skin and other mucous membrane surfaces—deteriorates when it is not supplied with adequate vitamin A.

As long ago as 1936, one of the world's great nutritionists, Sir Robert McCarrison, said: "When the food is deficient in vitamin A, the cilia slough off and the cells themselves lose their ability to secrete, thus becoming horny or keratinized, as it is called. Figure yourself what this means: no longer is this trapping, this propelling of harmful particles, whether of dust or bacteria or both, possible in the area so affected." McCarrison's observation has been confirmed countless times since.

As you might expect, vitamin A deficiency also weakens lysozyme defense. Clinical findings demonstrating this fact were reported by the World Health Organization in 1968.

Tears of children with xerophthalmia (pathologically dry eyes) were found to have greatly reduced lysozyme activity leading to reductions in the resistance of the eyes to infection. But the activity of the enzyme increased significantly after five to seven days of cod liver oil therapy.

Smokers Catch More Colds

In addition to making sure you have an adequate intake of vitamin A from fish liver oil, yellow vegetables and other rich sources, you can strengthen the healthy functioning of your respiratory system's mucous membrane by guarding it from abuse. If you smoke, you're actually paralyzing your cilia for as long as 30 to 40 minutes with each cigarette. A heavy smoker thus deprives himself of this valuable defense against infection—and statistics show that heavy smokers get heavier colds and get them more frequently.

For the same reason, avoid exposure to polluted air as much as practicable. Chemical pollutants in the air, such as sulphur dioxide, damage the cilia and attack the mucous membranes. Unfortunately you cannot entirely avoid environmental pollution. It's all around us. But stay clear of areas of heavy car traffic or concentrations of factory smoke when you can, and don't add to the hazard by using household pesticide or deodorant sprays.

Finally, remember that the lining of your respiratory system must stay moist. As you'll discover later in this section, over-heated American homes tend to be dry. And dry air inhaled into the respiratory tract parches the tissues, hindering the efficient working of the defense mechanisms.

91. Your Major Weapon Against Colds Is Vitamin C

Every winter, when sniffles, sore throat and headachy fever are all around, many fortunate and well prepared individuals manage to breeze through the colds season blessedly free of symptoms.

Many of those lucky ones take vitamin C every day for its protective effect. Knowing what we do today about this vitamin's role, such action should be practically routine among health-minded individuals. In fact, medical researchers now pretty well agree—some enthusiastically, some reluctantly—that vitamin C is indeed able to ward off, or at least minimize the severity and discomfort of colds and other respiratory illnesses. But they still don't agree on the amount of this nutrient that you should be consuming for best results.

For example, Dr. Terence W. Anderson of the University of Toronto reported in October, 1974, on a study involving 600 healthy volunteers. A number of the subjects received a relatively small dosage of vitamin C, amounting to only about 500 milligrams a week. But they increased their intake to 500 mg. *daily* at the first sign of illness. The remaining participants received a dummy pill, containing no vitamin C. According to Dr. Anderson, who is a professor of epidemiology and biometrics, the vitamin C group reported slightly fewer colds. More important, the colds they did get were less severe, resulting in 30 percent fewer sick days and less absence from work than the control group.

Take More When A Cold Hits
As a result of these findings, Dr. Anderson suggests that people seeking protection from colds don't really need more than about 200 mg. of extra vitamin C daily, "except possibly for brief periods during acute infection when gram doses (1,000 mg.) *may* be beneficial" (*Medical Tribune*, November 20, 1974).

There are, however, a number of very carefully devised and ambitious studies showing excellent cold-fighting results when

411

higher doses of vitamin C are used every day. Dr. John L. Coulehan and several colleagues tested the vitamin over a 14-week period at a Navajo Indian boarding school in Arizona. The experiment got underway in early February, near the height of the colds and flu season, and involved 641 children. Half received vitamin C in large amounts (one or two grams daily); the rest received placebo pills, containing a little citric acid.

The surprising results were published in the January 3, 1974 issue of *The New England Journal of Medicine*. First of all, the children receiving vitamin C had fewer observed sick days due to colds and other respiratory problems—about 30 percent less than among the controls. And the colds they did catch were accompanied by much less coughing and runny noses than were the other children's. But there was an additional bonus: the protection afforded by vitamin C extended beyond the respiratory tract. Children receiving vitamin C had fewer observed sick days *from any cause*—30 percent less than the controls, as a matter of fact. How could this be?

"Massive doses of vitamin C may increase resistance to certain infections, may mask symptoms through local or systemic actions or may indeed be virocidal (virus-killing) in some way," Dr. Coulehan and his assistants concluded. "There is no substantial evidence for any specific mode of action at present. . ." In other words, the doctors are saying that large doses of this nutrient can do us a world of good but they don't know why.

Even Dr. Anderson, who advises that 200 mg. of vitamin C offers a sufficient prophylactic effect, has helped supervise studies, involving thousands of volunteers, showing that a gram or more of vitamin C is not only very effective against colds, but perfectly safe as well. One four-month winter trial involving 818 volunteers clearly demonstrated that individuals taking one or two grams of vitamin C a day, and four grams at the first sign of a cold, suffered significantly less from the nagging miseries that often accompany a respiratory bout—mild and severe chills, fever of 100 degrees F. or more, and severe malaise. Also, their cold episodes tended to be shorter, and they missed fewer days of work than subjects who took no vitamin C (*Canadian Medical Association Journal*, September 23, 1972). No harmful side effects of any kind were observed.

All this would seem to confirm Nobel Prize winner Dr. Linus Pauling's contention, first published in 1970 in this book *Vitamin C and the Common Cold* (W. H. Freeman, San Francisco), that this nutrient is an easy and safe way to prevent or alleviate colds. Many doctors were quick to criticize Dr. Pauling for making such a statement. First, vitamin C's cold-fighting credentials were challenged, and once those were examined and admittedly found in order, a debate began about whether we really need *so much* vitamin C. Who is right?

There Are Average Numbers, But No Average People

Actually, it's probably closest to the truth to say that each side is partially right, because different people will need different dosages, depending on circumstances. Dr. Anderson, for example, very reasonably suggests that 200 mg. a day may be enough vitamin C for many normal, healthy persons who do not have a cold and are trying to avoid one. "If you take tissues that are not really saturated and give them some extra vitamin C," he points out, "you improve their resistance a bit. For some people, 100 mg. a day is enough to saturate. Giving them ten times the dosage won't improve their resistance any further. Having achieved this daily saturation, if you give extra doses when stress from a cold forces the leukocyte ascorbic acid (vitamic C) concentration down, then you can maintain saturation. Maybe this is the best combination—a little bit daily, and a big dose when symptoms first appear" (*Medical World News*, September 13, 1974).

It's important to realize, though, that Dr. Anderson is basing his advice on large experimental studies involving hundreds or even thousands of persons. Such statistics don't really answer the question of how much vitamin C is right for you. All they tell us is the *average* dosage needed to benefit a significant fraction of the group. Whether your needs fall above or below that average is another matter.

Dr. Roger J. Williams, the respected University of Texas biochemist, is aware of this problem. He points out that in the laboratory some young guinea pigs require at least 20 times as much vitamin C for good growth as others. In his book, *Nutrition Against Disease* (Pitman, 1971), Dr. Williams writes, "We need to recognize that each individual's problem (of getting enough vitamin C and other nutrients) is based upon his or her own requirements which are not set by any committee... The typical individual is quite different from the hypothetical average individual (who is not really an individual at all) ... Of necessity, for reasons involving inheritance, every individual has nutritional needs which differ *quantitatively*, with respect to each separate nutrient, from his neighbors."

Colds

This is why Dr. Pauling is also correct when he suggests that one to five grams of vitamin C per day may be necessary to prevent colds. Some people may need that amount. You may or may not. Dr. Pauling goes on to say, "There is evidence that some people remain in very good health, including freedom from the common cold, year after year through the ingestion of only 250 mg. of ascorbic acid per day. The requirements of a few people for ascorbic acid may be expected to be even smaller."

Now let's look at you. If you're just starting out on a daily regimen of vitamin C supplementation in hopes of avoiding future colds, Dr. Anderson's recommendations of 200 mg. a day might be a good guideline to follow. If, at this dosage, you should feel a sore throat, hoarseness or some other indicator of a cold. coming on, increase your intake as needed until symptoms disappear. Then instead of returning to your old level, experiment with a slightly higher dosage. Hopefully you will discover a level of vitamin C intake that either prevents all or most colds for you, or at least results in much milder colds. Chances are that level will be somewhere between the two extremes of 200 mg. and well over one gram.

Summer Cold?

Don't be fooled into thinking that the cold season is over just because the weather changes. Colds are caused by viruses, and they can strike at any time of the year that your resistance is low.

If you are one of millions of Americans who look forward to a special summer vacation, you just might find the high point of your year spoiled by a summer cold coming on when it's too late to change your plans. Fortunately, vitamin C can be just as effective preventing or easing summer colds as it is in winter.

As we saw in the last chapter, though, it's too late for prevention once you've caught a cold. Then your main concern is getting rid of the symptoms that are dragging you down—stuffy head, runny nose, burning eyes and raspy throat—and getting on with your summer fun. And the best way to fight a cold that has already arrived is by upping your intake of vitamin C.

Fighting a cold with a natural nutritional booster won't knock you off your feet even more than the cold itself does, the way that antihistamines and other drugs can work. Don't let the drugs make you spend your vacation in bed recovering from both the cold itself and the side effects of the treatment. The results of a 5-year study show that high doses of vitamin C can spare you the distressing symptoms of a cold while your body is fighting it off naturally at its own sure rate of speed.

According to Edme Regnier, M.D., your chances for dodging the misery of the common cold are good if you get to some vitamin C in time, and take enough of it often enough. Doctor Regnier was talking about the common cold in general, but his is especially good advice to the person prone to summer colds.

In a two-part article by Doctor Regnier published in the September and October, 1968, issues of the *Review of Allergy* (Volume 22, Numbers 9 and 10), the Salem, Massachusetts, physician fully described his five-year study of the successful application of high doses of ascorbic acid (vitamin C) and ascorbic acid with bioflavonoids in preventing and treating the common cold.

Every Three Hours, More Vitamin C

He tested 22 subjects, most of whom were adults ranging in age from 30 to 50. Five youngsters under 12 years were included, as well as a 73-year-old. In every case, the treatment with vitamin C in a high dosage successfully suppressed the symptoms of the cold.

How much vitamin C is needed to fight off a cold when early warning symptoms occur? As other researchers have noted, the amounts vary with every person, but Doctor Regnier found that when a cold strikes, the best way to treat it is with 600 to 625 milligrams every three hours. Four 200 mg. tablets, or 800 mg., taken every four hours did not keep the symptoms away as well as the established three-hour interval.

At bedtime, patients took 750 mg. of ascorbic acid so that they wouldn't need to disturb their sleep to take the usual dose on schedule. Then they were instructed to take another 750 mg. upon arising, before going back to their 600-625 mg. intake.

After three or four days of taking the high doses of vitamin C, the patients were able to reduce their intake to 375-400 mg. every three hours. If the symptoms recurred because the vitamin C dosage was reduced too soon, they simply went back to the original 600-625 mg. every three hours.

Those patients who suffered no setback, however, were given instructions to reduce the intake still more after two or three days at the "second stage" dose. Only 200 to 250 mg. were taken every three hours, and after a couple of days the interval opened up to from four to six hours between tablets. The ascorbic acid treatment could usually be discontinued after from ten to twelve days.

Too Much Better Than Too Little

Suppose the original high dose hadn't been reduced throughout the treatment? Doctor Regnier could see no objection to continuing the 600-625 mg. of ascorbic acid for the duration of the cold span. But he was trying to find to his satisfaction what the lowest effective dose of vitamin C would be in the treatment of a cold. He adds, however, "I have learned that it is advisable (and still safe) to err on the side of prescribing too large a dose of ascorbic acid in the later stages of a viral infection rather than too small a one."

Dr. Regnier was not concerned about identifying any particular strain of cold virus and testing the effect of ascorbic acid upon it. But his subjects lived widely enough apart—residing in Massachusetts, Pennsylvania and Hawaii—to give the vitamin C treatment a crack at a variety of cold viruses.

Just what does vitamin C do inside the body? It obviously earns its keep when colds threaten, but why? Doctor Regnier has speculated that there are two possible ways that vitamin C could fight colds and viral infection. One of these is to lessen the permeability of cell walls so that viruses cannot so easily penetrate them. The other is that ascorbic acid may decrease the permeability of the capillary walls. The effect would be to cut down the inflammation which spreads through the mucous membranes and vocal cords, manifesting itself as hoarseness. Lessening cell-wall permeability would prevent the spread of the invading organisms. Retarding inflammation would help alleviate the discomforting symptoms of a cold.

But what about preventing colds? Let us say that every day you walk from an air conditioned 72° office into a car that has been baking in the summer sun. The thermal shock depresses your metabolism and leaves you vulnerable—every working day. Is there anything that you can do to overcome this potentially cold-inducing situation? Doctor Regnier recommends a dose of 600-750 mg. of vitamin C to prevent that cold, with the same dose three hours later. Your chances of avoiding contamination after that are extremely favorable.

Four Years Without A Cold!

It really sounds as though, if you want to be free from colds, you should be getting considerably more vitamin C than the Recommended Daily Allowance of 45 mg. Again, how much you should take is your decision, but Dr. Regnier relates this observation about three nurses from J. B. Thomas Hospital in Peabody, Massachusetts, who took vitamin C supplements daily for four consecutive years.

Before they took the supplements they had caught colds frequently. But while they each took a supplement of 250 mg. everyday for four years, they did not suffer a single cold among them. Meanwhile, most of the other nurses working with them caught colds so bad that they were unable to work.

One of the three nurses had been taking doses of from 100-200 mg. daily for eight years before the doctor boosted her dosage to 250 mg. However, after the additional four years of the higher dose, the doctor asked her to stop taking the supplements. As a result, she caught two colds within one season, proving that a constant intake of vitamin C is essential to fight off colds, and that taking even 250 mg. daily for four years does not build up a lasting immunity to these infections.

If a summer cold should strike, you could hardly do better than to increase your intake of this nutrient. It is the best assurance you have that your cold will not keep you from boating, hiking, dancing or whatever your pleasure is, and that you will not be coughing and sneezing all over your fellow vacationers.

With large doses of vitamin C fighting on your side, maybe you can put colds out of season forever.

A Solid Cold-Prevention Program— Vitamin C And Wheat Germ

A world famous scientist reported in 1972 that for most of his life he "had always been the first to pick up any cold, and had almost died twice of pneumonia." But he had not had a cold for the previous 15 years, even though he was then 78 and presumably had less resistance to disease than he did when younger.

He learned about vitamin C? No, it's not that. This particular man is Nobel Laureate Albert Szent-Gyorgyi, the distinguished scientist who isolated vitamin C in 1930, who believed in it longer than any of us and who always made sure that he had plenty in his diet. One other nutritional element must be added to vitamin C to create a perfect defense against colds, he discovered. This other food that brings out the total protective quality of vitamin C is wheat germ.

In his book, *The Living State* (Academic Press, New York), Dr.

417

Szent-Gyorgyi states that he believes he owes to his combination of wheat germ and vitamin C not only freedom from colds in his later years, but also the very fact that he has lived as long as he has.

Dr. Szent-Gyorgyi describes how, after the isolation of ascorbic acid in crystalline form, he became aware that there seemed to be some element missing that would permit ascorbic acid to function with regard to human respiration the same way that it does in plants. Then in 1958, on the island of Jamaica, he was told by an acquaintance that a mixture of yeast and wheat germ eaten for breakfast every day had kept him from having colds for several years. Dr. Szent-Gyorgyi, being a chronic sufferer from colds himself, tried the same breakfast and found that after that he also had no colds.

Being the man he is, he was not content merely to accept a successful folk remedy. He made an intensive biochemical investigation and found that the only function of the yeast in the mixture was to split the glucosides in the wheat germ. Since the body is able to accomplish this without help, he decided to eliminate the yeast from his breakfast and found that the wheat germ alone is just as successful.

In a footnote, Dr. Szent-Gyorgyi states that his breakfast every day consists of a sliced banana, over which he pours about 2 ounces of wheat germ, adding milk. He also drinks tea to which he adds about a gram (1,000 milligrams) of vitamin C instead of lemon. In the afternoon he has another cup of tea, again containing a gram of vitamin C.

Two Ounces Or More Daily

By further investigation, the Nobel Laureate discovered a complex series of reactions between ascorbic acid and quinones produced by the splitting of the glucosides of wheat germ. The reactions were triggered by the manganese content of the wheat germ.

What it comes down to is that materials that are present in most plant foods to a very limited extent, are present most richly in wheat germ. Thus, Dr. Szent-Gyorgyi believes almost any plant food we eat will potentiate our vitamin C intake to some extent, so that vitamin C will have its beneficial effect. But to fully potentiate the large amounts of vitamin C recommended by him, by Linus Pauling and by growing numbers of other scientists, he believes that two ounces or more of wheat germ every day is a necessity. "My finding wheat germ useful against colds is not at variance with Pauling's statements," says Dr. Szent-Gyorgyi. "If one is deficient in two factors, administration of one of them may help to some extent, while full benefit may be derived only by taking the two in combination."

When the scientist speaks of "full benefit," he is talking about far more than merely preventing colds, important as that single activity may be.

Vitamin C, as is demonstrated biochemically in *The Living State*, functions as an antioxidant in relation to a wide variety of materials that we call "toxic" because, if they are permitted to oxidize within our systems, they initiate chain reactions that disrupt the normal orderly processes of life. There are hundreds—perhaps thousands—of such toxic materials. There are poisonous metals like cadmium and lead. There are toxins produced by harmful bacteria. There are the venoms of insect stings and snake bites. There are numerous viruses like the hundred or so of the common cold.

All these toxic hazards attack us in essentially the same way. They disrupt the normal healthful activities of the body when they are oxidized. Vitamin C prevents the oxidation. What the wheat germ does is to furnish the vitamin C with otherwise missing chemical elements that permit the vitamin actually to regenerate itself so that it is not used up the first time it functions as an antioxidant, but is able to perform the same protective role many times.

No wonder Dr. Szent-Gyorgyi declares in *The Living State* that: "I always felt that not enough use was made of ascorbic acid. 'If we lack ascorbic acid we develop scurvy. If we do not have scurvy, we have enough ascorbic acid.' So the argument ran; the logic was impeccable. The flaw in this argument is that scurvy is not the first symptom of deficiency. It is a sign of the final collapse of the organism, a premortal syndrome, and there is a very wide gap between scurvy and a completely healthy condition. Good health is the state in which we feel best, work best, and have greatest resistance to disease. Nobody knows how far we are from such a state. This could be established only by extensive statistical studies which are not available. Solutions to this problem are full of pitfalls. If, owing to inadequate food, you contract a cold and die of pneumonia, your diagnosis will be pneumonia, not malnutrition, and chances are that your doctor will have treated you only for pneumonia.

Colds

"Is our body such a poor mechanism that it has to break down every so often with a cold or other ailment? Or do we abuse our body, and feed it so poorly that its breakdown is comparable to the breakdown of an unlubricated engine? I am often shocked at the eating habits of people. What I find difficult to understand as a biologist is not why people become ill, but how they manage to stay alive at all. Our body must be a very wonderful instrument to withstand all our insults."

92. Does The Cold Weather Cause Colds?

Cold weather brings special health problems. Winter, with its icy winds and chilling dampness, seems to encourage illness. Certainly, colds reach their peak each year during the wintry months. But is it accurate to say that cold actually causes colds?

This is a debate that has gone on for centuries. Benjamin Franklin, arguing with future president John Adams, said no. On a winter journey, the two shared a room in an inn, where Franklin insisted on opening the window, to the dismay of his companion. Adams protested that the cold air would give him a cold. Nonsense, said Franklin, not cold air but recirculated air exhaled from their lungs was the thing to worry about. As Adams described the event in his diary, he finally went to sleep (with the window open) in the midst of the good doctor's lengthy and animated discussion of his theory.

Modern researchers still can't decide who was closer to the truth—Franklin or Adams. Experiments with 44 male volunteers at Baylor University College of Medicine in 1968 found little connection between getting cold and "getting colds." Drs. R. Gordon Douglas, Jr., Keith M. Lindgren and Robert B. Couch inoculated the men with a typical common cold virus, then exposed them to 39 degree temperatures while they were dressed only in cotton undershirts and shorts. In these experiments, involving healthy subjects, the researchers found no connection between colds and exposure to cold air.

But when subjects are in less than robust health, chilling *does* become a factor. Reporting on a monumental study involving 60,000 University of California students, Dr. Marshall C. Cheney noted in the *Practitioner* (December, 1952) that some students were resistant to colds, others were partially resistant and still others appeared to have little or no resistance.

This is what Dr. Cheney found about chilling: "Of no importance when agents of infectious colds are absent from the nose and throat, and in those who can 'take it,' chilling becomes a life

and death matter for susceptibles in crowded city areas . . ." Add
to this the fact that in winter people spend more time indoors in
stale air—where the cold virus has its best chance to circulate—
and you'll begin to see why the common cold is so much more
common in winter than in summer.

Being exposed to a virus is by no means the same thing as
being *infected* by one. At times a person can fight off infection.
Under other circumstances (lowered resistance *combined* with a
severe chill, for example), he can't.

Best To Play It Safe

Assuming, then, that both Franklin and Adams were at least
partially right, the following measures—in addition to taking
adequate vitamin C and wheat germ every day—are the best
insurance against colds:

Don't get overly fatigued. Many people find they are most
prone to catching other people's ailments when they are tired
and run-down. Get sufficient rest.

Regular, moderate exercise will not fatigue you. On the contrary, it will contribute to your stamina and improve your
circulation. While we're all familiar with the accounts of heart
attacks brought on by snow shoveling, we must remember that in
these cases it is not exercise, but *unaccustomed* exercise, carried
on beyond the person's endurance (and often after a heavy meal),
that leads to tragedy.

When winter infections are rife, stay out of crowds as much as
possible.

Wear sensible, outdoor clothing. Several layers of light clothing are better than one very heavy garment. Air is an insulator,
and the warm air between sweater and jacket, for example, will
give you extra protection. With several layers, you can discard
some of your wraps if the temperature rises or exercise begins to
overheat you.

If it's snowy or rainy, be sure to wear moisture-resistant clothing. Boots or rubbers, of course, are also called for. Wet
clothes conduct heat away from the body, and they should be
changed as soon as possible.

If you're going to stay out for a considerable length of time, you
can best keep your hands and feet warm by again following the
"layer" procedure. Two pairs of light socks are better than one
heavy one. An inner glove and an outer glove can keep your
hands toasty in freezing weather.

Make sure that your shoes are not too tight. Remember that poor circulation in the feet is a particular problem during exposure to cold, and that shoes that restrict circulation are a hazard.

93. Winter Air Needs Moisturizing—Dry Air Invites Colds

When the woes of wintertime are at their worst, and colds and sneezing and coughing are upon the land, did you ever stop to think how our cave-man-type ancestors managed to stay alive from November to March?

The strange fact is that before the invention of the house, man probably had much less of a problem with colds and the whole gamut of respiratory diseases than we do today, with all our insulation, aluminum siding and automatic thermostats. Ironically, a lot of the discomfort that too many people suffer in the winter is directly traceable to well-built homes and modern heating units.

One can go a step further than that, and state that by making the climate in the home just a little more like the climate in a cave, a tree, a dugout or a lean-to, one can not only expect to do less sneezing and coughing this winter—but be more comfortable as well!

To understand this peculiar situation, you have to be acquainted with two basic facts.

The first is that as air becomes cold, it loses the water vapor it ordinarily holds. Even if the cold air has just blown over the Great Lakes, it will still probably contain less moisture than stagnant city air on a hot, muggy day. Although the cold air has *access* to a lot of water, it is physically incapable of holding very much. Therefore, winter air is generally much drier than summer air.

If you are thinking that dryness is the problem with winter air, you're correct. But if cold air is dry air, wouldn't the cave man have suffered even more than we do? If the draft blowing into his bedroom was 20 degrees, wouldn't he be breathing air much drier than we are, sleeping in 68 degree comfort?

That's where the second fact comes in; there is dry air, and then there is *super*-dry air. Super-dry is the way air becomes in a home when cold air from the outside is heated in the house. A more accurate description might be to call it *thirsty* air, because it actively sucks out moisture from everything it touches in order to satisfy its thirst.

Technically, this is what the weatherman calls "relative humidity." This is a figure which expresses the percentage of water vapor in the air compared to the amount of water that the air is capable of holding.

Remember that when air is cold, it can't hold much water to begin with. But when the cold air from the outside enters a home and is rapidly heated, it suddenly takes on the ability to drink up much more water. If it came into a house with a relative humidity of, say, 80 percent, by the time it reached room temperature, that relative humidity will have dropped all the way down to something like 10 percent.

In other words, when air is cold and dry, it's more or less inert. But when it's *hot* and dry, it becomes "magnetized," attracting every drop of water in a house.

And when people breathe in such air, it actively and aggressively removes the natural moisture from the mouth, nose, throat and bronchial tubes. That's why people who live in unhumidified homes usually wake up in the morning with a dry, scratchy throat.

A Blizzard Outside, A Desert Inside

It is generally agreed that the ideal humidity for easy breathing is about 50 percent. Actually, unless there is a humidifier in the home, there is virtually no chance that the air in that home has anywhere near this much water in it.

For example, if the outdoor temperature is 20 degrees above zero, with an outdoor relative humidity of 35 percent, and the thermostat is on 72, the relative humidity of the air indoors is only 5 percent.

The mucous secretions that keep the mouth, nose and throat healthfully moist are composed of about 96 percent water. But when this water is dried out, the mucus becomes thicker and interferes with the action of the cilia, those tiny little rod-like cells that sweep dust, germs, and excess mucus out of the breathing apparatus and into the nose or mouth for removal. That is why people often have to "bring up phlegm" when they wake up in a dry home.

Vitamin A, as discussed earlier plays a vital role in maintaining the moistness and elasticity of the throat, bronchial tubes, lungs and all epithelial tissues. Also, vitamin C can give a huge boost to our natural resistance against the cold virus and other bugs. But beyond this, just how important is the question of super-dry air in producing respiratory problems, and what can be done about it? Dr. Charles S. Sale, a Norfolk, Virginia, ear, nose and throat specialist, is convinced that humidifying the home air is one of the best things a person can do to enjoy better health and comfort during the winter.

Typically, the wintertime relative humidity inside a home is from 3 to 10 percent. Dr. Sale says that the *ideal* humidity, as far as good health is concerned, is 40 to 50 percent. In a report in the American Medical Association publication, *Today's Health* (February, 1970), Dr. Sale explains that one of the basic functions of the membranes in the nose is to supply moisture to inhaled air so that it reaches a humidity of 85 percent in the lungs. What's more, "any alterations in the function of moistening will lead to disturbance in the nose, sinuses, ears, throat, and in certain cases, in the bronchial tubes."

Ordinarily, the nasal membranes are very resistant to penetration by viruses or bacteria. But Dr. Sale feels that the majority of the problems he sees during the winter months probably result from failure of the nasal membrane to maintain normal function—largely because of excessively dry air in the home.

Surprisingly, it turns out that when humidity in the home is maintained at about 50 percent, it has a direct effect on germs, as well as our mucous membranes. That's because when the air in the home is unusually dry, germs in mucus and saliva which are sneezed or coughed into the air may actually float around, maintaining their infectious potential, for several weeks. In contrast, with a relative humidity of about 50 percent, moisture in the air quickly clings to the germs and mucous particles and they settle to the floor where, Dr. Sale says, the germs soon die.

Humidifiers Reduced Soldiers' Colds

Dr. Abraham Gelperin, a preventive medicine specialist at the Abraham Lincoln School of Medicine in Chicago, set out to determine what significance properly humidified air has as a public health measure. His research, conducted at Ft. Leonard Wood, Missouri, and supported by the U.S. Army Research and Development Command, was published in March, 1973 in *Heating/Piping/Air Conditioning*.

Dr. Gelperin kept close tabs on about 800 soldiers living in eight barracks. In four of the buildings he had water lines installed into the furnace rooms so that humidifiers could be attached to the heating units. These units—which are also used in individual homes—operate by adding water vapor to hot air just as it comes from the furnace, so that the entire house or building receives humidified air.

From October through March, Dr. Gelperin found the number of medical visits necessitated by upper respiratory infections of soldiers living in the humidified barracks was 14 percent less than soldiers living in the unhumidified barracks. From January to March, the difference was a bit greater—18 percent.

Dr. Gelperin sees tremendous public health significance in this difference. He points out that if the soldiers in all eight barracks instead of four had been breathing humidified air throughout the winter, there would have been 151 fewer medical visits because of colds and similar problems.

The physician adds that military barracks (like office buildings) are in a sense unnatural because they bring together so many different people of different backgrounds, each bringing his own germs, which he proceeds inevitably to blow and sneeze at the others working in close proximity to him. When unnaturally dry air is added to this already strange situation, it isn't surprising that colds become rampant.

Cleanliness Is Important

Whether you are using a central unit attached to your furnace, or individual room humidifiers, the unit must be kept clean. The water in some humidifiers provides an ideal breeding ground for certain molds which can cause unpleasant reactions in hypersensitive individuals.

Joseph Gantner, an engineer and executive for a firm which manufactures humidifiers, reported that "it doesn't matter what kind of humidifier you have; if you let it get dirty, your efficiency decreases as far as getting water into the air, and the water that does get into the air could possibly be dirty."

Gantner said that his firm recommends that humidifiers be cleaned out with vinegar. Vinegar is an effective agent for killing microorganisms that might be growing in or around the humidifier. At the same time, its acidity helps cleanse the machines of dissolved lime which builds up as water evaporates.

If your humidification unit has a filter, the filter should be examined and vacuum-cleaned every week, and probably replaced several times a year.

94. Babies Don't Need Antibiotics For Colds

Usually a delightful, bright and alert baby, 16-month-old Laura just wasn't acting like herself. Laura's mother dated the change in the child from the time her pediatrician put her on an antibiotic for a sore throat. Laura got diarrhea from the antibiotic and a bad diaper rash. Then she got an earache and more antibiotics. The diarrhea came back, Laura lost weight and her interest in toys. Just when her earache seemed to be better, she developed another throat infection and was put on an escalated program of antibiotics that continued for six weeks.

What was wrong with Laura? A pediatrician who hadn't been doing his homework. Certainly Laura's pediatrician was kind and gentle and had her welfare at heart. But when he prescribed an antibiotic for her throat infection, he no doubt did not realize that he was doing the baby more harm than good.

Antibiotics wage war against bacteria—not viruses. What pediatricians sometimes fail to realize is that when they use antibiotics for the usual colds and upper respiratory infections of infants, they are using heavy ammunition for an enemy that isn't there. Because, according to an intensive study in Canada involving 4,700 infants, these infections, when they occur in children under three, *are rarely bacterial in nature.*

According to Drs. D. A. Stewart and H. Moghadam of the Hospital for Sick Children in Toronto, Canada, a child may have a positive throat swab culture and yet not be infected with the kind of bacteria which respond to antibiotics. Swabs were examined within an hour and any bacteria present were identified in the bacteriology laboratory. Every pediatrician should take note of the findings. For example, among 2,193 children with no evidence of infection, 77, or 3.5 percent, had a positive culture for Group A beta-hemolytic streptococcus. In 885 children who did have upper respiratory tract infection, only 14 had a positive culture for the same strain of streptococcus.

Drs. Stewart and Moghadam say that, "Much confusion exists about the necessity of using antibiotic drugs to treat upper respiratory tract infections in children, especially infants," (*Canadian Medical Association Journal,* December 9, 1972). Half of the children they examined showed clinical evidence of colds or other infection. The other half did not. But "there was no practical difference between the frequency of positive cultures from infected and non-infected children, suggesting that antibiotics were not required."

Before prescribing any antibiotic drug, the physician should take into account the available scientific data which, Drs. Stewart and Moghadam say, indicate that *most such infections are not primarily of bacterial origin.*

Although the B-hemolytic streptococcus is the main cause of pharyngitis (sore throat) in older children, it is seldom the cause in children under two years of age, it was pointed out by Mortimer and Boxerbaum in *Pediatrics* (36:930, 1965). But many doctors still use penicillin and other antibiotics to treat pharyngitis in infants. Indeed, say Drs. Stewart and Moghadam, "today it is rare for an infant with fever to escape being given these drugs for a 'sore throat' regardless of the cause." (*Canadian Medical Association Journal,* July 10, 1971)

Pharyngitis in young children is usually a viral, not a bacteriological infection, and yet the tendency to use antibiotics for these throat infections seems to be increasing. Why? Perhaps, say the Canadian doctors, because of "the doctor's doubts, the parents' anxiety or the pharmaceutical promotions." Also, because, "the physician is so pressed for time he often prescribes an antibiotic without looking for the true cause of fever, cough or runny nose. This is common practice but inexcusable and also dangerous. It may delay diagnosis of a more serious illness such as meningitis or urinary infection with severe consequences to the child.

"A proper history, a complete examination and appropriate laboratory procedures to facilitate diagnosis are the right of any sick child," they continue. "In most cases the 24-hour delay necessary to obtain a report of the culture is warranted. Pharyngitis or sore throat is rarely an emergency and delaying the administration of antibiotics for 12 to 24 hours, which is all the time that is necessary to identify the bacteria, will more often than not demonstrate that the antibiotic is not necessary."

Occasionally, the Canadian doctors say, for a baby who is very ill, prescription of an antibiotic is justified before the results of the culture are known. But, they emphasize, there is no justification for prescribing antibiotics over the telephone to treat coughs, fevers or colds.

It is hard, of course, for a mother whose sick, cranky baby is suffering from a cold, not to run to a pediatrician and hope that he will prescribe a wonder drug that will make her baby better. Unfortunately, as seen in the case of Laura, the wonder drugs have their limitations and their dangerous side effects.

95. That "Cold" Could Be An Allergy

Does this sound familiar: tight chest, a rattling when you take a deep breath, runny nose, recurrent earache, diarrhea, red and watery eyes, chronic sinus headache? If you think it's a cold take another guess. These are symptoms of cow's milk allergy, according to Dr. John W. Gerrard, a pediatrician of The University of Saskatchewan, writing in the *Journal of the American Medical Association* (November 7, 1966).

"One of the common problems facing both pediatricians and family physicians," says Dr. Gerrard, "is the child who seems to have one cold after another, each cold being followed by an attack of bronchitis or bronchopneumonia, often necessitating admission to hospital. The fundamental cause of the child's repeated respiratory tract infections frequently remains obscure . . . we have recently encountered four children whose predisposition to recurrent respiratory tract infection was relieved by the simple expedient of excluding cow's milk and dairy products from their diets . . ." No doubt there are many other children suffering in the same way, with worried parents who have tried everything to relieve them, missing the one basic cause of their problem, allergy.

Milk-Free Diet Brought Relief

The most alarming case described by Dr. Gerrard concerned a baby boy who caught a cold at two months and had to be admitted to a hospital with serious bronchitis. In the hospital he got worse in spite of oxygen and antibiotics. His lungs became increasingly congested, he ran a constant fever and was periodically unconscious. When, at last, he was put on a milk-free diet, he recovered quickly. His symptoms returned only when he drank ordinary cow's milk. From then on he was fed beef-base formula with vitamin supplements. Even a year later he suffered with nasal congestion and wheezing when he was given milk.

431

Colds

The family history disclosed that the mother, in perfect health, never drank milk. The father, on the other hand, loved milk and drank plenty of it. He suffered from chronic nasal congestion and bronchitis. He said he had always been plagued with respiratory discomfort, and could breathe through his nose only when he took nasal decongestants. He was raised on a farm and always drank at least a gallon of milk a day. When he consented to stop drinking cow's milk and eating dairy products, his breathing trouble cleared up completely in three weeks. Later, even small amounts of cow's milk or milk products—he was very fond of cheese—brought a prompt return of symptoms.

Dr. Gerrard described the case of an infant girl who was breast fed for six weeks, then put on a milk formula. At the same time a cold and bronchitis developed, and with it, abdominal distention. Her parents took her to the hospital. As soon as dairy products were excluded from her diet, her abdomen returned to normal, and her breathing cleared too. This child's father drank milk but had no symptoms. Her mother was also fond of milk, "but she had constant rhinorrhea (stuffed nose) complicated by frequent attacks of serious otitis media (earache) . . . the serious otitis media had always been thought to have been aggravated by pregnancy. Later it was learned that during pregnancy she had increased her milk intake, thinking that this was necessary for the welfare of her unborn child."

A 14-month-old boy suffering from persistent anemia lived on a diet composed almost entirely of cow's milk. At age 8 months he had become irritable and anemic, with constant nasal congestion, bronchitis and earache. Six months later when his anemia did not respond to oral iron therapy, he was admitted to a hospital. In the hospital it became apparent that with cow's milk eliminated, congestion and bronchitis cleared up. His stools were less frequent and his disposition improved. When milk was returned to his diet, all his trouble returned too.

The boy's mother drank between one and two quarts of milk a day. She experienced continual nasal stuffiness and bronchitis. The bronchitis had persisted since early adolescence. She was hospitalized, and while there, she stopped drinking milk. Within two weeks her symptoms cleared completely for the first time that she could remember. Following this she drank three quarts of milk, and within 24 hours her nose became obstructed, bronchitis returned, and her throat felt sore.

432

Dr. Gerrard does not say that all children and adults who suffer from chronic respiratory tract infections are allergic to milk, but the possibility of some form of allergy in such cases should not be ignored. In the absence of other disease conditions known to bring similar symptoms, the patients should be checked for milk allergy, along with intolerances to other foods.

Section 18
Constipation

96. What Is True Constipation? Few People Have It

The American public annually spends $200 million buying 800 different laxatives. This indicates that a great many people think they're constipated and that laxatives are what they need. In reality, relatively few people have true constipation, and laxatives almost always do more harm than good.

In general, it can be said that there are three basic causes of constipation. One is what doctors call "organic" disease, signifying that a specific condition, such as a physical blockage, injury, or other disease is causing the problem. Typically, this kind of constipation develops rather rapidly in people who ordinarily have not had any problem with bowel movements. This kind of change, occurring over a period of weeks or months, is a strong indication that a visit to a doctor, perhaps a proctologist, is in order.

Another kind of constipation is quite clearly due to stress, such as a radical change in the living habits or state of health. Typically, this kind of constipation will appear during a trip, in which you are eating strange food, sleeping in strange quarters, and moving your bowels in a strange bathroom. This kind of constipation does not automatically call for a trip to the doctor; neither does it indicate a need for a laxative. In a few days the condition will pass, and you will be none the worse for it. If the distress is really bothering you, the most knowledgeable doctors recommend one or two enemas with simply tap water or a couple of glasses of prune juice. This transient form of constipation often occurs during brief periods of hospitalization, and hospital staffs have been severely criticized for almost routinely prescribing laxatives for it. Too many patients, it seems, go home feeling that they *need* a laxative and continue taking one for several weeks. The frequent result is that they become psychologically, even physically, addicted to laxatives.

The third general kind of constipation is by far the most common, and is known as functional, or simply habitual constipation. This is what most of that 200 million dollars is spent for.

But what exactly is habitual constipation? A standard medical work, the *Cecil-Loeb Textbook of Medicine* (13th ed., Saunders, 1971), says that "Constipation ordinarily signifies the passage of excessively dry stools or evacuation less often than every other day." But it goes on to say that many patients expand the meaning of the word to include stools of small size or a sense of incomplete emptying of the rectum.

The idea that moving the bowels less often than every other day constitutes constipation is of course a controversial one. Many doctors believe that in some people, particularly those who may be very sedentary, or of an older age, or who simply don't eat very much, there is nothing at all abnormal about having only two or three bowel movements a week—perhaps even less in some cases. Unless the patient is suffering from a feeling of distress as a result of these infrequent movements, or has painful bowel movements in which hard dry stools are passed, he may not have constipation at all. He is simply on his own schedule.

97. Constipation Related To Disease

Most patients who go into a doctor's office to seek help with constipation typically do so only after years of trying to treat themselves. But they are not automatically going to get the help they seek from their doctor. In fact, many doctors cannot be counted upon to give even strictly medical help. Dr. Norman D. Nigro of Wayne State University School of Medicine, Detroit, told his fellow physicians at a panel presentation on constipation held at the 1974 AMA convention in Chicago that too many physicians lack adequate knowledge about either the significance or proper management of constipation. Some, he said, tend to dismiss it as something of no importance.

Doctors should be particularly alert (and the patient too!) if the constipation is of relatively sudden onset. After questioning the patient about any change in his life style, and giving him a physical examination, the doctor may then perform a digital examination of the rectum. The finding of no more than a few scant grams of feces indicates, according to the *Textbook of Medicine*, that habitual constipation is present. The next logical step is to search for local lesions in the area of the anus and rectum, which can be done with specialized tools such as the anoscope and sigmoidoscope. In many cases, a barium enema and X-rays will be administered, but Dr. Nigro warns that to avoid putting the barium above an obstructive lesion, the doctor should always visually examine the rectal area before giving barium.

Although serious conditions must always be ruled out, sometimes the medical problem may be as simple as weak stomach or back muscles, which may be caused by multiple pregnancies, neurological problems, or simply long years of inactivity. Ulcers or thrombosed hemorrhoids may sometimes be found, which would prevent relaxation of the anal sphincter. But such injuries are more often a *result* of constipation—through straining—than a cause.

The doctor (or the patient) is also well advised to check on any drugs the patient may be taking. Any medication, such as opiates (paregoric, given for diarrhea, is camphorated tincture of opium) which is designed to slow down nerve reactions, can be constipating. Certain antacid preparations which are nonabsorbable can also create constipation.

The physician also has a role to play in cases of fecal impaction. This is simply a large, hard mass of fecal matter which is lodged in the rectum. It is often accompanied by diarrhea, a watery waste that moves around the obstruction. The physician can break up the impaction with a rubber-gloved finger, and will follow this with an enema of cottonseed oil or some other softener, and follow this in turn with an enema of tap water.

Constipation And Heart Patients

Constipation, with its attending straining at stool, is a special threat to cardiac patients. In 1957, Dr. Norman Shaftel of New York told a symposium sponsored by the American College of Angiology that tests revealed that even in people with no previous history of heart disorder, straining produced important changes in heart rate, blood pressure and electrocardiograph patterns. Further, these changes closely resemble those which are seen in known heart patients.

Specifically, about 12 percent of straining episodes were found to be of sufficient intensity and duration to produce significant abnormalities. The frequency of such incidents, Dr. Shaftel declared, *is increased five times by constipation.* He was not able to state precisely how common death following strained defecation is, but he did say that it "is not rare."

Another aspect of the problem was revealed in an editorial in the *Lancet* (August, 1959), which reported that blood studies had shown "quite remarkable changes in the size of the veins of the limbs and of the flow of blood through them" during bathroom straining. These changes are much greater in constipation, and "may be sufficient to cause the mobilization of peripheral thrombi with subsequent embolization."

Constipation In Children

Probably the most common cause of chronic constipation among children is excessive milk drinking. It isn't so much that milk itself is constipating (in fact, milk often aggravates diarrhea) but that it tends to replace solids in a diet. (For the same reason, children who drink too much milk also become anemic.) If the child is drinking more than a quart of milk a day, his mother should cut back on the milk, and see that his appetite is filled with fresh fruits and vegetables and whole grain products. If the child won't eat enough of these foods to supply the calcium the milk was giving him, he should be given a calcium supplement.

Chronic constipation among children can be a source of recurring urinary infections. A study published in *Pediatrics* in 1973 by Drs. Neumann, de Domenico, and Nogrady revealed that children with these infections have three times the rate of constipation found in the general population of children.

The doctors put a group of children with a history of urinary tract infection and abnormal bowel habits on a regimen designed to eliminate constipation. The most important part of the program, it turned out, was the exclusion of all milk and milk products from the diet. Those who stuck to the regime had no more infections. In every case where there was a relapse, it was found that constipation was still present, usually as a result of reverting to milk.

The doctors explained that when the rectum is full, particularly in the small pelvic space of a child, there can be great pressure on the neck of the bladder. This in turn causes a back-up or retention of urine, which creates the right conditions for the multiplication of bacteria. These infections are much more common in girls than in boys, apparently because the presence of the ovaries makes the pelvic region even more crowded.

Significantly, at least one well known urologist has commented that the association between constipation and urinary tract infections is also found in adults. Prompt correction of constipation by a natural and safe means is therefore indicated in people of any age plagued with recurring urinary infections.

98. What Causes Habitual Constipation?

Once transitory changes of habit or physical illness are ruled out as causes of constipation, what is left? By far the two most common causes—which are often related—are failure of the normal defecation reflex, and a diet lacking sufficient roughage or fiber.

Obviously, many psychological factors can interfere with expression of the simple urge to move one's bowels. Some of these causes may stem back to childhood toilet training. Other people disrupt their normal defecation reflex by repeatedly failing to heed its call. After months or years of such a pattern of denial, the normal relationship between waste matter ready to move, nervous impulses, and muscular reactions leading to defecation becomes short-circuited.

Perhaps an even more common cause of failure of the defecation reflex is—ironically—stimulant-type laxatives, such as those based on senna seed or castor oil. The *Medical Letter* (Nov. 23, 1973) branded such products as "the least desirable laxatives," explaining that when taken regularly, they destroy the innate, normal defecation reflex with the result that "dependence on stimulant laxatives for evacuation may cause chronic constipation."

In light of the fact that such huge quantities of stimulant-type laxatives are sold, it is clear that a self-perpetuating cycle is involved. A person feels constipated, begins taking a stimulant laxative, and then becomes permanently constipated through the destruction of his normal defecation reflex, thereby becoming dependent on the laxative.

In addition, warns *The Medical Letter,* such preparations when given in doses large enough to relieve constipation can also cause cramps, diarrhea and fluid depletion. Chronic use can also cause a dangerous depletion in the vital mineral potassium, malabsorption and other disorders.

In addition, a strong laxative that "cleans out the system" removes not only the waste matter that should normally have been eliminated that day, but much of the still-liquid waste matter above it in the tract. Consequently, after such a purging, the person typically finds that he has no bowel movement for the next few days, and believing himself constipated again, takes more laxatives.

Despite all this, one well known senna-type laxative has for years been heavily advertised in major medical journals, with the probable result that many patients are taking this "least desirable laxative" on the recommendation of their physician!

Dietary Causes Of Constipation

Another common cause of constipation, often occurring simultaneously with an impaired defecation reflex, is a lack of adequate fiber in the diet. Basically, fiber is needed to give bulk to the waste, so that it can be expeditiously moved by segmental wave activity through the colon (up, over, down and out). Normally, mass propulsive movements occur once a day. But because the colon is much larger than a simple vessel designed to carry blood or urine, and contains segments (something like a long string of sausages), waste matter must obviously have sufficient bulk to be moved through this system.

Actually, most of the bulk in a feces consists of water, not food or food residue. But the water must be absorbed by the residue, and here is the problem.

Even when eaten in large quantities, foods such as cottage cheese, hard cheese, milk, and ice cream will not help matters any—because they contain no fiber whatsoever. And although few people realize it, meat contains the same amount of fiber as ice cream: zero. Likewise, sugar, which the average person consumes at the rate of two pounds a week, contains no fiber. Neither does soda pop, beer, coffee, tea, or other beverages. Orange juice contains only an insignificant trace of fiber (from the pulp).

Traditionally, bread has always been an important source of dietary fiber, but white bread contains only a tiny fraction of the fiber present in the natural wheat. When the bran and germ are removed from the grain, so is approximately 85 percent of the fiber. In other words, to get the same amount of fiber from a slice of white bread as you would from a slice of whole-grain bread, you would have to eat eight or nine slices of the white bread! (Actually, you would have to eat even more than this, because the slice of whole-grain bread weighs considerably more than the white bread, and the difference of 85 percent is calculated on a weight basis.)

Meanwhile, while Americans stuff themselves with meat, white bread, ice cream, cheese, soda pop, beer, cake, pastry, and other processed foods which contain little or no fiber, they are eating less and less of such fiber-rich foods as potatoes, cabbage, peas, beans, and fresh fruits and vegetables.

Consequently, no matter what the volume of the fiber-depleted food they eat, there is nothing for the water to be absorbed into in order to create the soft but firm bulk needed to facilitate easy elimination.

But what happens to the water in the bowels that is not absorbed by the food waste? The answer is that it is simply reabsorbed by the body through the wall of the colon. This removal of water is quite a vigorous process, with the result that when scanty waste matter moves sluggishly through the bowels, even the small amount of water that it has managed to absorb can be removed from it and returned to the body. By the time the waste matter reaches the rectum, it may be extremely compact and dry. It will also tend to be highly segmented or shaped by the contractions of the gut. In contrast, waste matter which contains generous amounts of fiber, and therefore of water, tends to be large, soft, and unsegmented.

Clearly, the answer to this problem is to somehow introduce more bulk into the diet, particularly the kind of bulk that will absorb and hold great amounts of water.

99. Wheat Bran And Other Foods To Conquer Constipation

Wheat bran, which is produced by the ton in the process of refining the flour, is certainly not the only source of natural food fiber. But it may well be the best. Unlike some other forms of fiber such as the fiber in nuts, wheat bran soaks up water like a sponge, increasing its weight approximately eight-fold when thoroughly moistened. At the same time, it is a very concentrated form of fiber, so it is easier to ingest than eating large amounts of fruits or potatoes. It is also extremely inexpensive.

But perhaps the best recommendation for bran is that it has actually been used and thoroughly tested by many doctors on great numbers of people. In every trial, it has proven remarkably effective in preventing and/or curing constipation. It will not do the trick in every individual case, but so far, doctors have yet to find any other food (or any substance, for that matter) that will help so many people, so effectively, so safely, and so inexpensively—a month's supply will average out to a cost of only two cents a day!

The idea that bran can abolish constipation is far from new. But until recently, it had more of the status of a folk remedy than of a medically-approved treatment. Its present wide acceptance as an unconstipating food can probably be attributed mostly to Surgeon Captain Thomas L. Cleave of the British Royal Navy.

Here is part of a letter published in the *Lancet* in 1962, from Dr. Harold Dodd: "Constipation is an ailment of so-called civilization and it can be greatly relieved by the way we live . . . . I cannot speak too highly of Surgeon Captain Cleave's prescription—one tablespoon of unprocessed bran daily. It restores to the diet what the miller has taken out. For several years I have practiced and prescribed a dessertspoon of unprocessed bran and one of unprocessed wheat germ daily. It is moistened according to taste with milk, gravy, soup, coffee, or fruit juice. In most patients it insures a daily formed stool as smooth as with liquid paraffin. . . . Patients with diverticulitis and subacute and chronic ulcerative colitis thrive on it."

In 1972, in the *British Medical Journal,* Captain Cleave himself gave a brief history of his early work with bran. As early as 1941, while he was Senior Medical Officer on a battleship, there was a scarcity of fresh food and vegetables and he "found such bran invaluable for correcting the constipation (of) the ship's company. . . . The sailors loved this stuff by comparison with purgatives. . . . I think it is a great tragedy of our present day age that, with the Medical Research Council showing at least 15 percent of the population to be on regular purgatives, this precious material is ever lost through the manufacture of white flour."

Bran probably got its biggest boost in the medical world in 1972 with the publication in the *British Medical Journal* of a study by Drs. Painter, Almeida, and Coleburn, who are respectively two surgeons and a physician. The primary purpose of their study of 70 patients (average age, 60) was to see what ameliorating effects bran would have on patients with diverticular colon disease. However, 28 of the diverticular patients were constipated before a few spoonsful of bran were added to their daily diet. After the introduction of bran, constipation was abolished in 15 patients and relieved in eight. Also of importance, the vast majority of the patients had to strain either always or sometimes when eliminating. After the bran, 80 percent were relieved of this condition. Also abolished or relieved in the great majority of the cases were cramping, abdominal pain, tender rectum, wind, heartburn, and incomplete emptying of the bowel.

Another study, by Dr. J. H. Cummings, published in *Gut* in 1973, held that with the addition of fiber to the diet, the stool is softer, and bulkier, usually resulting in an end to constipation.

Bran, it must be added, is not a laxative. It is rather a *normalizer,* or regulator of bowel function. The study by Dr. Painter and his colleagues proved this by demonstrating that chronic diarrhea is aided as much as constipation by bran. The bran apparently soaks up the excess water in the colon, and helps to form normal stools.

Some people object to bran on the ground that it is scratchy. Actually, once it's moistened, it isn't scratchy at all. It takes on the consistency of a sponge.

The kind of bran successfully used by these doctors is not the kind of bran that is sold as a breakfast cereal. This latter product is processed, and usually contains sugar. The doctors are unanimous in recommending unprocessed bran, which is a flaky-looking product available from health food sources.

When taking bran, it is best to begin with one or two teaspoons a day, always taken with some sort of fluid, and increase the amount until the desired effect takes hold. This may mean anywhere from two teaspoons twice a day to two or three tablespoons three times a day. At first, it can produce some wind and distension, but this condition almost always disappears within a week or two. It takes that long for your body to adjust to the added fiber.

A few people may not be able to tolerate bran. Or they may wish to get their fiber through different sources. This isn't very difficult. Fresh fruits such as apples, peaches, plums and pears are all good sources of fiber—and contain a lot of water as well. Eat the skins and all, but avoid fruits that have been sprayed with insecticides. If unsprayed fruit is not available, soak the fruit for a few minutes in 1/4 cup of vinegar diluted in a dishpan of water, and then rinse the fruit in clear water. This will remove 85 percent of the surface spray. Fresh leafy green vegetables such as cabbage and spinach are also valuable, as are foods rich in unrefined starch, such as white potatoes, sweet potatoes, pumpkins, squash, and carrots.

Dried fruits are also an excellent source of fiber, but they should be taken with plentiful fluids, soaked or stewed. Prunes, by the way, are valuable for their intrinsic fiber, whereas prune juice works its well-known effects because it contains a natural but as yet unidentified laxative substance. Because this substance works through a stimulating action on the bowels, prune juice should not be consumed regularly in place of real bulk.

Blackstrap molasses has a mild laxative effect which many people will not even notice. It is best consumed as a nutritional flavoring for milk, or as an ingredient in recipes, rather than for its laxative qualities.

100. Living Habits That Promote Easy Elimination

Food fiber is not the only answer to constipation. Regular exercise can be a great help. The more vigorous the exercise, the more it helps. Exercises which condition the stomach muscles and back muscles are particularly valuable, but a nice long walk every day will also help.

If the exercise makes you thirsty, as it ought to, take your fill of water. All the bran in the world won't solve your problem if you don't drink enough water to let it do its work.

Regularity of habits is also important. It's a good idea to regulate your bowel habits for the same time every day. A good time for this might be after eating a hearty breakfast which includes fresh or stewed fruit, an unrefined cereal product such as granola, wheat germ, or oatmeal, and some whole grain bread products. If that's too much cereal and bread, replace some of it with a few teaspoons of unprocessed bran.

Once in the bathroom, try to relax. Pick up a magazine or a book. Just make sure you aren't reading about constipation, because the idea is to take your mind off what you are doing. Stay put for about ten minutes, regardless of what happens. Repeat daily. Eventually, your colon will get the idea.

Speaking of toilets, it has been said that toilet bowls themselves cause problems by being too high. Critics say that feet should be planted firmly upon the ground to induce a proper bowel movement, and that toilets today tend to be too high. So if you want to, put a stack of old books under each foot, or keep a footstool nearby.

If all this sounds rather elaborate and artificial, it really isn't. What you are doing, from eating bran to getting yourself into a squatting position, is trying to get back to the kind of diet and living habits that mankind had for hundreds of thousands of years before the 20th century made him constipated.

Although current thinking places more emphasis on non-nutritive fiber than on vitamins in most cases of constipation, it is nevertheless true that many people have been helped nutritionally. The B complex seems to be the most important factor. Experimentally, when young men were deprived of thiamine, most of them became constipated. Most patients with pellagra, a severe deficiency of the B vitamin niacin, are also constipated. Brewer's yeast and rice polishings, both excellent sources of the B complex, have been used with success in treating constipation.

Nutritionist Adelle Davis believed, based on the research she read, that the B vitamin inositol is especially important in relieving constipation, and recommended blackstrap molasses as one of the richest sources of this vitamin—which is rarely, if ever, included in synthetic vitamin preparations. She also emphasized the need for plenty of calcium to relieve spastic colitis or spastic constipation caused by deficiency of this vital mineral.

Section 19
Diabetes

101. A Deadly Disease You Can Live With

Long before the Greeks found a word for it, diabetes (passing) was a plague in Egypt. In the world's oldest known medical document, dated 1500 B.C., Egyptian physicians referred to the symptoms. The word mellitus (honey) was added later by the Greeks, making the descriptive phrase diabetes mellitus—passing sweet—to describe the sweet urine passed by diabetics.

By the 19th century, scientists had learned that the mysterious disease that causes sweetness (which they then knew to be sugar) in the urine was somehow due to an abnormality of the pancreas. Von Mering and Minkowski were able to reproduce the characteristic symptoms of diabetes in a dog by removing his pancreas. It was a fortunate coincidence that several years earlier a biologist, Paul Langerhans, had become intrigued by peculiar clusters—islands—of cells in the pancreas, entirely unlike the other tissues of the gland. His discovery that the beta cells in the "Islands of Langerhans" produce the protein, insulin, had followed quickly. The relationship between difficulties in sugar metabolism and insulin production in the system was soon recognized. When, in 1922, Sir Frederick Banting produced insulin that could be injected to supplement what appeared to be a shortage of the hormone, the riddle of diabetes was presumed to be solved.

In the simplest terms, diabetes results when the body is unable to make full use of the carbohydrates (sugars and starches) we eat. Either because the pancreas does not produce enough insulin to process these sugars for storage or use in the cells, or because the insulin produced is less effective than it should be, the sugar (glucose) stays in the blood, accumulating there until it spills over into the kidneys and the urine. The body cannot afford this continued loss of valuable carbohydrates and eventually diabetes symptoms are likely to occur.

Insatiable Thirst Is An Early Symptom

The most blatant symptoms of diabetes are excessive urination, excessive thirst, excessive hunger, weight loss and weakness and fatigue. These symptoms are all rooted in the kidneys' efforts to remove excess, unprocessed glucose from the bloodstream. Ever-increasing amounts of urine are continually required to dissolve the concentrated glucose and get it out of the body. This unusual loss of fluid creates an insatiable thirst for more liquid to replenish the loss. The weight loss occurs because the body doesn't use the glucose; hunger follows when the body recognizes the need to fill in the weight loss. The lack of energy is the obvious consequence of lost glucose, normally the source of quick energy.

Experience has taught the modern physician not to wait for the obvious outward signs of diabetes. Samples of urine are tested for sugar content as a regular procedure in all but the most superficial general physical examinations. Many physicians administer the glucose tolerance test, where a specific amount of glucose is given when the blood is presumed clear of excessive sugar, to see if the body can handle the glucose normally. The most reliable diabetes test known today is laboratory analysis of blood serum for sugar content.

Once a diagnosis of diabetes has been made, the doctor and the patient join in a mutual effort to restore a carbohydrate balance in the system, all the while maintaining a good nutritional status. The ideal glucose concentration in the blood is normally 140 mg per 100 cc after meals. Diabetics rarely achieve this level, but they can function at near normal levels arrived at by diet, diet in combination with insulin, or by diet, insulin and drugs in certain severe cases.

In the early stages, the doctor determines whether a diet regulated to minimize carbohydrate intake will control the blood sugar levels in diabetes or whether insulin must be added. Doctors generally avoid prescribing insulin when diet can do the job because of the frightening reactions which can occur.

Insulin shock results from too much insulin getting rid of too much sugar at a time. Some sugar is essential in the bloodstream. Without it the body cannot function. If the blood sugar sinks too low in the diabetic, he suffers blurred vision, sudden weakness or dizziness, and eventually collapse. Diabetics usually carry a concentrated sweet or sugar cubes to counteract such an emergency.

During the early weeks of insulin treatment, swelling, particularly in the face, is common. Changes in vision also occur. In certain patients, a general allergic reaction to insulin creates serious consequences.

Diabetes Can Strike At Any Age

Anyone at any age can develop diabetes, but the disease occurs mainly in the middle and late years. Eighty percent of all diabetics are more than 45 years old.

Juvenile diabetes, affecting children or young adults, is usually too severe to be handled by diet alone. Doctors generally agree that insulin (sometimes in small amounts) is essential to control the disease in these cases. The amount of insulin required depends a great deal on the type of diet the child follows. If it is fairly strict, the necessary insulin is minimal. However, physicians tend to be permissive with diabetic children, requiring very little dietary restriction, relying on heavy doses of insulin to keep the sugar under control.

In handling the diabetic child, a great deal depends on the attitude of the family. Concern and responsibility without overprotectiveness are the watchwords here. The child should be taught to give himself the insulin injection. He should know the symptoms of insulin shock, and should be aware that it is important to test his urine for glucose content daily (do-it-yourself kits are readily available). Parents can help by serving foods that are within the bounds of safety dictated by his illness.

For older diabetics, the disease is referred to as maturity-onset diabetes, which is usually milder and does not progress as fast. Most of these patients can manage with careful diet alone, or, if they insist, with one of the oral drugs. In these patients, control of the diabetes is often less of a problem than how to handle the degenerative changes that have taken place. Heart attack, stroke, eye problems, and skin changes in the extremities because of poor circulation are common. Constant checking for changes is vital. Doctors urge older diabetics to pay careful attention to their feet. Infection in the feet can result in gangrene and eventual amputation. The feet must be kept clean and dry, and older diabetics are warned against breaking blisters, walking barefoot or engaging in other activities that might cause skin injury.

Diabetes is unwelcome at any age, but modern scientific advances have made diabetes a disease that can be lived with, and doors are opening to the ultimate control of the problem in all its phases. A diabetic willing to watch his diet and take the minimal precautions that any health-conscious individual would take anyway, can live virtually a normal life with virtually a normal life expectancy.

Perhaps the most encouraging, most convincing evidence of that outlook comes from the insurance companies. Diabetes patients are usually insurable. Insurance companies are generally willing to bet that diabetics who follow their doctors' advice will live to a ripe old age.

102. What Is A Diabetic Diet? Delicious!

Most people never get diabetes. The chances that you will ever have to walk the metabolic tightrope of this chronic disease are less than one in fifty. But if diabetes should strike, you would be doing yourself a great favor by following your doctor's dietary advice precisely.

A number of new research findings and recommendations by physicians indicate that a diabetic diet—conscientiously followed—can be a real life preserver. In fact, the diabetic who makes an extra effort to take care of himself is really a step ahead of his nondiabetic counterpart on the road to health. It's not surprising that a diabetic diet should be so beneficial. It *has* to be.

Delicious As Well As Healthful

First, let's clear up once and for all the widely-held notion that a diabetic diet has to be unappealing and harshly restrictive.

In the book, *Feast On a Diabetic Diet* (McKay, New York, 1969), naturalist and wild foods gatherer Euell Gibbons tells the story of his brother Joe, who was first diagnosed as a diabetic while in the Navy during World War II. After learning how to give himself daily insulin injections and follow a diabetic diet, Joe was discharged and sent home.

"Our paths diverged," writes Gibbons, "and it was many years before I saw Joe again. Then I was invited to spend a week at his home in New Mexico. I arrived, prepared to conceal my dismay at the way he must by now look, and all that he must have to endure on a diabetic regime."

Gibbons was in for a surprise! "I found that the years had changed Joe less than they had changed me," he writes. "My love of good food was beginning to show around my middle, but he was still slender and flat-stomached." That night the brothers dined on a delicate, herb-flavored consomme, broiled sirloin, asparagus spears, tossed salad, hot rolls, and for dessert, fresh melon balls.

"Dinner was a revelation," Gibbons discovered to his delight. But his pleasure turned to outright amazement as the wholesome, delicious meals continued. "Early in the week," says Gibbons, "I became aware of the curious fact that Joe was actually eating far better than he had before becoming a diabetic; indeed he was eating higher-quality food than 95 percent of the nondiabetics I know."

Weight Control Is Crucial

The most important factor in Joe's and every other diabetic's diet is weight control. By carefully calculating the proper daily calorie intake for their particular body weight and activity level and never exceeding it, diabetics are usually able to bring their weight down to an optimum level which is actually ten percent less than standard height-and-weight charts recommend. The reward for such diligence is great.

"The overweight diabetic who successfully peels off enough pounds to get his weight back to normal usually experiences a dramatic improvement in his condition. Indeed, the symptoms often virtually disappear," says Charles Weller, M.D. in his book, *The New Way to Live With Diabetes* (Doubleday, New York, 1966). "Weight reduction and control can bring this incurable disease closer to complete remission than any medication." In many cases, the newly slender patient can stop taking insulin.

One facet of the diabetic diet that almost everyone is familiar with is the strict ban on sugar. When diabetes strikes, the victim loses the ability, normally provided by the hormone insulin, to keep the sugar or glucose level in his blood within bounds. Depending on the severity of the disease, he may have to take insulin injections or oral drugs to get the glucose out of the blood and into the cells where it is needed. Too concentrated a source of sugar will quickly overtax the diabetic's insulin reserves and send the blood glucose skyrocketing out of control.

"One of the first dietary rules for all diabetics is to avoid all sugar and foods containing sugar, such as pastry, candy, soft drinks, etc. . ." says Dr. Weller. "Although giving up sweet desserts may be inconvenient for relatives of a diabetic, they can console themselves with the knowledge that apple pie and fruitcake are not essential to the human diet and, indeed, their excessive consumption can be dangerous." The wise diabetic chooses a dessert of fresh fruit.

Not All Carbohydrates Are Bad

While refined sugar and other simple carbohydrates like white flour must be carefully watched, diabetics are actually encouraged to eat more *complex* carbohydrates—the same bulky, fiber-rich unprocessed foods that all Americans should be eating more of. Vegetables are ideal. Spinach, asparagus, broccoli, cabbage, string beans and celery are among the so-called "Group A" vegetables which the American Diabetes Association says can be generously included in diabetic diets. Served raw, most "Group A" vegetables can be eaten almost without limit.

What makes these complex carbohydrates so special? "It's true that starch, honey, syrups, carbohydrates in fruit, vegetables, berries, and cereals all end up as glucose," writes Lawrence E. Lamb, M.D. in *Metabolics* (Harper & Row, New York, 1974). "The difference is in the speed with which the conversion is accomplished . . . Most of the bulky vegetables will delay emptying of the stomach and smooth out the absorption of sugars into the blood." Whole grain cereals also have this ability, he adds.

Because, as Dr. Lamb points out, "Diabetics are particularly prone to atherosclerosis with the complicating problems of heart attacks, strokes, and poor circulation to the feet," they must also limit the amount of fat in their diet. They are also urged to substitute polyunsaturated fats for the saturated type when possible. Fish and poultry are especially recommended, instead of fatty cuts of meat. Greasy, fried foods are discouraged.

Many diabetics eat smaller, more frequent meals, rather than the two or three big meals most people consume daily. Researchers have found that multiple frequent feedings tend to keep blood cholesterol levels lower.

Since diabetics eat less than most of us, they are advised to make every calorie count. Food supplements can help supply essential vitamins and minerals. Cod liver oil is a recommended daily vitamin A supplement for diabetics, Dr. Angela J. Bowen told a Southwestern Diabetes Symposium in San Diego (*Pediatric News*, June, 1974). Diabetics and others on low-fat diets often need supplemental amounts of this fat-soluble nutrient, and tasteless fish oil capsules are an ideal source, the Seattle, Washington, physician said.

She also recommended that diabetic patients be given a vitamin E supplement, ranging from 300 to 600 mg. (equivalent to approximately 400 to 800 I. U.) per day. Diabetics, like everyone else, need *all* the known nutrients, including 12 vitamins and 17 minerals, Dr. Bowen said. To be sure of getting the full range of trace elements and other nutrients, she encourages her patients to eat the widest possible variety of permitted foods, in addition to taking supplements.

Eat More Raw Foods

Diabetics who make an effort to eat more raw foods may be able to decrease or eliminate their need for insulin, according to Dr. John M. Douglass, of the Southern California Permanente Medical Group and Kaiser Foundation Hospital in Los Angeles.

One of Dr. Douglass' patients, an elderly man, had been taking insulin twice a day. When he started eating more foods in their raw, uncooked state, his insulin requirements began to fall. After four years he was able to get by with just 30 units of insulin a day.

A second patient, a young Mexican-American man, complained to Dr. Douglass that he would rather die than continue taking insulin "shots." By shifting to an 80 percent raw diet, he was able to control his diabetes with oral drugs alone.

What led Dr. Douglass to try the raw food regimen? "My rationale was that since early man lived entirely on raw foods, perhaps such a diet would be less stressful to the human system in general and less diabetogenic than a cooked food diet," he writes in *Annals of Internal Medicine* (January, 1975). Raw vegetables, seeds, nuts, berries, melons, fruits, egg yolks, honey, oils and goat's milk are the mainstay of Dr. Douglass' program. He theorizes that the interaction of enzymes normally destroyed by cooking may be responsible for the raw diet's effect.

When we also consider that most diabetics are advised to give up smoking, restrict their alcohol intake, eat less salt and follow a program of regular, moderate exercise, we can see that the diabetic approach to better health is a sensible one for nearly everyone.

103. Brewer's Yeast Has What It Takes To Normalize Blood Sugar

Far more than any other food, brewer's yeast may turn out to be the one single greatest nutritional support for maintaining normal body handling of sugar—and thereby preventing diabetes.

The key to the importance of brewer's yeast lies in its *biologically valuable* concentration of the trace mineral chromium.

It wasn't until 1973 that findings were published describing anything more than the chromium *content* of various foods. But, as nutritionists are learning, a food's content when broken down and analyzed in the laboratory may be extremely deceptive in terms of nutritional value for animals and humans. Molecules of a nutrient may be bound into chemical structures which are not biologically active and therefore have limited or no nutritional value despite the nutrient's prominence in a typical food-analysis chart. So it turned out in the case of chromium.

Dr. Walter Mertz (a pioneer in early chromium research in the 1950's and 1960's) and his colleagues at the Nutrition Institute of the U.S. Department of Agriculture in Beltsville, Md., tested selected food samples for both total chromium content *and* for biological value. For this latter test, tissue of laboratory animals was treated in the presence of insulin with measured quantities of a selected food, and an insulin-triggered reaction known to require chromium participation was measured. The investigators' results were published in the January/February, 1973 issue of the *Journal of Agriculture and Food Chemistry*.

Though in content certain foods had a higher chromium concentration than brewer's yeast (egg yolks, for example, and oysters), the amount of chromium with biological value was many times higher in brewer's yeast than in any other food. On a chart of relative biological values, dried brewer's yeast rated 44.88, while the next highest rating (for black pepper, of all things!) was 10.21. Calf's liver, American cheese, and wheat germ followed with relative biological values rated at 4.52, 4.39, and 4.05.

Insulin Can't Function Without Chromium

Doctors once thought that an inadequate supply of insulin, probably resulting from a faulty pancreas, invariably was the cause of diabetes. It is now realized that this explanation is much too simplistic. It has been found that many diabetic patients have normal amounts of insulin but somehow cannot utilize it properly. Dr. Mertz suggests that such diabetics may often be simply suffering from chromium deficiency.

Dr. Mertz and his colleague Dr. K. Schwartz first reported that laboratory animals require chromium for proper insulin function (*American Journal of Physiology*, 196: 614, 1959). Other investigators, including Dartmouth Medical School's famous trace mineral specialist, Dr. Henry Schroeder, confirmed the early findings. Rats made chromium deficient responded with abnormal glucose metabolism and soon developed disorders characteristic of diabetes in man. In the early stages these disorders could be reversed by feeding the animals trace amounts of chromium.

But does chromium have the same anti-diabetic effect in humans?

Yes, there is firm evidence establishing this fact.

Chromium Brought "Overnight Recovery"

The most dramatic proof of chromium's efficacy in promoting normal insulin action in humans occurred in a hospital in Jerusalem in 1966. A scientist from the U.S. Food and Drug Administration's Division of Nutrition and a local pediatrician were working with severely malnourished refugee infants, almost all of whom had (among their other woes) faulty glucose metabolism. Given small amounts of chromium in their diet, "infants made overnight recoveries from the inability of their bodies to use sugar," according to a press release issued by the FDA (April 16, 1966). Until that time, the FDA report added, "the role of chromium in the normal human diet had only been suspected."

An article in *Medical World News* (May 19, 1972), based on the report of Dr. K. Michael Hambidge presented at the 1972 meeting of the Federation of American Societies for Experimental Biology, states that the majority of elderly persons in the U.S.

have impaired glucose tolerance. In clinical trials, "as many as 50 percent of such patients have been restored to normal glucose tolerance on daily doses of 150 micrograms of trivalent chromium." (Trivalent chromium is the biologically valuable form of this mineral, such as is found in brewer's yeast.)

More recently, when biochemist Richard J. Doisy and co-workers at the Upstate Medical Center in Syracuse, N.Y., gave brewer's yeast extract to 12 elderly persons with impaired glucose tolerance (a major factor in maturity-onset diabetes), half regained a normal ability to metabolize their blood sugar within two months (*Medical World News*, October 11, 1974). Brewer's yeast also lowered the insulin requirements of some diabetic patients. Dr. Doisy says that everyone, not just diabetics, should be taking brewer's yeast for its normalizing effect on blood sugar.

As today's specialists in diabetes stress, there are undoubtedly many contributing factors to this disease which is so prevalent in industrialized countries. For example, laboratory rats can be made diabetic, their insulin-producing cells of the pancreas exhausted, by long-term feeding with excess sugar. Vitamin B_6 deficiency in humans can induce an abnormal glucose tolerance pattern similar to that of diabetes, and many diabetics show abnormal metabolites in their urine indicative of B_6 deficiency. Excess output of steroid hormones by the adrenal gland (and steroid drugs, too) are diabetogenic.

You can see that the problem is not simple. It goes without saying that chromium will be effective in treating diabetic symptoms only if a chromium deficiency induced these disorders. But, judging by the clinical results cited in *Medical World News*, perhaps half of all sufferers of this disorder may have brought on their illness by chromium-deficient diets; and chromium supplementation—the biologically valuable chromium contained in brewer's yeast—might reverse the disease process.

Deficiency Is Widespread In U.S.

Humans have higher chromium levels at birth than at any other time in life. It is possible that such a dwindling in chromium values is a normal physiological happening. But poor diet unquestionably plays a part. The older population in the United States has markedly low concentrations of tissue chromium, far more pronounced than those found in communities not yet consuming the chromium-poor refined foods of the "civilized" world—communities in the Far East, the Middle East, and Africa, for example.

Among trace mineral researchers, there is little question that widespread chromium deficiency exists in our country. Says Dr. Mertz, in an article appearing in *Food and Nutrition News* (December, 1966): "Chromium concentration in the average daily diet is approximately within the range of experimental rations leading to a low chromium state (50-100 parts per billion), and far below that of animal diets which maintain rats on a normal glucose tolerance (1,000 ppb and more)." In other words, the American public gets as little chromium in its food as rats deliberately made deficient to induce abnormal glucose metabolism. Judging by animal experiments, the American diet should provide at least *10 times more* biologically valuable chromium than it now does in order to insure proper insulin function.

Whole grains and seeds are a relatively good source of biologically valuable chromium—a fact which helps explain why the American diet, based so heavily on refined, mineral-stripped white flour, is chromium-poor. In wheat, much of the chromium is concentrated in the germ, so that wheat germ added to your cereal and puddings and casseroles and meat loaves is good chromium insurance. But brewer's yeast is far and away the best source of biologically valuable chromium.

Nature has supplied the human body with insulin. But, like all hormones, this one can't do its job alone. It needs the nutrients that a full natural diet supplies.

104. Vitamin E For Arterial Disease In Diabetics

Aside from the inability to maintain a safe glucose level in the blood, there are other challenges to survival that diabetics face. These problems involve the heart. Arteriosclerosis, for example, has become the major killer of diabetics, according to Dr. Edwin L. Bierman, one of the nation's leading researchers into diabetes and cardiovascular disease (*New York Times*, October 3, 1971).

Another researcher into this tremendous problem, Dr. Rachmiel Levine, of the City of Hope Medical Center, in Duarte, California, estimates that "seventy percent of deaths in diabetic patients are the direct result of vascular (blood vessel) disease. This is about two-and-a-half times the proportion of deaths from vascular disease among the nondiabetic population of all ages" (*Journal of the American Geriatrics Society*, November, 1971).

Dr. Levine pointed out that the vascular problems exist on every level from the capillary system all the way up to plaque formation on the aorta. "The introduction of insulin led to an enormous rise in the life expectancy of diabetic patients and has therefore revealed the width and extent and severity of the vascular lesions," he wrote. "For diabetes, insulin has shifted the center of gravity from glycosuria (presence of sugar in the urine) and coma, to the heart, the limbs, the kidney and the eyes."

A 1964 study prepared by the Metropolitan Life Insurance Company stated that of 2,634 deaths among diabetic patients at Boston's Joslin Clinic, 77.9 percent were due to cardiovascular-renal diseases. Coronary heart disease alone accounted for 53.3 percent of all deaths during this period (*The New England Journal of Medicine*, August 26, 1965). The article, written by Drs. Jean O. Partamian and Robert F. Bradley, goes on to point out that the mortality rate from acute myocardial infarction (heart attacks) in the general population is much less, varying from 15 to 47 percent.

No one knows for sure why diabetics have more heart problems, but the well-known English nutritional researcher Dr. John Yudkin has a plausible theory. He suggests "there might be a pathway through the pancreas: the glucose load leading to excess circulating insulin and this in turn, affecting lipid metabolism, a situation resembling a sort of prediabetes. Certainly," he continues, "researchers have known since the 1920's that diabetics suffer from coronary heart disease and vascular disorders far more often than normals do and that these disorders occur at younger ages. And patients with atherosclerotic heart disease often show impaired glucose tolerance."

It seems obvious that present measures to help diabetics are really only half-measures. On one side, the need for insulin to control blood sugar is recognized and dealt with. But on the other hand, the diabetic is running a greater risk from heart disease, and is certainly suffering damage to his circulatory system.

In an attempt to give diabetics a better-than-even chance of surviving the heart problems once blood sugar problems are under control, some medical authorities are taking a second look at vitamin E (alpha tocopherol).

Treatment Is Incomplete Without Vitamin E

During a talk to members of the Vermont Natural Food & Farming Association, Inc., (May 1, 1971), Dr. Evan Shute of the Shute Foundation for Medical Research in Canada pointed out that diabetes is more like *two* diseases.

"One disease is high blood sugar, treated by diet and insulin and all that sort of thing. All that does," he said, "is usher in the ugly second half of the disease, degeneration of blood vessels, and this is what kills. This is what knocks out the eyes and the kidneys and the heart and produces gangrene. This is where alpha tocopherol comes in to play. No diabetic is being treated at all unless he takes alpha tocopherol!"

In his book, *Vitamin E for Ailing and Healthy Hearts* (Pyramid, 1969), Dr. Evan Shute's older brother Wilfrid—a cardiologist also with the Shute Foundation—noted that in conventional treatment, it didn't matter whether or not the diabetes was mild, moderate or severe, or whether or not control was good or bad. *In no way was the progress of the vascular damage altered!*

After a number of years of successfully treating other cases with vitamin E, however, Dr. Wilfrid Shute writes: "Now we can confidently state that every diabetic must have adequate control of his disease through diet and insulin or another anti-diabetic drug so that he will not develop coma or hyperglycemia (high blood sugar) reactions.

Diabetes

"It is of equal importance that he have alpha tocopherol to minimize the result of his vascular involvement. All three are indispensable for effective treatment."

Extra vitamin E can also help. Writing in *Geriatrics* (May, 1974), Dr. Robert W. Hillman of the State University of New York Downstate Medical Center in Brooklyn, says that "diabetics with small-vessel disease of the extremities may benefit from a daily dose of 300 to 600 mg. of alpha tocopherol" (the same amount recommended by Dr. Bowen, which translates to approximately 400 to 800 I. U. of vitamin E).

Visual Deterioration Halted

Although results in restoration of sight to diabetics who have gone blind are not very good, there have been some spectacular results in earlier stages of the disease.

Dr. Shute describes the case of a 35-year-old patient he first saw in September, 1958. "He had been diabetic for 20 years. His eyesight was deteriorating, and he had had hemorrhages in both eyes for the past six years. His left eye was nearly blind. He showed other evidence of arteriosclerosis and had a three plus albuminuria, for example.

"On 600 units of alpha tocopherol a day, his eyesight began to improve within six weeks and was nearly normal in six months. His albuminuria was greatly decreased, and he was feeling really well.

"In June of 1962 he suffered a fresh hemorrhage in one eye, and his dosage of alpha tocopherol was promptly doubled. His eyesight returned to normal within two weeks. He admitted that he had become careless and had decreased his alpha tocopherol to 400 units a day. . . ."

Dr. Shute also reports that treating "the effects of vascular changes in the brain and retina is much less satisfactory than treating the relatively simple abnormalities in heart, kidney and extremities. This is to be expected, since nerve cells are so highly specialized and so extremely sensitive to anoxia (lack of oxygen)."

Any treatment with vitamin E that Dr. Shute prescribes for his diabetic patients is in addition to the insulin the patient normally takes. But this is not always the case, as some researchers have discovered. There are published reports that when the vitamin was administered in some cases, the need for insulin was eliminated.

In no way, however, can the suggestion be made to do away with insulin. It's needed. The millions of persons the hormone has helped cannot be anything but thankful for the chance to live fruitful, productive lives.

But it still makes good sense to try to combat that side effect—heart and artery disease—that accompanies diabetes. And it also makes good sense to take advantage of vitamin E's proven effectiveness for keeping a healthy heart and blood vessels.

105. Diabetics, Here's How To Save Your Feet!

A threat faced by every diabetic is serious foot trouble. From the moment the leg arteries begin to clog and the sense of touch is reduced, the feet are endangered. Yet, with proper care of the feet and dietary measures to maximize tissue health, the danger can be minimized.

First of all, why does a diabetic have to take special measures to protect his feet? There are many reasons, all involving the changed physiology of a diabetic. Chief among them is the narrowing of the arteries, particularly the arteries in the lower leg and foot. Many Americans seem to develop a certain amount of arterial clogging as they grow older, but in the diabetic, the process can be considerably faster. It may be because of the diabetic's abnormal metabolism of fats, or because of some alteration in the cells lining the arteries. In truth, doctors don't know, but they do agree that the process is generally most advanced in the legs and feet.

Often accompanying this reduced circulation of blood is a relative loss of nerve sensations in the feet. To someone with a painful corn on his foot, his freedom from pain might seem to be a blessing, but to the diabetic, it is a menace. That is because the diabetic is also extraordinarily prone to picking up infections. Also, any kind of damage to the skin is very slow to heal. A blister that would disappear from the heel of a healthy person in a few days may linger unhealed on the foot of a diabetic for weeks. The same with any minor sore, corn, cut or scrape. Resistance is very low, and when the warning signal of pain is also out of kilter, the danger is very real.

The chances of developing foot trouble are greater in persons who have had diabetes for a relatively long time, especially if the condition has not been cared for, and in diabetics who are overweight, or of relatively advanced age.

Gangrene May Develop

The ultimate danger from impaired circulation is gangrene. With the flow of blood to the feet choked off by clogged arteries, the cells do not receive the oxygen and the nutrients they need to repair normal wear and tear. And waste matters, like carbon dioxide and lactic acid, aren't carried away. The result is the death of the affected tissue, typically beginning with the part that is furthest from the heart—the toes.

In what doctors call "dry gangrene," the skin of the foot will become very dry, eventually like parchment, perhaps turning black. The dead flesh will resemble that of a mummy. Another form of tissue death is "wet gangrene" which results from infection. With the skin being so weak, and protective white blood cells all but absent from the area, bacteria rage through the affected tissue and hasten its complete destruction. In this form of gangrene, the foot is moist and foul-smelling.

The gangrenous area, full of bacteria and waste matter which threaten the entire body, usually must be removed. But along with the area which is obviously dead, surgeons often remove the surrounding area. This must be done because the cells adjacent to gangrenous flesh are usually in such poor health themselves from lack of fresh blood that they cannot heal the wound that results from amputation. So gangrenous toes or a heel may cost a person his entire foot, ankle, and possibly more. Sometimes a surgeon will try to save a person a few inches of tissue but will be forced to amputate again, higher, when the first amputation refuses to heal and exposes the patient to massive infection. A number of amputations may be performed, as the doctor tries to find the point at which circulation is sufficient to bring about healing.

Feet Need Daily Care

Most basic to foot care is the prevention of infection. And that means keeping the skin not just intact, but flexible, reasonably moist, and strong enough to repel the daily challenge of perspiration, bacteria and bruises. Careful daily inspection of the foot is a must. The diabetic should make a ritual of it, following the warm bathing of the feet. The diabetic may be unable to scrutinize his feet very carefully, for any number of reasons. If that's the case, he must get someone else to do the job, or see a podiatrist regularly. Podiatrists are specially trained to be aware of the problems faced by diabetics and how to handle them.

The following steps are recommended for the daily care of diabetics' feet:

1. Wear stockings that are color-fast, preferably white. Change them at least once a day. Wash new socks before wearing them.

2. Shoes should be pliable but offer some protection for the toes. You may find lamb skin exceptionally comfortable. Always use a shoe horn.

3. Wash the feet once or twice daily, with a neutral hypo-allergenic soap and warm water. Use an orange-wood stick for cleaning under nails. Don't cut toenails, file them straight across. Above all, be gentle.

4. Shun strong antiseptics. Be aware that irritations of the foot may be allergic in nature, and fungicidal powders may cause further irritation.

5. Don't attempt to remove calluses or corns either with chemicals or by cutting. Visit a podiatrist.

6. Never wear garters, not even nylon stockings with elastic tops. And don't sit with your legs crossed; this has the same strangling effect on your leg circulation.

7. Sitting in a chair all day with pressure against the femoral artery, will only aggravate your poor circulation. Give your feet as much exercise as you can, such as climbing stairs.

8. If you have diabetes and smoke, you might as well tie rubber bands around your ankles, because this is the effect that the toxins in smoke have on your blood vessels.

Vitamin C Speeds Wound Healing

Beyond washing, wearing shoes that are comfortable, and other common sense procedures, there is reason to believe that vitamin therapy can play an important role in preventing the degeneration of a diabetic's foot. With vitamin C, in fact, there is evidence—albeit indirect evidence—that this one vitamin can help the atherosclerotic condition of diabetic arteries while at the same time fighting infection and aiding in the healing in the skin of the foot.

The effect of ascorbic acid on healing major breaks in the skin has been well documented. Some of the major studies include those by Dr. David Klasson of New York, who showed that vitamin C taken orally and sprayed on the skin was the most effective treatment for victims of severe burns (*N.Y. State Journal of Medicine*, Oct. 15, 1951), and Dr. T. C. Hindson who demonstrated that vitamin C taken orally in the amount of about one gram a day was totally effective in clearing up "incurable" cases of prickly heat that had tormented patients for months with raw, itching skin (*Lancet*, June 22, 1968). Further, it is now a rather common practice for surgeons to administer ascorbic acid to speed the healing of surgical wounds. All of which strongly suggests that vitamin C may also be of benefit in healing the long-lasting sores and ulcers which diabetics are prone to get on their feet.

One researcher who has no doubt that ascorbic acid will go a long way toward putting some spunk into the limp resistance of the diabetic is Frederick R. Klenner, M.D. Commenting on 17 years of administering large amounts of vitamin C to diabetics, the physician states, "We have found that every diabetic not taking supplemental vitamin C could be classified as having sub-clinical scurvy. For this reason they find it difficult to heal wounds . . ." (*Journal of Applied Nutrition*, Winter, 1971-72). According to Dr. Klenner, the vitamin C supplementation he gave patients (10 grams a day) not only normalized their healing of wounds, but allowed them to make better use of their insulin, so that they needed less.

Another researcher, Dr. George V. Mann of Vanderbilt University, also believes diabetics need extra large doses of vitamin C. "The hallmark of chronic diabetes is accelerated vascular disease," he says (*Perspectives in Biology and Medicine*, Winter, 1974), and he suspects that the lesions that so often develop and impede circulation in the blood vessels of diabetics are a form of scurvy, or vitamin C deficiency.

Vitamin E Can Save Limbs

As we saw in the previous chapter, vitamin E probably has even more to recommend it as a protective nutrient for the diabetic. After three decades of research into alpha tocopherol, Dr. Wilfrid E. Shute came to the conclusion that therapy for the diabetic was not complete unless it included vitamin E along with dietary control and insulin. In his book, *Vitamin E for Ailing and Healthy Hearts*, the famed Canadian doctor says that many of his diabetic patients were spared from amputations of the foot or lower leg by taking large doses of vitamin E.

This is explained, he says, by the dual action of vitamin E in sparing oxygen within the affected tissue, and the opening up of collateral circulation, allowing more blood to pass through narrow arteries in the feet, thus washing the affected areas with nourishment.

Once gangrene has set in, surgeons usually amputate more than the immediately affected area. Dr. Shute says it is typical to amputate above the knee when the heel has become gangrenous.

With vitamin E, however, he has seen case after case where a sharp dividing line appears between living tissue and dead tissue, "as if a knife has been used." The result is that only a small area of the foot is lost, instead of an entire foot or half a limb.

Unfortunately, most of the clinical experience with vitamins and diabetic problems involves rather advanced symptoms—emergency cases, actually. How much more useful vitamins C and E (as well as better nutrition in general) would be purely as preventive, protective measures, can only be imagined.

Today's diabetic has at his disposal new arterial surgery techniques that may be able to save a foot or limb that would have been doomed a generation ago. But the saying that prevention is better than cure is especially true of the diabetic and his foot problems. In most cases, the complications that bring people to the surgery table could have been prevented by good hygiene. Good hygiene combined with protective vitamin therapy should do even more to eliminate foot problems as a threat to the diabetic.

Section 20
Diarrhea

106. Diarrhea—Some Natural Ways
To Control It

106. Diarrhea—Some Natural Ways To Control It

In most people diarrhea is only very rarely a condition which exists by itself. In perhaps 99 out of 100 cases, it is usually a symptom of something else, and it is extremely important to discover just what is causing the diarrhea.

When loose or otherwise abnormal bowel movements, often accompanied by mucous and other fluid-like substances, do not disappear by themselves in a matter of days, it is wise to have a thorough medical examination. Diarrhea could be the result of anything from a food allergy to a major disease of the colon.

Medical treatment such as radiation therapy or a regimen of antibiotics will often produce diarrhea because the normal bacteria in the gut are killed off by the medicines, easily allowing the food to drain through the gut, unchecked. Food poisoning is another common cause of sudden but short-lived diarrhea, and, ironically, serves the good purpose of purging the body of toxic bacteria as rapidly as possible. And, of course, anxiety can cause diarrhea just as readily as it can cause constipation.

Any form of diarrhea, even if it lasts only a matter of hours, depletes the body of needed nourishment. The nutritious foods you eat simply slide through your intestine, scarcely staying within the intestinal tract long enough for any nutrients to be extracted. As far as nutrition is concerned, it's almost as if you didn't eat anything.

Foods rich in unrefined carbohydrates, fiber and pectin help end bouts of simple diarrhea by "binding up" the foods you eat so they do not pass through the intestines as quickly, putting an end to diarrhea and giving your body the opportunity to obtain the nutrients of the food ingested.

Pectin is a substance similar in many ways to fiber-rich bran, being non-nutritive but highly useful in digestion. Carob flour, frequently used as a substitute for chocolate, is very rich in pectin and can be of considerable help in "binding" loose

472

bowels. A number of medical studies have proved its effectiveness. But carob is a nutritious food in itself, and it is possible that not only its pectin, but other nutrients such as magnesium are involved in its beneficial effects.

Bananas have long been used to treat diarrhea. Like carob products, they are rich in pectin, but also rich in magnesium, potassium, and other important nutrients. A classic article in the *Journal of Pediatrics* in 1950 by Dr. J. H. Fries claimed that bananas are better than other fruits, such as apples, in their anti-diarrheal action. Dr. Fries said that the pectin in bananas swells and causes voluminous, soft stools. He said, too, that the pectin absorbs unfavorable bacteria while promoting the growth of beneficial organisms. And because bananas are rich in potassium, they help replace minerals lost in diarrhea, while their easily digested carbohydrates help keep weight and energy levels normal.

For patients following a regimen of antibiotics, generous amounts of *Lactobacillus acidophilus* yogurt can be eaten. For an even more beneficial effect, tablets of *L. acidophilus* culture can be consumed along with whole and unprocessed yogurt. Coupled with the binding qualities of high fiber and pectin foods, these tablets will be of especial importance in enabling these beneficial bacteria to get established in the colon and help put an end to this form of diarrhea.

There are some cases of diarrhea in adults, however, which are chronic and habitual, much like habitual constipation. They may or may not be associated with diverticular disease, or other manifestations of the irritable bowel syndrome. The study by Dr. Painter and his colleagues which proved that a high fiber diet alleviated constipation showed that patients having chronic diarrhea, with half a dozen or more bowel movements a day, were helped by adding bran to their diet even more than those suffering constipation. Typically, the diarrhea sufferers, after adding small amounts of bran to their diets, had only one or two bowel movements a day.

Chronic diarrhea should always be medically evaluated before any regimen, dietary or otherwise, is begun. If it involves a malabsorption syndrome, there may be a long-standing vitamin or mineral deficiency which will have to be corrected. If the diarrhea is severe enough, it may be impossible to bring vitamin and mineral levels up to normal with the usual forms of supplementation.

Carrots Can Stop Diarrhea In Children

Next to respiratory disease, no other disease sickens and hospitalizes more infants every year than diarrhea, or gastroenteritis. And for every 100,000 children under the age of one who die every year, 29 of those deaths are attributed to diarrhea, according to Victor Cohn reporting in the *Washington Post* (September 14, 1974).

"In underdeveloped countries, this illness kills infants by the hundreds of thousands, according to World Health Organization figures. The lower U.S. death rate is probably due to better sanitation, better health and nutrition, and swifter and more advanced hospital care," reported Cohn.

Almost half of the infant deaths attributable to diarrhea, according to Dr. Albert Z. Kapikian of the National Institute of Health's Institute of Allergy and Infectious Diseases, are caused by a virus. "The rest," Dr. Kapikian said, "are caused by bacteria or, in some countries, parasites."

In any event, if your child has a simple case of diarrhea, his condition should be carefully observed since the large amounts of fluids lost through diarrhea, especially in severe cases, can develop into a dangerous state of dehydration in a matter of hours—very critical hours.

Carrots Curb Diarrhea

Much of the discomfort and devastation of childhood diarrhea might be averted if it were more generally known that one of the most effective remedies for this annoying condition might well be sitting on the pantry shelf. In almost every household where the cry of a baby can be heard, there are a few jars of strained carrots in the pantry. These carrots, according to a Connecticut pediatrician, can reverse the devastating effects of diarrhea which sometimes threaten infants with dehydration and even death.

The pediatrician, Dr. Carl L. Thenebe, who for the past two decades proclaimed the life-saving results he achieved with carrot soup in the management of diarrhea, was equally enthusiastic about the efficacy of carrots in any form. "There is no need now to go through all the rigamarole of making carrot soup. Baby food strained carrots are just as effective," he says. This is welcome news to the busy mother whose job is so much more frenzied when her baby has diarrhea.

Dr. Thenebe based his enthusiasm for carrots on his personal experiences. When a two-week-old boy was brought to his office, passing 16 watery green stools daily and vomiting his formula, the skin and mucous membrane of his mouth and throat were very dry, suggesting dehydration. Dr. Thenebe hospitalized the infant immediately and put him on the carrot regimen. The infant made a quick recovery. Another case concerned a little girl who was one year old when her mother brought her to Dr. Thenebe's office because she had been "out of sorts." She had had 13 watery green stools during the past 12 hours, and cramps. Within 24 hours after carrots were started, the abnormal stool frequency ceased. The child was like herself again and playful, her mother happily reported.

No Danger In Carrots

Dr. Thenebe used the carrot treatment in the hospitals and homes of over 600 sufferers of diarrhea (stemming from enteritis—inflammation of the intestines) without a known mortality. These cases included premature infants, epidemic diarrhea of the newborn, infantile diarrhea and diarrhea of older children. "I have also observed adults with acute enteritis and children suffering with acute colitis who were truly benefited by the carrots," he stated. "To date, I have not encountered a single child who was sensitive to carrots." In fact, he said, "I usually recommend that strained carrots be given to the infant before the addition of each new food. The buffering property of the carrots prevents the irritation sometimes caused by new foods."

Because of advances in medical hospital hygiene, and improved sanitation facilities in most communities, infantile diarrhea is no longer the devastating killer it was only 15 years ago in the United States. But even today hardly a baby emerges from the diaper stage without having had at least one bout with diarrhea which makes a wreck of his mother and leaves the child exhausted, weak, and wide open to secondary infections.

The use of carrots in the treatment of infantile diarrhea is by no means new. It was cited in the medical literature (*Journal of Pediatrics*, 1950) by Dr. P. Selander of Sweden who stated that carrots for this purpose had received many very favorable reports from Germany, France, Belgium and his own country, Sweden.

Little Known In U.S.

To treat diarrhea as early as possible after its inception, before the rapid loss of weight and fluids occurs, could be life-saving in itself. Some doctors say the best treatment is no food with only weak tea for 24 hours, then kaopectate, paregoric, or antibiotics when necessary. These remedies may stop the diarrhea but none of these can, like the carrots, enhance recovery by supplying the electrolytes that are so necessary to all bodily functions. When a severe diarrhea strikes, the circulating body fluids, particularly the blood, become depleted of water. The cells of the body are called on to make up the deficit. When these cells become dry, a state of dehydration exists. But that is not all. When the body's water is lost, there is an outpouring of the electrolytes or minerals which are so essential to the life of the cell—potassium, phosphorus, sodium, chlorine, calcium, sulphur and magnesium.

Carrots replenish the lost electrolytes and at the same time act to control their loss. By coating the inflamed small bowel, the carrots soothe the irritated colon and thus enhance healing. This soothing action appears to calm the excessive peristalsis which leads to a rapid disappearance of associated symptoms such as colic and painful straining.

These physiologic actions in themselves shorten the duration of the disease considerably. But carrots, according to a report of the Foundation for Chemical Research in Helsinki, Finland, have other remarkable qualities. Studies show that at least six antifungal substances are present in carrots implying that, in some cases of fungus-caused diarrheas, the carrots actually help to kill off the offending agent—much as an antibiotic would. It is well known that carrots are a rich source of vitamin A, the anti-infective vitamin.

Carrots, then, are not only an excellent food but also, when diarrhea strikes infant, child, or adult—a superior medicine. And isn't it comforting to know that one can go to the pantry instead of the medicine cabinet for a treatment which nourishes as it cures and, best of all—has no side effects!

Milk As A Cause Of Diarrhea

In many people an unfavorable reaction to milk takes the form of diarrhea. The diarrhea is sudden (it usually occurs within an hour of drinking the milk) and urgent. Sometimes a cramping abdominal pain and/or flatulence occurs without diarrhea, or may accompany it. Alarmingly severe abdominal bloating also occurs in some persons unable to tolerate milk.

A vital digestive duet, lactose and lactase, was named by

Marshall Sparberg, M.D. in *Medical Digest* (August, 1967) as the key to adult diarrhea from milk. Lactose is a milk sugar, but not one of the simple sugars that are rapidly absorbed by the body. Lactose is a combination of two sugars, glucose and galactose, and as such, it must be broken down by the enzyme, lactase, before the body can handle it.

Infants normally have plenty of lactase in the small intestine, throughout the time of maximal milk ingestion. Then the lactase level starts to dwindle. It decreases through childhood, until, as adults, many of us have lost lactase to below the point of effectiveness. An adult whose lactase level drops that low must stop drinking milk entirely, or be prepared to suffer the miserable consequences, stomach cramps and diarrhea.

Lactase must break down the lactose in milk before it reaches the colon. If this mechanism fails, as it does in many adults, the presence of lactose in the lower intestine is almost sure to cause diarrhea by one of two mechanisms: sugar there sets off an outpouring of water into the gut, with diarrhea the immediate result; if that doesn't do it, the fermentation of lactose in the colon causes lactic acid to form, and other products to break down. These tend to irritate the intestine and stimulate peristalsis, creating violent movement of waste solids and liquids through the colon.

Experienced physicians know that a patient's intolerance to milk rarely shows up in a casual interview. They watch for this possibility in every diarrheal disease, asking specific questions about when and how much milk is ingested. This is correlated with the character and frequency of the diarrhea. Some patients see the milk-diarrhea relationship on their own, but most people don't make the association; they can't believe their minimal use of milk could have such an effect.

Actually, for some patients, even the milk in coffee is enough to cause a diarrhea reaction. Some people who use a milk substitute for their hot beverages may find certain additives in them which may also cause diarrhea. A report in the *Canadian Medical Association Journal* (November 16, 1974), reported the case of a 72-year-old man who suffered from constant diarrhea for two and a half months. Medical tests performed on him in the hospital pinpointed a popular non-dairy creamer that he used to mix with his morning coffee as the cause of his diarrhea. The hospital investigators went one step further and stated that the exact cause of trouble in the creamer was carrageenan, an additive found in condensed and evaporated milks, as well as many popular non-dairy creamers.

Basically, most doctors agree that the best therapy for lactose intolerance is a milk-free diet. For people who have severe milk intolerance, Dr. Sparberg suggested a calcium supplement: bone meal may serve the purpose.

Section 21
Digestive
System
Ailments

107. The Digestive Channel

107. The Digestive Channel

The gastrointestinal tract is much like a tube that extends from the mouth through the body to the rectum. Food is taken into the mouth, broken down into a suitable form, and is then absorbed through the walls of the "tube" into the body tissues to nourish the cells.

The digestive process begins in the mouth, where food is chewed and mixed with saliva, a mixture of mucus and enzymes. The chewed food is swallowed and passes through the esophagus to the stomach.

Glands in the stomach walls secrete hydrochloric acid, several different enzymes and gastrin, a hormone. Each of these substances serves a specific purpose in digesting food. Some enzymes break down proteins, others work on fats, others attack milk sugars, and so on.

The stomach muscles contract to mix the food and the digestive secretions thoroughly. When the food mass has been broken down into a semiliquid state, called chyme, it is pumped out of the stomach and into the small intestine. More digestive fluids are secreted, and the chyme is broken down still further. Nutrients are absorbed from the chyme as it moves through the small intestine. The chyme then passes into the large intestine, where the final absorption of nutrients takes place. Water is absorbed from the remaining chyme, and this solid matter is excreted as waste.

Colitis, Enteritis And Ileitis

The three most common intestinal ailments—colitis, enteritis and ileitis—are all inflammations of the intestinal walls. Colitis occurs in the large bowel (the colon), ileitis is confined to the last section of the small intestine (the ileum) and enteritis can refer to an inflammation of only the small intestine or of the entire intestinal tract.

All three of these inflammations are characterized primarily by diarrhea which, if allowed to go untreated, can become so severe that ulcers form on the intestinal wall to cause pain and hemorrhaging.

Colitis, enteritis and ileitis can often be traced to anxiety, worry or stress. During times of severe stress, the body's stores of pantothenic acid are depleted. Experiments with animals have shown that enteritis and colitis can be produced in animals being kept on a diet deficient in pantothenic acid, even when the animals are not under stress. Since supplements of pantothenic acid will correct the deficiency and relieve the illness in animals, the person suffering an intestinal affliction should check his intake of this nutrient.

The severe diarrhea which accompanies these intestinal ailments leaves the intestines little time to digest and absorb food. Therefore, patients are usually deficient in vitamins A, B, C and E, protein, fat, potassium, magnesium and most other nutrients. Cutting down on food intake or eating only soft foods will not substantially diminish the severity of the diarrhea, and will encourage further nutritional deficiencies. Doctors should be sure their patients' diets are substantial and well balanced to speed recovery.

The entire vitamin B complex is especially important to improve digestion as well as to decrease anxiety. Because the first sign of deficiency of folic acid (one of the B vitamins) is damage to the intestinal walls, patients should be getting plenty of this vital nutrient. Extra protein is also needed.

A combination of good nutrition and some constructive emotional outlet to help the patient to deal with his anxiety combine to make an effective treatment for these intestinal disorders.

Heartburn

Heartburn is that familiar burning sensation sometimes called "acid stomach." It is often the result of eating too fast, or sitting down to a meal when emotionally upset or exhausted. Adults are likely to swallow air as they eat, particularly when they are tense and upset, much as babies swallow air when they nurse. If the swallowed air is not expelled, when it warms to body temperature it expands, and the force required to belch it can push stomach acid into the esophagus. The strong acid irritates the delicate esophageal membranes to cause discomfort—heartburn.

Antacids are no help to the heartburn sufferer. These preparations neutralize all the acid in the stomach and thus, interfere with digestion. The stomach reacts by secreting more acid to finish its job, and a vicious cycle is begun.

The best remedy for frequent bouts with heartburn is to eat

small meals often, instead of a few large ones. Eat slowly; sip cold liquids through a straw to avoid swallowing air. Try not to eat when you are exhausted or emotionally upset, or at least try to forget your problems at the dinner table. Be sure you are getting enough rest, and maintain a well balanced diet.

Gastritis

Gastritis is an inflammation of the stomach lining which most of us experience at some time in our lives. The illness causes an uncomfortable feeling in the stomach, nausea and vomiting. It is often accompanied by headache and loss of appetite. Gastritis in its occasional, simple form is usually brought on by eating too much rich food or overindulging in alcohol. It generally goes away in a few hours if nothing more is eaten.

Chronic gastritis is more serious, and can lead to ulcers if not corrected. The symptoms of chronic gastritis are many and persistent. The patient has no appetite, feels nauseous and may vomit mucus upon arising in the morning. He is fatigued and suffers frequent headaches. After meals there is a feeling of uncomfortable fullness and drowsiness which no stomach medication seems to relieve.

The illness can be brought on by many things. Habitual smoking and drinking are prime causes. Bolting meals, eating a lot of carbohydrate foods, drinking too much coffee or tea and constant use of aspirin can also contribute to chronic gastritis. Many times the upset occurs simply because of stress and nervous tension.

To relieve chronic gastritis, you must eliminate the cause. If worry is the motivating factor, in addition to trying not to worry so much, be sure your diet includes ample amounts of the vitamin B complex and calcium, both important to healthy nerves. Also, get plenty of rest, and refrain from eating spicy, hard-to-digest foods.

Dyspepsia

More commonly known as chronic indigestion, dyspepsia is among the most widespread types of stomach trouble. All of us know the symptoms of indigestion—a full, heavy feeling in the stomach, gas, heartburn, a gurgling, rumbling stomach and sometimes nausea.

Dyspepsia is usually of emotional origin. Anxiety, worry, disappointment—any type of psychological stress that upsets the nervous mechanism which controls the contraction of muscles in the stomach and intestines—can cause indigestion.

Secondary causes include excessive consumption of tea, coffee or alcohol, heavy smoking, a diet too rich in carbohydrates and habitual use of laxatives.

To avoid suffering dyspepsia, eat a well balanced diet. Cut down on sweets and other high-carbohydrate foods, coffee, tea, alcohol and milk, if necessary. Drink less liquids with your meals. And search out and try to eliminate the cause of your emotional stress.

Papaya And Peppermint For Better Digestion

If you could take a look inside your own stomach after a large meal, you would see a biochemical battleground, pitting the good guys (the digestive juices) against the bad guys (too much food and too much fat). And the good guys are getting the worst of it.

In the first place, the enzymes and hydrochloric acid in your stomach are having an extremely difficult time breaking up that mass of food. The digestive juices, which are produced by some five million glands lining the stomach, also have to work much harder on food that has a layer of fat around it. This is true of food that is naturally fatty, such as sausage, as well as foods that have been fried or otherwise doused in fat. And when the gastric juices can't break through all that bulk and all that fat, they call for reinforcements and more and more juices are secreted. Unfortunately, the additional acid, instead of limiting itself to attacking the food, also attacks your stomach, and may even reach up into the esophagus, causing acid indigestion and heartburn.

Eventually, if left alone, the food will slowly but surely be digested and your stomach will get back to normal. But waiting for this to happen is no pleasure.

So what do you do? First of all, resolve never to overeat again—knowing, of course, that you will. After that, start thinking about dessert. But make that dessert papaya.

Papaya, besides being one of the most luscious tropical fruits, has the extraordinary ability to actually help you digest the food mass in your stomach.

It does this chiefly through a group of enzymes known as papain. Among the constituents of this natural balm for bursting bellies are the proteolytic enzymes, alpha and beta papain, and chymopapain. A proteolytic enzyme is one that has a special function of breaking down protein. Chymopapain is an especially potent enzyme which helps break down *all* food in the stomach.

However, besides the alpha and beta papain and chymopapain, papaya has several supplementary enzymes—including amylase, lipase, and pectase. The presence of these accompanying enzymes is very desirable, because they increase the digestive activity of the main enzyme. Lipase, for example, specializes in breaking down fatty tissue, which in some cases prevents the protein-attacking enzymes from doing their work. So when papain enters the stomach, its broad spectrum of enzymes permits it to go to work immediately, and on many types of foods. It doesn't have to wait for the digestive juices to eat away one level of material before it gets down to work.

Although you may have heard about papaya and papain only recently, if at all, the food industry has known about its fantastic digestive properties for years—and has made good use of them. According to a Department of Agriculture research report, cited in a product information bulletin of the Wesley Laboratories, papain helps to digest connective tissues and muscle fibers, producing a definite softening of the meat. In 1955, this work led the federal meat inspection branch to approve the use of papain on retail meat cuts. From one point of view, this use of papain saves the housewife money by allowing her to buy a less expensive cut of meat, which through the tenderizing action of papain, becomes more palatable. But there is also an important health benefit to be gained by using papain in its concentrated powder form on meat.

The most expensive cuts of meat are naturally more tender for the simple reason that they have a very high content of fat infiltrating the muscle tissues. Meat like this comes from an animal which has not been permitted to get any exercise, and which has been fed very high-energy food, such as corn, wheat, sorghum and molasses, instead of being allowed to pasture on grass.

Inexpensive cuts of meat, on the other hand, are considerably tougher—but healthier for you—because they have less fat in them. They usually come from animals which have spent nearly all their lives on the pasture. We all know that lean meat is much better for us than fatty meat—and here's your chance to do something about it.

Buy the cheaper, less fatty cuts of meat and sprinkle papain on them as a tenderizer. Papain retains its activity for one to two hours at extremely high temperatures, while all other plant enzymes are quickly destroyed. In fact, it seems to actually do its work while the meat is cooking, rather than beforehand.

Of course, since papain is available in a number of different forms, there is no need to depend on someone else to inject it into your food. Nor is there any need to limit its use to beef. By simply eating some before a meal that you think is going to give you some trouble, papain will do its work right in your stomach.

The beauty of papain as a natural digestive aid becomes even more clearly defined when this enzyme is compared to commercial antacid preparations. The latter should definitely be avoided, as they pose both short-term and long-term risks.

For occasional indigestion, papaya makes a lot more sense than antacids.

Peppermint Soothes The Entire Digestive System

Although papaya is without doubt one of the most potent natural digestive aids, peppermint has long enjoyed a similar reputation. Nelson Coon in his book *Using Plants for Healing* (Hearthside Press, Inc., 1963), notes that peppermint has been used for a variety of ills since the time of the ancient Egyptians. He points out that peppermint—sometimes called brandymint, lambmint, curled mint or balm mint—is an extremely valuable herb for relieving pain that may arise throughout the length of the alimentary canal. It has also been used for abdominal cramps and has been found useful in diarrhea. It has long been used in combination with a number of other medicines to make them taste better and to alleviate whatever distress they may cause to the stomach.

Coon recommends brewing up the leaves and flowering parts of peppermint into an infusion. After the brew has simmered for a while, put a teaspoonful of what's left into a cup of cold water, and take as needed for the relief of flatulence, heartburn, and other digestive upsets.

In the *Complete Herbal* (Barre Publishers, 1972), Ben Charles Harris confirms Coon's advice and notes that peppermint helps eliminate hardening mucus from the alimentary tract—as well as the lungs. He says that the American Indians often used the warm teas of peppermint as an antispasmodic, and used it to stimulate the digestive juices as a cure for indigestion, colic and flatulence.

Probably the most popular way to get the benefits of peppermint is to enjoy a nice hot—but not scalding—cup of peppermint tea after dinner. Your taste buds will like it and your tummy will, too.

All herbs, including peppermint, taste best when they are used in a relatively whole state. And there is probably no herb that is more easily grown in a backyard than peppermint. It is amazingly vigorous and spreads so quickly that you'll think it's a weed. It's the perfect plant to establish in an area of your backyard or lawn that you don't feel like mowing. The leaves can be used throughout the summer to add a delightful mint taste to iced herbal tea. To keep a steady supply on hand, gather leaves early in the fall, put them in a pan, and bake them at a very low temperature until they are dry. Seal them in an airtight jar and you'll have enough for all winter. Herbalist Euell Gibbons recommends that it's best to dry all herbs simply at room temperature indoors. He says that this preserves their flavor, which stems from very volatile oils easily driven off by heat.

If you buy your peppermint in a store, try to get it loose—but sealed absolutely airtight. If you buy it in the form of teabags, remove the bags from the container when you've opened it, and keep them in a tightly sealed tin.

You'll find that papaya with a meal, and some peppermint tea afterward, makes a delightful and perfectly safe combination for better digestion.

Do You Have Enough Stomach Acid?

A good supply of hydrochloric acid in the stomach is vital for proper digestion of food. If the stomach does not secrete enough HCl, the digestion of protein and absorption of vitamin C are impaired, B vitamins are destroyed, and minerals are unable to reach the bloodstream. A surprising number of people are consistently deficient in hydrochloric acid. Not only do they suffer frequent digestive problems, but because of the loss of minerals, particularly calcium, their bones are brittle and slow to heal when broken.

Deficiency of hydrochloric acid may result from a low intake of protein and vitamins A and B. Lack of acid usually leads, in turn, to a decrease in digestive enzymes, and the muscle movements in the stomach which are needed to mix digestive juices with foods slow down. Therefore, digestion is seriously impaired. If the situation continues for an extended period, vitamin and mineral deficiencies may result, even when a well balanced diet is maintained.

To stimulate production of acid in the stomach, supplemental hydrochloride can be taken. The acid may be taken in dilute liquid form through a straw, but the mouth must be rinsed immediately after to prevent erosion of tooth enamel. Because of the dangers to the teeth, most physicians recommend tablets of glutamic acid hydrochloride.

Intestinal Motility

After eating, the muscles in the walls of the stomach and small intestine contract rhythmically to mix food with digestive juices, enzymes and bile. The movements also bring already digested food in contact with the absorbing surfaces of the intestinal walls. Contractions generally go on for several hours after eating. Without these contractions, food cannot be digested or absorbed.

A deficiency of potassium slows down intestinal contractions, sometimes to the point that the muscles become paralyzed. Potassium deficiency can occur after surgery, following a bout with diarrhea or prolonged stress, from taking drugs such as cortisone or diuretics, and from eating a lot of highly refined foods or too much salt. Insufficient potassium causes severe gas pains, and is usually associated with constipation.

To insure a good supply of this vital mineral, eat lots of fresh fruits and leafy green vegetables, and avoid overly refined foods. Potassium chloride can be mixed with table salt. Increasing consumption of foods rich in protein and B vitamins can also help stimulate digestion and absorption of important nutrients. Supplying the missing potassium or other nutrients usually restores intestinal motility within a few days.

Intestinal Bacteria

In the colon, bacteria extract nutrients from digested food, for transport to the rest of the body. These intestinal flora, called *Lactobacillus acidophilus*, must be present for proper assimilation of food. They also help supply the body with B vitamins. Supplementing the diet with yogurt or acidophilus milk encourages the growth of these bacteria. Vitamin C and pectin also prove valuable.

The colonic bacteria produce lactic acid to keep the intestines free of invading "bad" microbes, which cannot live in an acidic environment. If the friendly bacteria are destroyed or reduced in number, the hostile germs will infiltrate the colon to cause gas, odor and constipation.

Oral antibiotics kill the intestinal bacteria, and can cause deficiencies of B vitamins.

Vegetables with a high fiber content, such as celery, cabbage and carrots, stimulate the growth of intestinal flora. Conversely, a bland, smooth diet markedly decreases the amount of friendly bacteria.

Gas And Bloating

Gas is by far the most common digestive disturbance. Symptoms can be produced by either swallowed air, or gas formed by the action of putrefactive bacteria on various undigested foods in the intestines.

A bubble of air trapped in the stomach or in a loop of bowel can cause great distress. It causes distension of the viscera, thus stretching the nerve endings and causing pain, bloating and strange gurgling sounds. Those who eat rapidly and gulp their meals may trap air along with their food. Gum chewing, thumb sucking, poorly fitting dentures and so on, stimulate excessive production of saliva which must be swallowed—along with extra air.

If swallowed air does successfully pass the stomach, it may collect further down at the splenic or hepatic fixtures of the colon. The result is abdominal distress. It is the inability to remove normal or increased amounts of air which can lead to symptoms of gas.

Posture may also be important to the entrapment of air in the intestines. To obtain relief, take a stroll after meals, or try the following exercise. Lie on a flat surface. A bed is fine. Bring both knees up to your chest for a count of 10. Then try the knee-chest position while lying on your stomach. Doctors sometimes recommend heat, massage, or a gentle enema to relieve the condition. All of these methods have varying results.

Whatever its cause, doctors agree that excessive gas is a problem of no small proportions, one that sometimes sounds the ambulance siren in the dark of night because the pain it causes may be mistaken for heart pain. Dr. Manuel J. Rowen, a cardiologist associated with St. Elizabeth's Hospital in Elizabeth, New Jersey, says that "Gas causes pseudo angina. These . . . patients accumulate air in the gut. The pain it causes is referred to the precordium (the region over the heart or stomach). This they interpret as 'heart pain' " (*Western Medicine*, April, 1967).

Now, here's the good news. It has been found that pantothenic acid, a member of the vitamin B family which comes to your aid in times of stress, also comes to your aid to relieve intestinal gas and distension for which there is no physical cause. While air swallowing, as well as beans, cabbage, turnips, and carbonated beverages influence the gas we generate within ourselves, Dr. Rowen, Dr. Arnold Gelb and Dr. Jerome Weiss noted in *Western Medicine* that other factors influencing gaseousness are faulty digestion and gut motility. That's where the pantothenic acid comes in.

Experiments revealed that when pantothenic acid was given after surgery, there was a much shorter period of discomfort due to obstruction of the intestines which usually results from an inhibition of bowel motility, a condition known medically as ileus.

If you've ever had abdominal surgery, you know how wretchedly painful ileus can be. In its mildest and perhaps most common form, ileus causes post-operative distension with accompanying wind pains and abdominal discomfort. This may follow the simplest operation, possibly not even involving the abdomen. In its severe form, fortunately rare, the intestines become completely paralyzed, all function ceases and the patient's life is in grave danger.

In a double blind study of hospital patients suffering from gas pains, Drs. Nardi and Zuidema found a significant difference between the controls and a trial group receiving a pantothenic acid supplement. Those who got pantothenic acid were able to expel trapped gas in an average of ten hours (*Surgery, Gynecology & Obstetrics*, 112:526; 1961). Compare their happiness at relief from abdominal distress with those who did not get pantothenic acid and suffered gas pains for 77 hours. Another boon to patient, hospital and hospitalization insurance or the patient's bankroll was the fact that length of stay in the hospital was much shorter for those who got the pantothenic acid (two days against 14 days). No adverse effects were observed.

How Pantothenic Acid Works

By what magic does pantothenic acid work to achieve this blessed relief from the distress which usually accompanies surgery? It seems that without pantothenic acid, a very important substance called acetylcholine cannot be produced. Acetylcholine is a chemical which transmits messages at the nerve endings. Without it, the nerves cannot control motor and secretory intestinal activity. It has, in fact, been found in experimental animals, that after a period of stress, the acetylcholine reservoir in the body is diminished (*British Medical Journal,* September 14, 1963). However, if pantothenic acid is given, the acetylcholine level may be increased by as much as 50 percent. This was determined by Lynch, Spurgeon and Worton (*Journal of Applied Nutrition,* 11:117, 1958).

These experiments suggest that the stress of abdominal operations produces a depletion of the supply of acetylcholine, which in turn causes a varying degree of intestinal atony or loss of motility in the intestinal muscle, and that the administration of pantothenic acid, by preventing such depletion, also prevents the development of ileus.

But what about the person who hasn't been anywhere near the operating room and still suffers all the distress of "burbulence"? What can pantothenic acid do for him? Since pantothenic acid is a component of the co-enzymes concerned in the formation of acetylcholine, unless we get enough pantothenic acid to prevent the depletion of acetylcholine, we're going to lose gut motility, a condition which is related to the ileus suffered by post-operative patients, a condition which sets the stage for "burbulence."

How much pantothenic acid do you need? This depends on you and your chemistry. Dr. Roger Williams states in *Nutrition Against Disease* (Pitman, 1971) that "some may have much higher needs than others." The Food and Nutrition Board of the National Academy of Sciences—National Research Council recommends a daily intake of 10 milligrams. But your requirements, especially if you're suffering with "burbulence," may be considerably higher. An increased need for pantothenic acid seems to run in families and some families have been shown to require as much as 20 times more of this vitamin in order to maintain health than others, Dr. Williams points out.

Carlton Fredericks, Ph.D., reported in his *Newsletter of Nutrition* (October 1, 1972) that "250 milligrams daily has not only been reported to relieve postoperative gas pains, but to prevent them. My recent observations," he says, "suggest that those who are troubled by intestinal gas and distension for which no physical cause has been found sometimes respond to pantothenic acid—so much so that I am persuaded that these people have an elevated requirement for the vitamin, difficult to fulfill even with a reasonable choice of foods."

Where Do You Find Pantothenic Acid?

It was once thought that because pantothenic acid is distributed so widely in foods, the chances of developing a serious deficiency were slight. But since the growth of food processing and other vitamin-damaging influences on the food supply, available vitamins in our foods decrease every year. Pantothenic acid is present in the germ of all grains. It is therefore sacrificed when flour is refined and not restored in the enrichment farce. We should, therefore, make certain to use those foods which are particularly rich in pantothenic acid in order to prevent even a marginal deficiency. Nutritional yeast, liver, wheat germ, kidney, heart, salmon and eggs are among our best sources of pantothenic acid.

If the windy syndrome is causing you discomfort and embarrassment, try getting more exercise and more pantothenic acid (also known as calcium pantothenate) and chances are you will no longer feel like Ogden Nash when he wrote, "I feel as unfit as an untuned fiddle, and it is the result of a certain turbulence of the mind and a certain 'burbulence' in the middle."

Ameba, Worms, And Other Intestinal Parasites

Animals kept on diets deficient in protein or vitamins A, B_1, B_2, biotin, folic acid, or other nutrients have been infested with many types of parasites, including trichinae, obtained from undercooked pork, and trichomonas, which can grow in the lungs or intestines as readily as in and around the vagina. When these parasites have been implanted in healthy animals on an adequate diet, however, infestations have not occurred.

Medication Will Not Permanently Destroy The Parasites

If the animal is kept on a deficient diet, reinfestation quickly occurs. But the invaders gradually die out when the diet is made highly nutritious. Both parasites and worms infest animals deficient in vitamin A, whereas well fed controls remain free of infestation.

Although intestinal parasites are surprisingly common, there seem to be no studies showing the effect of dietary improvement on humans infested with them. It is known that a high intake of refined foods, particularly sweets, which supply little or no nutrients yet satisfy the appetite, can cause individuals to become susceptible to pinworms which thrive on sugar. Research does indicate, however, that when any type of parasitic infestation is present, the diet should be unusually adequate and refined foods strictly avoided. Yogurt or acidophilus milk appear to be especially helpful in cases of amebic dysentery and perhaps all intestinal infestations. In addition, every effort should be made to maintain a sufficient supply of stomach acid to destroy many parasites obtained from food. A physician must determine when vermifuges should be used, but often such medication imposes severe stress and is unsuccessful.

Section 22
Diverticulitis

108. Diverticulitis—It's Our Most Common Bowel Ailment

If you are past the age of forty and always have been accustomed to eating a standard diet primarily consisting of low fiber and refined carbohydrate foods, chances are one out of two that you will eventually experience the pain and distress of diverticular disease of the colon. The outlook becomes even grimmer in the later years; diverticular disease strikes nearly seventy percent of the people past the age of seventy.

The general course of the disease begins with persistent constipation, sometimes altered by diarrhea, and soon involves nausea, vomiting, abdominal swelling, cramps and pain in the lower left side. Chills and fever add to the general feeling of sickness. If the condition worsens, complications may develop, affecting the bladder, small intestine and uterus. Hemorrhage and rectal bleeding may ensue, and in extreme cases the result is death.

Diverticular disease has become the most common bowel ailment of our times, reaching almost epidemic proportions in the United States and other Western nations where overly refined foods play a major role in the diet. Because of the general nature of its symptoms, encompassing an entire array of vague abdominal ailments, the medical profession has been rather slow to recognize diverticulosis as a disease in its own right.

Medical researchers are now convinced that diverticular disease of the colon and a closely related ailment known as spastic colon, or the irritable bowel syndrome, have long been the target of equally erroneous therapy. For many years, it was the general practice to prescribe a low-residue, soft diet for people with these conditions. Today, it has been reliably established that this popular treatment does nothing more than reproduce the same physiological insult which created the disease in the first place. What diverticular patients need, in fact, is a diet high in fiber from whole grains, vegetables and fruits.

Nevertheless, there are many people who are still operating on the outdated advice that they must scrupulously avoid foods high in fiber, because they will supposedly irritate the tender lining of the colon and trigger cramping and pain. This *seems* to make sense, but to understand why it really doesn't, you have to understand the nature of the physical problems involved in the irritable bowel syndrome.

How The Disease Is Caused

The basic lesion in diverticular disease is the diverticulum, a pea-sized balloon poking through the muscular lining of the lower bowel. As one recent British text puts it: "Literally, a diverticulum means a way-side house of ill-fame and these way-side houses certainly live up to their evil reputation." Actually, it is not so much the diverticula themselves that cause trouble, but the inflammation which occurs when food particles become lodged in these sacs, often along with bacteria. Then the condition is known as diverticulitis.

The causation of diverticula was graphically explained by Drs. Denis Burkitt and Neil S. Painter in an article for the *British Medical Journal* (May 22, 1971). According to the physicians, both pioneers in the study of diverticulosis, waste matter is normally moved through the sacs of the lower gut by waves of muscular contraction. When the bowels are relatively full of waste matter, as they are in primitive peoples on high fiber diets, the muscles surrounding the membrane lining of the intestines need to contract only slightly to move it along. But when waste matter is scanty, and compacted, as it is in those eating a highly refined diet, the muscles have to contract with much greater force to create the pressure required to keep things moving. It is something like squeezing a tube of toothpaste; when the tube is full or near full, only slight pressure will expel the toothpaste. But when the tube is nearly empty, you have to squeeze and squeeze to get it out.

Drs. Painter and Burkitt explained that when the intestines contain only scanty waste matter, they must contract to the point where they form individual bladders or segments, closed on one end and open on the other, in order to empty themselves. The most intense contractions take place in the sigmoid colon, just before the rectum, which is lined with powerful muscles. But the human intestine was not designed to handle this kind of intense pressure. The result is that the bowel lining gives way to the pressure and balloons through weak places in the muscular lining, especially in the highly-stressed sigmoid colon. This is very similar to the process in which a segment of the entire gut is forced out through the muscular wall of the abdomen under great stress to form a hernia.

Old Treatment Clearly Counter-Productive

Here is what Dr. Franz Goldstein, chief of the Department of Gastroenterology at Lankenau Hospital and Professor of Medicine at Jefferson Medical College of Philadelphia, said about diet and the irritable bowel syndrome: "Low-residue diets tend to constipate. In chronic colonic afflictions, especially in ulcerative colitis, the irritable bowels syndrome, and diverticular disease, low-residue diets, though frequently prescribed, are clearly counter-productive and are actually contra-indicated in the latter two conditions" (*Journal of the American Dietetic Association,* June 2, 1972).

Dr. Goldstein went on to say that what is true of diet in relation to diverticulitis is also probably true of "the extremely common functional disorder known as 'spastic colon' or the 'irritable bowel syndrome'." This condition, he noted, may be a forerunner of diverticular disease, explaining that "the two conditions often cannot be differentiated on clinical or radiological grounds and seem to blend into one another until the complication of diverticulitis arises."

A diet high in roughage, or indigestable fiber, is therefore indicated as a good means of preventing the formation of both "spastic colon" and diverticulitis. But what about people who already have this condition? Wouldn't the high-residue diet cause them distress? Theoretically, it could, depending on the kind of fiber they eat. Eating a lot of seeds and nuts, which have not been thoroughly chewed, could conceivably cause problems. However, when fiber is eaten in the form of bran, the outer coating of the wheat kernel, there are no problems. In fact, eating unprocessed bran now seems to be the best thing that a person with such bowel problems could do for himself.

The reason for this is simple: bran actually absorbs about eight times its own weight in water, which according to surgeon T. G. Parks "results in the passage of more bulky, softer stools, particularly in patients previously troubled with constipation" (*Proceedings of the Royal Society of Medicine,* July, 1973). Dr. Parks, who has given bran to a number of his patients with diverticular disease, said that this kind of stool is precisely what might be expected to prevent formation of high-pressure segments of the bowel from which diverticula can explode.

Another test of bran for patients with the irritable bowel syndrome was described in the *American Journal of Clinical Nutrition*, 1974, by Dr. Joseph L. Piepmeyer of the United States Naval Reserve. Dr. Piepmeyer selected 30 patients with the irritable bowel syndrome for a trial of bran. These patients, he said, all had the irritable bowel syndrome, typified by a cycle of constipation followed by the passage of hard, small stools, followed in turn by diarrhea. Many of them had varying degrees of wind, and frequently suffered some abdominal bloat and cramping.

Each of the patients was instructed to take eight to ten rounded teaspoons of unprocessed bran every day, either alone or mixed with other foods. They were also warned that there is an "adjustment period" of from one to four weeks when taking bran, and they should not discontinue it if at first it made them gassy or gave them diarrhea.

It is interesting to note that Dr. Piepmeyer also took the time to explain to these patients the importance of roughage in terms of the anatomy of their bowels, and to describe to them exactly what wheat bran is, emphasizing "the uniqueness of unprocessed bran versus other cereal products."

After four months on bran, 23 of the 30 patients reported improvement in their symptoms. Four patients withdrew from the study because they didn't like the taste of bran, so of those who actually took it, 90 percent improved. As was expected, their stools increased in volume and there was also a "marked decrease in abdominal distention and cramps which was associated with some decrease in anxiety."

An earlier major study on the effects of bran on people suffering from diverticular disease was published in the *British Medical Journal* in 1972 by Dr. Neil S. Painter and colleagues. Reporting on a clinical trial which lasted several years, the three doctors declared that of seventy patients with *severe* diverticular disease of the colon, 62 enjoyed marked relief of symptoms through a program of dietary change. The patients were instructed to take some unprocessed bran every day, but also were told they could add other forms of food fiber to their diet from fruit, vegetables and whole grain bread. In addition, they were all told to reduce their intake of refined sugar in any form. Among the symptoms which were relieved in the great majority of cases were constipation, severe colic, abdominal pain, tender rectum, wind, heartburn, nausea, bloated feeling, and incomplete emptying of the rectum.

Surgery . . . Or Bran?

In severe cases of diverticulitis, when the patient is in great pain, and the diverticula become infected or even perforated, surgery may be recommended. However, there is a tendency to think of surgery as a *definitive* treatment for many serious disorders, but all too frequently, at least in diverticulitis, it doesn't quite work out that way.

Doctors attending the fifth biennial congress of the International Society of Colon and Rectal Surgery in 1974 heard from Dr. Adam N. Smith, consultant surgeon at the University of Edinburg in Scotland, the results of a long study designed to determine how beneficial bowel surgery was, and if a dietary change could influence the outcome.

Dr. Smith explained that "if high intraluminal pressure (inside the segments of the colon) is one of the predisposing factors in the genesis of diverticular disease, it follows that operations for this condition may be judged effectively in terms of colonic motility (pressure-creating contractions)."

He therefore decided to test the long-term usefulness of bowel surgery performed on diverticular patients by measuring the resultant drop in colon pressure. He did this with two groups of patients. One group had had a portion of their incompetent tract removed in an operation known as a colon resection. The other group were patients who had what is known as a longitudinal myotomy, a relatively new operation in which some of the muscles which create the motility or contracting effect are surgically cut.

Dr. Smith and his colleagues devised a method of measuring intraluminal pressure of the colon by placing a number of surgical balloons into the bowel and recording the extent of muscular contractions. From this work, they found that colon resection patients had no reduction at all in motility or pressure following surgery. Although the sigmoid colon portion of the bowel had been removed in these patients, the problem simply moved higher up in the bowel.

In the patients who had a myotomy, an operation involving the cutting or dissection of muscle tissue, there was a considerable reduction in intestinal muscle activity following surgery. However, Dr. Smith and his colleagues found that this reduction only lasts for about a year. After that, it starts climbing again, so that after three years, it is very nearly back to what it was before surgery.

Having determined that both surgical techniques for diverticular disease leave much to be desired, the Scottish surgeons then set out to see what the course of improvement would be if bran were added to the post-operative diet. Five myotomy and five resection patients were put on a daily dose of 20 grams of unprocessed bran in addition to the normal diet. (This works out to about four tablespoons of bran a day.) The patients were monitored for five years, during which time they were repeatedly subjected to tests to measure intraluminal pressure. And here is what the doctors found:

Among the myotomy patients, who with surgery alone typically experienced only a one-year improvement, *the bran diet kept the pressure down during all five years of observation.* In fact, Dr. Smith said, "the colonic activity fell even lower than it did with myotomy alone and has been well maintained."

With surgery alone, patients who had undergone a colonic resection experienced not even a temporary drop in pressure. But with a few tablespoons of bran every day, the drop in pressure was significant and well maintained throughout the five years. "In light of our findings we advise giving patients bran either after resection or a myotomy," Dr. Smith concluded.

There is no doubt that in some instances the bowel has become so damaged or infected that it must be surgically removed to prevent the waste products of the intestine from polluting the bloodstream with dangerous bacteria. However, there is good indication that—at least in some cases—a bran regimen given to diverticulitis patients can actually make surgery unnecessary.

This was one of the conclusions of the earlier studies by Dr. Neil Painter. "Twelve patients who suffered from painful diverticular disease had recurrent attacks of severe colic and *might well have come to surgery,*" Dr. Painter said, ". . . In four the colic was relieved and in seven it was abolished by the bran diet. None came to surgery despite the fact that formerly they had had attacks of severe pain. One woman of 50 had had three attacks of left renal colic . . . she was placed on a bran diet and had no further pain for two years. Occasionally she experienced mild cramps . . . . this disappeared when she doubled her intake of bran for a few days. *Thus even severe pain which might have led to surgery will respond to a high-residue diet.*"

Dr. Painter added that he is frequently asked if bran doesn't irritate the bowel. His answer: "In not one of the 62 patients was the appetite made worse by bran. This suggests that the widely held view that so-called 'roughage' irritates the gut is not founded on fact; bran when moist becomes 'softage'."

Section 23
The Ears and Hearing

109. Hearing Loss: America's Foremost Chronic Health Problem

Hearing loss is considered America's foremost chronic physical impairment, affecting more than the total number of people handicapped by other diseases which limit a person's ability to function normally, such as arthritis, poor vision and heart disease.

According to the latest United States Public Health Service study, more than 19 million persons are afflicted with hearing disabilities, including 3.5 million school age children. In a study conducted by both the New York University Deafness Research and Training Center and the National Association for the Deaf, independent researchers concluded that there were actually 203 deaf persons for every 100,000 population segment in the United States (*New York Times*, Nov. 21, 1974). The study pinpointed "regional pockets" of deafness located throughout the country, with the Northeastern states having the lowest incidence of deafness and the North Central states having the highest.

Dramatic Increase In Hearing Difficulties

Hearing impairment can result from a number of causative factors, either independently or in combination with each other. Difficulties can result from the damage done by high fevers caused by viral infection; external accidents which can damage parts of the inner ear; the extreme accumulation of earwax, also known as ceruminosis; deterioration due to aging, considered by many to be the leading cause of deafness in this country; dietary deficiencies which hinder and restrict the nutritional maintenance of the delicate and specialized tissues within the inner ear which receive and transmit sound to the brain's hearing center; and congenital defects.

Some researchers, however, are concerned with the causes of the dramatic rise in the number of people suffering from hearing impairments, since the last widescale survey on deafness, conducted over 40 years ago, showed that less than half the present number of people were suffering from hearing loss. Hearing experts speculate on a number of reasons for what to them was a "surprising increase": a better means of general medical treatment which now enables people to survive diseases which would ordinarily have killed them in the past but now leave them with physical disabilities as an aftermath, such as the hearing impairment caused by meningitis, once considered a fatal disease; a sizeable increase in the incidence of congenital deafness, largely the result of the increasing number of marriages among people with this form of deafness; and the increased length of life expectancies, since gradual hearing loss, or presbycusis, is associated with aging. "It is estimated that 10 percent of the people over the age of 50 have presbycusis," reported Dr. Robert H. Mathog in *Geriatrics* (August, 1974).

The increased use of certain drugs such as quinine, some antibiotics and aspirin is considered a cause of the increase in nationwide hearing difficulties, especially in the case of tinnitus (ringing in the ears). "I can't tell you how many people lost their hearing in this manner (the consumption of drugs), but we do know that drugs affect hearing," said Dr. Jerome D. Schein, who heads the New York University Research Institute and is director for the National Census of the Deaf Population.

The increasing number of loud and harsh sounds of environmental noise is recognized by many experts as a major contributing factor to the increase in hearing difficulties. "Noise levels in American cities have doubled in 10 years and in some places are 64 times higher than 15 years ago. With the noise increase has come evidence of increased hearing loss," reported an article in *Family Health* (January, 1974). This sonic pummeling has not only become a part of our personal environment, but it has become the leading industrial hazard for workers. "Noise induced hearing losses are our most common occupational disease," reported Dr. Harold R. Imbus, Medical Director, Burlington Industries, Greensboro, North Carolina (*Medical Tribune*, Nov. 27, 1974).

110. Perceptive And Conductive Deafness

Hearing quality depends, to a large extent, upon the efficient working of the eighth cranial nerve, which carries sounds from the inner ear to the brain. However, various other parts of the ear apparatus may be involved in hearing impairment too. This type of damage, in which an obstruction of the transmission of sounds prevents them from traveling to the receiving center of the inner ear, is known as conductive deafness. In these instances the minute skeletal structure within the middle ear may still be transmitting sounds to the inner ear, but the ability to distinguish these sounds is definitely diminished. Cases of conductive deafness, such as otosclerosis (a spongy overgrowth of bone in the inner ear, limiting the monitoring of sound vibrations), accumulations of earwax (cerumin), obstructing boils in the ear canal and instances of ear drum damage can often be alleviated.

Nerve deafness, or perceptive deafness, is a much more serious problem, involving the actual receiving mechanism somewhere in the inner ear, the neural pathways from the inner ear to the brain, or the brain center itself. The gradual loss of hearing associated with old age (presbycusis), congenital problems of deafness, damage done to the inner ear by certain drugs, the ravaging effects of infectious diseases such as mastoiditis, where the pus which results from untreated infections of either the outer or inner ear, destroys the inner ear's mastoid cells and delicate bone, Meniere's disease (a frustrating tryad of symptoms involving vertigo, hearing loss and tinnitus) and the damage caused by excessive noise are all forms of perceptive deafness.

There is some evidence that a lack of B vitamins may be a very important cause of perceptive deafness. In *Nutritional Disorders of the Nervous System* (Williams and Wilkins Company), Dr. John D. Spillane cites deafness as one of the symptoms of beriberi and pellagra. These vitamin B deficiency diseases have killed hundreds of thousands of people in parts of the Far East and in our own South due to a combination of poverty, ignorance and poor food patterns.

Owing to the poor mental state of many patients with advanced pellagra, it is difficult to evaluate their hearing loss. However, Dr. Spillane was able to confirm the following percentages: five cases of deafness out of 46 patients; eight cases out of 60 patients; and seven cases out of nine patients.

Of beriberi (caused by deficiency in thiamin, another of the B vitamins) Dr. Spillane explains that deafness is probably uncommon in well-advanced cases and may be unnoticed in the acutely ill patient. However, he believes that the auditory nerve is mainly involved in the mild latent form of the disease. In other words, individuals suffering from a mild deficiency (just as many of us undoubtedly are) might notice the "nerve deafness" without the other symptoms of beriberi.

Dr. Spillane tells of prisoners of war who had beriberi because of the inadequate diet in the prison camp. Many of these suffered temporary deafness. Of 38 Chinese women being treated for polyneuritis (another symptom of vitamin B deficiency), two were deaf and seven had persistent tinnitus or ringing in the ears. There is little doubt that lack of vitamin B may be related to many cases of tinnitus.

In a number of cases of neuritis found in Jamaica, the symptoms were numbness in feet and legs, difficulty in walking, incoordination of muscles, deterioration of vision and deafness. The deafness was perceptive and it was found when these patients were autopsied that the auditory nerve, which carries sound impressions from the ear to the brain, had deteriorated greatly, presumably due to lack of vitamin B. Among prisoners of war tinnitus was a common complaint, frequently followed by gradual deafness. The deafness usually afflicted both ears and began with a feeling of "fullness" in the ears.

111. Can Gradual Hearing Loss Due To Aging Be Prevented?

How many of us have had to speak slowly, loudly, enunciating carefully to be understood by an aging person?

Presbycusis, a sensory-neural type of progressive hearing loss, affects many people as they get older. The highest tones are usually the first to go, but the loss is usually so minimal that the individual shrugs it off. Gradually, the impairment gets worse. So slow is the usual rate of hearing loss, it may take years to notice that it is happening. Difficulty in understanding conversation is interpreted as the other person's poor enunciation. Only after perhaps ten years or more does it suddenly become apparent—the sense of hearing is being lost.

Repeated Exposure To Noise Harmful

What causes this gradual hearing loss? Scientists warn that prolonged exposure to noise of 85 decibels is one of the primary hazards to ear health. At a symposium of the American Association for the Advancement of Science held in Boston in December, 1969, Dr. Samuel Rosen, Clinical Professor of Otology (Emeritus) at Mount Sinai School of Medicine in New York, reported that "Loud sounds can make tiny blood vessels contract, and that repeated exposure lengthens the time it takes for them to relax again. So a noisy life might lead to injury to arteries, and to an increase in fatty materials in the bloodstream that makes arteries clog up in the heart or brain . . . Even for people who work in noisy places, 'you may forgive or forget it, but your arteries never will.' "

But even in a world where the assault of noise becomes more intense year by year, should the ear degenerate merely because it is 65 years old? Must membranes stiffen, and physical and chemical processes break down at that age?

Aging: A Result Of Vitamin Deficiency

Dr. G. F. Taylor, writing in the *International Journal for Vitamin Research* in 1968, concluded that the classical signs of aging can be stopped by an increase in the intake of vitamins B and C. Vitamin deficiency, then, is a significant factor leading to a slow down of body processes, such as a loss of hearing in old age.

Vitamins B And C Improve Hearing

Years ago, Dr. G. Gordon, who was treating anemia, nervous exhaustion and digestive disorders, gave his patients at the Hard-of-Hearing Clinic of the Medical College of Alabama brewer's yeast, liver extract, vitamin C, and glutamic acid (a constituent of protein particularly needed by the brain) and discovered hearing improvement in 76 percent of them. The largest gain, Dr. Gordon found, was in hearing high tones. Patients realized that they were once again able to understand what was being said because the consonants, spoken in high tones that they could not hear before, were now distinct (*Journal of the Medical Association of Alabama*, 1948).

Vitamin A And Otosclerosis

Otosclerosis, a conductive type of deafness in the aged, blocking the sound waves from entering the inner ear, is another major cause of hearing impairment. In this process, explains Dr. Robert E. Rothenburg in his book, *Health in the Later Years* (New York, 1964), "the bones surrounding the middle and inner ear tend to become hardened and overgrown; this will result in interference of the transmission of sound waves."

Because otosclerosis is a disease that fixes the middle ear bones so that they cannot vibrate sound, some doctors rely on surgery for improvement. A stapedectomy either removes the malfunctioning stapes, which is then replaced by a stainless steel or plastic filament, or frees the stapes of adhesions so it can vibrate normally. A fenestration—an operation in which a hole is drilled into the bone so that sound waves can pass through to the inner ear—might also restore hearing.

Once otosclerosis is established, surgery appears to be the only remedy. But must this condition occur? Research performed by the renowned Sir Edward Mellanby in 1934 demonstrated by experiments with laboratory animals that a lack of vitamin A causes an overgrowth in the small bones of the ear, thereby preventing the transmission of sounds. On the same trail, Dr. M. Joseph Lobel reported the results of treating 300 hard-of-hearing patients with injections of vitamin A in the *Archives of Otolaryngology*, May, 1951. Of the 300 patients, 249 indicated their hearing of conversational tones had improved.

The Ears And Hearing

At a symposium on Metabolic Functions of Vitamin A at the Massachusetts Institute of Technology in November, 1968, Dr. Oswald A. Roels of Columbia University reported findings that a lack of this vitamin causes cell membranes to break down. Vitamin A regulates the stability of the walls of tissue cells and he concludes that much of the aging process is due to a vitamin A deficiency.

High-Fat Diet And Poor Hearing Linked

In a study of the Mabaan tribe of Africa, Dr. Samuel Rosen, an ear surgeon at Mt. Sinai Hospital, concluded that diet, as well as quiet, is a factor in preserving hearing. He learned that they had no high blood pressure nor artery hardening, no malnutrition nor deficiency diseases—and virtually no deafness. The Mabaans ate very little saturated fat, he discovered, and their diet consisted mainly of fruits, vegetables and nuts.

Dr. Rosen pursued the relationship of coronary heart disease to hearing loss in countries used to high-fat diet such as Finland. Patients residing in two mental hospitals whose cholesterol levels were being studied were given hearing tests by Dr. Rosen. Those patients in the experimental group (who were on a low-fat diet) had "better hearing throughout the entire audiometric range than those in the control hospital" who were on a typical Finnish high-fat diet. (*Archives of Otolaryngology*, 82: 236-243, September, 1965.) "Indeed," the report continued, "the 50- to 59-year-old group in the experimental hospital had significantly better hearing than the group ten years younger in the control hospital. The difference in hearing in the two hospitals parallels the difference in the incidence of coronary heart disease."

Inner Ear Problems And Cholesterol

Dr. James T. Spencer, Jr., reported in *The West Virginia Medical Journal* (February, 1974) that many cases of inner ear disease could be successfully treated by putting patients on a high nutrition, low-fat diet similar to that prescribed for heart patients. In fact, Dr. Spencer said, hearing loss and other inner symptoms may actually be forerunners of heart disease.

As an assistant clinical professor of otolaryngology at West Virginia University School of Medicine's Charleston Clinical Division, Dr. Spencer examined patients with hearing loss, ringing or fullness in the ears, vertigo and other symptoms of inner ear problems. Staggering, nausea, vomiting and headaches were also present in some cases. Laboratory analysis revealed that 46.6 percent of the subjects were suffering from elevated cholesterol levels, triglycerides or similar fats in the blood. Abnormal glucose tolerance indicative of diabetic patients or a pre-diabetic condition was evident in 87 percent of the patients, and 80 percent of the subjects were overweight to the point of obesity.

Putting the emphasis on what he calls "good basic nutrition," Dr. Spencer altered the patients' diet to restrict fats, refined sugars and starches, and concentrated sweets. He also urged all overweight patients to reduce their weight to an ideal level. The majority of those who conscientiously followed his instructions reported significant improvement. "Phenomenal gain in hearing has resulted with as much as 30 decibel improvement in an affected ear," Dr. Spencer reported. Ear discomfort, vertigo, headaches and other symptoms were also relieved as blood lipid levels fell.

There was an added bonus. "In addition to these improvements," he reported, "these patients generally improve in appearance from weight loss, exhibit or admit to having more energy, and feel more youthful. They are very grateful patients."

Any diet that corrects proteinemia must also be assumed to be beneficial for the heart and arteries: "While treating the patients' inner ear disorder," he noted, "simultaneous improvement in their general health and increased longevity can be expected to follow."

Fat in the diet presumably affects hearing by accumulating in the blood vessels feeding the hearing apparatus. In such a case, while a low fat diet would help, vitamin E should help too. Vitamin E protects against the deterioration of body fats. Peroxidation of fats (the interaction of oxygen and fat) is often called a major factor in the aging process. In preventing the "excessive oxidation of cellular lipids," the process known as aging can be retarded (Dr. A. L. Tappel, *Nutrition Today*, Summer 1968).

112. Our Ears Need Better Protection From The Noise Around Us

Dr. Samuel Rosen did a lengthy study of the hearing ability of the Mabaans, a primitive tribe of the southeastern Sudan, which was discussed in the preceding chapter. He discovered that these people could hear sounds and noises at the age of seventy with the same efficiency and discrimination as the average American youth of eighteen. Heretofore, it had been an "accepted and established fact" that loss of hearing came naturally with old age. In fact, there is a technical name for such loss, *presbycusis.*

Now we must ask how much hearing, if any, is lost "naturally" through old age and how much loss is preventable? Is our environment systematically damaging our ears? The answer is an unequivocal yes. Our sound environment—the noise to which each of us is subjected—is an ever present danger to the hearing acuity of us all.

Noise impairs hearing. As a case in point, consider Gerald J. of Dubuque, Iowa. He was young, vigorous, and well educated with a two-year Associate degree in Building Maintenance and Management. But he lost his first job becasue of a hearing impairment.

An otological examination proved that Gerald had incurred a severe hearing loss. Although he had received a disability pension from the Armed Forces for his hearing impairment, the military service had merely increased his disability, not created it. In Gerald's own words, "When I was a boy I worked long hours driving a tractor in the fields. My father, an extremely frugal man, refused to install a muffler on my machine. Consequently, my hearing was bombarded from twelve to fourteen hours daily with the wild vibrations of a three foot straight pipe. Even though I suffered more hearing loss in the artillery, my hearing was pretty shaky before I entered the service."

It has been estimated that more than half of the industrial

machines in the United States are capable of creating a hearing loss. Any worker who mans a machine which bumps, grinds, pounds, or hammers either wood, metal, or rock is working in surroundings which may place his hearing in jeopardy. Specifically, this means workers in mining, construction, farming, heavy industry, and transportation.

Lawn Mowers Cut Hearing

The householder and do-it-yourselfer may also incur hearing loss from impact sounds. Ethel B. of Sycamore, Illinois, started her power lawn mower for the weekly grass clipping season. Dr. Darrell Rose, Audiologist at Colorado State University, administered a hearing test immediately before and after her weekly ritual. Ethel complained of a slight ringing in the ears but reported no other physiological symptoms, even though her forty-five minute exposure to the din of her power mower had created a temporary 15 decibel loss in her hearing.

Of course, "temporary" is the key word in Ethel's case history. Many hearing losses caused by impact sounds tend to be temporary, and a good rest in relative peace and quiet will restore much of the hearing which was lost. Unfortunately for householders like Ethel, however, the ephemeral hearing impairment tends to become more and more permanent as exposure continues.

In the past, lawn mower companies had placed power machines on the market which had been carefully engineered to run more quietly than most models. These sound-reduced machines had been advertised, left on the market, and ultimately removed and discontinued. The reason? No one wants to buy them. Most males who buy such appliances equate noise and power in a direct ratio. If the lawn mower makes an ear splitting racket, the householder reasons it must have "zip." On the other hand, if the machine is relatively quiet, he concludes that it couldn't possibly have the power to do the cutting he wants.

Dr. William Shearer, Director of the Speech and Hearing Clinic at Northern Illinois University, pointed out, "Even those who have careers in offices may incur a permanent hearing loss. Workers in large complexes such as a city room of a newspaper or a large insurance office constantly face the whine of computer reels, the clack of electric typewriters, the jangle of telephones, and the buzzing of communication systems. These sounds beat against each other to build into a crescendo of noise which can do damage to the sensitive membranes of the inner ear. In any one day there isn't much of a hearing loss, but over a span of time, such as four or five years, there may be a decided loss."

How Sound Wears Out The Ear

How does sound damage hearing? That which we perceive as sound is in reality changes in air pressure. In order for the human ear to hear a sound it must change air pressure at least 40 times per second (this means 20 cycles per second—there are two changes in air pressure for each cycle). If, however, the air pressure changes more than 40 thousand times per second (20,000 cycles per second) the sound is too high for the human ear to hear.

Sound is transmitted through the three ear parts: the outer ear funnels sound waves to the eardrum; the middle ear passes the vibrations through three bones commonly known as the "hammer," "anvil," and "stirrup;" the middle ear bones vibrate the fluid in the cochlea, which has tiny hairs protruding from the walls. The hairs translate the vibrations into electrical energy and send impulses to the brain, which interprets them as noise or sound.

Low frequency sounds are dealt with throughout the path of the inner cochlea, but high pitched sounds are analyzed by the ear at the front of this organ. Consequently, the area where the high frequency sounds concentrate tends to wear out first. When the ear is bombarded by too many high pitched, loud noises, the hair cells in the inner ear are destroyed, and once lost, can never be replaced.

A hearing loss may be stated in decibels. For instance, if a sound must be raised to 15 decibels above the standard for an individual to hear it, he is said to suffer a 15 decibel hearing loss.

A decibel (*deci* meaning ten; *bel* in honor of Alexander Graham Bell) measures the smallest amount of sound which the human ear can distinguish. Actually, the human ear is so delicate that at certain frequencies it can discern sound that moves the eardrum only one-tenth the width of a hydrogen atom. But decibels must be considered in conjunction with loudness, pitch, and intensity. Loudness denotes how loud the listener perceives the sound; intensity means the amount of energy being used at the sound source. Pitch affects the listener in a unique way. Certain high frequency sounds are recorded by the brain as louder than lower frequency sounds with the same intensity. For instance, a 20 decibel sound at 1,000 cycles per second (cps) would be equal in loudness to 40 decibels of sound at 200 cps.

One of the unexplained phenomena concerning sound is the human reaction to it. It seems that males tend to endure lower frequency sounds better; females seem to be more comfortable with the higher frequency sounds.

When is hearing protection needed? The booklet entitled, "Industrial Noise and Hearing Protection," published by Employers Insurance Co. of Wausau, says: "If a worker is subjected to many hours per day of noise which is in excess of 85 decibels . . . the use of ear protection devices is recommended." The American Medical Association uses the more conservative figure of 90 decibels.

What of sounds in excess of 90 decibels? In a booklet entitled, "Guide for Conservation of Hearing," written by the Callier Hearing and Speech Center in Dallas, Texas, are listed maximum time exposures to various sounds to remain within the safety zone of hearing conversation. For instance, if the sound to which you are exposed is 90 decibels, the exposure should be limited to 120 minutes per day; a 100 decibel exposure should be limited to fewer than 25 minutes; at 120 decibels, your exposure should be under five minutes per day.

A decibel isn't a straight line measurement, by the way. The risk to your hearing at 120 decibels isn't just one-third greater than the risk at 90 decibels; according to recent research, it's nearly 100 times as great if high frequency sounds are prominent.

Signs Of Hearing Loss

How can you tell when you start to lose your hearing? Dr. Darrell Rose explains it this way, "The soft, high pitched sounds go first; the rustle of clothing or chirping of a cricket, sometimes even the songs of birds. Many don't notice a hearing loss, however, until family members complain about the volume level of the stereo or TV set. But sooner or later, a severe hearing impairment will affect the voice frequency range—then the high pitched sibilants (such as the letter 's') will start to be garbled and conversations will appear mumbled."

Without complicated scientific instruments, how can you tell if noise is loud enough to do damage? If you must shout to someone only a few feet away to make yourself heard over the din or racket in the background, the noise level is high enough to cause potential damage.

Sudden loud noises also create stress and nervousness. These are the kinds of sounds that often occur when they are least wanted or least expected, such as the banging of garbage cans in the early morning, or the explosive "boom" of a supersonic plane.

Health Is Damaged In Other Ways

Some medical practitioners claim that repeated sudden noises can work on an individual and create a state of nervousness which can lead to ulcers. There may be some truth to the allegation, for Dr. Claude Fortier, at the University of Montreal, subjected rats to the intermittent noise of a shrill siren. As a result of the noise bombardment, he found the rats had suffered atrophy of the thymus gland, the overstimulation of the adrenal glands, and gastric ulcers.

Other experiments have shown that a sudden door slam can raise a man's blood pressure higher than the result of a shot of morphine. Even the plaintive cry of a baby has doubled the amount of blood pumped by the heart. The increased oxygen which is consumed with the rising blood pressure results in restlessness, nervousness, and in some cases, exhaustion.

Dr. Darrell Rose states, "Biologically, unwanted noise gives about the same kind of symptoms as fear. An unexpected or unwanted sound can cause the pupils of the eye to dilate, mucous membranes to cease secreting, skin to take on a pallid look, adrenals to secrete heavily, and many of the internal organs to spasm."

People normally dream about four or five times each night. But Dr. Julius Buchwald of the Downstate Division, New York Medical Center stated that if these dreams are disturbed by unwanted sounds a person may suffer from paranoidal delusions, psychoses, hallucinations, suicidal and homicidal impulses and nightmarish memories. Not to mention, of course, that interrupted sleep can cause irritation, fatigue, and tension. Awake, many people might not be aware of the noise around them, but annoyance builds up, resulting in frayed nerves and outbursts of anger.

What To Do About It

If the public would insist upon it, noise from the mechanical monsters of construction would not be a problem. For instance, a new pile driver shakes piles into the ground by vibrations, not banging. It's faster, quieter, and costs about the same. Air hammers have mufflers available but few contractors use them because they don't have to. As for riveting, steel girders could be welded together just as well. Blasting on construction sites may be muffled by special steel mesh blankets weighing several tons each. They not only reduce much of the unwanted sounds of blasting, but they confine debris to a small area.

Noise along highways may be prevented by the installation of deflectors and new concepts in highway landscaping. Routing the airlanes along people-free strips of land will reduce the noise of air traffic. Further air noise reductions may be made by a change in flight patterns. Supersonic flight over populated areas should be prohibited.

Soundproofing a home is a step in the right direction to control sound. All walls, even those not facing the periphera of the home, should be insulated. Acoustical tile installed on the ceiling, carpets on the floor, long draperies, upholstered furniture, double glazed windows, and felt or rubber mats under all appliances help reduce the sounds or blanket them. Furnace rooms can be lined with acoustical tile and flexible connections may be installed between units and ducts.

It should be noted, however, that although acoustical tile helps to keep a room quiet, it does little good in an apartment when the impact sound comes from the room above. The best way to combat such sound is to talk the landlord into installing carpet in the upper room.

Installing weather stripping on the inside doors may reduce sounds within a home as much as 25-30 decibels; without it, sound will likely be reduced only 10 decibels.

Support legislation for reasonable sound abatement programs. Memphis, Tennessee, decided it was going to become a quiet city. It took them two years, but they made it and were dubbed for the next fourteen years as the quietest city in the United States. The secret of their success was a two year educational program to acquaint the citizens with what they were trying to accomplish. This was followed by a period of issuing summonses in a fair but firm program and increasing education concerning noise. At first the citizens objected to the tickets issued as a mere nuisance, but later they cooperated with the city ordinance and accomplished an enviable record.

Even with realistic sound controls we may not be able to preserve the same levels of auditory acuity as Dr. Rosen reported for the Mabaans. But we can come a lot closer to them.

113. Loud Music Impairs Hearing

If your teenage child or grandchild is addicted to loud popular music, the nerve-shattering volume at which he plays his records may be a serious matter. Every day, young people are permanently damaging their hearing by subjecting themselves to too many decibels of musical din.

It doesn't matter whether it is called rock-and-roll, hard rock or acid rock. When it is performed live, it comes out only one way—loud. And because the music is amplified electronically to such a high intensity of sound, it is slowly turning young people deaf.

Frederick L. Dey, M.D., Ph.D., reported in the February 26, 1970, *New England Journal of Medicine* that tests among 15 men aged 18-25 with normal hearing showed that loud music can indeed be hazardous to your child's—or anyone's—ear health. The experiments indicated that a temporary shift in the threshold of hearing induced by any loud noise was pushed beyond the point of rapid recovery when the music was played too loud for an extended period.

According to the results, two persons out of a hundred listening to music at the 100-decibel (db) level would show slow recovery rates from the damage to their ears, and at 110 db, 16 percent of the people listening would suffer adverse, and probably permanent, damage to their hearing. (The decibel is a unit of measure that expresses the relative intensity of sounds.)

To understand comparative intensities of decibel values, consider that normal conversation registers 60 db, a loud motorcycle, 110 db, an overhead jet plane, more than 115 db, and a hydraulic press, 120 db. A rock band amplified to its peak is charted at a loud 120 decibels of intensity.

The investigators have determined that a person's hearing faculties are temporarily reduced (the threshold is raised) when the ears are subjected to loud noise. But hearing should recover from the effects of loud noises two minutes after the noise has stopped. They call this standard recovery time the Temporary Threshold Shift two minutes, and abbreviate it TTS_2.

516

Two Hours Can Damage Hearing Forever

A person's hearing can safely tolerate a threshold shift of as much as 40 decibels for as long as two minutes. Anything more than that involves a risk that the hearing will not fully recover. Using their experimental findings as a base, the investigators showed that a person exposed to loud music being played at 120 decibels for two hours encounters a TTS_2 ranging from 35 db to 44.9 db; in other words, levels that exceed the safety limits.

The Discotheque Is A Blast

George T. Singleton, an ear, nose and throat specialist at the University of Florida, measured sounds inside a dance hall and found that anybody directly in front of the band was blasted with 120 db of sound, and even in the middle of the dance floor 106-108 db was the average. The testers had to move 40 feet outside the building before the decibel level dropped to 90.

At the Houston Speech and Hearing Center, Dr. James Jerger found that out of a five-man combo, none of whom had reached his 23rd birthday, three members showed a slight but permanent loss of hearing, and one of them had suffered a 50 decibel temporary loss.

Music No Longer Soothing

We do know that the world is becoming a noisier place in which to live. City dwellers' ears are almost incessantly assaulted with unwanted noises, both indoors and outside. Even farmers are liable to ear damage as noise levels from tractors and power saws pass the danger point. A simple modern convenience such as air conditioning brings with its comfort the price of a constant hum, at best.

Just when it seems we should be seeking quiet places for relaxation and enjoyment, many people, especially most of the young people, have developed a craving for quite the opposite. Rock music sets a mood by drowning out everything around it to the point of even numbing the audience.

What makes the noise from rock music so dangerous is that the damage comes disguised as entertainment. People have always turned to music to divert and soothe themselves, and loud music is nothing new. What is new is the electronic amplification of the instruments to decibel levels intolerable to the healthy ear.

You should warn your youngsters that hearing seriously damaged by loud noises cannot be repaired.

114. Earwax: A Common Cause Of Deafness

Earwax, or cerumen, as the professionals call it, is a very common cause of deafness among Americans. Yet it is a problem all too commonly overlooked by doctors, according to Dr. James Kawchak (*Journal of Occupational Medicine*, Vol. 3, No. 1, 1963).

A Natural Barrier To Infection

Under normal circumstances, earwax is not a curse, but a natural aid. The thousand or more modified sebaceous and sweat glands located in the outer part of the ear canal continuously secrete cerumen, and for a very definite reason. The light yellow substance, composed of water, fats, free fatty acids, cholesterin and lecithin, performs functions essential for maintaining good hearing. It lubricates the skin, preventing a dry, crusty, infection-prone ear canal, and it traps bacteria, dust and even insects, eventually packaging the foreign substances into a compact little ball.

The role earwax plays in preserving our hearing can't be overestimated. A minor infection such as a pimple, which we would ignore in most parts of the body, would threaten us with total deafness if it occurred in the ear canal. What's more, the passage from the ear to the brain is short and direct, and a serious ear infection can be life threatening. Without earwax, these dangers would be far more common than they are. Even cerumen's role in eliminating dust from the ear is of great importance. Dust on the tympanum would eventually produce distorted and muffled hearing. The result would be similar to allowing dust particles to pile up on an exposed phonograph or radio speaker.

Vigorous Jaw Movements Help Dislodge Cerumen

Ordinarily, once the cerumen lining the ear canal is sufficiently laden with dust and other impurities, nature takes over to excrete it from the ear. The wax dries into flakes, and the motion of the lower jaw in talking, yawning, but most important, in eating, massages the ear canal in such a way as to move the cerumen along toward the outer ear. During sleep, the dry wax simply falls out.

The increased pollution of our environment has had a very pronounced effect on hearing difficulties caused by the excessive buildup of earwax. Under normal circumstances, the ear eliminates earwax spontaneously, but dust and dirt particles in the air often adhere to the natural waxy substance, creating a substance which is no longer a defense against infection, but an infecting and troublesome substance itself, which is not easily expelled.

But, perhaps even more significant in the current prevalence in hearing difficulties caused by the excessive accumulation of earwax is the change in our eating habits. Not too many years ago, a snack meant a raw carrot, an apple, a couple of slices of green pepper, a pear—good fresh foods high in nutrient and fiber. Meat, too, was tough and chewy. So was bread. Every meal was a challenge for the jaw muscles.

That kind of workout provided precisely the sort of stimulation for the ear canal required to keep it free of excess cerumen. Today's pablum-type diets, centering as they do around foods highly processed, beaten and boiled into submission, offer little challenge to jaw muscles. One result is likely to be a build-up of earwax and creeping deafness.

Dr. Kawchak gave such an example from his own practice: A 34-year-old woman, a secretary in a large office found it more and more difficult to use the telephone at her right ear. There was a feeling of "blockage," and sound in general was muffled. Her symptoms had been building up over a three-year period. Otoscopic examination revealed the right external auditory canal to be completely blocked with cerumen. An audiogram was taken and showed a highly significant hearing loss. Once the ear was cleaned, the blocked feeling disappeared, and a second hearing test showed dramatic improvement.

Although deafness is typically associated with the aged, cerumen-related hearing problems are no respecters of age. Young children frequently suffer a cerumen build-up practically from birth.

Symptoms Of Impacted Cerumen Are Varied

Deafness is only one of many possible symptoms of ceruminosis. Another might be tinnitus, a buzzing, ringing or roaring sound in the ears. Some people may develop a severe earache, and if the wax gets lodged beyond the isthmus of the ear, it could cause a reflex cough. Dizziness is a fairly common symptom. Many people report an annoying kind of echo sensation, in which the sound of their own voice seems strange. According to Ralph Peimer, M.D., writing in the *Eye, Ear, Nose and Throat Monthly* (December, 1960), if the cerumen which protects the ear by entrapping bacteria isn't eventually excreted, it will serve as an excellent medium for the bacteria to grow in. Even fungi have been found actually growing in cerumen.

A report published in the *Journal of the American Medical Association* (January 5, 1970) went so far as to link excess cerumen accumulation with disturbances in the behavioral patterns of mental health patients. According to the report, more than 1,700 patients, or 42 percent of the hospital population, failed a hearing test. That was far in excess of the 10 percent failure rate expected in the general population. "The majority of those who failed had impacted cerumen in both ears. . ." reported the *Journal*. It added, "In some cases, cerumen was impacted to an extent that general anesthesia was necessary to remove it."

The most interesting part of the study was the effect that removing the cerumen had on the patients. With their improved hearing, 50 of the patients were promptly rehabilitated and dismissed from the hospital. According to Dan F. McCoy, chief of the hospital's speech and hearing department, "If you can eliminate even a little hearing loss, or an infection, frequently you will get great changes in behavior."

A finding like this warrants concern as to how many children who are having problems in school may have a hearing problem—perhaps impacted cerumen. Or how many older people who are thought to be "senile" because of impaired alertness are actually suffering from a hearing difficulty.

Many Popular Treatments Useless Or Dangerous

Most ceruminosis treatments down through the years have proved useless—if not downright dangerous. Some prescription drugs, particularly those containing hydrogen peroxide, have been known to irritate the skin of the ear canal. Salt water and olive oil have also been tried without success.

At one time, propylene glycol was thought effective, but in 1947 it was tested by Dr. B. H. Senturia and his colleagues (*Laryngoscope*, 57: 633-656). The chemical was found to cause a rapid swelling of the wax, which could produce severe pressure and pain, and would, of course, make removal of wax more difficult. Water, too, often does more harm than good by causing the wax to swell rapidly.

The most dangerous earwax "treatment" of all involves the cotton-tipped swabs which people often poke and jab into their ears. Herbert Silverstein, M.D., wrote about some of the resulting injuries in *Transactions of the American Academy of Ophthalmology and Otolaryngology* (May-June, 1973). After studying 27 patients who were treated at the Massachusetts Eye and Ear Infirmary and the Children's Hospital in Philadelphia for ear injuries, Dr. Silverstein wrote, "The most common object causing damage to the tympanic membrane and ossicular chain was a cotton-tipped applicator (13 cases)."

In addition to hearing loss, these patients suffered dizziness, bleeding, vomiting, and often severe pain. Not only is the risk of permanent ear damage high in using the swabs, but the swabs are not effective; any wax that can be dislocated by them is on its way to falling out of the ear of its own accord anyway, and the harder wax is only compacted more deeply in the ear by pressing the swab against it.

Fortunately, ceruminosis can be treated in simple and safe ways. In some cases, a switch to foods that require hearty chewing may in itself shake the wax loose and solve the problem. At the very least, this should help prevent the problem. If the wax is too hard to be dislodged even by vigorous chewing, glycerol is one of the few substances which can soften it without causing the wax to swell. Some preparations available without prescription are little more than glycerine and antiseptic and will serve the purpose.

Only in severe cases is medical intervention necessary. On the other hand, anyone even slightly concerned about his hearing should not hesitate to have an examination. By all means, it ought to include exploration of the inner ear with an otoscope, for that is the only way a cerumen plug blocking the ear can be detected.

115. Meniere's Disease

If you can picture yourself on a small boat battling the high seas with a roaring gale pitching the craft from breaker to breaker, you have some indication of the sensation of seasickness that is the lot of hundreds of thousands of people in this country who suffer with Meniere's disease.

Meniere's disease is an affliction of the inner ear which includes the following symptoms: the loss of hearing; ringing in the ears; dizziness and nausea, frequently accompanied by vomiting; the distortion of sound and a feeling of pressure in the inner ear. The disease, whose symptoms were first collectively described by Prosper Meniere in 1861, usually strikes sufferers between the ages of forty and sixty, and more frequently strikes men than women.

The dizziness varies from simple unsteadiness to violent, whirling vertigo. A natural or induced sleep while the patient is suffering from an attack seems to take care of all unpleasant symptoms. The patient awakes feeling refreshed and healthy.

It is believed by some researchers that Meniere's syndrome is due to a hemorrhage of the small, delicate parts of the inner ear known as the semicircular canals. Others suggest some imbalance of fluid and pressure in the inner ear. One treatment consists of giving the patient 50 to 100 milligrams of niacin (a B vitamin) about 20 minutes before each meal. Low salt intake is another remedy used by physicians. Some doctors have found that if their patients give up smoking many of the unpleasant symptoms stop.

A Vitamin Therapy That Helps

A thorough-going study by a physician of high standing describing a successful vitamin therapy for Meniere's disease was published in the *Archives of Otolaryngology* (Volume 75, page 220, 1962). The physician, Dr. Miles Atkinson, an otologist, was at that time on the faculty of New York University and has since retired.

Dr. Atkinson believed that there was an association between Meniere's disease and migraine headaches. "Meniere's disease is migraine of the ear and migraine in Meniere's of the occipital lobe," Dr. Atkinson stated. The association between migraine and Meniere's disease is no new observation. Meniere himself referred to it. But, according to Dr. Atkinson, the relationship has not received the recognition which would appear to be its due.

Both, according to Dr. Atkinson, are the result of a vasospasm (spasm of the blood vessel) and a subsequent vasodilation (stretched blood vessel) which leads to an increased flow of blood. In the Meniere syndrome, it is the primary vasospasm which produces the outstanding symptoms, the sudden acute vertigo which comes on abruptly and lays the patient low, while a secondary vasodilation, which results in the accumulation of fluid in the labyrinth of the ear, produces the secondary effects which are often by contrast relatively minor—the headache, the general malaise, the transient hearing loss of the early attacks. Thus, vertigo is the predominant manifestation. According to Dr. Atkinson, it is best treated by seeking to prevent the spasm of the blood vessel.

Vitamin B Deficiency

It has long been recognized that nicotinic acid (vitamin B_3) is effective in controlling Meniere attacks in the vasoconstrictor group, and it was assumed that this was due to its vasodilator action. But Dr. Atkinson suspected that some of the beneficial effects achieved with B_3 were due to its properties as a vitamin. He found severe chronic vitamin B deficiency in Meniere patients.

"Then comes the question, routinely asked by critics and by those to whom the conception of chronic vitamin deficiency is new or unacceptable—why the deficiency, particularly in a prosperous and well-fed country such as the United States?" Dr. Atkinson said, "I have no certain knowledge as to why such deficiencies arise, but we do have a number of suggestive leads. For instance, it is common knowledge that the diet of a great many people is far from ideal—the rich eat too much fat, and the poor eat too little protein, and the in-betweens eat too many carbohydrates. Some eat too much in order to comfort themselves; others eat too little in order to fashion themselves. The diet records of most of the patients I see in my office make dismal reading."

But intake is only one aspect of nutrition, Dr. Atkinson insisted. "What about absorption? This may be interfered with by gastrointestinal disease, for example, and by many drugs. Of the drugs, antibiotics are at the present time the most significant offenders because of their widespread use. The first Meniere attack frequently follows upon some illness in which antibiotics were liberally used. Always when antibiotics are given," Dr. Atkinson maintained, "vitamins should be given at the same time. How often is this done?"

Some sufferers may find relief by replenishing their intestinal flora through the addition of yogurt or buttermilk to their diets—a simple expedient well worth trying. Others, however, may not. Each one of us is a metabolic individual. Some of us do not manufacture any B vitamins in the intestine. Those with liver disease do not utilize or store vitamins sufficiently. The incidence of gallbladder disease in patients with Meniere's is twice that of the general population, Dr. Atkinson has observed. In order to overcome deficiency in these patients, a high dosage of vitamins over long periods of time has been found to be *essential*. Moreover, maintenance therapy to prevent recurrence is necessary for years, perhaps to some degree even for life, or relapses will occur.

This suggests something more than inadequate intake, rather some defect in utilization of the B vitamins, due perhaps to a metabolic fault. Dr. Atkinson does not overlook the fact that there are other possible causes for this neurovascular dysfunction. He suggests allergy, eye strain, alcohol, tobacco, stress and strain of mind and body as factors which may serve as triggers in particular cases.

Dr. Atkinson's therapy included both injection and oral administration, in order to gain control as rapidly as possible. Injections, he points out, must be intravenous because the solutions used in the dosage necessary are painful if given intramuscularly or subcutaneously. Injections are given daily for the first one or two weeks, then three times weekly until a large measure of control has been established, usually to a total of 60 to 70 injections. Dr. Atkinson found that 60 is about the smallest amount that will produce adequate control in Meniere's disease. Oral therapy is given together with the injections, again to the maximum dose compatible with response and tolerance. This is continued thereafter for several years.

Dr. Atkinson used both nicotinamide and nicotinic acid. Nicotinamide has no vasodilator action, only the vitamin effect, and thus can be used in high dosage without producing any unpleasant flushing. But, in the treatment of the vasospastic group of Meniere's cases, nicotinic acid in addition is essential to achieve success. Nicotinic acid also has a vasodilator effect, and Dr. Atkinson points out it is tempting to assume that this must be the reason for its effectiveness in a vasospastic condition. But, it may not be as simple as that. Nicotinic acid has at least one other action that we know of; reduction of the blood cholesterol level if given in very high dosage. It may have others. However that may be, adequate dosage of the three main fractions of the B complex, together with nicotinic acid, has been found to control Meniere attacks. But it takes time.

116. Understanding The Misery Of Tinnitus

Describing the misery of tinnitus (ringing in the ears) is not easy, so few persons who suffer from this malady ever get the full measure of sympathy to which they are entitled. Because they do not have great pain, or a visible wound, the victims are expected to overcome the discomfort they experience by sheer willpower. The truth is that they seldom can. There is actually a physical basis for most tinnitus, and one can no more will it away than talk oneself out of a broken leg.

Various Sounds Heard

In its advanced stages, the sound is constantly there—all day, all night. There is no time in the patient's conscious moments that he does not hear what has been described variously as: ringing, buzzing, a noise like a waterfall, a jet of steam, a saw or an engine, a splash, ringing of bells or the telephone, chirping, grasshopper or cricket sounds. To sleep you must always overcome the wretched noise. The sounds are persistent; you hear it during a conversation, if you are listening to music or watching television, reading or working. This distracting, distressing, maddening noise is ever present.

The condition, as discussed in great detail by Dr. Jean-Pierre Taillens in *Review Medicale de la Suisse Romande* (80/2:65-78) indicates an abnormality in the auditory canal at some point along its course. The where and why create a serious problem for the doctor. Sometimes the reason is insolvable, the causes can be many and/or unrecognizable.

The Pulse Is Noisy And Is Heard By The Ear

In nature, absolute silence does not exist. Normally the ear detects the sounds of the internal life when external sound is absent. An illustration of this, reported by Dr. Taillens, is that the noise one hears when holding a conch shell to the ear is actually the echo of the sound of the blood stream running through the capillaries of the cochlea (a spirally tube which is a part of the inner ear). One researcher (Békésy) claims that the minute sound of the constant spontaneous movement of the cells of the body is enough to stimulate a resonant vibration in the ear. The cells move in a range of one ten-millionth of a millimeter. This might give some idea of the extreme delicacy of the auditory make-up we have, and at the same time help us realize the possible loudness of the ringing sound discussed here.

The types of tinnitus fall into three general categories. The first is "exotic" or "periotic." This comes from disorders of organs near the auditory apparatus. These sounds actually have an observable physical basis. The doctor, using a stethoscope, can hear them as well as the patient. One cause of these noises is the contraction of one of the ear muscles, or alternating contractions of the soft palate, of the tongue or the uvula. Another is chronic catarrh (an inflammation of the mucous membrane) which can cause hollow noises, like snapping when swallowing, due to the separation of the congested tubular wall. Noises also may occur at the movement of the jaw bone.

Vascular noises are truly the most common of all, and result from some physical incapacity. For example, sufferers of pernicious anemia or chlorosis are likely to hear a whirring sound of the jugular vein, like a turning wheel or a loud noise. Persons suffering from impairment of the heart, or carotid, or from arterial trouble near the ear get a noise connected with the throbbing of the pulse. It occurs at regular intervals along with the pulse beat. Combinations of arterial and venous disorders can also occur, having manifestations in the persistent sounds of the inner ear.

Any Disorder Can Cause Tinnitus

The second type of tinnitus is called "entotic tinnitus." Here the sounds are heard only by the patient; they are completely subjective. The sounds are accompanied by deafness, which is an important factor in diagnosis. In the external ear, accumulation of wax, foreign objects, bony growths, and the like often cause dizziness and tinnitus. When any of these is removed, the symptoms disappear.

Where the middle ear is concerned, just about any disorder can cause tinnitus—that includes all types of infections and inflammation. The same is true of the inner ear; however, the possible sources of the trouble involve many parts of the body and make tracing it very difficult. Tumors of the acoustic nerve cause tinnitus; in Meniere's disease even cutting the cochlear nerve won't stop tinnitus and no one seems to know what will. Certain glandular disorders can cause tinnitus and so can high blood pressure.

Drugs Can Cause Tinnitus And Deafness

There are some commonly accepted causes of tinnitus. The internal ear is an organ which is most sensitive to poisons of all kinds. Tinnitus is often one of the first symptoms indicative of and preceding deafness due to poisoning. One of the poisons which can cause such injury is quinine, often used as a medicine for malaria. Another is salicylate, a part of most aspirin compounds. It can produce a congestion of both the middle ear and the labyrinth, where a bloody discharge can be noted. If the drug is stopped early enough, said Dr. Taillens, tinnitus will disappear; if not, the noises can persist indefinitely. There is room here for speculation on chronic arthritis and headache victims who saturate themselves with aspirin. How many have experienced tinnitus and not been aware of the reason?

There is a long list of drugs which can bring on acute tinnitus when given in large doses: barbiturates, aureomycin, streptomycin, therapeutic arsenic, cocaine, opium and their derivatives. Some persons are especially susceptible. Stopping the drug is often the only effective remedy against this condition.

Deafness and tinnitus can result from exposure to certain chemicals. These can be aniline, arsenic, benzene, mercury, lead, carbon monoxide, illuminating gas, phosphorus and sulphur. Gas station attendants are exposed to lead and carbon monoxide frequently; dry cleaners are constantly breathing the toxic benzene fumes.

Clue To More Serious Ailments

Tinnitus and deafness often act as a clue to other serious systemic defects. Diabetes, chronic nephritis and a faulty fat metabolism are three such conditions. One should have one's blood examined for sugar, urea and cholesterol count if tinnitus occurs. Virus infections are also likely to result in this type of ear trouble.

One aspect of tinnitus has especially intriguing overtones—reflex tinnitus. It's a sort of sympathetic reaction to the strangest types of stress. One reported case had tinnitus relieved when the patient had his glasses adjusted; another had a denture refitted with a resultant tinnitus cure; still another responded to the enlarging of a tight collar. Reflex tinnitus can probably be caused by anything from an aching tooth to an arthritic joint.

The final type of tinnitus, "central tinnitus," is the most frightening, actually the most serious of all. The victim hears sounds of all kinds which seem to be coming from the central auditory canal. They are intolerable and violent. They spread over everything and echo throughout the head. The noises are heard in both ears which hampers any classification of the cause. Furthermore, the noises resist everything and persist over a similar sound produced by the audiometer, even with greater intensity than ordinary subjective tinnitus. Such a condition is often the sign of the development of a serious disorder, and calls for a complete neurologic examination.

It should be noted that there is such a thing as auditory hallucination. While this condition persists the patient hears articulate sounds, bits of phrases or melodies remembered from times past. The problem of auditory hallucination had long been considered a psychiatric problem, but recent studies have shown it to be a normal part of the formed auditory hearing loss in some older individuals suffering such ear diseases as tinnitus.

In an article in the *Journal of the American Medical Association* (February 10, 1975), entitled "Musical Hallucinations in Deafness," researchers reported on two elderly patients who thought they were "going crazy" because they were hearing distinct musical tunes of many years before that no one else could hear. The researchers, noting that reported cases of such auditory hallucinations were extremely rare, assured the two individuals that the sounds that they were hearing were purely physiological in nature. "Treatment," according to the researchers, "consists mainly of assuring the patients of the benign and nonpsychiatric character of the disorder."

117. Some Practical Suggestions For Choosing A Hearing Aid

Professional advice on whether to try a hearing aid is encumbered with several shortcomings: it is based on hearing tests conducted in a soundfree booth remote from the actual sound environment in which people live; it subscribes to a rigid, numerical criterion as to the extent of loss necessary to justify use of a hearing aid; it takes insufficient account of an individual's lifestyle and objectives; and it takes for granted that every patient is severely and permanently embarrassed at the prospect of wearing a hearing aid.

Millions of Americans who would benefit greatly from the amplification provided by hearing aids are dissuaded from seeking them. Only some two million Americans own hearing aids, when at leat ten million could profit from them. And the incidence of hearing impairment is rising, as people live longer and our environment becomes noisier.

Admittedly, hearing aids are fragile, frustrating, ugly, overpriced implements. The quality of sound they provide approximates that of a cheap transistor radio. Their promotion and advertising stress concealment rather than service. Their price is outrageous, though the average hearing aid costs hardly more to build than a portable radio. A prominent professor of otolaryngology in New York, who wishes more of his patients used aids, refers to hearing aids as "Volkswagens priced like Cadillacs."

Nevertheless, hearing aids provide amplification of sound that millions need and aren't getting. Not only is an amplification system vital to their hearing, but it provides an important element of prevention. For often, people who hear badly don't try very hard to hear, and hearing that is not used deteriorates.

Do You Need An Aid?
As a rule, hearing professionals—the otolaryngologists and audiologists—base their judgment of a patient's need for an aid on

an audiogram. This is a test of how well one hears pure tone signals transmitted at various frequency ranges, usually between 125 and 8,000 cycles. If a patient's hearing in his better ear averages 40 decibels or more below normal at the "speech frequencies" of 500, 1,000 and 2,000 cycles, he is likely to be told that a hearing aid is indicated. If the loss is between 20 and 40 decibels, he is almost always told that his loss is "not serious," and he can "get by okay" and does not need an aid.

There are some variations to this guide. A patient with a severe or profound loss in one ear, but good hearing in the other, might be advised to try an aid. People with losses which are about the same at all frequencies are more likely to be led to an aid than people with sensory neural (nerve) losses, which are invariably greater in the upper than lower pitches. People with severe noise tolerance difficulty will be steered away from aids.

But in most cases, the 40 decibel criterion is followed quite closely. Clearly, however, losses of less than 40 decibels are serious for people who earn their living with their ears—lawyers, musicians and auto mechanics are prime examples. Indeed, with normal conversation conducted at about 60 decibels, losses less than 40 decibels interfere with normal family, social and business life.

A person cannot, then, blandly accept the "objective" criteria followed by the hearing professionals. If you suspect you have a hearing loss, by all means have your ears examined by a physician and your hearing tested by an audiologist. But however reassuring their evaluation might be, do not dismiss the idea of trying a hearing aid if your ears don't serve you well at home and work. Be especially alert to whether or not you misunderstand words you feel you are hearing but still don't get because of inattention. Mishearing words is often a sign, not of inattention, but of a sensory neural loss in which sound is heard but not understood. Word discrimination tests, conducted like audiograms in a sound-free booth or very quiet room, are too "clean" to provide accurate information on how well one comprehends words in the real world.

If you decide to get a hearing aid, heed your own experience and observations with various aids as much as the advice of the audiologists or hearing aid dealers who counsel you. This is not only necessary because of the unreal auditory environment of centers and showrooms but because there are few conclusive findings on the best type of aid an individual should use.

Hearing professionals and hearing aid dealers often, quite innocently perhaps, advance pet theories as scientific fact.

Types Of Hearing Aids

Hearing aids are mostly classified in terms of where they are worn: "behind the ear," "in the ear," "body" and "CROS." CROS is an acronym for "contralateral routing of signals," a system that picks up sound on one side of the head and transports it, usually via wires enclosed in eyeglass frames, to the receiver on the other side.

It is generally believed that body aids are the sturdiest and provide the best tone control, that CROSes are usually the best for people with high frequency losses, that behind-the-ear aids are the most comfortable and provide the best sense of sound directionality, and that in-the-ear aids are the least disruptive to a wearer's psyche, because they are widely advertised as the least conspicuous and provide relatively modest decibel gain.

Tips On Getting An Aid

The hearing impaired individual ought to do a good deal of foraging and decision making on his own. Consider applying the following guidelines in your search for a hearing aid.

First and foremost, do not reject the possibility of using a hearing aid merely because you are told your loss is not serious enough. Only you can decide how serious it is to *you*.

Do not emphasize to an audiologist or dealer any embarrassment you might feel about the prospect of wearing an aid. If you do, they will be more likely to suggest that an aid is not needed or to recommend an aid on the basis of its concealability rather than performance.

If you have a high frequency loss, make it clear to the audiologist or dealer that you want to try a CROS, even if you do not already wear spectacles. Many hearing professionals and merchants do not advise patients with good vision to try a CROS because they anticipate resistance to the use of spectacle frames that house the CROS's electronics system.

Do not be confused by the profusion of styles and brand names that abound in the hearing aid field. Hearing aid manufacturers are essentially assemblers of parts and the great majority of them buy the major parts—the microphone, amplifier and earphone—from only a few component makers. Thus, aids with similar decibel gain and parts positioning are much like one another whatever brand name they bear.

Insist on trying an aid for at least two weeks before buying it. Try it in a variety of aural situations; in restaurants, at work, at parties, at movies and in quiet conversation. Plans that permit a one month rental before purchase are standard procedure throughout the hearing aid field. Do not patronize a dealer who will not permit such a trial period or guarantee in writing a full refund if within 60 or 90 days you find the aid not to your liking. *Never forget that an aid cannot be judged in the quiet of a hearing center or showroom.* If you eventually decide to buy an aid you have rented, the rental fee should be applicable to the purchase price.

Do not assume that aids of the same brand name and style will be the same. In many cases, quality control of aids is poor and frequency response, gain and distortion characteristics can vary among aids that are supposed to be identical.

Bargain for a much lower price than dealers will ask. As a rule, dealers charge nearly four times the amount they pay for an aid. State health and welfare programs customarily pay dealers 10 to 20 percent above cost, and dealers are delighted to get the business. You might have trouble obtaining such a reduction, but most dealers will take 10 to 25 percent off list without much pressure.

Try several aids before giving up on aids altogether or accepting one you consider inadequate. It is often particularly difficult for people with sensory neural losses to find an aid that provides reasonable tone quality and worthwhile improvement of word discrimination.

If you insist on trying a number of aids, it is quite possible that you will be pressured, subtly, by your audiologist and dealer to accept an aid they maintain is the best you can possibly find. This pressure frequently takes the form of implications that your determination to hear as well as you can actually reflects emotional instability; that in short, the locus of your problem is in your personality rather than your ears.

Obviously, hearing and emotions affect one another. The inability to hear well can often be accompanied by tension about misunderstanding conversation or not hearing danger signals that in turn can intensify hearing difficulties. But this does not justify acceptance of an insufficient hearing aid without a firm effort to find the best. If a conscientious search does not locate an aid that pleases you as much as you think it should, you will at least know that you have tried.

Once You've Purchased Your Hearing Aid

Be patient if, when you first try an aid, you find the new and extra sounds it brings you irritating and disconcerting. People whose hearing impairment is severe or whose losses are long-standing are especially likely to find squeaking doors, rustling papers and raspy voices hard to tolerate when they first try a hearing aid. This fact underscores the importance of obtaining an aid in the early stages of a loss.

If your first hearing aid is successful, consider supplementing it with another that can serve you in specific situations. For example, if you decide to use a behind-the-ear aid for your left ear, consider trying, in addition, a CROS with a right side pick-up and left side earphone to use when you are driving. Audiologists usually frown on the use of different aids, unless one is amplifying both ears at once, but several people with complicated high frequency losses enjoy using more than one aid.

Finally, we come to the subject of embarrassment. It is unfortunate that today aids are designed and advertised for their ability to conceal rather than relieve a hearing loss. It is certainly true that a great many people are embarrassed by hearing aids, but there is nothing in history or human nature to indicate that these feelings are deep rooted or permanent. In the 19th and early 20th centuries many people used obvious, ornate ear horns and cornets. Within the past decade, glasses have ceased to bear a stigma and have become fashion accessories. Whatever might be best for you, the important point to remember is that the objective of hearing aids is to improve the way you *hear*. And they help.

Section 24
Emotional and Nervous Disorders

118. New Light On Mental Disturbance

Sigmund Freud once compared the flare-up of a neurosis to an electric light in the ceiling. You can study it for years, he said, and never understand what makes it go on or off until you find the controlling switch on the wall. He went on to say that the problem of the psychiatrist is to find the switch.

Since the time of Freud, psychiatry has flowered into an important specialty in the practice of medicine. Its practitioners are numbered in the tens of thousands in the United States alone, and many millions of people have undergone some form of psychiatric treatment. Yet as the experience and knowledge of the psychiatric profession expand, it has become increasingly clear that along with the successful treatments there are failures. Many people with behavioral problems simply do not respond to psychiatric techniques. The psychiatrist does not always succeed in finding the right switch merely by probing the emotional history of the patient's infancy and early childhood.

It has now been demonstrated clinically that the reason for some of these failures, perhaps for many of them, is that the therapist has been looking for the switch in the wrong place.

If Drugs Affect The Mind, Why Can't Vitamins?

The assumption underlying nearly all of psychiatry and psychoanalysis is that troublesome or deviant behavior is a result of deep emotional problems which the patient does not recognize or understand. There are few exceptions to this general principle. All psychiatrists realize that brain damage and drugs such as LSD can cause mental and behavioral aberrations. And there is a growing realization that schizophrenia, the most severe psychiatric disorder, is profoundly involved with metabolic abnormalities. Everything else is essentially caused by emotional difficulties, psychiatrists claim. In addition, psychiatrists will also tell you that a great many physical symptoms are the result of emotional difficulties, and they will readily undertake to "treat" people suffering from asthma, headaches, dizziness, loss of appetite, rashes, obesity, drug and alcohol addiction, and a host of other conditions, by discussing their emotional problems.

Many physicians find it quite convenient to agree with this point of view, and will quickly refer to a psychiatrist any patient who fails to respond swiftly to prescribed medication. Often a referral is made before any medical treatment is even tried, because the symptoms which the patient has do not fall into a pattern which is named in some medical text. ("Headaches? Cold feet? Can't stand to be in the house? There is no such disease, Mrs. Smith. Your symptoms are *psychosomatic*. Let me refer you to Dr. _____ .")

But now, researchers are reporting that psychiatric patients are very frequently deficient in certain vitamins, especially those which are found in fresh fruits and vegetables, such as folic acid and vitamin C.

Often, it is found that the problem with psychiatric patients, including those labeled "senile," is not simply a vitamin deficiency, but a vitamin *dependency*. In other words, these people, for some poorly understood reason, develop an abnormal need for a certain nutrient. There are numerous reported cases of patients improving only when very large amounts of nutrients are administered regularly. In fact, this is the basis of megavitamin therapy for schizophrenia. Schizophrenics, it has been found, very often require huge amounts of niacin and vitamin C, along with lesser amounts of other nutrients, in order to normalize their brain chemistry.

Out Of Touch With Reality—Or Hard Of Hearing?

There is still more medical evidence that the standard psychiatric approach to mental disease overlooks some basic physical problems. One such problem is impaired hearing. As reported in the *Journal of the American Medical Association* (January 5, 1970), Mr. Dan F. McCoy, chief of the Speech and Hearing Department at Elgin State Hospital in Illinois, discovered that more than 1,700 patients in that institution, or 42 percent of the population, failed a hearing test. The failure rate which could be expected in the general population is only 10 percent. Most of those who failed the test had impacted earwax. Removal of the wax often revealed other problems, such as infection, cysts, and perforated eardrums.

"If you can eliminate even a little hearing loss, or an infection, frequently you will get great changes in behavior," Mr. McCoy said. It's bad enough that the patient cannot hear what the psychiatrist is saying, but imagine the impression on the psychiatrist when the patient seems to be staring into space, or making some inappropriate response. No doubt, he interprets this as just another symptom of mental illness, never suspecting that the poor man or woman just can't hear what he is saying!

And in fact, after treatment by an otologist, more than 50 patients from Elgin improved to the point where they were placed with families outside the hospital.

How Valid Is Psychiatric Practice?

An editorial in the *Journal of the American Medical Association* for March 21, 1964, begins with this statement: "Psychiatry and psychoanalysis today have not lived up to their well-advertised and hoped-for promise. One has only to talk to disappointed patients and confused and frustrated therapists to ascertain this." And no wonder!

In view of all the evidence that every so-called "psychiatric" symptom in the book can be—and often is—produced by factors which have nothing whatever to do with emotions or the patient's childhood, the question arises: just how valid, in medical or scientific terms, is the practice of psychiatry?

Certainly, there seem to be cases of mental disturbance which are caused by emotional factors, shocking experiences, and parental conflict or abuse. But do such cases account for the vast *majority* of psychiatric cases, or only the minority?

Although much remains to be learned about mental illness, at this point in time it seems far more fruitful to assume that mental illness is often physical in nature. A small but growing number of psychiatrists are aware of this.

119. Schizophrenia And Megavitamins

For the mental patient, there is often more relief in vitamin B therapy than in years of psychoanalysis, shock treatment, tranquilizers and institutionalization. Consider the heartbreaking true story of a girl we'll call Joan. Shortly after she graduated from a fashionable girls' college, her parents noticed that she began to do strange things, such as repeating simple motions innumerable times, and endlessly wiping imaginary spots from mirrors. She became troubled by hallucinations of various kinds. A psychiatrist quickly made a diagnosis of schizophrenia, which was confirmed by several other specialists.

Joan was placed in a hospital where she was given a series of electrical shocks and put on heavy doses of tranquilizers. The result of this more or less standard treatment was that she became catatonic, a detached state of virtual immobility and speechlessness. More specialists were called in and her family tried a new hospital. But Joan's condition only deteriorated, until she was totally withdrawn from reality. Over a period of five years, she was in and out of seven hospitals, running up bills of nearly $230,000.

Finally, her parents found their way to a psychiatrist who had been experimenting successfully with treating schizophrenia as a metabolic disorder. His examination revealed that Joan's mental symptoms were the result of chronic pellagra, a niacin deficiency disease caused by malnutrition.

It was discovered that just before she graduated from college, Joan had decided to go on a crash diet, and a doctor had prescribed amphetamines as part of the regimen. She cut down so sharply on food that she was losing 12 pounds a week, with the result that her body was depleted of vital nutrients, including niacin, which is essential to the normal functioning of the brain.

Joan's pellagra and her schizoid symptoms finally disappeared as a result of a carefully supervised diet, fortified with heavy doses of vitamin C, niacin, and other vitamins in the B complex.

But Joan's mind remains scarred by those five nightmare years in mental hospitals.

Joan's family can't help wondering how many other children may have been mistakenly committed to mental hospitals throughout the country. They hate to think that the anguish they had to endure is being repeated. When they confronted the doctors who treated Joan, it was explained that the tendency of amphetamines to produce schizophrenic symptoms was not generally known to the medical profession until very recently.

Help Was Available But Ignored

What the psychiatrists didn't tell Joan's parents is that the link between severe psychiatric symptoms and niacin deficiency was forged 10 years before Joan was born! At that time, in the late 1930's, it was discovered that niacin was the specific cure for pellagra. And one of the chief symptoms of pellagra is mental disturbance, beginning with irritability and sleeplessness and progressing to a "toxic confusional psychosis with symptoms of acute delirium and catatonia" (N. K. Horwitt in *Modern Nutrition in Health and Disease,* Wohl and Goodhart, ed., 1964).

More pointedly, in 1965, the year before Joan became ill, journalist Gregory Stefan published *In Search of Sanity* (University Books), a gripping first-hand account of how he struggled with schizophrenia for four hellish years, during which time he was treated by a dozen of America's top psychoanalysts. Like Joan, he also underwent shock treatments and took powerful tranquilizers. Nothing helped until he heard about a psychiatrist in Canada who had reported success using huge doses of niacin to treat schizophrenia. He began taking this vitamin in large amounts himself, and in short order, his symptoms vanished. For the first time in years, he said, it was no longer "a struggle to get through each day without blowing my brains out."

And as if this wasn't enough to alert the psychiatric world, in 1966, the year that Joan became ill, Drs. Abram Hoffer and Humphrey Osmond first published *How To Live With Schizophrenia* (University Books, Revised Edition, 1974), in which they gave numerous case histories of effective treatments with niacin, and reported on large-scale double-blind confirmation studies. Unfortunately, most psychiatrists throughout the country continued to ignore niacin. One reason, according to Dr. Osmond, was that they refused to admit that a vitamin in massive doses can have therapeutic value.

Today, many people are familiar with the "megavitamin therapy" which Drs. Hoffer and Osmond first began using back in 1952. Dr. Linus Pauling, the brilliant biochemist and winner of two Nobel Prizes, calls it "orthomolecular psychiatry," meaning that the doctor goes about his work by adjusting nutrition so that the right molecules wind up in the right place, permitting the complex chemical reactions within the brain to proceed normally. Hundreds of psychiatrists are now using this approach, most of them reporting that when megavitamin therapy is used along with more conventional therapy, their success rate is *doubled.*

Schizophrenia—A Detective Story

Dr. Abram Hoffer, a psychiatrist from Saskatoon, Canada, does not restrict his treatment to traditional methods such as electroconvulsive shock, tranquilizers and psychoanalysis. Dr. Hoffer pioneered in the use of large doses of niacin (vitamin B_3) or the related compounds nicotinic acid and niacinamide, to treat mental illness.

Dr. Hoffer is convinced that, although schizophrenia manifests itself in psychiatric problems, it is really a disease caused by abnormal body chemistry. Schizophrenia is in this view actually a physical, not a mental, disease.

Dr. Hoffer has several reasons for believing this. First, symptoms can be switched on and off by regulating the drugs or vitamins used. Even if the medication is mixed into the patient's food or drink so that he does not know he is receiving it, the results still occur. This would not be true, of course, if the illness were "all in the patient's head."

Secondly, hallucinatory drugs such as LSD produce effects very similar to the symptoms of schizophrenia. The inference is that another chemical, this one produced in the body, causes "true" schizophrenia.

Third, schizophrenia seems to be hereditary. If an identical twin becomes schizophrenic, there is an 85 percent probability that the other twin will become schizophrenic too, even if they were separated at birth and reared in different families. This eliminates the possibility that the illness is the result of inability to cope with environmental factors, and suggests that it results from an inherited biologic factor.

For these reasons, Dr. Hoffer and his assistant, Dr. Humphrey Osmond, have treated hundreds of schizophrenic patients metabolically with much success. In their book, *How to Live With Schizophrenia*, they outline the details of their megavitamin or orthomolecular therapy. For most patients, Dr. Hoffer prescribes three grams of vitamin B$_3$ and three grams of vitamin C daily. Dosages are increased if necessary. Often this is accompanied by 250 to 1,000 mg. of pyridoxine (vitamin B$_6$) and 100 to 3,000 mg. of thiamine for depression. Vitamin B$_{12}$ and folic acid may also be prescribed in some cases.

Chemical tranquilizers, anti-depressants and other conventional therapies are also used, as needed.

Sleuthing For Chemical Clues

The scientific detective work that led these two researchers to niacin therapy makes a fascinating story. Before going to Saskatchewan in 1951, Dr. Osmond had experimented in London with mescaline. This prime hallucinatory drug, derived from a Mexican cactus plant, has a chemical structure similar to that of adrenalin. While playing back a recording of effects produced by mescaline in a volunteer, a colleague who was a severe asthmatic remarked that sometimes when he took large doses of adrenalin for his asthma, he experienced similar effects—a feeling of unreality and distorted visions. Remembering that the writer Aldous Huxley, after taking mescaline, commented that the schizophrenic is like a man permanently under the influence of mescaline, Osmond and Hoffer picked up the clue. They soon found another. A Canadian physician told them that during the war, for lack of adequate supplies of normal adrenalin, a pinkish kind sometimes had to be used during anesthesia. When patients recovered, they had hallucinations and other disturbances.

Adrenochrome is a chemical derived from adrenalin. When adrenalin decomposes, it may form adrenochrome. Perhaps, they reasoned, adrenochrome is the hallucinogen in pink adrenalin. If so, it might be that under normal circumstances in the body, adrenalin decomposition goes through an adrenochrome stage of brief duration and is then oxidized, but that in schizophrenics the stage might be prolonged because of a metabolic defect. The schizophrenic, they suspected, may not have the necessary body chemicals to dispose of the poison rapidly enough to prevent intoxication and bizarre symptoms.

Osmond became the guinea pig. Ten minutes after taking an injection of adrenochrome, he noticed the ceiling in the laboratory changing color. Outside, he found the corridors "sinister and unfriendly" and was unable to relate distance and time. After a second injection, he reported: "I felt indifferent toward humans and had to curb myself from making unpleasant remarks."

Speculating that inability to metabolize adrenochrome might be the culprit in schizophrenia, the two investigators began a search for some method of treatment. Their search led them to nicotinic acid, a form of vitamin B_3. At that time, nicotinic acid had been used in what was then considered large doses for delirium and also for repression. Did the nicotinic acid neutralize adrenochrome? Would it reduce the production of adrenalin? Would it relieve the frightening symptoms of schizophrenia? It was worth a trial. The results, of course, are now history.

Schizophrenia—'A Genetic Biochemical Disturbance'

Dr. David Hawkins, medical director of the North Nassau Mental Health Center in Manhasset, New York, is a slender, mustached man with twinkling eyes and a gentle voice. He is co-editor with Dr. Linus Pauling of the book, *Orthomolecular Psychiatry: Treatment of Schizophrenia* (W. H. Freeman, 1973). Seated behind his desk in his quiet office at the suburban center, he discussed orthomolecular psychiatry, popularly known as megavitamin therapy.

"Orthomolecular psychiatry regards schizophrenia as a genetic biochemical disturbance. The functioning of the brain is dependent on its composition and structure, on its molecular environment," he explained. "We consider biochemical defects to be primary in causing mental illness and our emphasis is on biochemistry and nutrition. Disturbed family relations and personal conflicts may contribute to the patient's illness, but psychodynamics is not our primary treatment approach. First we treat the psychosis, then we help the patient adjust to life."

Orthomolecular psychiatry believes that mental illness can result from a low concentration in the brain of any of the following vitamins: thiamine, niacin, pyridoxine, B_{12}, biotin, ascorbic acid or folic acid.

But the basic biochemical defect (or defects) that causes mental illness has not yet been determined. "Scientists are working on it," said Dr. Hawkins. "Maybe we'll have the answer in 10 or 20 years. Orthomolecular psychiatry is pragmatic, empirical. The point is, it works."

"We haven't discovered why it works, but we have clinical proof that it *does* work. Orthomolecular psychiatry is a promising branch of medicine, and the public is making the decision in its favor," said Dr. Hawkins.

No less an authority than Nobel Laureate Dr. Linus Pauling has been impressed by these results. "I feel that it is the duty of every psychiatrist to add megavitamin therapy to his armamentarium," he stated in *Schizophrenia,* Second Quarter, 1971.

Noting that we have in our bodies a blood-brain barrier designed to keep undesirable molecules and contaminants out of the brain, he suggested, "This barrier may also sometimes operate to keep good molecules out of the brain. I have thought that it might well be that the value of megavitamin therapy for some patients is the result of their having a blood-brain barrier that is operating too efficiently, in such a way that even though in the peripheral tissues the concentration of vitamins may be essentially optimal, there could still be a local avitaminosis in the brain itself."

A Life-Long Illness Brought Under Control

Jerry Witt (not his real name) is a personable young man of 27 whose psychosis has been arrested but who continues to see Dr. Hawkins weekly for psychotherapy. He had a turbulent history of mental illness which manifested itself in early childhood with nightmares, hyperactivity and hypersensitivity to sound. Always bright, he was at the top of his class without effort until he reached sixth grade. Then he retrogressed and couldn't concentrate on his studies.

"I began to have hallucinations—the Japs were always attacking me. . . . My family spent a fortune to try to help me. For years I saw psychiatrists three times a week, while I was going in and out of different private schools. . . . I was 17 when I became involved in drugs and I would just kind of disappear for weeks at a time," Jerry says.

No psychiatrist ever told his parents that he was schizophrenic, but they always believed his illness was biochemical rather than psychogenic, since their other two children functioned well.

Then Jerry's mother heard about orthomolecular psychiatry through her rabbi and after a violent episode, Jerry was admitted to Brunswick Hospital under Dr. Hawkins' care. Megavitamin therapy was initiated and Jerry was put on a high-protein, low-carbohydrate diet. When he returned home after two months, he showed considerable improvement. He got himself a job and stayed away from drugs. However, his illness is of long standing and Jerry has deep-rooted psychological problems. While the schizophrenia is definitely under control, he still finds concentration difficult.

Is the chronic patient more difficult to help? Yes, says Dr. Hawkins. A patient who has been withdrawn for years will acquire bad habit patterns and superimposed disabilities. When the disease is caught early, the response is better.

From Visions Of Terror To A Bright Future

Lilly is an example of a schizophrenic who took ill suddenly, began orthomolecular treatment within a year and made a dramatic recovery. Lilly, an attractive young lady with cascading dark hair and shining eyes, is now 31 years old and single.

"About six years ago," she said, "I had a romantic breakup. It broke me up, too, and I went into a deep depression. . . . Then I began to have hallucinations. Things would seem to blow up in front of me and change colors. A white man would become black. Eerie voices were stalking me. I tried not to pay attention, but it got to the point where I couldn't concentrate, and I finally lost my job as a secretary.

"That was it . . . I panicked," said Lilly. "I went to a psychiatrist for a couple of months, but psychotherapy and tranquilizers didn't help. I was so miserable, I left home. When I came back, my mother told me about megavitamin therapy and begged me to try it. She had read about it in a newspaper article."

Soon Lilly had an appointment at the clinic. Dr. Hawkins asked no psychological questions about her childhood or family. After a series of tests, he prescribed huge daily doses of vitamins B_3, B_6, C and B_1, plus the high-protein, low-carbohydrate diet. In two weeks, her hallucinations ended.

Lilly went back to work and found "the best job I ever had." She appears confident and well integrated. She sees Dr. Hawkins only twice a year. Lilly realizes she must live with her problem all her life—like an obese person or a diabetic. She has never skipped her vitamins, but when she goes off her diet, she becomes "nauseous and headachy."

Test Scores Reflect Improvement

One fascinating study which not too many people are familiar with was reported by Drs. George Watson and W. D. Currier in the *Journal of Psychology* (49, 1960). This study is unusual in several respects. First, it involved the use of placebo pills along with vitamin pills. Estimation of improvement was not left solely to clinical observation, but was also gauged by the standard psychological test known as the Minnesota Multiphasic Personality Inventory (MMPI). Also, the amounts of vitamins given were much smaller than those usually administered to psychiatric patients. Whereas Dr. Hoffer usually begins with a niacin dose of at least three grams a day, and sometimes five or 10 times this much, Watson and Currier used a little less than one gram a day, but along with 31 other vitamins and minerals in generous amounts. *The entire B complex was used in this formula,* including thiamine, riboflavin, pyridoxine, B_{12}, folic acid, pantothenate, inositol, and choline, along with the niacin.

The patients, consisting of 30 unhospitalized emotionally disturbed subjects, were first given placebos or dummy pills. Seven improved, six got worse, and seventeen showed no change. Their average reduction in total test scores on the MMPI (the higher the score, the more serious the mental disturbance) was only 4.4 points, which is not considered significant (average total score was about 220 points).

When the vitamin supplements were substituted for the placebos without the knowledge of the patients, and administered for the same length of time, 22 subjects improved, two became worse, and six were unchanged. Average reduction in the MMPI score was 17.13 points. This was considered a significant improvement. And when vitamin therapy was continued for a longer period, success was even more impressive: 24 were improved, five unchanged and only one worse. Average reduction in MMPI score was 26.77 points, considered highly significant.

One of the subjects was a 29-year-old man who had a history of progressively increasing illness over a 12-year period. He had gone the usual route of analysis and tranquilizers, but nothing seemed to help his paranoid schizophrenia. In his first interview with the investigators, he said that his behavior was "controlled by a machine in outer space. Sometimes the machine holds me down in the bed and won't let me get up." He also reported that there was a voice in his head that talked constantly. To make matters worse, he reported continuous pain in his bowels, stomach, legs, and a throbbing in his head. His score on the MMPI at this time was 253.

After two months on the experimental vitamin tablets, he told the doctor: "The machine is me. Looking back, I didn't recognize it before. This thing has to be in my own head—it couldn't possibly be outside." After several more months he stated: "I've felt better this month than I have for a long time. The pains all over have diminished. I have not been awake at night like I used to be." And while "the voice" used to keep him awake for hours when he went to bed, he now reported that he fell asleep within 15 minutes. His mother reported that her son was now "beginning to act like he did before becoming ill," and that he had "gone to the library for the first time in several years and was studying physics." After two years of treatment, his MMPI score had dropped by 76 points. While he was not considered to have fully recovered, he had certainly made impressive improvement.

A Month Of Vitamins Ends Years Of Illness

Another case was that of a 47-year-old woman who had been under psychiatric care for several years and had been taking a variety of tranquilizers. When first seen, she told the doctors that during the acute periods of her illness, "I felt I had two minds." Her husband was the cause of this condition, she believed. It was learned that her two sisters also suffered from mental illness.

After only a month of taking the B complex-rich vitamin supplements, she reported: "I am better, much better. I feel better than I've felt in seven or eight years. I never expected to feel this good again." Her score on the MMPI dropped 35 points. Seven months later, her MMPI score was a normal 163, and she told the doctors: "I'm fine, wonderful. My husband is fine. I can never understand how one person can interrupt a home life like I did."

A Vitamin Dependency

Watson and Currier make this final observation: "These studies indicate that some states which are psychologically diagnosed as functional mental illness, and at the same time are not accompanied by clinical evidence of nutritional deficit, *apparently involve unsuspected nutritional deficiencies, and may be helped by appropriate nutritional therapy.*"

This is a crucial point. Generally speaking, we can distinguish between two different kinds of vitamin deficiency. The most common kind of deficiency is simply failure to eat (or sometimes, absorb) a "normal" amount of the vitamin. This amount can vary from individual to individual, but the variance is usually in the realm of requiring two or three times the amount that someone else requires for good health.

The second kind of deficiency involves a pronounced

biochemical abnormality, and may require hundreds or even a thousand times the usual amount of one or more vitamins for normalization. It is really a *dependency,* rather than a deficiency. This is not to say that the individual is actually using this amount of vitamins in the normal way. In some cases, the extra amounts are required so that a faulty utilization mechanism can simply latch on to the amount it needs. It is something like pitching a thousand balls at a very clumsy batter so that he can successfully hit at least one.

In other cases, huge amounts of vitamins are needed in order to block a biochemical reaction which is producing toxic products, such as adrenochrome.

Full Range Of B Complex Works Best

Niacin is the backbone of megavitamin therapy, but the related B vitamins are essential to success. Child psychiatrist Dr. Allan Cott made this clear in an article in the journal *Schizophrenia* in 1971 (3; 2). Dr. Cott writes that over a period of five years he treated 500 children afflicted with childhood psychoses, hyperactivity, and brain injury with the orthomolecular approach and found this treatment to show much greater promise than any other which has been tried. He notes that his results are being "duplicated by many physicians and clinics, by the Institute for Child Behavior Research and the New York Institute for Child Development." As for the vitamins which he uses, he states: "In those cases in which positive results have been obtained, treatment included niacinamide or niacin, ascorbic acid, pyridoxine and calcium pantothenate used in massive doses." He adds that he also frequently uses riboflavin, thiamine, vitamin E and folic acid. *Five of these substances, besides the niacin, are members of the B complex family.*

Dr. Cott points out that pyridoxine, or B_6, is involved in five different inborn vitamin dependency conditions. "Many parents and physicians reported significant changes in psychiatric cases when only pyridoxine was used in massive doses," he says.

Many investigators have reported success using pyridoxine as an anticonvulsant both for infants and adult epileptics. Dr. David Coursin reported in a 1954 issue of the *Journal of the American Medical Association* that he gave a dosage of 100 mg. of pyridoxine intramuscularly to 100 patients with various illnesses relating to the central nervous system, with excellent results, especially in patients with brain disorders.

Thiamine, or vitamin B_1, has long been known to be essential to a healthy nervous system. As early as 1939, it was shown that patients deprived of thiamine become confused, irritable, depressed, and fearful of impending disaster. Dr. Tom Spies in 1943, in the *Association for Research on Nervous Disorders* (Vol. 22, p. 122), told of 115 patients eating a diet low in thiamine. They became timid and depressed, but within 30 minutes to 20 hours after receiving supplementary vitamin B_1 they became pleasant and cooperative.

Dr. Cott did not mention vitamin B_{12} as among those which he administers, possibly because the young children he deals with have no great need for it. Older persons, however, are often in dire need of B_{12} supplementation, as we'll see in a later chapter.

We Have Come A Long Way

Our present knowledge of psychiatric disorders and how they can be ameliorated by dietary means might be compared to the degree of understanding of physical illness and vitamins which existed several hundred years ago, when it was first discovered that scurvy could be cured by drinking the juice of lemons or limes. Psychiatric disorders are far more complicated than simple scurvy, but we at least know that niacin and all the related B complex factors (along with megadoses of vitamin C) somehow bring about relief. How these vitamins do their work is not yet fully understood. Yet, this must not deter us from appreciating their effectiveness.

Schizophrenia remains the single most common cause of hospitalization in the United States. So we are fortunate indeed that we have come as far as we have. It is a great day in medical history when Dr. Cott can report that one of his young patients who had multiple daily seizures for two years became seizure-free after only three days of megavitamin treatment, and remains seizure-free four years later!

And we know we have come a long way indeed when Dr. Hawkins can report that after the adoption of orthomolecular methods, the number of yearly visits required per patient dropped from 150 to just 15! (*Orthomolecular Psychiatry: Treatment of Schizophrenia*, edited by David Hawkins and Linus Pauling, Freeman and Company, 1972). Dr. Hawkins further states that by adding megavitamin treatment to other techniques used at the clinic, he has been able to *double* the recovery rate, halve the hospitalization rate, and virtually eliminate suicide among a group of patients whose suicide rate is ordinarily 22 times that of the general population!

A Physician Must Guide Therapy

Megavitamin therapy is not something that you can do yourself. It must be carried out under the direction of a qualified medical psychiatrist. In most cases, these psychiatrists use megavitamin therapy along with other modalities. In addition, the vitamins and the amounts used are generally custom-tailored to the individual. Shock treatment has multiple biochemical effects and, supported by megavitamins, the improvement can be dramatic. Hormones, antidepressants, and tranquilizers are used when necessary. Phenothiazines (tranquilizers) are often prescribed, but quickly reduced to maintenance level.

Psychotherapy is not ignored. Emotional upsets affect the brain chemistry which will aggravate the biochemical problem. While the patient is psychotic, psychotherapy is merely supportive. When the patient is no longer plagued by perceptual distortions, the orthomolecular psychiatrist will help him resolve his personal problems.

No serious side effects from megavitamin therapy have been reported, but large doses of niacin can sometimes cause a "flushing" syndrome. This is usually controlled by temporarily switching from niacin to niacinamide. In any case, therapy must be carried out under the watchful eye of an experienced doctor.

It is worth remembering, though, that good nutrition, particularly with respect to the B vitamins, is essential to *everyone's* mental health.

120. Megavitamins For Disturbed Children

Megavitamin therapy is also being used successfully in treating childhood schizophrenia, a developmental abnormality that seriously interferes with a child's functioning in all areas of his life. In the past, psychotherapy was the most common treatment and its results were questionable. The use of drugs altered the behavior disorders by sedating or tranquilizing the child, but the effect was merely stop-gap. With megavitamin therapy, the improvement in children is even more impressive than in adults. Children whose treatment begins between three and nine years of age have a fine chance of recovery.

Dannie's Doing Fine Now

Dannie, an alert 12-year-old who wants to be a dentist, is a schizophrenic who has made a remarkable recovery on megavitamins. Though he always had a sleeping problem, was shy, uncoordinated and would sometimes talk to himself, his parents chalked up his increasingly erratic behavior to the stress of moving into a new neighborhood. They never thought there was anything wrong with him—just the usual problems of growing up. However, when he was eight years old and in the second grade, his teacher noted the discrepancy between his obvious intelligence and his low I.Q. score. He was subnormal in abstract thinking.

"On the advice of the school psychologist, we consulted a pediatric psychiatrist, who suggested psychotherapy and said that a long-term treatment would probably be necessary," said Dannie's mother, a nurse. "We turned it down.

"Then we read a newspaper article about the North Nassau Clinic, and we took Dannie there. He was immediately put on vitamins, and we noticed an improvement within a month.

"Dannie is now outgoing and relaxed," his mother continued. "He's developed a sense of humor and appears to be well accepted by his classmates. He rides a two-wheeler like the other kids on the block and, best of all, his report card is sprinkled with

A's. Right now, he is taking vitamins C, B$_6$, and nicotinamide."
How often does he see the doctor? "About nine times a year."

Disturbed Children Need Niacin

According to Dr. Abram Hoffer, whose highly successful orthomolecular therapy for schizophrenics was described in the
previous chapter, both the "problem" child who fails to do well
in school and the schizophrenic confined to an asylum are
victims of vitamin B$_3$ (niacin) deficiency. In effect, they are
suffering from a form of pellagra; their illnesses are different *in
degree only.*

In 1968, Dr. Hoffer decided to try treating antisocial, disturbed
youngsters with large doses of niacin and ascorbic acid (vitamin
C). As he reports in the journal *Schizophrenia* (Second Quarter,
1971), the majority of children recovered with such therapy.

One 9-year-old boy, Peter, had suddenly become hostile,
irritable and fearful about a month before seeing Dr. Hoffer. He
complained of visions and other perceptual illusions. He was
even afraid to take a bath for fear he might drown himself.

Peter was given 1.5 grams of nicotinamide (a form of niacin)
and ascorbic acid daily. Here is Dr. Hoffer's own description of
the results: "After one month he was slightly better. After the
third month he was even better . . . His performance in school
had improved substantially. . . After seven months he was
normal."

Twenty-four of 38 children recovered while taking niacin,
relapsed within a month when a placebo (sugar pill) was
substituted, and then recovered again when the vitamin therapy
was renewed.

Improvement was achieved *without* the benefit of any traditional psychotherapy whatsoever; he relied on from three to
twelve grams of niacin and three grams of vitamin C daily. "In
every case good nutrition was emphasized," he added.

How dramatic was the children's recovery? "I should emphasize that by 'well' or 'recovered,' I mean they are free of
symptoms and signs, are performing well in school, getting on
well with their families and with the community," Dr. Hoffer
reported.

After 24 such successes, Dr. Hoffer became convinced that
many mentally disturbed children are simply vitamin B$_3$ dependent. "In principle," he says "it is the same as labeling every
person who recovers on vitamin doses of vitamin B$_3$ as having
suffered from pellagra or subclinical pellagra."

Pellagra Symptoms Have Been Forgotten

Why haven't other psychiatrists and psychologists recognized the startling similarities between the ailments? "Unfortunately, psychiatrists are no longer familiar with the clinical manifestations of pellagra," Dr. Hoffer says. "When the older literature is examined, it is clear that the best model of schizophrenia is pellagra. It is so good that for many years psychiatrists in mental hospitals could not distinguish between them.... long before pellagrins became psychotic they suffered from tension, depression, personality problems, fatigue ...." In other words, subclinical pellagra could easily be mistaken for mental illness.

Just how thin is the line that divides the "disturbed" child from the pellagrin, and the pellagrin from the schizophrenic? "It is entirely quantitative," says Dr. Hoffer. "Pellagrins require vitamin doses and schizophrenics require megavitamin doses. But even this distinction is not absolute.... There is thus a quantitative continuum from pellagrins who fail to ingest vitamin doses of vitamin B_3, say 50 mg. per day or less, to chronic pellagrins who require up to one gram per day, to acute schizophrenics whose needs are three to six grams per day.

"The group who require 50 mg. per day or less will develop pellagra if their diet is deficient. The group requiring over one gram per day will develop schizophrenia since no modern diet will provide this amount of vitamin B_3."

Dr. Hoffer believes that the "disturbed child syndrome," like schizophrenia, runs in families. "My data shows that vitamin B_3 dependency is inherited," he said. "In more than 100 families that I have examined in the past 10 years, I find that if one parent is vitamin B_3 dependent, one quarter of the children also will be. If both parents are vitamin B_3 dependent, one will expect more than three quarters of the children also to be vitamin B_3 dependent. There has been no generation gap."

121. Fasting Can Control Schizophrenia

While Americans have been learning to correct abnormal metabolism by administering vitamins, a Russian scientist has pursued a different path and also obtained good results.

The Soviet treatment for schizophrenia—controlled fasting—which has improved 64 percent of the patients treated, was reported by psychiatrist Allan Cott, M.D., in the publication *Schizophrenia* (First Quarter, 1971). His findings are particularly significant in that they are the result of a trip to the Soviet Union to see the Russian physician, Dr. Uri Nickolayev, who has been using and refining this technique through 23 years of research and clinical experience.

According to Dr. Cott's report, the fasting therapy requires that the patients, who usually volunteer for the treatment, stop eating solid foods for 20 to 30 days. However, the fasting is done under close medical supervision. Patients can drink as much water as they want, but no less than a quart a day. Exercises, including outdoor walks and breathing exercises are an essential part of the treatment, and must be performed for a minimum of three hours every day. Baths, showers, enemas and massages round out the daily regimen.

The typical patient, after 28 days of fasting, loses 15 to 16 percent of his starting weight, but is not starved. Far from it. Instead, his skin color and muscle tone improve. Most important, though, his mental outlook changes remarkably for the better.

A 22-year-old male patient told Dr. Cott, through a translator, what it's like to undergo the controlled fasting therapy. This man, who had first shown schizophrenic tendencies when he was 14 years old, described how he felt before, during and after the treatment.

"I felt full of apathy," he said. "I was not concentrated and when reading, I had to read a line over and over. When I spoke to people, I couldn't remember what I said. I felt a complete weakness in my muscles. When I was punished by being isolated when I was in the Army, I refused to eat for three days and found that I felt better. I then decided to fast or eat very little. I read about the fasting treatment in *Science and Life Magazine* and applied to Professor Nickolayev for treatment after my discharge from the Army.

"From the first to the fifth day I had headaches. On the fifth day my feelings of tension left and a feeling of indifference appeared. My feelings changed rapidly until the 18th day. On the 19th day I became restless and had to pace around the room. On the 20th day I felt that something changed . . . inside, and that there was something in my head and it had to come out. After that I felt better.

"I Felt Joy For The First Time . . ."

"On the 21st day I felt like I was covered with a sack. By the twenty-second day I began to feel better. I felt the sun, the air, the forest and I no longer felt alienated. The next day I felt like exploding and all my hostile feelings returned. The doctors felt that the return of these feelings was an indication that the fast should be stopped. The fast was terminated on the twenty-seventh day, but I had a very poor appetite. My appetite gradually improved and my spirits improved. I felt joy for the first time in a long while."

Progress throughout the treatment is measured as the patient passes through six stages, three during the fasting period and three more in the "recovery period," during which he begins to eat again. The first three stages of treatment are marked by the patient's initial hunger and excitability, followed by loss of appetite and diminished reflexes until, according to Dr. Cott, "after a period of depression, the physical and mental condition of the patient suddenly improves; he feels stronger and is in a better mood. This marks the beginning of Stage III . . . During this stage the tongue gradually loses its white coating, the odor of acetone (from his breath) disappears, the patient's complexion improves and psychotic symptoms recede." By the time the patient reaches the end of the third stage, his internal biochemistry has leveled out and his appetite is restored.

Professor Nickolayev describes the mode of action of the therapy as follows:

1. While leading to acute exhaustion, fasting serves as a powerful stimulus to subsequent recuperation.

2. Fasting ensures rest of the digestive tract and the structures

of the central nervous system. This rest helps to normalize function.

3. Acidosis provoked by fasting and its compensation reflects a mobilization of detoxifying defense mechanisms which probably play an important role in the neutralization of toxins associated with the schizophrenic process. As the acidosis decreases, the blood sugar level rises. The pH of the blood remains constant after acidosis decreases. Other parameters of the blood continue to remain constant. Insulin levels become normal. The biochemical dynamics during fasting are the same for mental illness and for normals.

Low Protein Diet During Recovery

During the recovery period, as the patient begins to eat again, he is kept in the hospital for as many days as he had fasted. Starting out with fruit juice mixed with water and taken by spoon, the patient gradually adds salt-free fruits, vegetables and milk to his diet, adding cottage cheese, brown bread, honey and a porridge of grits towards the end of the week.

However, meat, eggs and fish are not allowed, and meat may not be eaten for at least six months. Even then, only very little is allowed. One of the reasons for this particular restriction is that schizophrenics have more protein in their bodies than average persons. After the fast brings the protein level down to normal, a rise in it would probably cause a relapse.

As the patient begins the first week of the recovery period, he is again irritable and lacks strength. Next, he becomes easily excited, and finally, as he enters Stage III of the recovery period, he becomes normal again and steadily improves physically and mentally.

Patients report that hunger subsides by the second or third day after they stop eating, and appetite disappears by the fifth day. Dr. Cott says that, "Many patients request that their fasting period be extended to insure the permanence of their improved state." The voluntary treatment ends if the patient decides to break the fast.

Dr. Nickolayev has found more than 64 percent of the schizophrenics treated to be helped by this therapy. After their release, patients eat a restricted diet or else suffer a relapse. When a patient leaves the hospital, he is advised to fast for from three to five days, but not more than a total of ten, at various times throughout the month. The patient knows when to stop fasting, for that is when he regains his appetite, his tongue becomes clean and symptoms disappear.

The report of such a simple, drugless and apparently quite effective treatment for schizophrenia is little short of sensational. Now Americans who suffer from schizophrenia may receive the benefit of this new kind of therapy, thanks to Dr. Cott's report about the Russian treatment. And his willingness to investigate a method of healing practiced in a different part of the globe is highly significant.

All too often medical advances suffer from the closed minds of practicing doctors who shut out any indication that the way they have been practicing may not be the very best way. Because of this, many people suffer needlessly from their doctors' self-imposed ignorance of up-to-date medical findings.

Will Combined Therapies Work Even Better?

Fortunately, Dr. Cott, who has successfully treated hundreds of mentally disturbed children with large doses of vitamins, has not fallen so utterly in love with his own chosen method as to be blind to the merits of any other. Dr. Cott believes that the Russian approach may also prove valuable to his patients. Therefore, he and his associates are trying fasting therapy whenever orthomolecular treatment proves unsuccessful, adding megavitamins to the fruit and vegetable diet prescribed for the recovery after fasting.

As we have seen, the controlled fasting therapy is also a means to allow a patient's biochemical imbalance to return to normal. This would lead us to believe that a combination of two methods, each aimed at producing the same result, would be a desirable amalgamation.

This international exchange of medical knowledge and experience which resulted in the disclosure of the highly successful Soviet controlled fasting therapy gives American doctors a new means of treating the dreadful disease of schizophrenia. But Dr. Cott's trip has also left its mark on Russian soil.

He reports that Professor Nickolayev has since written to inform him that he will administer high doses of megavitamins during the recovery stages immediately following the fast, and also when the patient resumes a full diet of fruit and vegetables. Dr. Cott added, "He feels that with the addition of the megavitamins to his fasting therapy his unit can improve the results in those patients who are not helped fully by the fast."

122. Reaching The Autistic Child

The autistic child does not respond to his environment. If he is autistic from infancy, he does not learn to talk. If autism develops later, he simply stops talking. He does not respond to others, and seems not to see or hear them. He is completely withdrawn.

This personality disease of children has proved so untreatable that it has caused much despair in medical circles. But at a conference of the Canadian Schizophrenic Foundation held in Toronto in May, 1973, Dr. Bernard Rimland unveiled a remarkably successful treatment.

Dr. Rimland, a research psychologist from San Diego, told the Toronto meeting a compelling story of the results of high vitamin dosages with a group of such children. Dr. Rimland's experience with megavitamins goes back to 1965 when Drs. Osmond and Hoffer were interviewed by a *New York Times* reporter whose story described the results they were getting in successfully treating adult schizophrenics with massive doses of vitamins. A number of parents with autistic children read the article and in desperation decided to try the vitamins on their own. In most instances they had tried psychotherapy which proved to be totally useless.

Home Treatment Sometimes Worked

"Shortly after this," said Dr. Rimland, "I began to get letters from parents describing the results of these experiments they had tried. The *Times* article was not explicit enough to tell the parents what kinds of vitamins to use and what dosages, so there was quite a variation in vitamins and dosages. As I read these reports it became evident that some children had shown remarkable improvement on the vitamins. The parents were reporting good results when the vitamins were taken and a resumption of symptoms when they were stopped."

This sparked Dr. Rimland's interest and he decided to make a survey of all parents on his mailing list at the Institute for Child

Emotional And Nervous Disorders

Behavior Research. About 60 parents responded and Rimland found that there were four vitamins that were outstanding in their positive effects. These were niacinamide (B_3), pantothenic acid, B_6 and vitamin C. As the megavitamin proponents steadily emphasize, vitamin C and the B vitamins are water-soluble and there is no danger of overdose because the body simply throws off what it doesn't use.

On the basis of these reports, Rimland and his staff designed a special vitamin formula and then enrolled about 300 children in a nationwide study. They required that any child taking part had to be under medical supervision, and this created some difficulty because most physicians turned out to be anything but eager to have anything to do with the vitamin therapy program.

Rimland said, "One family with two autistic children said their doctor was adamant in his refusal to let us enroll their two children in the study. This doctor was so determined not to be taken in that he wrote Nobel Laureate Linus Pauling, who had offered to respond with a personal letter to any physician asking about the validity and safety of our study. When the doctor got a personal reply from Dr. Pauling, he reluctantly agreed to let the children take part. It turned out that the two children improved so much that the doctor wrote us a letter asking if the family's three other children could be enrolled in the same study to see if their learning disabilities would improve. It was interesting to see this extremely skeptical physician change his mind this way."

The study was designed so that the children were on the vitamins for a three month period and then off for one month to see if there was a deterioration. Then treatment was resumed for a short time to see if their behavior would again improve. Depending on the child's weight, dosages were one, two or three grams a day of vitamin C, the same amount of niacinamide, 150-450 mg. of B_6 and 200 mg. of pantothenic acid, plus a high potency multiple B vitamin tablet.

Both parents and physicians were asked to complete a form periodically, giving their observations on the child's improvements relating to speech, alertness, sleeping and eating habits, tantrums and other kinds of behavior. Before beginning the study, each of the parents had completed a detailed form on the child's birth history and medical background and this information was recorded on a computer tape. Dr. Rimland then turned the computer tape over to several university computer centers and asked them to apply a new type of data analysis called computer cluster analysis. This is designed to learn if there are certain subgroups among these autistic children and sort each subgroup into a special cluster. In some instances there is a genetic vitamin dependency. An improvement in these children can be predicted. In other cases there might be destruction of brain tissue from a viral infection. These children would not improve with the vitamins.

Results Judged Independently

After Dr. Rimland and his staff assembled all the information, they gave it to three judges who independently examined the data to decide whether each child had improved or not on a scale from 99 to 0. In cases where the judges did not agree, the case was discarded. In cases where the judges were sure the child had improved a great deal, the child got a score of 99. If the improvement was not spectacular, he got an 80. Where there was probable improvement, he might get a 40. A zero meant the child not only had not improved but had actually deteriorated.

After the computer clustering had been completed and the scores assigned, the results showed that well over 50 percent of the children improved significantly and about three percent got worse on the vitamins. Most important from the scientific standpoint, the children differentiated by the clusters responded differently to the vitamins. "In each case," said Dr. Rimland, "these were primarily the evaluations of the parents who were observing the children every day." Improvement showed in reduced tantrums, increased alertness, improved speech, better sleep patterns, greater sociability.

One mother wrote, "We are on the 31st day of the vitamin study and I want to discuss the changes that took place these last three days. I am too excited about it to wait for the next period. For the past two days Susan has been doing a lot of talking, initiating conversations, asking questions, commenting on everything she hears around her."

At Dr. Rimland's suggestion, some of the parents who had not seen significant changes during the study were asked to double the dosage of B_6. One mother who did so wrote: "Now this has made a difference. She is very eager to do things . . . at slight suggestion ready for almost anything. Eager to play basketball in front of the house. Hasn't printed her name or numbers for over a year, but doing it now. I can't emphasize enough that she has refused to do anything these past months. Even my husband who is a disbeliever says she has improved these past four days."

Another parent said, "Elsie has been on the doubled B_6 and has shown great improvement . . . she is sharper and more aware of the outside world . . . we lit our Chanukah candles and she surprised us all by singing a Chanukah song from beginning to end."

In this connection Dr. Rimland said, "It is my feeling that of these vitamins for children, B_6 will be found to be the most important. Some of the children respond very well to niacin or niacinamide but in the most dramatic results we've seen, particularly the classical cases of autism, they have proven to be B_6 responsive."

On the other hand, when the vitamins were stopped, a parent wrote after ten days of no treatment: "William seems to have withdrawn into himself, no longer exhibiting the lively interest in the world around him that had marked the previous month. His newfound willingness to cooperate and obey such directions as he understood disappeared rapidly. His old repertoire of mannerisms and bizarre hand motions and positions, which had been waning, reasserted itself with a vengeance."

The three percent of the children in the study who got worse became irritable and difficult to manage. They were extremely sensitive to sound and would cover their ears when there was a loud or shrill noise. In some of this group bed-wetting returned. These problems were so severe that many were taken off the vitamins when the parents could no longer tolerate the behavior.

Dr. Rimland approached a number of medical people to see if they could find an answer to the problem, but without success. During this period he got a call from nutritionist Adelle Davis, who had served as a consultant in the design of the study. She asked what nutrients they were using. When Dr. Rimland told her, she said, "Well, how about the magnesium?"

Dr. Rimland recalled, "I laughed in a guilty and embarrassed way because I knew she had recommended magnesium and said, 'Adelle, I decided not to use magnesium because we already had a whole handful of pills and we couldn't ask that another five or so pills be added to that. Besides, we weren't convinced that the magnesium was that important.' "

She said, "You're going to have problems."

"What kinds of problems?" Dr. Rimland asked.

"Bed-wetting, sound sensitivity and irritability," replied Adelle Davis.

"She hit right on the button just exactly what was happening with a segment of our study group," said Dr. Rimland. "This results because when you give B_6 in large quantities it interacts with magnesium in such a way that magnesium is taken out of other body systems. So, if the child happens to be marginal in the amount of magnesium the body stores, then B_6 takes essential magnesium and you have a magnesium-deficient child. We immediately informed the parents whose children had developed these side effects to add magnesium and they reported that the side effects went away, in some cases overnight."

There are also failures, of course. Not all behavior problems stem from vitamin dependency. There are diseases that affect the brain. Allergy should probably be investigated as a possibility.

Yet many autistic and otherwise disturbed children have responded to nutritional therapy, and that is remarkable for a disease that for decades has not responded at all to dozens of attempted treatments. More doctors should learn about it. There are autistic children everywhere, but few doctors who have even an inkling of what to do for them.

123. Psychosis, Or Vitamin B$_{12}$ Deficiency?

Medical literature abounds with articles by physicians and psychiatrists explaining how individual nutrients or groups of them have proven highly successful in restoring mental health, often in very severe cases. B$_{12}$ is a good example of a vitamin which has repeatedly been shown to have amazing therapeutic effects. A report in the June 27, 1959, *Journal of the American Medical Association* related the case of a 44-year-old housewife who was admitted to a mental hospital on a diagnosis of severe mental breakdown. She had hallucinations and delusions. Intramuscular injection of vitamin B$_{12}$ quickly restored mental balance.

Note that this report was published in 1959. Since then, many other reports in major medical journals concerning the efficacy of B$_{12}$ have been published. One might think that this would be enough to alert psychiatrists to at least try B$_{12}$ therapy in all cases of mental breakdown. But this is far from being the case. The *Medical Journal of Australia* (Nov. 11, 1972) carried a communication by Dr. Douglas Vann concerning an 84-year-old woman who was languishing in a geriatric ward of a hospital. Her condition was "grossly psychotic and demented." Dr. Vann then gave her intramuscular injections of B$_{12}$ plus the related B vitamin, folic acid. "The response was an unexpectedly rapid return to intellectual and behavioral normality, but with almost complete amnesia for the period of psychosis and dementia," Dr. Vann says.

Drs. Smith and Oliver related in the *British Medical Journal* of July 1, 1967, the story of a woman who apparently was well nourished, but depressed. Four days after entering the hospital, she became confused, had delusions and hallucinations, and could only be kept in the hospital while tranquilized. She was given injections of vitamin B$_{12}$, and within 24 hours her mental condition started improving, and within a few days her mental symptoms were normal.

Deficiency Damages The Brain

The New York *Herald Tribune* on February 17, 1959, quoted the highly respected Dr.Victor Herbert of New York's Mount Sinai Hospital as placing the blame for many patients being committed to mental hospitals on brain damage resulting from a lack of B_{12}. However, the mental changes which may occur as a result of such a deficiency are quite difficult to diagnose because the symptoms so closely resemble those of authentic mental illness.

The *British Medical Journal* of March 26, 1966, stated editorially: "It is true that vitamin B_{12} deficiency may cause severe psychotic symptoms which may vary in severity from mild disorders of mood, mental slowness, and memory defect to severe psychotic symptoms including agitation, depression, severe confusional and hallucinatory states, and paranoid behavior. Occasionally, these mental disturbances may be the first manifestations of B_{12} deficiency ..."

A dramatic instance of how vitamin B_{12} alone can sometimes help in psychiatric disorders was described by Dr. H. L. Newbold, writing in *Orthomolecular Psychiatry* (1; 1, 1972). The patient was a 33-year-old Ph.D. candidate who had suffered a psychotic breakdown two years before Dr. Newbold saw him. At that time, he was completely out of touch with reality, felt a kind of snapping sensation in his head, and perceived space as being greatly foreshortened, which made him feel like a midget. He was hospitalized and given tranquilizers, which controlled the worst of his symptoms, but he still felt very lethargic, lonely, and insecure, and work on his Ph.D. thesis was impossible. He underwent psychoanalysis, but it failed to help him very much.

Chemical analysis showed that his serum level of B_{12} was very low. Following two injections of hydroxocobalamin, a form of B_{12} which can only be given by injection, the patient "spoke of a remarkable improvement of his condition. At that time his memory was much improved and he found that he was learning well. He was participating in class activities, and for the first time in two years, was hard at work writing his Ph.D. thesis." During the next five months, the patient maintained an excellent level of improvement. There were only two exceptions, Dr. Newbold says. They occurred when it was attempted to give injections only once every 10 days, instead of twice weekly. The result was that the patient quickly became tired and depressed. Apparently, he was not suffering from a simple deficiency, but rather a kind of *dependency* state.

Nerve Destruction Comes First, Then Anemia

Pernicious anemia is the symptom most closely associated with B_{12} deficiency. But the mental damage caused by a lack of this nutrient may occur quite some time before anemia develops, according to a study by Dr. Oded Abramsky, a member of the Neurology Department of Hadassah University Hospital and Hebrew University Hadassah Medical School in Jerusalem, Israel. And the results can be devastating—and irreversible.

Writing in the *Journal of the American Geriatrics Society* (February 1972), Dr. Abramsky describes the cases of three B_{12}-deficient patients. From his case studies, he has concluded that "mental or psychiatric manifestations such as mental apathy, fluctuations in mood, memory disturbance, paranoia or frank psychosis may more often precede the blood changes (of anemia) by a number of years." In addition, Dr. Abramsky continues, there may be changes in the nervous system—and hardly of the beneficial variety. They may include such problems as soreness and weakness of the limbs, diminished reflexes and sensory perception, changes in temperature in parts of the body, difficulties in walking, stammering, and jerking of limbs.

What makes this vitamin so important is its effect on myelin, the protective sheath that covers the spinal cord and other elements of the nervous system. Although your need for vitamin B_{12} is generally minute—the Council on Foods and Nutrition of the American Medical Association says that your body requires only two to ten micrograms a day (a microgram is 1/1000 of a milligram)—if that small amount is missing from your diet or is absorbed improperly by your system, the result may be disastrous. The myelin sheathing will begin to disintegrate, and with it your nervous system and possibly your mental health.

According to Dr. J. MacD. Holmes, writing in *Medical News Magazine* (April 1967), mental symptoms appear in more than 50 percent of the cases afflicted with myelin lesions. He says these symptoms range from mild disorders of mood, mental slowness and memory defects through delusions, paranoid behavior and sometimes violent hallucinations.

Early Diagnosis Imperative

The terrifying point made by Dr. Holmes'article is that "Vitamin B_{12} deficiency may never be considered until psychosis is far too advanced to respond to treatment. It must be emphasized that the cerebral disturbance may sometimes precede other symptoms for many years, and early diagnosis is imperative if treatment is to be effective." The longer a B_{12} shortage exists, the less likely the patient can be returned to normal.

For some people, increasing their intake of liver and other B_{12}-rich foods may not be enough. That's because there is another substance in your body that is vitally important for the absorption of B_{12}. It's usually referred to as the intrinsic factor, or Castle's factor, and is a mucoprotein synthesized in your stomach—when all is going well. The intrinsic factor is the material to which B_{12} binds itself so that it may be absorbed through the stomach lining and into those parts of your body where it belongs. There are, however, a number of people who are missing or are underproducing this important factor. For them, vitamin B_{12} injections are an absolute necessity.

For most of us, the basic problem is to insure against a B_{12} deficiency. The best answer is a steady supply of vitamin B_{12} through a carefully planned diet. Desiccated liver can conveniently provide the nutrients that appear in whole liver—including the elusive vitamin B_{12}.

So, take no chances! Do not allow this deficiency to start. Of all the vitamin deficiencies, this is about the most difficult to reverse, and is irreversible once it has gone too far.

124. Minerals That Heal The Mind

If you were to visit San Francisco psychiatrist Richard A. Kunin, you might get a haircut instead of a head shrink.

It isn't that Dr. Kunin is skilled in creating new hair styles. His skill is far more valuable—creating new personalities out of tortured ones. The lock of hair which Dr. Kunin snips is used to give him some clues as to what minerals are lacking in the patient's body. For, as Dr. Kunin has discovered, the minerals we don't get in our foods can make all the difference in the world in the way we feel and function. Besides discussing a patient's hang-ups, Dr. Kunin takes a sample of hair for spectrophotometry.

Hair analysis is not exactly new to some physicians, but in the field of psychiatry it is certainly an innovation. Hair contains higher concentrations of minerals than any other body tissue. With the results of these tests, Dr. Kunin learns quickly if mineral deficiencies are triggering a patient's symptoms. If they are, dietary habits will get more attention than dreams.

Many people have absolutely no conception of what constitutes a good diet, Dr. Kunin explained. Patients who come to him suffering depression or psychotic episodes "have a history of gross or severe dietary indiscretion and poor diet" for either months or years. This, compounded with the stress of some loss in their life situation or the stress of starting some major undertaking, "has taken more out of them energetically and biochemically than they had to give," he says. The result is a mental breakdown.

As you have probably surmised, Dr. Kunin is a rare phenomenon—a psychiatrist who recognizes the importance of nutrition to the mind as well as the body.

Dr. Kunin confesses that he himself is a convert to the need for knowledge of nutrition in the practice of psychiatry. When he was a student at the University of Minnesota, he was indifferent to the whole thing and actually walked out of a nutrition lecture when the chief surgeon of the university hospital went overtime. He himself was malnourished, as many students are, he says. His interest in learning about nutrition's role in mental health was stimulated when patients told him about their own experiences. Then he started digging into the works of the pioneers of megavitamin therapy, Drs. Hoffer and Osmond.

Hallucinations Halted

His first success with a patient using nutritional therapy induced him to dig even deeper into every aspect of the subject. This patient, he recalls, was "a flamboyant hallucinator, and paranoid." She was overweight and her fifth husband was an alcoholic. "The possibility of a metabolic factor in her prolonged hallucinatory state prompted me to give her niacinamide (vitamin B_3). The response was dramatic. She'd been having visual and auditory hallucinations off and on for four years. Now, after four days' treatment with niacinamide, she was so much improved that her friends were commenting on it. And in a week she was almost well. That case made me take greater notice of metabolic factors in schizophrenia."

Another one of Dr. Kunin's patients, D. M., was a 24-year-old school teacher. For a year D. M. had been having attacks of anxiety and dizziness with a rapid, irregular pulse. Although he maintained a high-protein, low-carbohydrate diet, and quit smoking and drinking, he did try marijuana several times, and found that it aggravated his symptoms. These symptoms became so severe that he ended up in the medical ward of a hospital. His attending doctor felt that the symptoms must be psychosomatic because he was suffering with headache, tightness in his chest, hyperventilation, a racing pulse, muscle tics and general weakness. But to Dr. Kunin, changes in pulse, muscle tics and weakness suggested low potassium levels. This was confirmed subsequently by hair analysis for trace minerals—only 14 parts per million of potassium against a normal of 37 to 170 ppm. D. M. responded promptly to supplementation with potassium chloride solution. In addition, Dr. Kunin encouraged him to include more potassium-rich foods in his diet—vegetables, bananas, oranges and some grains.

Another patient who got a new lease on life with his change in diet was a 47-year-old former intelligence agent. Eight years earlier he had been put on drugs because of muscle spasms and arthritis. He lost his job and his wife. His sexual responsiveness worsened year by year, leading to depression with suicidal tendencies. This gentleman had been scrupulously avoiding animal fats because of fear of heart disease. He ate no egg or liver. He relied heavily on skim milk and cottage cheese. His vegetable intake was a small salad without dressing. He was taking Dilantin, an anti-convulsant, because of seizures following withdrawal of barbiturates several years earlier. He drank about six ounces of hard liquor every day. Dr. Kunin's nutritional program for the man included a dolomite supplement to replace magnesium losses. He was also started on folic acid to protect against antifolate activity of the Dilantin. Dr. Kunin advised him to include liver, eggs and nuts in his diet. The patient followed these suggestions carefully and five months later reported that he was no longer depressed and that his sexual responses were normal again.

"It's not easy," Dr. Kunin confides, "for a physician to switch from the traditional pill approach to nutritional therapy.

"It means a lot of night work, perusing books and articles. Knowing where to go for information is a key factor—it's hard to know where to turn in this field because the sources are not obvious at first." Dr. Kunin started by reviewing his biochemistry, then attended many biochemistry seminars, culled the textbooks on endocrinology and metabolic diseases, reviewed physiology and dug through the medical literature for new developments.

As a result of his intensive studies, Dr. Kunin devised a chart which is a valuable aid in tracing processes to determine what dietary factors are missing which could cause a particular psychiatric problem. The chart reveals at a glance how even a seemingly small lack, such as the lack of a trace mineral, can stall a metabolic process vital to health and lead to a state of depression, a migraine headache, or a schizophrenic seizure.

Magnesium For Emotional Stability

Magnesium, for example, interacts with many enzymes. This may be why the lack of magnesium has been implicated in such diverse ailments as kidney stones, osteoporosis and emotional instability. In fact, it was pointed out by French scientist M. L. Robinet, in a study of suicide statistics and geological maps, that more people commit suicide in areas where the magnesium content of the soil is low.

"The use of magnesium permits one to support adversity with more serenity," Mr. Robinet concluded in the *Bulletin of the Academy of Medicine* published in France (1934).

It was the importance of such minerals to the dynamic interchange of all nutrients that made Dr. Kunin aware that many conditions, including the inability to cope, might be better treated with nutrition than tranquilizers or Freudian psychoanalysis.

The clear connection between the trace minerals and mental health has also been delineated by Dr. Linus Pauling, who said in *Science* (1968), "The micro-nutrients, the trace elements when they are deficient, are clinically associated with mental deficiency and mental illness."

Dr. Carl Pfeiffer, of the New Jersey Neuro-Psychiatric Institute in Princeton, has extensively researched the need for trace substances in successfully treating schizophrenics. He reports success using zinc, manganese, calcium, lithium, or cobalt in combinations and quantities designed to meet the requirements of the individual.

In a published symposium, *Orthomolecular Psychiatry*, Dr. Pfeiffer describes the unfortunate consequence of foods grown on poor soil coupled with processing methods that further rob them of crucially important mineral elements. As just one example, Pfeiffer writes, "Nuts are a good source of trace elements, but the metals promote rancidity, so the peanut butter will not have as long a shelf life if the trace metals are allowed to remain in it. Our modern hydrogenated peanut butter never turns rancid! What happened to the trace metals?"

Organic Food For Mineral Nutrition

To help avoid the pitfalls of depleted foods, Dr. Kunin recommends that his patients include organically-grown vegetables in their diet.

"When you're eating natural foods," he says, "you're eating nature's own package." Dr. Kunin believes that organic vegetables, because of the way they are grown, may contain plentiful trace minerals in a form easily absorbed by the body.

Sometimes, however, just eating enough mineral-rich foods isn't enough—the prolonged use of diuretic drugs, for example, can bring about serious mineral depletion. The use of diuretics, Dr. Kunin recalls, led one patient to the psychiatric ward suffering from delirious psychosis. "I found a full grown case of pellagra complete with scarred tongue, rash on the ankles and dementia," Dr. Kunin recalls.

While most physicians are not familiar with this kind of

nutritional therapy, Dr. Kunin feels that this kind of information can be most helpful to them. And perhaps the best way for them to get it is from their patients. "Most doctors will be interested," he says. "They do like to know that people are interested in taking care of themselves, and the inquisitive and informed patient also helps the doctor to be more receptive to developments in this field."

125. Bone Meal Can Relieve Anxiety

The patient, a 13-year-old girl named Mary, had a long history of anxiety. Her tensions created problems in making and keeping friends. Insomnia plagued her every night, and the fatigue which resulted compounded her nervousness. Taking a test at school was torture. All her tensions, apprehensions and irritability developed into a constant morbid fear.

Many psychiatrists would have delved deep into Mary's past in an attempt to uncover some traumatic emotional experience, perhaps while she was being toilet trained. But Mary's psychiatrist, Dr. John Wozny at the Department of Educational Psychology of the University of Alberta, had a hunch. He had seen research indicating that there is excessive rise in lactate levels (lactate is a normal metabolic product) in patients with anxiety neurosis, and Dr. Wozny knew that calcium binds with lactate, thereby neutralizing it. With the permission of her parents, he put Mary on a high-calcium diet. "Twenty-three days later," Dr. Wozny reported, "great improvement was recorded . . . Mary indicated that she felt better, had managed to overcome some peer group problems in school, was getting a full night's sleep, and had managed to reach the point where she had a downright willingness to enter into school test situations."

Aware that one case history cannot prove a theory no matter how positive the results, Dr. Wozny also tested his theory on a fourteen-year-old boy named Larry. Larry also had anxiety problems, with a long record of ineffective therapy. His condition was coupled with a nagging symptom of stiff neck muscles, which Dr. Wozny believed was due to his highly nervous state. However, once on a high-calcium diet, Larry's work in school began to improve. He reported that his stiff neck was feeling better, and the problem eventually disappeared. But Larry went even further to demonstrate the effectiveness of the high-calcium diet. "After twenty-three high-calcium days," Dr. Wozny said, "it seems (Larry) came to doubt the relative effectiveness of what was going on, and applied good scientific principles to his problem. Without telling anyone, he went off his diet to see if what we had been doing was just chemical nonsense. I saw him in my office on the twenty-sixth day, and Larry was a very chagrined young man. His stiff neck had come back with a vengeance. A hasty return to the calcium regimen restored a trouble-free muscular condition. Larry and I were most impressed."

Better Than Psychotherapy?

Mary and Larry yield pretty good testimony on the effectiveness of calcium in solving their troubles. But can calcium actually take the place of psychotherapy? Can calcium really help the apprehensive woman who has to look under her bed before she can go to sleep, the irritable father who constantly yells at members of his family, the nervous employee who believes with no justification that others are plotting for his job? There is indeed a good chance that calcium can help in many of these cases because of its ability to enter into a chemical association with lactate (or lactic acid). Scientists have shown that it is an excess of lactate in body chemistry that causes much of the anxiety, nervousness, irritability, tension and fear that plague many of us today.

Two psychiatrists, Drs. Ferris Pitts, Jr. and James McClure, Jr., at the Washington University School of Medicine in St. Louis, demonstrated the role of lactate in anxiety reactions in a study which is truly historic in importance (*New England Journal of Medicine*, December 21, 1967). Their well-designed experiment involved nine normal controls and nine patients diagnosed as suffering from anxiety neurosis. The patients accepted as clear-cut sufferers from anxiety displayed a variety of unmistakable symptoms: feelings of impending doom, fears of insanity, fears of heart attacks, smothering or choking sensations, difficulty in breathing, etc., and had been troubled by these symptoms for at least two years.

Injecting both patients and controls with lactic acid, Drs. Pitts and McClure found that, without any psychic stimulus whatsoever, the lactic acid brought on anxiety attacks in all nine patients, and also in two of the well controls!

Calcium Prevented Anxiety Attacks

The psychiatrists reasoned that since lactic acid is a normal metabolic product, the only way to control an excessive level is to introduce a substance which can neutralize it. This is where calcium comes in. In further investigation, they tested this hypothesis, administering lactic acid to both normal and anxiety patients with, in some cases, the addition of calcium to the lactic acid. They found that the lactate alone caused anxiety attacks in 13 out of 14 anxiety patients within a minute or two after the infusion started, and also in two out of 10 normal subjects. One of the normal subjects described his symptoms as "palpitation, tightness-lump in the throat, trouble breathing, shuddering sensation all over, can't stop shaking feeling . . . I'm very apprehensive and jumpy." But where calcium was administered with the lactate, anxiety symptoms for the most part did not occur.

Explaining his own success with the technique, Dr. Wozny says, "It appears that calcium enters into a chemical association with lactate (forming calcium lactate) in such a way that it binds lactate into a physiologically inactive form and reduces its capacity to produce anxiety reactions." But while many elements can combine with lactic acid, the capacity of calcium to inhibit lactate's effect on our nervous systems lies in its role in nervous impulse transmissions. Simply stated, calcium ions reside at the ends of nerve cells (termed synapses) and maintain electrical connections and communication between nerve cells. In a healthy nervous system, calcium combines with lactic acid around the sensitive nerve endings, preventing the acid from irritating the nervous system. But if too much lactic acid is present in your system, or if there are insufficient amounts of calcium available to perform its neutralizing role, the result is anxiety.

Lactate Is Produced In The Muscles

Where does all this lactic acid come from? Lactic acid is a normal product of glucose metabolism. Glucose undergoes a chain of reactions in our cells which gives us the energy to carry on our everyday affairs. The glucose in our systems comes from glycogen which, in turn, comes from the carbohydrates which we consume. The glycogen is stored in our livers and is broken down to glucose as the need arises.

In the normal course of events, and in the normal metabolism of glucose, lactic acid is not produced to any great extent. However, when energy must be produced fast—for example when a runner takes a sprint—the cells in his body metabolize glucose and produce energy without using oxygen. This metabolism of glucose under anaerobic conditions is termed glycolysis, and the end-product of glycolysis is lactate. When the lactate builds up, the result is fatigue. Therefore, it is inevitable that there will be lactate in everyone's blood, and periods of heavy exercise or simple muscle tension will produce even larger amounts of lactate in your system.

It is only when too high a level of lactate is reached that problems develop. But if plenty of calcium is available, the lactate will not have its unpleasant effects.

It is indeed a vicious cycle which prevents many of us from truly relaxing and enjoying life. When muscle exercise or tension produces enough lactate to induce anxiety states, the anxiety leads to greater muscle tension, which produces more lactate, and so on. But this cycle can begin not only with muscular stress, but also with mental stress, because psychic tension can cause enough tension in our muscles to produce an excess of lactic acid. Unless our intake of calcium is high enough to counteract the lactic acid build-up, anxiety results. It is therefore imperative that we all get enough calcium to keep from being trapped in a vicious cycle of stress.

Bone Meal For Natural Calcium

How can we insure optimal levels of calcium in our bodies? Take daily supplements of bone meal tablets. Bone meal, the pulverized long bones of young beef cattle, contains all the natural bone minerals with calcium predominant. But in addition to calcium it also contains phosphorus, magnesium and other trace minerals in the proper proportions to aid the body in its absorption and utilization of calcium.

Vitamin D is another nutrient necessary to make certain that the calcium in bone meal is put to good use. Without vitamin D, calcium will not be properly absorbed through the intestinal tract into the bloodstream. You can get bone meal tablets with vitamin D already added to them, or preferably you can secure your vitamin D from a capsule of either halibut or cod liver oil.

We already knew that calcium is necessary for the good health of our bones, our hearts, our teeth and our muscles. But patients like Mary and Larry have taught us another valuable lesson: if we keep our diets high in calcium we might save ourselves a lot of mental anguish—from tension, apprehension, nervousness, irritability, dizziness, numbness, trembling, faintness, palpitation of the heart, even intense fear and feelings of impending doom. All are symptoms of anxiety.

126. Improve Your Moods— Without Tranquilizers

A junior executive at a Hollywood studio was asked by his boss to make a speech to an important group of movie exhibitors. It was a prestigious assignment. His performance would have an important effect on his career. The young man began to chew his nails and worry about his speech. His wife, seeing him upset, induced him to take some tranquilizing pills. They worked like a charm; his worries just melted away. When the big moment arrived, the speech was still unprepared. But our junior executive was not the least bit nervous. He spoke off the cuff. His remarks had no continuity, no punch, and made no sense. The speech was a complete flop. The young man, however, did not realize that he had made an utter ass of himself and was grinning happily when he sat down.

Many of us are grinning happily as we goof life's big moments. One reason is we are living in a pill-popping period. Little pink pills to dispel the blues, little green pills when the kids are bugging us, little purple pills to turn down our motors so we can sleep, little orange pills to get us going in the morning. Shame of shames, we even give pills to school children. And not content to have infiltrated the schools, the drug companies are now going after those children who are still at home—the pre-schoolers. "If your child is into everything, if he is a little rascal," the voice on the radio purrs, "you should discuss this with your doctor. Your little rascal may need something to calm him down."

Today some doctors will prescribe a tranquilizer almost as frequently and as casually as they prescribe aspirin. There are now more than 60 different brands of tranquilizer drugs to help you shut out the realities of existence. Their soporific names have become household words—Valium, Librium, Equanil, Harmonyl, Librax, Repoise, Serentil, Solacen, Miltown, Thorazine, and many others. Their names deliberately seduce you. They all play variations on the same theme. If something is bothering you, don't find the cause and correct it. Take a tranquilizer and you won't give a damn. Even if these pills did not have dangerous side effects—even if they did not cause a swing of the pendulum into states of deep despair, or even if they didn't cause dangerous metabolic changes in your body—which they do, the whole philosophy of taking a pill to change your mood is wrong.

After all, what is life if not feeling? To the extent that you lessen feeling and awareness, to that extent do you diminish life?

Can you savor joy if you have never experienced sorrow? Can you experience the exhilaration of an audience's applause if you never suffered a qualm or sweated over your presentation?

There are times when the suffering is so acute and unbearable that these medications are justifiable. And that is what their original purpose was—for the treatment of institutionalized mental patients.

Serenity Or Suicide?

But use of mood altering drugs has now invaded every aspect of American life. As many as 220 million prescriptions were written for them in 1970. Two out of every three adult Americans use them, at least occasionally. Drug manufacturers spend an estimated 800 million dollars a year, spreading their persuasive advertising over the pages of widely-read scientific journals and medical magazines directed to doctors. The ads advise the doctor to prescribe a happy pill for women who are tired of doing the dishes, for the single girl who is tense and overanxious, for the elderly patient who suffers with insomnia, loss of appetite, agitation, crying, apprehension. This is usually followed by a full page of warnings, precautions, and adverse reactions that are in no way related to harmony, solace and serenity.

After the initial upswing which these tranquilizers bring, there is often a sharp descent into the pits of despair. Numerous suicides have been recorded in the medical literature from meprobamate (chemical name for the 'mild' tranquilizers Miltown and Equanil), and the actual number is thought to be much greater (*Medical Letters on Drugs and Therapeutics*, December, 1960). These so-called tranquilizers also cause drowsiness, chills, nasal stuffiness, extreme fatigue, and sometimes fever, weakness and diarrhea. They also can cause liver damage and the shaking disease, Parkinson's. None of these conditions contribute to extended periods of happiness.

Valium and Librium, the first and third most often prescribed drugs, are equally dangerous. Hundreds of suicides and tempted suicides have been linked to these tranquilizers, according to a report in the Washington *Post* (January 31, 1975). More than 20 million prescriptions a year are written for Valium alone.

B Vitamins Do It Better

Doctors who have never really made a study of nutrition do not seem to realize that many conditions for which a tranquilizer is prescribed could be far better handled by improving the nutrition to include a plentiful supply of the B vitamins. These nutrients are vital to the health of our nerves and to our ability to handle stress.

Tension and nervous problems can be symptoms of wrong eating. We in America consume far too many "empty" calorie foods. Not only do these foods contain no vitamins of their own, they rob our personal vitamin bank account. When we eat natural carbohydrates, the vitamins we need are supplied by the food itself. But when we eat refined sugar or white flour products, our bodies must steal the B vitamins needed for their processing from muscles, nerves, and other organs. Obviously, if we eat large quantities of refined sugars and starches, we induce a B deficiency, especially B_1 (thiamine), which can cause fatigue, nervousness, constipation, and other unpleasant symptoms.

Many of us are going on cockeyed reducing diets. We lose weight—true. But we also lose our tranquility. The more protein we consume, the more vitamin B_6 and magnesium we need to metabolize it. A deficiency of vitamin B_6 can trigger a tic, a twitch, or a tremor. It can cause tension, insomnia, irritability, quarrelsomeness—the very symptoms which induce millions of people to reach for a tranquilizer.

Where do you find vitamin B_6? You won't find it in ordinary white bread from which the wheat germ and bran have been removed. You will find it in nutritional yeast, blackstrap molasses, wheat bran and germ, liver, heart, and kidney. Bear in mind that much vitamin B_6 is lost in cooking, canning and exposure to light and long storage.

If you get your B_6 from natural sources of the B complex, you will also be getting pantothenic acid, which is essential to your ability to handle stressful situations. One of the most recently identified fractions of the vitamin B complex, pantothenate is present and important to every single cell of your body. Its tremendous assist in situations of stress is due to the fact that it is absolutely essential to the smooth functioning of your adrenal glands. Without pantothenic acid, adrenal glands just don't express their usual "fight or flight" reaction. A lack of pantothenic acid can cause your adrenal glands to go on strike, to lie down on the job and refuse to produce cortisone and other important hormones. Without these hormones, you simply cannot operate on all cylinders, and you are particularly vulnerable to any situation that causes stress. And let's face it, life is made up of stresses. Pollution in the atmosphere, the unavoidable additives in our food, unpleasant noises, a cranky boss, a house full of kids—these are all stress situations which pantothenic acid can help you face much more effectively than a tranquilizer.

Look for pantothenic acid in the same foods that contain the other B vitamins—rice bran, brown rice, wheat germ, soybeans, salmon, egg yolk, peanuts, and especially nutritional yeast.

Another fraction of the B complex that will help you see the silver lining behind every cloud is thiamine (vitamin B_1), sometimes called the "morale" vitamin, because without it your nerves tend to fray.

Thiamine For Mood Stability

Early signs of thiamine deficiency are so commonplace that they are frequently ignored—a lack of energy and constant fatigue. A person who is deficient in thiamine neither eats well nor sleeps well, and tends to be cross and irritable.

If you have any of these symptoms, don't reach for a tranquilizer. Look to your thiamine intake just as a precaution.

Much of the irritability in people who give you a hard time at the shopping centers or on the highway might be traced to a deficiency in this essential nutrient. "Many groups do not receive adequate amounts of thiamine," says Miriam E. Lowenberg in *Food and Man* (John Wiley & Sons, Inc., 1968). "Often, dietary lack of thiamine is not so great as to cause definite illness, but the intake is not enough for good health."

Mood changes are sometimes the first indication that this vitamin is lacking. If your memory has become faulty and your concentration poor, start immediately to increase your B_1 intake. If you feel unstable emotionally and overreact to the normal stresses and strains of everyday living, if you blow a fuse at the slightest provocation, these are some of the redlight warnings of thiamine deficiency.

Thiamine therapy usually brings dramatic recoveries, even after the deficiency has advanced to the stage of beriberi—the name given to extreme thiamine deficiency many years ago. Back in the 1890's, Dr. Christiaan Eijkman found he could give chickens polyneuritis (beriberi in man) by restricting them to a diet of polished rice. He could reverse the process and cure them when he fed them the natural unprocessed brown rice. That's a clue for you. Never use processed rice. Brown rice is inexpensive, easy to prepare, delicious, and rich in the "morale" vitamin. "The cereal grains are a good source of thiamine," Dr. Lowenberg said, "but the thiamine is in the germ and outer coatings so that we find cereals such as white rice and white flour have lost their thiamine." Thiamine is water soluble so the more water you use in cooking, the more thiamine you are losing. It is destroyed by high temperatures.

If you are pregnant, nursing, facing surgery or a big day at the office, these are stressful conditions that call for more thiamine. If the children are struggling with exams, or the love of your life with an income tax return, they will all be much more cheerful about it if they have plenty of thiamine working for them. Put out a dish of sunflower seeds for them to snack on. Seeds are a wonderful source of all the B vitamins.

Magnesium For Sound Nerves

An undersupply of several other nutrients can affect your personality, your charisma, and the way you face each day. If you are even mildly deficient in the mineral magnesium, you are apt to be highly nervous, irritable, quick to pick a quarrel, uncooperative, withdrawn, surly, apathetic or belligerent. Dr. Willard A. Krehl says that magnesium deficiency unquestionably causes changes in nerve conduction, transmission at the myoneuro junction and muscular contraction (*Nutrition Today*, September, 1967). The British medical journal, *Lancet*, (October 1, 1966), reports that mental apathy and depression are caused by a thiamine deficiency which in turn can be caused by a magnesium deficiency.

Foods rich in magnesium include nuts and seeds, dolomite, bone meal, some meats (especially liver which contains concentrates of all the minerals), eggs, fruits and vegetables—preferably organically-grown.

Happiness, someone once observed, is like a butterfly. The more you chase it, the more it will elude you. But if you turn your attention to other things it comes and softly sits on your shoulder.

Emotional And Nervous Disorders

Don't chase happiness with mood-changing pills. That is the road to misery. Instead, turn your attention to improving your nutrition and some day, when you are hardly thinking about it, you will sense the butterfly of happiness sitting softly on your shoulder.

127. Breaking The Chains Of Depression

The most widespread emotional illness in the United States is depression. More than four million persons a year are treated for it with anti-depressant drugs. Many, many millions more never seek help because they are not aware that depression is a mental illness.

Yet each year an estimated 60,000 of them are so burdened by their depression that they take their own lives.

Very often the victim of depression swings in a predictable cycle to the other end of the pendulum—mania, or exaggerated exuberance. Mania, too, is an emotional illness.

The pendulum may swing every few weeks, or perhaps only once a year. Yet, inevitably, the victim rebounds from periods of extreme enthusiasm, energy and boisterousness to moods in which the slightest effort requires more energy than he can muster, or his head is constantly splitting with pain, and life seems dark and hopeless.

Writing in the November 23, 1964 issue of the *Journal of the American Medical Association*, Nathan S. Kline, M.D., gave the five most common symptoms of depression: (1) feelings of sadness; (2) fatigue; (3) loss of interest in social environment; (4) self-neglect; and (5) insomnia, especially in the early morning hours.

Only when a person suffers these symptoms, when he is at the very bottom of the depressive cycle, when his emotions are in tatters and he feels he can't face one more day, will he seek psychiatric help. Then, what help can he expect?

Anti-Depressive Drugs Ineffective

British psychiatrist Colin Brewer offered a partial answer to that question in a letter published in the April, 1969 issue of *The Medical Journal of Australia*. Referring to tricyclic compounds and monoamine oxidase inhibitors, both widely-used anti-depressants, Brewer says, "It has been frequently claimed that these drugs can cure depressive illnesses, especially in the early stages . . ."

But, he says, "despite their widespread administration, the number of admissions for depression has increased steadily. In the United Kingdom, the increase since 1958 has been about 300 percent and this seems to have been a familiar experience in comparable societies."

The reason these cases are growing is simple, says Brewer: "Anti-depressants do not work; or rather, they do not work very often." Only about 15 percent of the population suffering from depression will show a specific response to these drugs. And those who do respond probably have a genetic basis for their illness. Yet, no attempt is made to limit anti-depressant therapy to these particular patients.

"The trouble," says Brewer, "is that the label 'depression' almost invariably leads to the administration of 'anti-depressants' in a truly—and terrifyingly—Pavlovian fashion."

Mania Controlled With Lithium

If it's difficult to treat the depressive state with drugs, why not treat the manic phase instead? Many psychiatrists work under the assumption that since mania is at the opposite end of the pendulum, any treatment which could eliminate the mania would also eliminate the depression.

One substance which is apparently effective in treating mania is the toxic trace mineral lithium. In 1949 Australian physician John F. J. Cade was carrying on research with the mentally ill when he found that excited animals can be calmed by oral doses of lithium.

His first human test was with a man who had been hospitalized for years because of violent manic-depressive episodes. Three weeks after Dr. Cade began treating him with lithium, the patient was moved from the locked ward for violent patients to the convalescent ward.

Cade reported the results of further tests in the September, 1959 issue of the *Medical Journal of Australia*. He reported that manics responded marvelously to lithium. But those suffering only from depression showed no improvement.

Today, lithium is prescribed by many psychiatrists. Most of them are in agreement that the mineral is effective in eliminating mania—but mania is only a part of the manic-depressive cycle, and not the most troublesome one at that.

Shock Treatment As A Last Resort

What's left for the manic-depressive? Two more standard treatments are psychotherapy and shock treatment. Psychotherapy can be effective only in the relatively small number of cases which are the results of a patient's emotional inability to deal with problems. Electroshock treatment is still extremely controversial. Some psychiatrists claim it is the equivalent of the Middle Ages custom of drilling holes in people's heads to let out the evil spirits—and no more effective. Others claim it is the most effective method available for dealing with mental illnesses.

If the patient is lucky, he will respond to the anti-depressants, or the lithium, or to psychotherapy or to shock treatment. He will soon be back at the job, picking up where he left off, feeling fine. And his recovery will sometimes be permanent.

But this happy ending is far too rare. In literally millions of cases, the manic-depressive becomes a permanent victim of what Montreal psychiatrist David J. Lewis calls "a sickness that feeds on itself and that can warp the personality, disrupt the family and, at its worst, end in self-destruction."

For them, the pendulum never stops swinging: exuberance—dismay; laughter—tears; hope—despair; enthusiasm—exhaustion.

B$_{12}$ For Depression After Childbirth

Still others manage to escape this gloomy picture through a special kind of nutritional therapy.

In 1968, a 23-year-old woman in Yonkers, New York, had her first baby. Although usually cheerful and emotionally stable, she became very depressed, apparently without reason, within a few days of delivery.

Her case is far from rare. So common is depression following childbirth that doctors consider it a normal reaction. But in some cases the problem becomes severe—and sometimes it becomes serious enough to require psychiatric hospitalization.

The young mother was not depressed because of the new responsibilities of caring for her child, though that often causes the illness. Nor was her illness a reaction to drugs, although antibiotics and sulfonamides can induce depression in sensitive individuals. Even viral infections seem to produce depression in some people, but that was not the cause of the illness in the young woman.

In fact, the true cause would have gone undiagnosed and

untreated by the vast majority of doctors, psychiatrists and psychoanalysts now practicing in this country. The woman simply lacked one of the substances needed by her brain in order for it to function properly.

The substance was vitamin B_{12}. She was given large doses of the nutrient, and within two days improvement was noticed. Within a week, all symptoms had disappeared.

How many cases of depression following childbirth result from vitamin B_{12} deficiency? No one can answer that because no one has ever investigated it.

Six-Month Depression Cured In Days

Pregnant women are not the only ones so afflicted. A 53-year-old housewife had suffered for four years with intermittent numbness and tingling in the arms and legs and a weakness of the hands. In the final six months before she was hospitalized at Croydon General Hospital, Surrey, England, the woman said she felt very depressed.

She appeared well nourished and fit, but upon careful examination it was discovered that she was lacking in vitamin B_{12}.

The doctors treating her decided to give her injections of vitamin B_{12}. Within two days there was some slight improvement in her condition. After 48 hours the improvement was marked, and within a few days symptoms had completely disappeared. The case was reported in the July 1, 1967 *British Medical Journal*.

Vitamin B_{12} has brought equally dramatic results in treating dementia, psychosis and other severe mental disturbances. Such cases are described in an entire chapter on B_{12} elsewhere in this section.

Strange as it may seem, manic-depression may actually be a blessing, a warning that a vitamin B_{12} deficiency exists and that, if not corrected, the deficiency will irreversibly damage the central nervous system.

128. "Super Oxygen," A Promising New Treatment For Senility

As we get on in years, we don't learn new things as easily as we did as youngsters. And we have odd little memory lapses. What town *was* that, where we spent our vacation two years ago? Is it *e* before *i* or *i* before *e* except after *c*? And what *is* the name of the girl our grandson married—a perfectly familiar name, right on the tip of the tongue, but for the moment unrecallable?

It's not necessarily a sign you're getting senile, if your mind plays tricks on you like that. Highly competent men and women, holding responsible jobs at the peak of their careers, are subject to similar lapses as they reach the years of 50 and beyond. You might say that this slight deterioration in the brain's functioning is a human "norm."

There is reason to believe, however, that it doesn't *have* to be a norm. Furthermore, it appears probable that the graver brain deterioration seen in senility is a treatable and perhaps preventable disease.

Getting More Oxygen To The Brain

One of the most dramatic—and controversial—developments in the treatment of senility is hyperbaric oxygenation, in which the patient is exposed to pure oxygen under high pressure (OHP) in a special chamber. The rationale is that senility is often caused by a deficiency of blood flow to critical areas of the brain, with subsequent poor oxygenation of these vital tissues. In the elderly person with excellent mental and physical health, there may be only a seven percent decrease in the blood flow to the brain, whereas patients with narrowed cerebral arteries or other organic brain disease may have as much as a 20 to 25 percent decrease in blood—and therefore oxygen—flow to the brain (Alvan L. Barach, M.D., *Journal of the American Geriatrics Society*, September, 1970).

The classic study using hyperbaric therapy to treat senility was carried out with 13 elderly male patients, all of whom had been hospitalized for many months, and in some cases for several years, because of symptoms of senility. Ruled out from participation in the experiment were any patients exhibiting heart, respiratory, or metabolic difficulties which might pose a risk under OHP treatment. As described in the *New England Journal of Medicine* (October 2, 1969) by Dr. Eleanor A. Jacobs and three colleagues, the patients were first given three standard tests designed to evaluate efficiency of memory, concept formation, and presence of physical brain damage. Arterial blood samples were also obtained and tested for oxygen.

Each of the 13 was treated for 90 minutes twice a day, for 15 days, with hyperbaric oxygen. At the same time, five other patients were used as controls, and although put into a chamber, breathed a mixture which was nearly identical to ordinary air.

When all the patients were retested, an average of 12 hours after coming out of the chamber, those who had been breathing pure oxygen showed remarkable increases in their scores, while the control patients had no significant change. In the experimental group, the mean average score on the Wechsler Memory Scale went from 76 to 103. The average score on another test went from 10 to 41, and on the third test from 25 to 49.

Blood samples taken during the test showed a very marked increase in the amount of oxygen in the blood of those breathing the pure oxygen, while the control subjects had no increase at all. This seemed to establish a very clear relationship between increased oxygenation of the brain and mental performance in elderly senile people.

Improvement Lasts Longer Than Expected

Now for the big question: is this improvement temporary or permanent? And the answer, although not clear, is intriguing.

The researchers point out that it is well known that increased levels of oxygen tension in the blood diminish very quickly, returning to normal in about 30 minutes. And oxygen levels in the brain, which burns up a relatively tremendous amount of oxygen, are probably normalized much sooner, they point out. But the tests which revealed improvement were given an average of 12 hours after oxygenation, which means that the improvement lasted at least 24 times longer than can be explained by the presence of extraordinary amounts of oxygen in the brain.

Dr. Jacobs and her colleagues point out: "It is not likely that the treatment modifies basic degenerative processes, but we know of no other form of therapy that offers statistically significant improvement of function." And they add that it is possible that administering pure oxygen without any increased pressure might have very similar results. In their words: "Much remains to be learned about the practical value of hyperoxygenation and senility."

Four years later, Dr. Jacobs was quoted in *Medical World News* (January 5, 1973) as reporting that she and her associates had increased the number of patients treated and studied to 75, and commented that "Our experiments show that improvement persists longer than we would have expected, but we aren't sure how long. . . . We believe oxygenation merely acts as a biochemical activator of the central nervous system and we're trying to find out what's being activated and by what."

Younger Patients Can Also Benefit

Meanwhile, other researchers are also studying OHP treatment for senility, and some are reporting promising preliminary results—although most improvement seems to be only short-term. In addition, the treatment seems to be of very limited usefulness for people in their 70's or 80's, or when senility is not resulting directly from arteriosclerosis. Dr. Erie Kindwall, director of the Department of Hyperbaric Medicine at St. Luke's Hospital, Milwaukee, says, "Our best successes come with the younger patient who often refers himself to us saying, 'I just can't seem to recall or think the way I once did' " (Allentown *Evening Chronicle*, February 7, 1973).

Dr. Jacobs and her colleagues agree that hyperbaric oxygen's implications for mental health are not necessarily confined to elderly people who have become senile. As they point out: "It has been shown . . . that memory and learning curves peak at an early age: between 15 and 20 years. Thus it is likely that many people in functional stages between those of peak learning and gross senility are undergoing slow, but progressive and measurable decreases in memory and learning."

What the researchers imply is that for the great mass of people—all those between youth and extreme old age—there has been noted a rapidly increasing tendency for atherosclerosis—arterial narrowing because of plaque forming on the inner walls of the blood vessels. One of the earliest and most predictable results is a diminished supply of blood to the brain, which can cause the brain to receive less oxygen than it requires. A minor manifestation of slight oxygen insufficiency would be the annoying memory lapses referred to earlier—or the inability to think through a new set of problems as quickly as in earlier years.

All of us, in other words, might conceivably improve our memories, our capacity to learn, and our protection against senility in old age by health measures that increase the amount of oxygen reaching the brain tissue.

Pure Oxygen Is Dangerous

But hyperbaric oxygenation is not without its dangers. In amounts not very much greater than those used therapeutically, excess oxygen becomes toxic to certain enzyme systems, and can damage eyes, lungs, and even the central nervous system. In short, great caution must be used with OHP both in selection of patients to be treated and in monitoring the heart, blood and nerves before, after, and preferably during treatment.

Nevertheless, hyperbaric therapy is worth knowing about, if for no other reason than that pressure chambers are being installed in more and more hospitals and there is an increasing likelihood that a doctor (or an acquaintance) may suggest that you undergo such treatment.

Probably the most important reservation about the use of OHP for senility was expressed by Dr. Edwin Boyle, Research Director of the Miami Heart Institute in Florida, who points out: "We have 25 million old people; how are we going to treat them in the few OHP units around? The studies show we'll have to take another look at senility and try to find more effective therapy" (*Medical World News*, January 5, 1973).

From a practical point of view then, it seems that the most important discovery to come out of the experimental use of OHP for senility is not simply that it works temporarily, but that the degenerative process known as senility is not irreversible. More important, by implication, it may also be preventable. But as Dr. Boyle points out, we now have to find a more efficient way of improving blood circulation and oxygen delivery to the brain.

Recent research indicates that such a practical technique may already exist. Many senile persons, some of them badly deteriorated, have been pulled back from the abyss of confusion and helplessness by nutritional supplementation. Nutritional treatment is at least potentially more efficient and much less expensive than hyperbaric oxygenation. Yes, it is still in the experimental stages, but there has already been a great amount of pioneering work done, and the results published in scientific journals. In the next chapter, we will take a close look at this method of preventing and treating senility.

129. Senility Is Not
A One-Way Street

The problem of declining mental abilities as age advances is one that leaves many—perhaps most—doctors with a baffled awareness of inability to cope with the situation. Whether or not there is cerebral arteriosclerosis involved, the simple fact is that as age advances, all too often a narrowing of the peripheral blood vessels—the tiny capillaries spreading their network throughout the brain—reduces the supply of oxygen available to the brain tissues. The result is confusion, disorientation, and failure of memory in the oxygen-starved cells of the brain.

It is as a direct result of this decline in aging minds, more than any other single factor, that nursing homes everywhere are becoming crowded with elderly people who are not organically ill, but are simply unable to take care of themselves.

Two Types Of Senile Forgetfulness

According to Dr. V. A. Kral, of the Gerontologic Unit of McGill University's Allan Memorial Institute of Psychiatry in Montreal, senescent forgetfulness may be one of two types (*The Canadian Medical Association Journal*, February 10, 1962). In the first or "benign" form, the subject may be unable to recall relatively unimportant data and parts of an experience, while remembering the experience itself. At another time, the previously missing details will be recalled, but *others* will be forgotten. "A typical example of this type of memory impairment," writes Dr. Kral, "was found in a woman of about 80 who remembered that she had attended, some years ago, the wedding of her son in a New England city, but was unable to remember the name of that city. When asked again on another occasion, she remembered the name of the city."

In the second or "malignant" form of senile forgetfulness, the subject fails to recall even recent events, and this loss leads to confusion, disorientation and "senile dementia." "For example," continues Dr. Kral, "had the lady mentioned above suffered from this type of memory impairment, she might have forgotten the wedding of her son which she attended and not only the name of the city where it took place."

He labels the latter condition "malignant" because such patients "have a significantly higher death rate and shorter survival time" than other subjects of the same age. The problem appears more physiological than psychiatric in origin. "Our data tend to show that the type of memory dysfunction in the aged can be taken as an index of the general health of the individual," Dr. Kral states.

Is this mental confusion and disorientation—so common among many of the elderly—an unavoidable part of aging? M. L. Mitra, medical assistant at Nether Edge and Winter Street Hospitals in Sheffield, England, doesn't think so. Instead, he believes that much of what passes for "senility" is simply the result of easily avoidable deficiency diseases—particularly too little of the B vitamins and vitamin C in the diet. A simple change in eating habits, rather than commitment to a nursing home, could be the happy solution for thousands of the aged.

"Nutritional deficiencies are being recognized with increasing frequency in the practice of geriatric medicine," Mitra reported in the *Journal of the American Geriatrics Society* (June, 1971). "Among elderly people in countries like Great Britain it is not uncommon to see 'subclinical' vitamin deficiency, in contrast to the frank avitaminosis seen in less affluent countries." The reason? "Like people in some developing countries, many of the elderly tend to live entirely on a diet consisting of potatoes and a few slices of bread and jam."

All Confused Patients Were Vitamin-Deficient

To illustrate his point, Mitra presented 28 case histories of patients admitted to a hospital geriatric unit in a "confused state" over a six-month period. After measuring the level of ascorbic acid (vitamin C) in the leukocyte layer or "buffy coat" of their blood and running pyruvate metabolism tests (P.M.T.) to determine B vitamin abnormalities, he found that all the patients had at least one thing in common: a vitamin deficiency. Many were 80 years of age or older and had been living alone. For most, fixing a balanced, hot meal for themselves alone every day was "just too much trouble." Seventeen were found to be suffering from thiamine/vitamin B complex deficiencies; two others had pellagra (a niacin-deficiency disease). Seven patients had low serum levels of vitamin C, and two others had mixed vitamin deficiencies.

F. B., 88 years old, lived alone and ran her own lodging house. She was admitted to the hospital because of severe dehydration and a confusional state. She had been taking chlorpromazine, a central nervous system depressant, while at home, but the confusion had persisted. When her P.M.T. results proved abnormal, an oral dosage of concentrated vitamin B complex solution was prescribed. Her confusion disappeared. She regained her mental faculties and was able to return home.

R. M., 76 years old, also lived alone. Admitted to the hospital because of opthalmoplegia, a paralysis of the eye muscles, she suddenly became very confused. So severely confused, in fact, that her doctor made a provisional diagnosis of Wernicke's encephalopathy—a degenerative disease of the brain in which the gray matter becomes inflamed. But Mitra suspected something much simpler; the woman's P.M.T. values were strikingly abnormal, suggesting a B vitamin deficiency. Sure enough, after she received injections of concentrated B complex, her mental state improved so dramatically that she was discharged within a fortnight.

N. H., 72 years old, lived alone on an old-age pension. She was admitted to the hospital in a confused state with a painful case of dermatitis. Doctors diagnosed pellagra. Treated with B complex, "she became a different woman," Mitra reported. "When she was discharged, she was normal except for osteoarthritis of the knees. She has not required any further hospital admissions."

In some cases, faulty diet was only part of the problem. "Increased metabolism due to infection may deplete vitamin B complex in the body," Mitra added. "The water-soluble vitamin B complex also may be washed out in heavy diuresis caused by diuretics. A large number of our patients were treated with these commonly prescribed drugs."

Entire B Complex Involved

For Mitra, the pieces were beginning to fall together. P.M.T. values—used to diagnose the earlier cases—generally reflect thiamine (vitamin B_1) levels. But the P.M.T. readings were also abnormal in the case of pellagra (a vitamin B_3 deficiency). And that wasn't all: "Deficiency of folic acid (another B vitamin) may be associated with the confusional state," he noted, "and deficiency of vitamin B_{12} is a known cause of dementia."

Since all the B vitamins are derived from the same natural sources where they are always found together, the treatment seemed obvious: massive doses of concentrated B complex solution, either injected or taken by mouth. And the results were more than gratifying. In case after case among the aged patients, confusional states improved or disappeared, as the case histories testify: "She became much quieter and easily manageable . . . the patient was discharged home as a mentally normal person . . . she became oriented . . . he became his 'normal self' again," and so forth.

"Confusional states, if treated at an early state with B vitamins, may clear up," Mitra concluded.

But for other confused patients, the deficiencies included more than just the B vitamins. Some were found to be suffering from a shortage of vitamin C.

R. C., 95 years old, lived with her bachelor son who was employed full-time. She had been treated with diuretics for congestive heart failure. Entering the hospital in a mild confusional state, she complained of intense bone tenderness and multiple bruises—common indicators of vitamin C deficiency. After treatment with a gram of vitamin C daily for two weeks, her mental state improved to the point that she could be discharged home.

In case after case, massive doses of vitamin C (as much as two or three *grams* a day for three to six weeks) brought similar results.

For Mitra, the lesson seemed obvious. "Confusion is extremely common in the elderly and is often a therapeutic challenge to the clinician," he concluded. *"Confusion of acute onset is more often due to a physical illness than to an underlying psychiatric disorder."* (Emphasis added.)

Niacin Opens Narrowed Vessels

How are vitamins able to exert such a beneficial effect? One clue is provided by research conducted at the New England Hospital in Boston. A report by Franklin I. Shuman, M.D., of that hospital, with Ronald I. Goldberg, M.D., published in the *Journal of the American Geriatrics Society* (June, 1965) claimed good results with 66 percent of elderly patients with enfeebled mentalities, fair results with 25 percent more, and poor results in only eight percent of the cases.

The basic successful therapy was the administration of nicotinic acid (vitamin B_3) in combination with a high potency multivitamin supplement.

The reason for the success of this vitamin treatment was not pinpointed, but the authors stated that "The vasodilatory (opening the blood vessels) action of nicotinic acid is well known, and indeed this vitamin has been used for many years for this purpose. Its effects apparently are due in part to cerebral vasodilation, which counteracts the effects of cerebral sclerosis."

Mental Deterioration Is Not "Normal"

As Dr. Robert E. Rothenberg has noted in his book, *Health In Later Years* (New American Library), "Acute mental deterioration rarely occurs among normal older people before the eighties." Yet all too often, friends and relatives reluctantly interpret a confusional lapse, a loss of memory, or even a growing tendency to repeat oneself as the first signs of an inevitable, full-blown case of senility in a loved one.

But what is the real basis of the acute mental confusion, forgetfulness and hostility which we lump under the label of "senility"? How many of the elderly are victims of subclinical malnutrition with its accompanying symptoms of senility? And how many more have been . . . or will be . . . committed to nursing homes or geriatric hospitals where efficiency-first, large scale cooking methods that rob foods of vitamins B and C may merely serve to perpetuate their confusional states? As M. L. Mitra observed in his report, many of these people are "victims of social neglect—a circumstance that is common, particularly among the elderly."

No one doubts that the families of those aged individuals want to do the *right* thing. But unless they can convince their loved one to improve his or her diet, to eat more fresh fruits and vegetables and unprocessed foods, in addition to taking natural supplements (especially those that supply vitamins B and C), their efforts will be in vain. With better nourishment, many a septuagenarian (and octogenarian, for that matter!) would find that recurring mental confusion, agitation and memory loss needn't be an inseparable part of aging.

It would certainly be a tragedy if a family reluctantly decided to send a "confused" or "senile" loved one off to a nursing home, when all that was really needed to keep that person healthy, independent and alert might be vitamin supplements and a wholesome, hot meal daily.

130. Vitamin E And The Retarded Child

A minute isn't long. But every time a clock ticks off five of them, a retarded child is born somewhere in the United States. Each and every year, more than 100,000 babies—or approximately five percent of all children born in America—are born afflicted in this way.

Most children born retarded will remain that way until death. Cures are unlikely. Can anything at all be done for them?

Twelve-year-old Tommy screamed and moaned most of the time. He was irritable, morose and he fought like a steer when any of the nurses or hospital personnel at Ontario Hospital School, Orillia, Ontario, Canada, tried to give him the help and nursing care this mentally retarded child had to have. Doctors prescribed every sedative and tranquilizer they could think of to calm Tommy down, but nothing seemed to improve his disposition.

Because there was nothing left to try, desperate doctors began giving him 400 units of alpha tocopherol (vitamin E) four times a day. In a few days time, according to M. Houze, M.D. and other specialists at the hospital, "He became less irritable and more quiet, and as time passed, he actually began to like and respond to nursing attention." In less than two months Tommy looked better physically, and was easier to feed. In another month he began to laugh when tickled—something no one could remember him doing before. The calming effect vitamin E had on Tommy lasted. Rather than a disturbing factor in the ward, he became a pleasant addition to hospital society.

Appetite And Disposition Improved

Donny, a boy of three, had extreme behavioral problems. He had to be wrapped up in a sheet in order to be fed. Sometimes he would vomit most of what he ate, making it necessary to feed him by tube. For most of his waking time he cried. Aside from drugs, every known type of tonic and vitamin had been tried on Donny to no avail. Then tocopherol treatment was begun—400 units four times a day. In less than a month his appetite and disposition improved greatly. He began to eat willingly and even asked for second helpings. "Of late, he has become one of the best-liked children in the ward."

Tommy and Donny were part of a study reported in the *American Journal of Mental Deficiency* (Nov., 1964). Twenty mentally retarded boys were divided into three age groups: those under 10, those between 10 and 13, and those over 13 years of age. For six months, the first group received 400 I. U. of vitamin E twice a day; the second group, three times a day; and the oldest group, four times a day.

Officials were astounded at the results. "As early as two weeks after treatment began, some intellectual and behavioral improvement was noted by the teachers in half of their subjects, more frequently in the children of the second (10 to 13 years) group. The fact that these patients were brighter, more alert and more cooperative made their care and management easier." The doctors noticed no improvement in the I.Q. of these children, however, and the most severely retarded children did not show any apparent response. The principal value of vitamin E in these cases was its calming effect, impressive enough, considering the disappointing results with the best and newest tranquilizers and sedatives.

No Child Remained Unimproved

More recently, the Chief of Child Psychology at the National Institute of Public Health, Buenos Aires, Argentina, reported impressively on his results with vitamin E used as a treatment for mentally defective children. Dr. A. del Guidice wrote, "We have treated many complications in our infantile psychotics . . . no child remained unimproved when properly treated. Generally we have begun treatment with 200 to 300 milligrams of vitamin E daily, increasing over a period of as long as six months to doses approximating 2 grams daily—depending on the age of the child and his type of disease. Vitamin C was also given in doses of 500 to 1500 milligrams daily. It was added because of my belief that it reinforces vitamin E—it being clear, always, that the latter is the basic item."

Among the case histories reported by Dr. del Guidice was that of a twelve-year-old girl, a congenital idiot who exhibited aggressive impulses which called for physical restraint almost all the time. She shouted and cried for no apparent reason, and was extremely moody. The girl could not speak properly and could not understand questions. She was unable to manage her own toilet routine. Six years of orthodox medical treatment had brought no improvement.

In 40 days of vitamin E therapy she made more progress than in all of the previous six years. Within a year she was fairly subdued, sat correctly and watched her surroundings calmly. She lost her babbling, crying and aggressiveness, and sat at the table and ate by herself for the first time.

A three-year-old patient of Dr. del Guidice stuttered and suffered from an inferiority complex that was so severe she couldn't even play with her brothers and sisters. On the third day of tocopherol therapy she showed improvement. After three months of tocopherol treatment she was completely free of stammering, could recite three verses of a poem with ease and fluency, and played happily with other children.

Doctors continue to bemoan the lack of an effective treatment for the mentally retarded. How many children might be saved from life in an institution by the use of vitamin E? Many? None? A few? Let's test it. If your child were one of these, wouldn't you want to know for sure?

131. Minimal Brain Dysfunction—Now There's Hope

What causes minimal brain dysfunction? It is believed that there may be a biological or chemical change in the brain tissue that results in poor function. The brain, a most complicated organ consisting of millions of cells with intricate connections, may be injured either before, during or after birth. Among the suspected causes of injury are incompatible RH factor in mother and child, poor nutrition, inherited defects in the genes, technical problems at delivery, trauma and infectious diseases. Recent studies relate pollutants in our air, food and water to brain damage.

It is estimated that about five percent of American children are afflicted with a minimal brain dysfunction. It manifests itself with difficulties in learning and making social adjustment. The child is often late in walking, talking and toilet control. He may have perceptual difficulties, reversing letters or skipping lines. Sometimes he can't distinguish right from left. He may have a hearing problem, and the subtleties of sound elude him. He may find it difficult to communicate and is repetitive in speech. Often learning to ride a bike is a Herculean task. He rejects baseball because he is awkward with a ball and bat. Nothing can hold his attention for long and he dissipates his energy in all directions like a lighted sparkler.

Of course, every child has growing problems and time may be the healer. But when several of these symptoms plague a child, minimal brain dysfunction is suspected, and early investigation is indicated.

From Dunce To Scholar In Two Years

How far can a child go—a child with a brain dysfunction?

Ron, immature and sad-eyed, was the scorned classroom

dummy in the fourth grade of his suburban school. He couldn't sit still in his seat—he would wriggle like a Mexican jumping bean until he ended up sprawling on the floor. He was disruptive, destructive, impulsive. He had a memory like a sieve and his attention span was about as long as a T.V. commercial.

Ron is now in sixth grade and is miraculously up to grade level. Why the dramatic improvement in his learning ability? Ron is also a respected member of the class football team and an enthusiastic Boy Scout. What's the secret of his social acceptance after years of being an outcast?

The answer to both questions is a program that improves the functioning of the brain—diet therapy and vitamins coupled with sensori-motor exercises.

Until he was 10 years old, Ron had all the symptoms of minimal brain dysfunction. Uncoordinated and plagued by perceptual problems, he couldn't concentrate and he couldn't learn. Out of frustration, his behavior became erratic.

Ron's parents stopped at nothing in their attempt to quicken his apparently slow mind and quiet down his super-charged body. Let Ron's mother tell the story: "We knew in our hearts that he wasn't stupid, that there was something else wrong. We helped him every night with his homework. His father thought he was lazy and stubborn but punishments and bribes were to no avail. Even the neurologist we took him to could find nothing wrong.

"Just about when we were accepting the fact that Ron was slow, we heard about the New York Institute for Child Development. The day we took him there was the turning point of our lives. After a battery of functional, neurological, biochemical and educational tests, they discovered that Ron was hypoglycemic and had a perceptual disorder. They prescribed a high protein, low carbohydrate diet and megavitamins. They gave him eye exercises. The family pediatrician scoffed, but within six months Ron's report card improved. He's calm now and he can concentrate. In one year, he jumped two grade levels in reading, arithmetic and spelling. What more can we ask for?"

Twelve-year-old Ron is happy, too. Offer him a piece of chocolate and he turns it down. "I'm sticking to the diet and the vitamins. School is easier for me now. The teachers and the kids don't pick on me anymore. I'm doing fine, getting better and better."

The Chemistry Of Achievement
And Underachievement

While the New York Institute for Child Development treats the severely brain-injured as well as those with minimal brain dysfunction, their primary thrust is with the underachiever and their results are impressive.

Alan C. Levin, M.D. medical director of the Institute and a member of the American Academy of Pediatrics, glowed as he discussed the program in his pleasant office at the Institute at 36 East 36th Street.

"More than three quarters of all children seen here have a basic biochemical problem or a physical problem, such as poor visual, motor or auditory function. When a child comes here, he is put through a series of biochemical and neurological tests, including tests for low blood sugar, allergies, thyroid malfunction, hormone and trace mineral deficiencies. Visual, auditory and tactile perceptions are evaluated. The Institute treats the child, guides the parents and keeps in touch with the school. About 80 percent of all the children show marked improvement, often within weeks. Many will reach their normal class level, depending on their I.Q., of course."

The program is triple pronged: a diet regimen plus sensori-motor therapy and treatment aimed at whatever other physical disorders are indicated. Dr. Donald L. Gutstein, the Institute's nutritionist, explained how they evaluate a child's dietary needs. "The diet regimen is determined by assessing the biochemical tests, monitoring for food allergies and reviewing the child's dietary habits. Specific allergies are uncovered by charting the child's behavior and food intake throughout the day. Also, we ask the family to record for one week everything the child eats, and from this we estimate the protein and carbohydrate content and the food additives."

The diet prescribed eliminates refined sugar, refined flour and food additives. All preservatives and artificial sweeteners are excluded. The child is instructed to eat high protein, low carbohydrate meals and protein snacks. Fresh, raw juices and vegetables are encouraged.

In addition to the diet, specific vitamins and minerals are usually prescribed, initially consisting of B_3, B_6, C, E, pantothenic acid and calcium, the dosage being determined by the levels found on the tests and by the child's age and size. When allergies are noted, complete avoidance of the food or foods is mandatory.

Just as important to rehabilitation, says director Judith Dowd, is sensori-motor therapy, since all these children have difficulty coordinating at one or more developmental levels. They may have problems hopping, skipping, eye tracking, handwriting, ball catching. Therapy includes balance training, gross motor organization (lateral and cross lateral movements on command), fine motor organization (eye and finger exercises) and eye-hand organization (overhead ladder and eye-hand tracking). All exercise programs are designed individually according to the needs of the child. They are administered at the Institute but home programs are prepared for youngsters who cannot attend sessions in New York.

How Laura Recovered Her Self

Many of these children have high I.Q.'s. Laura is a cute nine-year-old perfectionist with a peaches and cream complexion, whose native intelligence withered under the burden of a malfunction of her adrenal glands, low blood sugar and perceptual disorder. Not too long ago, she lagged far behind her classmates in reading and writing because she reversed letters and skipped lines. Her sickly skin tone worried her parents who believed it was an indication of a physical disorder. Though a timid child who spoke in whispers and hid behind her mother's skirts, she shattered her family with constant crying spells and her inability to sleep.

"We finally discovered that her emotional and learning problems were biochemical in origin and we stopped using the Freudian umbrella," says Laura's mother, who took her child from doctor to doctor in an attempt to help her. "The New York Institute for Child Development found the causes of her difficulties. With the change in her diet, the megavitamin supplement, and the sensori-motor program, there was soon a noticeable change in her personality as well as in her school work. Instead of getting up at the crack of dawn, she now sleeps nine hours a night and has to be awakened. She speaks up now and participates in discussion. Her coordination is better and there is improvement in her vision, although she still needs visual training.

"When Laura goes off her diet and eats junk at a party, she may get a crying jag. Then she starts reversing letters and her reading comprehension suffers. But this condition improves after she resumes her diet. Laura is now in the fourth grade and keeping up with her classmates."

The interaction between mind and body is an intuitive gut wisdom probably as old as mankind. Oriental philosophy postulated that the mind controls the body. But the body also controls the mind, and the vanguard of the medical profession is treating brain dysfunction through biochemistry. They believe that nutrition to the brain affects the nervous system which controls the learning process.

"We are aware that the approach to this problem is multifaceted," said Dr. Levin. "The treatment involves a medical, nutritional, functional and educational assessment. We've treated over 1,500 children and we know that our therapy works. Parents, teachers and the youngsters themselves have moved from a hopeless acceptance of their learning disabilities to a positive, dynamic program. Of course, the earlier you get a child the better, because psychological problems inevitably follow learning problems."

If nutrition is so effective with the brain dysfunctioned, will it also increase the learning ability of the normal child? William T. Mullineaux, Clinical Director of the Institute says *yes*. "We believe that harmful food additives, white flour and excessive sugar are the culprits that upset the normal functioning of the brain. We tested the effect of controlled food and vitamins on normal children in a Harlem nursery and found a 20 percent increase in I.Q. over a period of a year. There is no doubt that diet affects learning performance."

Nutrition appears to be a powerful aid in helping normal youngsters achieve their potential as well as an important weapon in attacking the learning problems of the brain dysfunctioned. The New York Institute of Child Development is showing the way.

132. Stuttering Can Be Overcome

His face reddens and contorts, his eyelids flutter, his speech muscles mobilize. The stutterer is tense; he is afraid to speak. He has been through this before and anticipates his stuttering. He hears the staccato sounds of an obstinate word and senses the impatience—possibly even scorn or pity—of those who are listening. The harder he tries not to stutter, the more difficult it is for him to avoid it. He is caught in a self-perpetuating cycle in which he becomes more and more frustrated in his attempt to speak clearly.

Why does he stutter? Is stuttering a psychoneurosis, an inherited disturbance in the central nervous system, a bad habit, or a combination of these? The experts still don't agree. Not too long ago stuttering was believed to be the result of forcing handedness—for example, forcing a left-handed child to use his right hand. The possible link between handedness and stuttering led London researchers, Drs. Gavin Andrews and Mary Harris, to conduct a study of 80 stutterers of whom 56 were right-handed, 21 were ambidextrous and three were left-handed. But in analyzing 80 nonstutterers, 52 were found to be right-handed, 23 were ambidextrous and five had experienced a change in handedness. This and similar findings helped to discredit the old theory that associates stuttering with handedness.

What probably lay at the bottom of this tradition was the knowledge that speech is controlled by the dominant cerebral hemisphere and that the dominant hemisphere, or side, of the brain was on the left in right-handed people and on the right for left-handed people. According to Franklin Brook, speech therapist and author of *Stammering and Its Treatment* (London, 1957), "Lack of cerebral dominance is believed to be much more frequently associated with incidence of stammering." In other words, neither the left nor the right side of the brain dominates the stutterer's speech, which results in his inability to speak normally.

Dr. John Paul Brady, a psychiatrist at the University of

Pennsylvania School of Medicine, whose approach to the treatment of stuttering was described at the 124th annual meeting of the American Psychiatric Association in May of 1968, offers additional insight into the nature of stuttering. "The disorder called stuttering may be viewed as consisting of two components which continuously interact: an abnormal speech pattern (dysfluency) and anxiety or tension in a variety of speaking situations" (*American Journal of Psychiatry*, December, 1968).

Anxiety Sustains Stuttering

Abnormal speech patterns are first noticeable in children two to six years old. Children this age often have difficulty expressing themselves. Speech is new to them, and it's not uncommon for them to stumble as they try to put what they are thinking into words. The primary stammerer, often a nervous or high-strung child, has speech that is a little more cluttered than is usual for a child his age. But although he hesitates and repeats words more frequently than his playmates the child is neither aware nor anxious about his difficulty in expressing his thoughts. He doesn't try to avoid stuttering but merely accepts it when it occurs. While three to four percent of all children stutter, they often outgrow it, and stuttering persists in only one out of a hundred. The child who is a primary stammerer may come out of it by himself, but sometimes professional help is needed. However, the best way to help a child overcome his handicap is not to treat it as such but try to keep him *unaware* of his speech disorder.

From ages six to eight the condition develops into what is known as secondary stammering, persisting often as a result of over-anxious parents who have caused the child to be self-conscious about his speech imperfections. They are frightened by the prospect of their child's growing up to be a stutterer. They fear he will be socially unacceptable and that stuttering will be a block to any vocation they have hopes of for him. So the child is coached whenever he opens his mouth with "encouraging" remarks such as "Don't talk too fast" or "Take a breath and think before you speak." They hope this will break him of the habit, but unfortunately, it has an inhibiting effect on the child. He becomes self-conscious, worried that he will stutter, afraid to speak. He becomes tense and, inevitably, he stutters.

Even the lucky child with knowledgeable parents who ignore his early tendency to stutter, still has to get by in the playground where his friends will tease him when he stutters.

The adult stutterer usually has no trouble speaking alone or to animals or children too young to evaluate the quality of the stutterer's speech. Social situations are his downfall. He knows he stutters. He becomes anxious about speaking. He stutters again. If his condition is not severe, however, only stress situations or those that create much tension and anxiety cause him to stutter—for example, if he is called upon to speak in front of an audience. If his condition is severe, it is almost impossible for him to speak to others, regardless of the situation. A mere "good morning" from a neighbor might trigger an embarrassed, muddled response.

It is regrettable that not all adult stutterers attempt therapy. Many attribute their impediment to "nerves" and try to live with it, however unhappily.

Today's therapists, who understand that stuttering is aggravated by the selfconscious stutterer's attempt to avoid stuttering, often use treatment that distracts the speaker from hearing his own voice when speaking. Dr. Colin Cherry, whose therapy was described in the November 21, 1955, issue of *Newsweek,* asked stammerers to read simple texts while they were deafened by loud noises heard through headphones. In 24 out of 25 cases improvement was "remarkable." The one exception was a man who worked in a noisy environment and therefore was not distracted by the din heard through the headphones.

Mannerisms Become A Crutch

As a stutterer tries to control the stuttering he anticipates, his speech is accompanied by muscle tenseness sometimes resulting in grimaces, trembling (either in the lips or in the whole body), coughing and fist-clenching. Also, the stutterer often speaks rapidly in an attempt to get the words out without any further embarrassing delay, which only contributes to more stuttering. When the difficult word is at last released, the stutterer "rationalizes" subconsciously that his behavior has helped him through one tough spot so, no doubt, it will help him again. He continues to twitch, tremble or repeat whatever mannerisms he may have.

Realizing how much the stutterer relies on stuttering behavior to "help" him speak, some therapists use negative reinforcement, or punishment, whenever their patients exhibit these mannerisms. The minute the stutterer coughs, for example, to fill in the time while he is bracing himself for a difficult word just ahead in the text he is reading, the therapist shouts "wrong!" or pushes a button that gives the patient a shock. Although it may seem cruel, the fact is that by being punished, the stutterer learns not to lean on the behavior to which he is accustomed and in time to abandon it completely. By getting rid of the mannerisms, he conquers half the disorder.

Three-Part Therapy Works Best

But the efficacy of using only this method—or only psychotherapy—is questioned by other therapists, such as Dr. Brady, who feel that it is not sufficient treatment to keep the stutterer from falling back again into the old pattern once he is outside the therapist's office. A more significant treatment of adult stuttering, Dr. Brady feels, consists of three techniques of behavior modification: *speech habit retraining,* use of an *electric metronome* and *systematic desensitization.* All three methods complement each other and can be administered in varying degrees depending on the severity of the condition. Speech habit retraining and the use of the metronome help to rectify the stutterer's abnormal speech patterns, while systematic desensitization gradually alleviates the anxiety and tension provoked by speaking situations.

In retraining speech habits, the therapist asks the patient to read in a slow, relaxed manner. When a block comes along he is not to struggle with it, as he customarily does, but must stop and go back to an earlier, easier point in the text. If the therapist discovers that the patient is reverting to his old speech habits, i.e., speaking rapidly, over-tensing his speech muscles or struggling with a difficult word, he flashes a red light, a signal to the patient to relax and start over again. As the patient acquires fluency, his reading rate is accelerated to a normal 150 to 200 words per minute. Later on, the patient can put down the book and try conversing with the therapist. Both reading and conversing with some kind of a signal device can be continued at home.

Since the tendency of the typical stutterer is to speak rapidly, the metronome is a useful tool that forces him to slow down to the pace it sets, thereby retraining his rate of speech. The patient is given first a desk metronome, the kind pianists use, and must pace each syllable of his speech to the regular beat of the instrument. At the start of his retraining, the stutterer's speech is paced with a 60-beat per minute speed and as his fluency increases, the rate is set at 100 to 120 beats per minute, a tempo that puts his speech in the normal range. As the patient continues to improve, the desk metronome is replaced by an electronic metronome, built into a small hearing aid and worn behind the ear. This battery-operated device has two controls which vary its rate and volume. If the patient has trouble, he can slow the rate of the metronome, and as he becomes more confident, he can lower the volume until the ticking can no longer be heard and he is on his own.

Dr. Brady reports that the wearing period varies from weeks of use by one patient to perhaps permanent use of the metronome by another.

Shrinking Sensitivity

What about those stutterers who can't cope with high stress situations despite speech habit retraining and the use of a metronome? These are the stutterers who need extra help to get them through difficult speaking situations, which produce in them immense anxiety and tenseness. In introducing his therapy, Dr. Brady cites a technique developed by J. Wolpe (*Psychotherapy by Reciprocal Inhibition,* Stanford University Press, 1958), which is known as systematic desensitization and is particularly helpful to those stutterers suffering neurotic disorders. In order to reduce the sensitivity of the stutterer so that he is able to face situations that ordinarily create extreme anxiety, the patient is asked to imagine a series of speaking scenes beginning with the least tense and proceeding to what is the most tense for him. In Dr. Brady's program, the patient not only imagines but actually ad libs his way through each scene, as though it were actually taking place.

Out of an estimated two million stuttering Americans, there might be an Aristotle, a Darwin, a Winston Churchill among them, who, with treatment and encouragement, can rise above his handicap just as those great historical figures did. Even one of the leading authorities on speech therapy, Dr. Wendell Johnson, was himself a stutterer until he was 37 years old. Stutterers come from all walks of life, from all levels of intelligence. With the promise of this new approach to the treatment of stuttering, perhaps freedom of speech can at last be enjoyed by all.

133. A Hyperactive Child Needs Nutrients, Not Drugs

A prominent psychiatrist, practicing in New York City, has found that by shunning drugs and administering large, therapeutic doses of certain vitamins to children with hyperactivity, he has gotten even better results than have ever been claimed for the dangerous amphetamines. In effect, he points out, he has found a way to improve or cure the health problem responsible for the learning disability, instead of merely masking the problem and leaving it untreated, which is what drug administration does.

The man who has spoken out against drugging hyperactive school children is Allan Cott, M.D., whose use of megavitamin therapy to treat psychoses was described in an earlier chapter. Dr. Cott is psychiatric consultant to the New York Institute of Child Development and maintains his own private psychiatric practice as well. He says that he would like to eliminate use of Ritalin and the amphetamines, the two types of drugs that have gained notoriety in calming hyperactive children. He says that their quieting effect wears off too soon and that they may produce dangerous side effects. Besides, he says, the child's real problem is not the hyperactivity (that is but a symptom), but an internal biochemical disorder that responds to massive doses of vitamins B_2, B_3, B_6, C and E, as well as to a change in diet.

Exchanging Old Symptoms For New
While those who back behavior-altering drugs for children claim that the problem ends with the onset of adolescence, they are speaking only about the hyperactivity. Dr. Cott found that adolescence only brings on slightly different symptoms.

"Actually," he says, "the first group of children I saw who had learning disabilities were adolescents who weren't doing well in junior high school or in their late elementary grades. They were perfectly normal children, in schools for normal children. They just couldn't learn and they couldn't concentrate. Their mothers remarked about them that they would try to read, but after a few mistakes would get up, uneasy. Taking a long history on these kids, I found that the outstanding symptom that they suffered earlier in life was hyperactivity, even though by adolescence the hyperactivity was, for the most part, gone."

What made Dr. Cott decide to try large doses of vitamins in reducing hyperactivity in children?

"I've been treating psychiatric disorders, that is, mental illness, with the use of massive doses of vitamins for a number of years," he says. "I found such good results in the treatment of adults that I extended its use to the children in treating childhood mental disorders. The improvements were more marked than in adults, and produced more dramatic results.

"One of the things that I found while I was treating these children was that as their illness began to recede and was at least under reasonable control, their hyperactivity, which is one of the major symptoms of all children who suffer from any kind of emotional disorder, subsided. As the hyperactivity subsided, the children were able to begin to learn."

Then a mother brought her 19-year-old son, a college student, to see Dr. Cott. This case was to be a turning point in the treatment of hyperactive children with vitamins.

Reading Had Been Agony

"The boy and his mother told me that he had, with the exertion of the greatest kind of effort, gotten through high school and into his first year of college. They came to see me when he came home for the Christmas holidays," Dr. Cott recalls. "He said that his friends would finish their day's homework in about two hours or so, while he frequently would have to work eight hours to do the same work. Because reading, concentration and comprehension were very difficult, he would have to read a paragraph over and over before he could absorb the meaning.

"I put him on massive doses of vitamins, those suitable for an adult of his height and weight, and about two months later received a letter from his mother. I forwarded it to the American Schizophrenia Association so that they could have it on file, if they wanted, because it was a kind of testimonial for orthomolecular therapy that I hadn't seen anywhere before.

"You see, here was a 19-year-old boy, and for the first time in his mother's memory of him, he would sit and read a book with pleasure. Up until that time, reading had been agony for him.

"I began speaking about him to the staff of the Institute. They began to work with the vitamins. When they had seen a sufficient number of cases in order to have a fair sized sample, they were astonished, just as I had been, at the results that they were getting. They then set up a department for the treatment of learning disabilities, combining their standard methods of treatment with the use of the vitamins. A thirty pound child might receive one gram of vitamin B_3, 200 milligrams of B_6, one gram of C, and 400 to 800 units of vitamin E. As a result, they saw a marked upswing in rate of child development.

Vitamins Need Time To Take Hold

"In the meantime, in my own practice, I continued treating these children I saw who had learning disabilities and always got the same results. If the parents were persistent and stuck with the medication, the children began to improve. The parents who tried it and got very little results were the parents who had given it up much too early. It's not like a drug."

That is, the vitamins require a longer time to take hold because they are building up a healthy cellular foundation, step by step, and not just eliminating symptoms the way that the drugs do. Rather, the slower working vitamins actually take hold inside the body where there is a demand for more of a nutrient than, perhaps, the diet can provide. Either the nutrient wasn't in the food, or the food couldn't be absorbed properly by the body. Once inside, the vitamins have staying power. Their effect is felt for a long time afterward because they encourage basic biochemical changes in the child, which may mean the reduction of hyperactivity and a new ability to sit down, learn enthusiastically, and work constructively. And they have no side effects.

Don't drugs do the same thing? Drugs do indeed slow down the child's overactivity. But they are unwelcome guests who, when they visit, do more than that for which they were invited, and then leave you to clean up the consequences.

Drug Therapy Is Fashionable But Dangerous

Dr. Cott says, "Ritalin, as you know, is in great vogue now. The amphetamines, they come around again and again just like hypnosis; it runs in about 10 to 20 year cycles as popularity advances. The amphetamines and other stimulants hold the same kind of cyclical interest for medicine. But the use of amphetamines and Ritalin on children really infuriates me. Ritalin and amphetamines do, in many children, cut down the hyperactivity. Actually, the use of these medications was begun on an empirical basis because it was found in the treating of disturbed children that if you gave them a tranquilizer, it would stimulate them. A sedative would stimulate, whereas a stimulant like Ritalin or the amphetamines would tranquilize them. They began using it for this reverse effect that it produced.

"Both these stimulants interfere with sleep, they interfere with appetite, and I would certainly not use Ritalin or the amphetamines in an adolescent because they are addicting. When one uses Ritalin or the amphetamines in learning disabilities, one is then committed to keep these drugs going for several years at least. I don't know how long some of the doctors who are treating them would keep them on the drugs.

"Frequently the child's disturbance is so great that he is in imminent danger or the parents are in imminent danger of having their child expelled from school. I find it necessary to use some medication, some drug. Most often I will use something like Mellaril in small doses, because Mellaril seems to be one of the few tranquilizers which do not give the adverse effect. Except in a rare case, I find Mellaril to be a benefit. The use of Ritalin or the amphetamines for a short period of time would be acceptable in extreme cases, but not over a long period of time."

Dr. Cott says that the children usually show a noticeable response to the vitamin therapy within weeks or months, and after that the initial improvement continues, often for years. The reasons, he says, are that the vitamins get at the basic disorders.

Vitamin therapy, then, simply reinforces the child's diet with nutrients which he should be getting all the time. Dr. Cott believes that a nutritious diet is most important, not just to the hyperactive child, but to every child. While some hyperactive children need massive doses of specific vitamins, others—as we'll see in the next chapter—are suffering because of substances in the food that they eat every day.

134. Food Additives Trigger Hyperactivity

Chemical additives, especially artificial flavors and colors, in processed convenience-type foods are causing learning and behavior problems in children, according to prominent allergist Dr. Ben Feingold of the Kaiser-Permanente Medical Group in San Francisco.

A big problem facing modern educators is the so-called hyperactive child who is unable to sit still and concentrate long enough to learn in the classroom, says Dr. Feingold. In California, the number of affected children rose from two percent to an average of 25 percent in just 10 years, he reports, paralleling a sharp rise in food additive consumption by the American public.

By taking away the junk foods, Dr. Feingold has been able to cure childhood hyperactivity quickly and dramatically in many cases. "We can turn these children on and off at will," he observed, "just by regulating their diet."

Hyperactivity Traced To Salicylates

The allergist makes crystal clear that the common denominators—the villains—for most hyperactive children are *salicylates*.

The low molecular makeup of these chemicals enables them to be quickly broken down and absorbed by the body, where they may interfere with the functioning of the prostaglandin family. And this causes considerable biochemical confusion for some people—even mayhem! Aspirin is 77 percent salicylate but is far from being the only source of this allergenic chemical.

The salicylates, in addition to being a component of various drugs and occurring in some foods naturally, are used in a vast array of additives, particularly as artificial coloring agents and artificial flavorings.

They appear as antioxidants, leaveners, thickeners—the list is practically endless, Dr. Feingold points out.

So people with really serious salicylate sensitivity, such as many hyperkinetic children, are in deep trouble, unless they're alerted to the situation and can avoid the offenders.

Bottled beverages, candy, ice cream, dessert powders, cake and frosting mixes, baked goods and sausages usually contain salicylates. Natural sources include tomatoes, plums, berries, grapes, apricots, wine, wine vinegar, tea—a complete list is to be found in Dr. Feingold's comprehensive book, *An Introduction to Clinical Allergy* (Charles C. Thomas, 1973). "It took me two years to write and is based on 40 years experience," he says. "I've put everything I know into it in the hope that people in the health professions, for whom it's meant, will understand the enormity of the salicylate problem." But as the title indicates, the whole field of allergy and sensitivity is encompassed.

Fantastic Results From Home Cooking

What's brought "fantastic" results, to use Dr. Feingold's own word, with the disturbed children, is a diet kept as free as possible of all salicylates. But it takes some doing to get mothers to revise meal planning and preparation in this age of convenience foods. The Feingold regimen requires "starting from scratch" and switching completely to "home cooking."

But because hyperactivity is such a baffling problem to everyone involved, parents who come to Dr. Feingold are usually willing to try anything and fully cooperate.

He immediately takes the youngsters off drugs which have been prescribed in a desperate effort to bring them under some degree of control when they disrupt entire classrooms or their home life.

Then the patients are given the elimination diet he took 18 years to develop. And in two or three weeks, Dr. Feingold says, they're well on their way to "normal" behavior and often show increased scholastic ability within a month's time. Many of these children have high I.Q.'s, but hyperkinesis tends to disrupt their attention span and learning process.

If there's deviation from the special Feingold diet, though, the disturbance syndrome immediately returns. So parents are admonished to "religiously" follow the diet regimen, which means that 80 percent of all food additives must be eliminated from menus. And since there are some 3,200 artificial flavors alone, in addition to all the other additives, that takes some doing!

Most Meals Are A Chemical Disaster

Compare this regimen with the typical diet of most children and adults. Dr. Feingold describes an average child's breakfast as being a meal to bring shudders to the knowing: a cereal loaded with nonessential flavors and colors, added to entice the child's appetite; a beverage, either chocolate or other drink, most of which are rich with various artificial flavors and colors; pancakes made from a mix, or frozen waffles laced with tartrazine dyes to make them golden yellow; or frozen French toast.

Further, says the allergist, a concerned and conscientious mother often gives her child a chewable synthetic vitamin tablet that may be artifically flavored and colored.

Then to cap the ironical situation, which is tragic as well, Dr. Feingold says, "a child may be given a dose of the hyperkinetic control drugs before he gets off to school. And there he may ingest hot dogs, luncheon meats, ice cream and various beverages having reactive chemicals. He's particularly likely to drink Gatorade, which sturdy athletes on TV are always encouraging kids to select. This, Feingold asserts indignantly, "is poison for many—it's loaded with tartrazine! Is it any wonder that our children are jumping out of their skins and failing to learn?"

One of Dr. Feingold's most startling exhibits is a graph projected to show the annual increase in dollar value of the output of artificial flavors and soft drinks, which parallels a graph for increased incidence of hyperkinesia and learning disabilities among schoolchildren in the U.S. Both graphs cover a ten year period, and both are headed rapidly upward.

A logical question here is—shouldn't the FDA be concerned about this sensitivity to additives that Dr. Feingold has clearly demonstrated? To this, the allergist answers an emphatic "yes." He has made appeals to FDA officials to not only thoroughly test the offending chemicals, but to clearly identify them on labels, not just as being artificial colors or flavors, but what they are, precisely. Such a study would be comparatively simple, he says, because all the chemicals in question have similar structures.

"I say that if all these thousands of flavorings and colors are so closely related in structure, they *all have to be eliminated*," insists Dr. Feingold. Just removing Red dye No. 2 from the market isn't by any means enough. The aniline colors used in hair dyes, he adds, can cause very serious consequences.

Dr. Feingold is urging the FDA and manufacturers to make

products available which don't contain the offending chemicals at all.

Needless Chemicals Pose Needless Risks

"I'm certainly not a nihilist," he says. "As the world's population grows and as our food supplies have been built up in vast quantities, technology and industry have had to find ways to preserve foodstuffs, to keep them insect free." But while all additives can't be condemned out of hand, he believes that many of them really aren't essential. The function of flavors and colors, for example, is merely cosmetic.

"There has to be a balance. We just can't go on increasing the chemicals in the diets of people throughout the planet. Where will it all end if we continue on such a course?" Dr. Feingold wonders. In 1970, more than 3,735,000 pounds of aniline dyes were certified for use in foods, drugs and cosmetics. This is a 15-fold increase in 30 years. What the figures might be on the flavoring agents, considering they're even more widely used, and more varied, one dare not try to guess.

Dr. Feingold adds: "We just don't know the long range effect of the thousands upon thousands of chemicals we're ingesting altogether. There are studies of the toxicity they set up in animals. But what do they do to humans?"

Dr. Feingold's work has centered almost exclusively on the salicylate sensitivity of hyperactive children. Thousands of them are afflicted with this disturbance in the U.S. alone. And calls for help are coming in from everywhere—letters from Puerto Rico, South Africa, Germany—all over. Dr. Feingold says, "We're hoping our program will advance sufficiently so that school systems will move into it throughout the country and throughout the whole world someday."

How extensive the use of additives in foreign lands, Dr. Feingold doesn't know. In France, he says, only 300 are permitted. He wants to get details from other countries, since this will have an important bearing on his work.

Dr. Feingold is also hoping that health professionals will be inspired by *An Introduction to Clinical Allergy* to join in the research on the effects of chemicals in foods so that "we'll have definitive answers to the tremendous problems being created."

(Dr. Feingold also presented his theories in a book intended for the layman, *Your Hyperactive Child*, published by Harper and Row, 1974.)

According to Dr. Feingold, there are as many as 15 different additives in a single cake mix and "you can add a few more for the prepared frosting."

Hopefully, Dr. Feingold says, the word about salicylates will become increasingly publicized. And if even a few mothers can be persuaded to avoid chemical-laden foods, there will be fewer disturbance problems in children to come.

135. Allergies Unhinge The Mind

Is it true that the vast majority of people with mental and behavioral problems, and those with strange "psychosomatic" symptoms are really suffering from their emotions?

Consider this case from the joint files of two New England physicians. The patient, a teenage girl, was racked by depression and suicidal tendencies to the extent that she had to be hospitalized four times during her adolescence. Despite psychiatric attention, she became increasingly withdrawn. Shock treatments were tried but they proved useless. During her last period of hospitalization, which lasted three years, her condition was worse than ever—she had become almost completely withdrawn from reality.

At this point, it was decided to subject her to "provocative testing"—in which extracts of suspected allergenic substances are administered. Not on the skin, as most allergy tests are, but injected or placed under the tongue, where the substance is quickly absorbed. Her physicians, psychiatrist Dr. William Philpott of South Attleboro, Massachusetts, and allergist Dr. Marshall Mandell, director of the New England Foundation for Allergic and Environmental Diseases in Norwalk, Connecticut, learned a great deal from these tests. As described in an article in the *Roche Image of Medicine and Research* (February, 1972), they discovered that the girl was extremely sensitive to several substances. Saccharin made her dizzy, nauseated and anxious. Chlorine, even in concentrations weaker than those in drinking water, made her depressed and afraid to swallow. Lamb meat produced confusion and crying.

Diet Restriction Ends Mental Illness
Her doctors reported that "once these allergens were removed, the patient regained her equilibrium and was eligible for discharge. There has been no recurrence of symptoms since she left

Fuller (the sanitarium) and she is now preparing to enter college."

It would not be unreasonable to conclude from this case history that had the girl been tested for allergies at the age of 13, she might well have been spared all those agonizing years in institutions.

Is this case just one in a thousand? No, says Dr. Mandell, who has helped more than 200 patients with mental symptoms by eliminating allergens from their diet and environment. The trouble is that only a handful of doctors are aware of what is called the Chemical Reaction Syndrome, and how to test for it.

Here is another revealing case history, which Dr. Mandell reported on at the Second International Congress of Social Psychiatry held in London on August 8, 1969. F. D. was a 38-year-old man with a history of childhood asthma and hives. More recently, he had been complaining of severe fatigue, mental confusion, nervous tension and frequent "virus infections." The man was told by a psychiatrist that emotional stress was the underlying cause of his troubles, and that his poor health was due to poor resistance which was the consequence of his unresolved mental problems.

Allergic To 15 Different Foods

Eventually, the man was referred to Dr. Mandell, who administered injections of 21 different food extracts. No less than 15 of these tests evoked "psychiatric" responses. Wheat, for example, made him tense, restless, and produced loud abdominal rumbling. Coffee made him lightheaded and extremely tired. Milk made him dizzy, confused, and gave him a sore throat and "blocked" ears. His fingertips became cold and white. He was also allergic, it turned out, to chicken, eggs, peas, corn and other foods.

Dr. Mandell comments: "It was readily shown that his entire problem was a food allergy syndrome . . . his illness was not of psychic origin and his recurrent misdiagnosed syndrome could not possibly be successfully treated by therapy based on psychiatric concepts. He has been well for one year without any medication or allergy treatment; he avoids the major test-incriminated foods and restricts his intake of minor offenders."

Here is a case typical of so-called mental disturbances of children. A 10-year-old girl came out of the girl's lavatory in school in an extremely confused and disoriented state. When she staggered back to her classroom, she walked into the wall. She did not know who her teacher was, and when her mother was summoned, she did not recognize her, either. Many of the teachers were certain that the girl was psychotic, while others suspected that she had taken some drug in the lavatory.

Fumes Caused Mental Disturbances

What in fact had happened in the bathroom was that the girl had been exposed to the fumes of an antiseptic-deodorant cleaning solution containing pine oil. Tests by Dr. Mandell revealed that the girl was allergic to the chemicals in the pine oil, as well as a number of other chemicals. Prior to the bathroom incident, this girl had been under treatment for asthma and hay fever, and had great difficulty concentrating in school. Among other things, tests revealed that she was highly allergic to methyl alcohol, which was the solvent in the ink used in the school duplicator. When given papers which had been produced by this machine, she became nauseous, dizzy, developed a headache, and was unable to concentrate on her lessons. The same thing happened when she was given felt marking pens to work with, because she was allergic to the toluene solvent in the ink.

Ultimately, it became necessary to replace the gas stove in her home with an electric one, and to remove from the house many powerful chemical cleaners, which had also been causing the girl trouble. When this was done, and some precautions taken at school, the girl greatly improved.

One of the most interesting cases of allergy recorded by Dr. Mandell involved a 33-year-old woman who was extremely hostile and emotionally upset. Soon after she began talking to the doctor, she decided that she could not bear another minute in his office. She had to have a chocolate bar on the way home. In fact, what she really needed was to have one immediately. Dr. Mandell persuaded her to take an allergy test. He placed under her tongue a concentrated extract of chocolate. The patient was not aware of what was contained in the medication. Within a few minutes she became very warm and then very cold. Her speech became slurred, and she was "acutely anxious and confused," to quote Dr. Mandell. Having established that her emotional symptoms were an allergy related to the chocolate, he then gave her another very dilute dose of the extract under her tongue. Within 20 minutes she was smiling, and commenting on how much better she felt.

Chemicals Shock The Brain

"Ecologic mental illness is an important facet of man's total reaction to his natural and synthetic environment," says Dr. Mandell. He suggests that the brain should be considered as a complex shock organ, since many of the environmental contaminants are very common hydrocarbons such as gasoline fumes, tobacco smoke, and natural gas fumes which people contact from day to day. The brain which has the richest blood supply of the body aside from the heart itself, is exposed to these contaminants on a regular basis.

Dr. Mandell does not claim that all mental and emotional problems can be overcome by allergenic treatment. He only suggests that tests for allergies should be among those procedures used when physiological factors in a case seem to indicate that something more than psychogenic causes may be present.

Dr. Mandell has considerable concern for persons who may have committed crimes or been involved in serious traffic accidents because of some allergic reaction. "It would be a shame," he says, "if such persons were confined to mental institutions, some of them perhaps even in catatonic states being fed through stomach tubes with the very foods to which they are allergic."

In a world where chemicals, synthetics, pollutants, and additives of all kinds are encountered in virtually every moment of existence, the potential for mental disturbances arising from ecological factors is awesome. From the work of Dr. Mandell and Dr. Philpott, we already have a fairly good idea of what hypersensitivity to these allergens can mean in terms of misdiagnosis, the savings of a lifetime spent on useless psychiatric treatment, and the waste of human potential. It is still much too early to state with confidence exactly what proportion of so-called "psychiatric" disorders are a result of allergy, except to say that it is certainly significant.

Section 25
Emphysema

136. Emphysema Is Slow Suffocation

Take a deep breath and hold it. Then let it out slowly. It feels good, especially if your lungs are in good shape. But, if you have emphysema, every breath your body takes is pure misery. And that misery is repeated every time you have to breathe.

The onset of emphysema follows no set pattern. Sometimes it begins in childhood with a series of respiratory infections accompanied by difficulty in breathing and early chronic bronchitis. Or it may appear later in life as a slowly developing airway obstruction, finally becoming recognized by the age of 30 or 40.

Regardless of when it is diagnosed, medical authorities have come to recognize the malady as a health menace of potentially epidemic proportions in the United States today. Yet emphysema is a disease whose name is hardly known to the general public. It is something new. Our forefathers did not become debilitated and finally die of their inability to expel stale air from their lungs. The current plague of emphysema is unlike anything known to history. Each year there are at least half a million new cases of emphysema coming under medical care, according to the Department of Health, Education and Welfare. The Social Security system pays out well over $100 million a year in disability benefits for people crippled by emphysema. In 1970 the disease was a primary cause of 30,000 deaths and a contributory cause of another 60,000. And emphysema is increasing its hold on the public faster than any other disease—four times faster than lung cancer and faster even than heart disease.

Emphysema is vicious. Breathing is labored. The patient can't expel enough stale air to take in enough fresh air. Victims work hard to breathe, even while asleep. Every day brings frequent coughing attacks. The heart has to work overtime to pump blood through a damaged pair of lungs.

Linked To Cadmium Pollution

The cause of emphysema has been considered "unknown" although it is generally recognized that the incidence of disease rises with air pollution levels and that it must be related to the deposit of foreign particles in the lungs.

To pinpoint the cause of emphysema is obviously an urgent objective of medical research. In 1973, for the first time, specific information emerged. Two studies published simultaneously in the *American Review Board of Respiratory Disease,* one from Boston University School of Medicine and the other from Washington University Medical Center in St. Louis, both pointed to the mineral cadmium as one important cause, if not the sole cause of emphysema.

Cadmium is a mineral that has long been known to be highly toxic to human beings and that has no value whatsoever in human metabolism. Yet the substance is released into the air by numerous industrial processes, and has become an almost inescapable pollutant. An exposure amounting to only a few micrograms a day—a few thousandths of a tiny milligram—is enough for cadmium, over a period of years, to begin showing its health-destroying and sometimes lethal effects.

During autopsy examinations of people who had been afflicted with emphysema, Dr. Russell N. Hirst, Jr., of Washington University found high amounts of cadmium in the lung tissue. He also found that the extent to which the incapacitating disease had developed correlated closely with the amount of cadmium the lungs contained.

Dr. Gordon L. Snider of Boston University approached the same question in a totally different way, spraying aerosols containing small amounts of cadmium into the air being breathed by laboratory rats. The cadmium-polluted air, he found, induced emphysema in the rats.

The discovery that emphysema can be caused by the accumulation of cadmium in the lungs would help explain the well-established link between cigarette smoking and the development of emphysema. An enlightening study in the *Lancet* (February 5, 1972) which stems from the Clinical Pharmacology section of the Boston Veterans Administration Hospital, points the finger at cigarettes as a major source of cadmium accumulation in the human body. The study, which is a statistical analysis of autopsy findings, finds that smokers accumulate more cadmium in their bodies than nonsmokers, and "in addition, the accumulation in smokers is related to the number of pack-years smoked. It is concluded that tobacco constitutes a major source for cadmium accumulation in man."

Once emphysema takes hold, there is no cure from this debilitating disease that turns a once-healthy individual into little more than a wheezing vegetable, unable to do even the simplest of tasks, such as walking, without the most difficult effort. But as you'll see in the chapters that follow, there are at least two lines of research that offer promise. One is a series of exercises. Although it can't be considered a cure, it allows emphysema sufferers to lead more or less normal lives by getting their lungs working more efficiently. On the other hand, research shows that better nutrition may prevent emphysema from developing in the first place.

Stale Air Is Trapped Inside

Emphysema is relatively easy to picture. Think of an upside down tree inside your chest. That's a "bronchial tree." The trunk is the windpipe. From it extend two main branches, called bronchi. One goes to the left, the other to the right. From each bronchus, smaller offshoots branch off by the thousands. These are called bronchioles. At the end of these are nests of bubble-like air sacs called alveoli. There are millions of them and if they were spread out they would cover an area of about 800 square feet—approximately the equivalent of two tennis courts.

In the daily operation of the lungs, a person breathes in about 600 quarts of oxygen and exhales an equal amount of carbon dioxide. At the alveoli, blood and inhaled air are separated by only a very thin membrane which allows oxygen and nitrogen to diffuse into the bloodstream and carbon dioxide and other gases to pass into the alveoli.

In emphysema, the walls of those air sacs begin to break down. This results in groups of ruptured air sacs combining to form larger sacs which tend to trap carbon dioxide-containing air inside the lungs. Also, the lungs begin to lose their elasticity. In addition, some of the bronchioles which ordinarily pass air upwards and outwards, become partially blocked, making exhalation even more difficult.

Strangely enough, inhalation is not blocked. But as more air comes in from outside and becomes partially trapped, the increased pressure causes larger air traps, called bullae, to form inside the lungs.

So, as a result of emphysema, the patient finds himself with a pair of lungs filled with stale air he really can't exhale. He feels as if he can't catch his breath, when in fact, his lungs are nearly filled with air, albeit bad air. The problem is to get it out so fresh air with oxygen can be brought in. Otherwise, the oxygen level keeps dropping throughout the body because the alveoli can't do their vital work.

As the disease progresses, the bronchial tubes and windpipe degenerate, growing flabby almost to the point of complete collapse. The emphysema patient must literally squeeze the air from his chest. This causes problems because expelling air too forcefully puts a heavy strain on the alveolar walls. Like balloons which have been inflated too long, they lose flexibility and wrinkle when deflated. However, in a normal person, exhalation is a passive act. Air leaves the lungs because of an elastic recoil. The relief is automatic—something done all day long, something we hardly ever think about—until something starts going wrong.

Chronic emphysema has been around for a long time, although never so apparent as it has been since about 1960. In fact, emphysema was relatively unknown until industrial pollution began to blanket the nation in the 40's and 50's. It has gotten worse—much worse—more recently.

Because of the growing air pollution, emphysema has become so prevalent that one doctor, Dr. Russell S. Hastings, a professor of pathology at the University of Southern California, maintains that everyone over 12 years of age has it.

At a January, 1971 meeting of clinical pathologists in Houston, Dr. Hastings said he had examined thousands of lungs and found no really "clean" lungs. "I believe that everyone over 12 has emphysema. I know I can't find a normal lung in anyone over that age."

137. Vitamins That Protect The Lungs

In the present state of the medical art, emphysema is incurable. Because it is a degenerative disease—and scientists generally believe that no way will ever be found to regenerate dead tissue—there may never be a cure. Fortunately, there is increasing evidence that a good diet, adopted soon enough, will make it far less likely that you will ever develop emphysema.

For protection of your lungs, vitamin A and E are the best defense against visible and invisible air pollutants that saturate our environment. New evidence has emerged which points out the protective role played by those vitamins in the face of contaminants invading the human lungs.

According to researchers from Battelle-Northwest's Nutrition and Food Technology Research Section in Richland, Washington, vitamins appear to play a much more vital role in safeguarding lungs from the ravages of air pollutants than has been generally realized.

In their research on pollutants, vitamins and lung health, Dr. Daniel B. Menzel and his associates at Battelle concentrated on the pollutants nitrogen dioxide (NO_2) and ozone (O_3). Nitrogen dioxide is spewed into the atmosphere whenever coal, oil or gasoline are burned. Ozone is produced when nitrogen dioxide is exposed to the sun's ultraviolet rays and interacts with hydrocarbons and other gases to form photochemical smog.

Ozone is so poisonous that when it is in the atmosphere at the level of .35 parts per million, Los Angeles school authorities are warned not to let children jump, skip and run during recess hours.

Functions As An Antioxidant

The key to vitamin E's protective role against NO_2 and O_3 is the nutrient's antioxidant property. That is, it inhibits oxidation which is the chemical result of oxygen's combining with another substance. When attacked by nitrogen dioxide or ozone, both the unsaturated fatty acids which are bountifully present in the lung tissue, and vitamin A, another material that oxidizes readily, are protected by vitamin E's presence.

Protection of vitamin A—that is, conserving it rather than having it destroyed through oxidation—is essential for the maintenance of healthy mucus-secreting lung tissue.

When vitamin E protects these substances from oxidation, it prevents the formation both of dangerous hydrogen peroxide—a toxic and cell-killing material—and of "free radicals," unattached molecular fragments which are highly destructive to every cell with which they come in contact.

The Battelle researchers set up an experiment to determine just how well vitamin E functions to protect the lungs from the damaging oxidation of pollution. Two sets of rats, one on a vitamin E-deficient diet and the other on a diet supplemented by vitamin E, were exposed to air polluted by NO_2. Subsequently their lungs were analyzed. It was found that those deficient in vitamin E had significantly lower levels of unsaturated fatty acids in their lung tissues than did those protected by vitamin E supplements. In other words, the breakdown through oxidation and formation of toxic materials had been significantly halted by vitamin E's presence.

In another experiment, two sets of rats—again one deficient in vitamin E and the other well-supplied—were exposed to a stream of air containing 1 ppm of ozone. Those deficient in the vitamin showed early signs of pulmonary stress and soon died; the other group survived twice as long in the ozone atmosphere. Dr. Menzel published these results in the *Journal of Agricultural and Food Chemistry,* March, 1972.

Even though its potency as a lung protector has been thus demonstrated, vitamin E is not believed to play a specific role in building lung health. All it does is preserve the purity of other materials—chief among them vitamin A—which do directly enter into the health of the lung tissues.

Essential For Mucus Production

A leading authority on vitamin A, Dr. Luigi M. DeLuca of the Massachusetts Institute of Technology, has frequently stressed that vitamin A is essential to the lung's lining—or epithelium. It is not just the lungs, but mucous membranes throughout the body—the mouth, the entire respiratory tract, the gastrointestinal tract—that require vitamin A for maintenance of the mucus-secreting mechanism.

Emphysema

The flow of mucus, and the waving motion of the mucus-bathed cilia—microscopic hair-like projections—are the respiratory system's primary defense against invading microorganisms and pollutants from the atmosphere. Beyond this consideration, the lung itself must remain moist and lubricated by mucus in order to properly perform its function of exchanging new air for old.

Dr. DeLuca postulates that vitamin A "steers" the epithelial cells to differentiate (that is, specialize) into mucus-producing cells. In laboratory animals, he noted, squamous (scaly) cells instead of normal mucus-secreting cells tend to develop when vitamin A is absent from the diet.

Protected by sufficient vitamin E, vitamin A can go about its work. It will not *cure* emphysema, however. Once the degeneration has set in, it is going to remain for life.

138. Exercise Makes Breathing Easier

The idea that exercise—not resignation and stagnation—is the proper road to helping emphysema victims was first explored in 1961 and 1962 by Dr. Harry Bass, who was then at the University of Alabama Medical Center. Increasing numbers of people with emphysema were being seen at the center.

Dr. Bass wanted to test his theory that exercise under carefully-controlled conditions, and with close medical direction, might cut down on the total disability which seemed to be the fate of emphysema victims.

His patients trained against a progressively increased exercise load every day. Two of seven men, previously unable to work, were able to return to their jobs. His results were not clear, however, because oxygen was administered to the patients, in addition to the exercise.

When Dr. Bass transferred to Peter Bent Brigham Hospital in Boston, he devised a more carefully controlled study. Riding a stationary bicycle loaded with sophisticated electronic circuitry was the only prescribed exercise. As the patients improved their ability to pedal, however, they automatically started walking more. In fact, each patient wore a pedometer which recorded this new-found mobility.

Learned To Use Oxygen More Efficiently

In a report in the *Journal of the American Medical Association* (December 23, 1969), Dr. Bass summarized nine years of work in what is considered a controversial area.

Eleven patients with chronic obstructive lung disease had completed an 18-week program of graded bicycle exercises: Dr. Bass' measurements showed the training was an effective form of therapy, although not necessarily the end-all in therapy.

The 11 patients entered the exercise program after thorough medical screening. All had chronic obstructive lung disease with dyspnea (difficulty in breathing) while walking at an ordinary pace on level ground or while washing or dressing. But they were motivated to lead a more active life.

Dr. Bass said that all patients felt better at the end of the 18-week program and had increased their activities of daily living.

Tabulated results of the program showed some improvement in the functioning of the lungs. "My patients all have a decreased pulse rate and use oxygen more efficiently," Dr. Bass said.

"Many of these people had been housebound except to sit on the porch. Now they can take walks and go to the movies."

Why the improvements? "I am still uncertain," Dr. Bass replied. "It is probably a combined heart, lung, and total body effect.

"It may be that by decreasing the pulse rate the heart may do as much work with less effort. This is still speculation."

Since then, Dr. Bass has had even more remarkable results. One of his patients, a 50-year-old suburban Boston housewife with a history of chronic lung disease dating back 20 years, could walk a few feet—on one of her good days. She was essentially bedridden.

"By clenching my hands so hard the nails cut into my palms, taking a deep breath, and pushing off with a lung full of air, I could get across the hallway," she said. Less than a year after beginning the exercise program she reported her condition in these words:

"Last week I was driven into Boston, got out of the car and entered an office building, walked down a long hallway to the elevator bank, took an elevator to the 10th floor. I traveled down another hall, entered an office and there spent an hour talking. I then descended to the street and was driven home. I had no trouble and stayed well within safe physical limits. I still had a margin of strength."

Another man, a laborer who was previously working half a week, was able now to put in a full week's work, after exercising.

Such research has resulted in techniques to help make life more bearable for the emphysema patient. They offer no cure, but positive aids in reducing discomfort and panic-producing experiences stemming from a dyspnea attack.

Patients Taught New Ways To Breathe

More and more physical therapy departments in hospitals around the country are introducing courses in breathing retraining, the net result of which is to generate confidence in the afflicted individual and enable him to become more active.

Instead of being chained to an oxygen tank, people are able to return to once-simple tasks like light housework, walking, climbing stairs, and shopping.

Many of these programs involve simple exercises, although not necessarily the stationary cycling used by Dr. Bass. It is impossible to give here a general exercise program that will be adequate for all—or even most—people. For victims of emphysema, either too little exercise or too much can be dangerous. Each condition is unique, and each exercise program must be individually tailored by a doctor.

Often the patient is first taught the necessity of relaxing neck and shoulder muscles. Then diaphragmatic breathing exercises start—forcing air out, clear to the base of the lungs, so fresh air can be brought in. There are also specific exercises for strengthening abdominal muscles.

Pursed-lip breathing is another favorite—by forcing the air through nearly-closed lips, the bronchi, bronchioles and windpipe open wider to let the air out.

Patients learn to coordinate exertion with expiration (exhaling). They breathe out when they stoop to tie a shoe or take a step up the stairs. Activity is encouraged within limits, of course, and under doctor's instructions. If a dyspnea attack threatens, the patient is taught to sit down, hands on legs, head far forward, and breathe out.

Learning how to breathe effectively and with minimum effort pays big dividends to the person whose lung capacity has been reduced and virtually lost through disease. Many have learned to do it, throwing off breathing habits of years and following the simple rules taught by doctors and therapists. The beauty of it is—no matter if substantial portions of the lungs have been destroyed—life can still go on at a reduced pace.

It isn't easy at first—it takes plenty of self-discipline—but it's worth the effort, say those who've been through the mill!

Section 26
Epilepsy

139. Ancient Myths Yield To New Medical
Knowledge

139. Ancient Myths Yield To New Medical Knowledge

From biblical times, individuals have been afflicted with "seizures"—mysterious fits during which they fell to the ground and foamed at the mouth. Perfectly normal, happy, intelligent people the rest of the time, they suddenly appeared to have been bewitched when a seizure overtook them. Seizures, being unpredictable, often occurred in public, to the horror and fear of onlookers. Thus, during past ages, a whole tradition of the supernatural grew up around epilepsy. Plainly these sufferers were possessed of demons. Why else would they froth at the mouth, twitch convulsively and be unaware of what had transpired after they awoke from the sleep that follows epileptic seizures?

As superstition waned and people ceased to believe overtly in witchcraft, some other notions grew up to explain the phenomenon of epilepsy. Perhaps, since this disease seemed to be hereditary, it was caused by sins of the parents. It led to insanity, people said, or it led to feeble-mindedness. It was caused by masturbation, they said. Epileptics became criminals, they said; they should not marry or have children. In fact, laws were passed in many states forbidding the marriage of epileptics.

Today, medical learning has wiped out once and for all every single one of these misconceptions about epilepsy. However, much of the old superstition remains in those dark, unexplored corners of people's minds where are hidden all the silly fallacies we hate so much to give up, because giving up the fallacies means that we have to make an effort to think our way through to the truth. So the families of some epileptics still conceal the disorder from their friends and neighbors. Epileptics themselves may feel shame, as though there were some terrible disgrace attached to epilepsy which does not apply to diabetes, arthritis or tuberculosis, for example. Yes, incredible as it seems, there are still individuals in our enlightened twentieth century who whisper dark, shameful gossip about those who suffer from one of the most mysterious and dread disorders—epilepsy.

Social Stigma Is Disappearing

Fortunately, there is evidence that such discrimination and prejudice against epileptics is becoming more and more the exception to the rule. A Gallup Poll conducted at five year intervals in behalf of the National Institutes of Health revealed that in 1949, only 45 percent of all Americans believed epileptics should have equal employment opportunities. In 1974, that figure had increased to 81 percent (*The Washington Post*, May 16, 1974).

In 1949, 24 percent of those interviewed said they would object to their children going to school or playing with epileptic children. Only five percent still felt that way in 1974.

Almost anyone to whom you mention epilepsy will tell you that it is an uncommon disease. So it is surprising to find that there are approximately three million epileptics in this country. The majority of these people are able to lead almost normal lives.

What is epilepsy? Medical researchers still do not have all the answers to explain this mysterious disease. We do have an instrument which will diagnose epilepsy—the electroencephalograph. "Encephalo" means "brains" and "graph" means "writing," so this jawbreaker of a name refers simply to an instrument which records the electrical workings of the brain in writing. The brain, like the heart, gives off electrical currents. In using the electroencephalograph, the patient merely sits while electrodes are attached to his head through which his brain's electrical currents are recorded. The brain of an epileptic records a different kind of pattern from that of a non-epileptic.

The Types Of Epilepsy

There is pretty general agreement on the different kinds of epilepsy. *Petit mal* (meaning *little sickness* in French) is a form of disorder which is much more common in children than in adults. Seizures generally are quite frequent—in fact there may be hundreds in one day. They last only a few seconds and may be overlooked, because they may give no indication except for a slight hesitation or confusion. The child may drop whatever he is holding, or he may fall and immediately get up. There may be rhythmic twitching of the eyelids or eyebrows. *Petit mal* attacks are usually worse in the morning hours and they usually grow less frequent and less serious as the sufferer grows older.

Grand mal (big sickness) is what most of us mean when we think of epilepsy. The patient becomes unconscious and falls.

Saliva may appear on his lips. He may cry out (although he is not feeling any pain). His muscles tighten into a spasm or convulsion, and he twitches violently for a minute or two. Actually the seizure does not last long, although it may seem long to the helpless observer. During an attack of *grand mal*, the patient may mimic normal movements. He may appear to be beckoning with his fingers. His eyes or head may turn to one side or another, as if he were actually looking to that side. He may get up after the attack and feel dull and drowsy for a time, or he may go into a deep sleep and sleep for hours.

Many epileptics have a warning when they are going to have an attack. It is called an "aura" by physicians. It may be a strange feeling in the stomach, a dizzy feeling or an unpleasant odor that the patient believes he smells.

Not many, but some, cases of epilepsy are caused by damage to the brain either at birth or later in life. In the other cases, the disorder is called "functional" or "idiopathic," meaning that a physical examination reveals nothing wrong with any organ. However, it is possible that functional epilepsy may result eventually in injury to the brain or other parts of the body, if seizures are frequent.

The difference between an epileptic seizure and a "faint" is that the first is a disturbance in the brain, while the second involves a sudden lowering of the blood pressure, which causes the patient to become unconscious. A faint generally has some outside immediate cause—the sight of blood, bad news, etc. But an epileptic convulsion comes without any such circumstances.

At present, drugs are given which are at least partially effective in relieving epileptic convulsions. Dilantin and phenobarbital have proved to be effective in many cases. However, as with all drugs, there are side effects and sometimes very serious ones, which necessitate the closest supervision by the physician and constant testing to make certain that these side effects are not fatal.

Vitamin B₆ Can Prevent Seizures

In some cases, there is a more natural means of controlling the disease. To the infant suffering from these violent seizures, vitamin B_6 can be the blessed key to a normal life. Infantile spasms are sometimes relieved by daily 50 to 100 mg. dosages of B_6, and improvement in some chronic epilepsy cases has been noted with 200 to 300 mg. doses of the vitamin, says Dr. David B. Coursin of St. Joseph's Hospital in Lancaster, Pa. Such convulsions can be the result of an inborn error of vitamin B_6 metabolism, he told the fourteenth annual meeting of the American Society for Clinical Nutrition, held in May, 1974, in Atlantic City, N.J.

Dr. Coursin is a nationally recognized authority on this subject. It was he who proved, with the use of an electroencephalograph, that injections of B_6 could stop a baby's convulsions and prevent them from recurring.

Since then, Dr. Coursin's findings have been confirmed by other doctors, and also by laymen. In July of 1971, an Osceola, Wisconsin man, Harry T. White, reported that his young son had suffered *petit mal* seizures for three years. Anticonvulsant medications were ineffective, and he decided to give vitamin B_6 a try. "It worked," he reported. "One week after administering B_6, our boy was seizure-free of *petit mal*."

Mrs. Joleen Nightingale of Medford, Oregon, reported similar improvement in her son. "Our sixth child, baby Jason, began having seizures at 6 months," she wrote us. "Shortly after awaking he would go into a series of convulsions, which would leave him irritable and very tired.

"He underwent the usual tests at the hospital and had a definite brain wave reading of *idiopathic centrencephalic epilepsy*.

"He became so dull and uninterested, and slept so much it broke my heart—having three or four series of convulsions a day.

"I took him to two specialists. One insisted that he would need to take Dilantin every day for the rest of his life—the other, phenobarbital.

"My husband (bless him) said they were both dangerous crutches which could not actually affect the epilepsy, and have actually produced worse conditions in some.

"We had to find something harmless, and natural."

Brewer's Yeast Brought Improvement In Five Days

Then Mrs. Nightingale came across a magazine article telling about epileptic patients who had been helped by vitamin B_6. "I knew we had to try it!" she said.

"I put two tablespoons of brewer's yeast (a good B vitamin source) a day in his bottle. Within five days he showed a growing, gradual improvement. He was going all day without a single seizure, then two days, four days—I was thrilled!

"I told the doctor and he said I was 'grasping at straws'. When the brewer's yeast was gone, I began giving him 10 mg. tablets of B_6 daily. All of a sudden this child quit his twitching at night (sleeps all night), began perking up mentally, regaining what he had forgotten and learning again. His red, drowsy little eyes sparkled and he squealed with energy. But best of all, these arms have cuddled a serene little boy—without seizures.

"Only twice have I detected the slightest trace of the old pattern. His eyes would water and he would blink, but no rolling of his eyes in the head, no arms flying, chest heaving—just a blink. *Something prevents it.*"

There is also evidence that vitamin D helps control epileptic seizures. This was demonstrated in an 84-day study involving 23 epileptic patients at the Glostrup Hospital in Denmark. All had been taking anticonvulsant drugs for periods of from three to 17 years with only limited success. But when vitamin D supplements were administered, the frequency of fits was reduced by one third, according to Dr. Claus Christiansen and colleagues (*British Medical Journal*, May 4, 1974).

Section 27
The Eyes

140. The Eyes Can Reveal Health Problems

We tend to take good vision and normal eye health for granted. For that reason, few of us really understand how much sound vision means to us until our eyesight is seriously impaired, either through injury, neglect or disease. Perhaps we take the elementary textbook analogy of the human eye to a camera too literally, considering the eye a mechanical instrument which can be readily repaired if something goes wrong. Certainly, surgeons have developed some pretty remarkable techniques for repairing the eyes: they use lazer beams to "patchup" tears in the retina, and freezing techniques to repair other parts of the retina; they insert artificial lenses to replace those made useless by cataract conditions; and they reconstitute pressure within the eyeball itself by injecting synthetic fluids under rather delicate circumstances. But these are considered stopgap measures at best. The eye and the camera have only elementary functions in common; no camera, no matter how complex and sophisticated, could possibly duplicate the myriad organic functions that the human eye is capable of.

The Eye Mirrors Body Health

Like every other organ in the body, the health of the eye is dependent on sound nutrition, proper care and exercise. And like the other organs, the eye often reacts to physical ailments in other parts of the body. Pain and soreness of the eye often results from illnesses such as influenza, viruses, colds, certain fevers, allergies, shingles, migraine headaches, various forms of neuralgia and sinusitis.

Certain nutritional deficiencies show up in the eyes long before they begin to affect the rest of the body seriously. An alert physician can spot these latent nutritional shortages in the course of a thorough examination of the eyes. For example, a haziness in the back of the eye, unrelated to any distortion of color vision or to enlargement of blind spots, can be caused by inefficiency of the optic nerve due to a deficiency of one or more of the major B vitamins.

141. Various Types
Of Blindness Explained

There are varying degrees of blindness ranging from residual reduction in vision to total loss of sight. Residual reductions in sight allow limited visual ability only with extremely powerful corrective lenses, and this is accompanied by aggravating periods of eyestrain. Victims of such severe visual impairment are considered "functionally blind," unable to read standard print even with the aid of eyeglasses.

Of the 9.6 million people in the United States with some form of visual impairment, 479,000 individuals are designated as being legally blind, according to the National Society for the Prevention of Blindness, Inc. (NSPB). Legal blindness is defined as the inability of a person to see no more at a distance of 20 feet than a person with normal sight can see at a distance of 200 feet, usually phrased in ocular terminology as a vision which does not exceed the visual acuity of 20/200. The term "legal blindness" is used primarily to determine eligibility for public assistance and income tax allowances.

The most tragic aspect of this category of blindness, which claims more people every year, is that more than half of the new cases could be prevented with current medical knowledge and techniques.

Aging And Blindness
The incidence of blindness, or total loss of vision, like all other visual impairments, increases alarmingly with advancing age, according to NSPB statistics. Here are some facts on various types of blindness and aging:

Cataract, the leading cause of blindness, accounts for 16 percent of all reported cases of blindness. Although the prevalence of cataract steadily increases after middle age, 75 percent of all people over 65 years of age develop the condition to some degree.

Glaucoma, is second among causes of reported cases of blindness. Nearly all cases occur in people over 35 years of age. The disease can be successfully treated if diagnosed in its early stages, but it is especially dangerous because glaucoma is sometimes painless and symptomless in the early stages.

Diabetic Retinopathy, a disorder of the blood vessels, accounts for 10 percent of all the cases of blindness reported in this country. It only affects diabetics, usually older people who have had diabetes for ten years or more.

Retinal Changes are associated with aging and account for 13 percent of the reported cases of blindness. Over 80 percent of these cases involve damage inflicted on that part of the retina adapted for viewing objects distinctly, nearby or at a distance. The retina contains rods, cones and other vital nerve cells and fibers. The posterior part of the retina is where the sensation of vision is first initiated.

Vascular Disorders, which appear more frequently in older people, account for eight percent of all the reported cases of blindness in the aged. According to *Transactions* (March-April, 1974), the official journal of the American Academy of Opthalmology and Otolaryngology, "Three different scientific studies show that hypertension and allied circulatory disorders are closely related to vision loss caused by blockage in the branch veins transporting blood (to the eyes)." The researchers said the best way to avoid the problem is to monitor the blood pressure regularly, keeping it within normal limits as much as possible. This is especially important, they said, if the persons are over 50 years of age.

Other physicians have stressed the importance of sound nutrition, emphasizing foods rich in vitamin E, to stop the deterioration of visual sensitivity due to impaired circulation. It's well known that vitamin E oxygenates the tissues and exerts strong anti-clotting powers. The circulatory blockage in the arteries in and around the eyes is not unlike the hardening of arteries in other parts of the body, slowing function and causing the sense organs to behave more sluggishly.

142. Protect Yourself Against Cataract

A. J. Street, O.D.

The lens of the eye is a precisely formed yet flexible structure containing 65 percent water and 35 percent organic material, chiefly protein in solution. The transparency of the normal lens is remarkable, considering its plastic nature. Its ability to keep the eye in focus automatically is a feat which cannot be duplicated by the finest man-made optical instruments.

Like all parts of the body, however, the lens can suffer from neglect and abuse. Given improper care the clear transparent lens material may turn milky and dark, become opaque, and suffer the physical changes known by the dreaded name "cataract."

The word "cataract" has a curious beginning. In its English origin the word was used to describe floodgates, or at least some type of heavy iron gate. How it came to describe an ocular disease is not known, but the transfer of meaning is clear. The "gate" that closes on the pathway of vision can be complete or partial. In most cases it shuts out at least a portion of usable sight.

Eye Structure

Before discussing disorders of the lens, it is important to know a little about its composition and function. The refracting (light bending) system of the eye is a dual one, composed of the cornea and the lens. The cornea is a clear, slightly oval window in the front of the eye whose optical function is to focus on the retina the essentially parallel light rays coming from distant objects. Since it is the first optical barrier to light entering the eye, the cornea furnishes about 75 percent of the eye's total refracting power.

The crystalline lens is an auxiliary refracting system within the eye whose power is but one-fifth that of the cornea. In a sense its function resembles that of the fine tuning adjustment on a television set. Light rays coming from relatively near objects, that is, closer than twenty feet, are not parallel in nature. It is the job of the lens to make minor adjustments in the refraction of the cornea that will compensate for the change in light rays and thus continually maintain a precise retinal focus regardless of the distance of the object being viewed. To do this, the lens must be flexible and must change shape as required. It is slightly convex when the eye views distant objects, becoming highly convex when the eye looks at near objects.

The ability of the lens to change shape, and therefore its refracting power is called accommodation. It is governed by the action of three tiny groups of muscles, the ciliaries. The ciliary muscles act automatically, on signal from the subconscious region of the brain. Their well-coordinated contractions loosen the suspensory ligaments holding the lens in place and thus give it the freedom to relax and assume a more convex shape during accommodative action.

The lens is composed of epithelial cells, the same cellular substance that forms the surface skin of the body. As cells are continually added throughout life, the formation becomes layered, the newest cells on the outside of the lens body compressing those laid down earlier, until the inner lens structure resembles that of an onion.

Proper accommodation depends on continued lens flexibility. Sometimes when a person reaches about 40 years of age the central layers of the lens, now quite compressed by the continual arrival of new epithelial cells, become firm and inelastic and begin to resist the shape changes necessary for adequate accommodation. This is the condition known as presbyopia, or far-sightedness of age, wherein the eye can see perfectly at a distance but becomes increasingly unable to see near objects.

The crystalline lens is a completely bloodless structure, having no direct contact with the circulatory system of the body. It is composed mainly of soluble protein and water and is surrounded within the eye by the aqueous humor, a water-like fluid filling the anterior third of the eyeball. The lens obtains its nutrition from the aqueous humor which, in turn, is linked directly with the blood. Any interference with the uptake of nutrients by the lens can cause tissue death and loss of transparency of the lens substance.

Cataract And Nutrition

Research workers investigating the etiology of senile cataract, the specific form of opacity associated with advancing age, have found a marked change in the protein content of cataractous lenses. In contrast to normal lenses, which contain about 35 percent soluble protein, lenses showing advancing opacification contain increasing amounts of insoluble protein, and decreasing amounts of the soluble variety. Apparently a shifting balance in the soluble/insoluble protein occurs in the senile cataractous lens, with the soluble protein diminishing more rapidly than the insoluble increases. Thus, not only is there a change in protein type, but an actual loss in total amount as well.

Other changes in lenses with advancing senile opacities are lowering of the water content, i.e. drying out of the lens in certain forms of cataract, and a decrease in the amount of ascorbic acid (vitamin C) found in the lens.

However, it would be difficult to attribute cataract solely to a deficiency of vitamin C. Although the aqueous humor and lens normally contain a high concentration of this vitamin, and the levels fall rapidly during the onset of scurvy, cataract is not one of the effects of the disease. Furthermore, large doses of vitamin C given to persons with cataract have never resulted in absorption of the opacity to any degree. For these reasons most doctors decline to attach any great significance to the correlation between lowered vitamin C and the onset of cataract.

Vitamin D also has been found indirectly involved through calcium metabolism in cataract formation. Long before confirming animal studies were made, abundant clinical evidence showed a close relationship between tetany, a disease of calcium deficiency, and a particular type of zonular cataract found in young children. Numerous laboratory workers have since been successful in demonstrating similar lens changes in animals maintained on a calcium-poor diet.

One of the most thorough studies was that of Dr. Goldmann, in which he induced periods of tetany in dogs by withholding calcium in the diet. In this way he was able to produce subcapsular opacities during the periods of calcium deprivation. In the intervening tetany-free periods new clear fibers were laid down in the lens. By repeating the process several times, Dr. Goldmann was able to observe alternating layers of opaque and clear lens fibers, indicating an obvious relationship between subcapsular cataract and the calcium deficiency of tetany. Experimental studies by Drs. Swan and Salet produced cataract in 49 rabbits which were maintained on a low-calcium diet. Inasmuch as vitamin D is essential for proper calcium metabolism, it is believed to be an important agent in prevention of zonular cataract.

Stages Of The Disease

Once cataract begins to develop it passes through three recognizable clinical stages, *incipient, mature,* and *hypermature.* The incipient stage shows small opacities that may pass undetected for many months or years because of lack of visual acuity involvement. Often this stage can be identified only with the aid of the ophthalmoscope or the slit lamp. Both instruments are used routinely by the optometrist and ophthalmologist in the examination of the eyes.

The mature stage of cataract is characterized by opacification of individual lens fibers and a gradual extension of involvement across the entire face of the lens. Vision begins to decrease, and the individual may complain of fogginess and haloes around lights. It is during this stage that removal of the cataractous lens is most often recommended. If removal is delayed until the hypermature stage, the lens contents may become liquified, vision entirely obscured, and the success of any subsequent operation jeopardized.

During the mature stage the vision acuity is often the determining factor in timing the removal of a cataract. The individual who depends heavily upon the use of his eyes, for instance, will naturally be the first to notice the lack of clarity and will be the first to seek medical assistance. Conversely, the person who has no specific visual demands, as is the case with many older persons, will not be troubled by a mild lack of vision and may get by very nicely until a later stage of development. Since cataracts develop at different rates in different people, some may never find a need for surgical removal of the lens, even though they must adapt to some mild clouding of vision.

Surgical removal of senile cataract is a fairly simple procedure. The operation is usually done under local anesthesia, and the patient is often out of bed in a few days. In a typical operation an incision is made near the corneal margin. A small triangular aperture is cut in the periphery of the iris to allow free aqueous circulation after removal of the lens. The suspensory ligaments holding the lens in place are cut, and the lens deftly removed from the eye through the corneal incision.

Enlargement Of Images

Removal of the crystalline lens creates a refractive deficiency, making the affected eye extremely far sighted. Plus power spectacle lenses must be used to make up the deficiency if the individual is to see well again. Since the spectacle lens must be positioned several millimeters distant from the crystalline lens' former position within the eye, a sizeable amount of retinal image magnification is found to occur.

If the operation has been binocular, that is, on both eyes, the abnormally large appearance of objects is not a problem. Since all things are changed equally, the patient soon adapts to his new environment. Should the operation be uniocular, however, with usable vision remaining in the unoperated eye, the magnification difference will make impossible the use of both eyes simultaneously, without incurring double vision. In these cases, a wiser choice may be to forego the operation until vision becomes poor in the better eye, or, if for physical reasons the operation is essential, to correct the resultant monocular farsightedness with a single contact lens. Since the contact lens can be placed very close to the original lens site, very little magnification results from the correction, and the two eyes may be used together in a normal fashion.

A new approach has been tried in the correction of aphakia (absence of the crystalline lens). Rather than rely on spectacle or contact lens correction of the acquired refractive deficiency, surgeons have, in a few cases, replaced the cataractous crystalline lens with a new lens made of plastic. The plastic lens, with a refractive power equal to that of the removed lens, is sutured into the site formerly occupied by its organic counterpart. Any refractive error caused by cataract surgery is thereby automatically eliminated. The new lens cannot accommodate, however, and the patient must wear spectacles for reading.

Most surgeons who have used this technique feel it holds great promise, but must be perfected before it will be successful in large numbers of cases. One problem encountered with the new lens concerns its rejection by body tissues. Whenever a particle of foreign matter lodges anywhere within the body, antibodies surround it in an effort to expel the intruder. Dramatic examples of tissue rejection have been seen in heart transplant operations. In the case of the eye, the substitute lens must be made from a material that will not trigger antibody reaction and cause rejection of the new optical correction.

Of course, prevention of cataract is much to be preferred to its surgical removal. To improve your chances of keeping healthy eyes, start now to improve your nutrition. Be sure your diet includes sufficient vitamins and minerals, especially riboflavin, vitamin D, vitamin E (which improves the blood supply), and calcium. Have your eyes examined regularly, and remember: a well nourished body is a healthy body, and the rewards of good health are great.

143. Riboflavin Deficiency Encourages Cataract

It is well known that a deficiency of vitamin B_2 can cause cataracts in both animals and in humans. Dr. P. S. Day in experiments conducted at Columbia University produced cataract in every single one of the rats deprived of riboflavin in an otherwise perfect diet. If the diet continued, eventual blindness resulted and further successful therapy was impossible. However, Dr. Day found that adequate amounts of riboflavin given before the point of no return caused the cataract to be reabsorbed and the eyes returned to normal in every respect. When these same animals were put back on a riboflavin-deficient diet, the cataracts returned, according to Donald Stewart McLaren in his book *Malnutrition and the Eye* (Academic Press, New York and London).

Does this B_2 therapy also help humans threatened with cataract? According to the work of Dr. Sydenstricker of the University of Georgia and University of Georgia Hospital, it most certainly does. Dr. Sydenstricker first tried vitamin A on 47 patients all of whom were suffering eye disorders. Although vitamin A is of value in treating many types of eye disorders, it did not produce the desired benefits on Dr. Sydenstricker's patients, 18 of whom had opacities which usually indicate the formation of a cataract while six had fully developed cataracts.

The 47 patients were then given 15 milligrams of riboflavin daily. This was the only therapy used. Within 24 hours, there was dramatic improvement. In practically every one, there was an end to the symptoms of itching, burning of the eyelids, sensitivity to light, faulty vision and general eye weakness. Those who were not helped within the first 24 hours were relieved within the next 24 hours. After nine months on riboflavin therapy, even the cataract patients became normal in every respect. The cataracts had been reabsorbed.

To prove the efficacy of B_2, Dr. Sydenstricker put a few of the cured patients back on a riboflavin-deficient diet. The same eye symptoms soon returned. Again they were corrected by therapeutic doses of riboflavin.

There are two phenomena, then, that are accepted by the medical profession as valid. It is well known that a high galactose diet causes cataracts. It is also well known that a deficiency of vitamin B_2 causes cataracts.

What is not so well known is that galactose is an antagonist of B_2 and causes riboflavin deficiency. Dr. S. Lerman writing in the *Archives of Opthalmology* (65, 181, 1961) reported that excessive amounts of milk sugar or galactose *increases the need for vitamin* B_2. The Johns Hopkins scientists were well aware of the role of B_2 deficiency in the causation of cataracts. But they said, "In such states, lens changes are accompanied by a wide variety of other manifestations such as loss of weight, inactivity, and inability to reproduce . . ."

144. Microwave Ovens Can Cause Cataract

Microwave ovens may cook a potato in five minutes, a rib roast in half an hour, and an egg in thirty seconds, but their time saving qualities certainly do not outweigh the dangers they cause to your health, especially the health of your eyes.

A disorder commonly linked to microwave radiation is cataracts. Doctors still dispute whether the microwaves themselves cause the cataracts, or whether they elevate the temperature of the eye to a point where the heat causes the cataracts (Symposium of the Biological Effects and Health Implications of Microwave Radiation, Sept., 1969). Nobody argues that the cataracts are there because microwave exposure caused them—directly or indirectly.

"That microwave ovens are manufactured to stringent safety standards does not make them harmless," noted Dr. Milton M. Zaret, a respected New York City eye surgeon and microwave specialist. "Although these appliances have been used since 1950 without reported injuries, it has been discovered that the initial signs of microwave cataract are asymptomatic and may not appear until years after the exposure has occurred. Further, if the patient delays obtaining an eye examination until he has failing vision, the etiological signs may be masked at that time by cataractous changes in the lens substance. Before accepting the idea that no injuries are attributable from ovens, we should be given evidence that specific types of microwave injury were sought and found to be absent."

An occupational exposure of 10 milliwatts of radiation per square centimeter (M.S.C.) is the "permissible" standard set by the American National Standard Institute. But as Dr. Zaret said in March of 1972, "This presupposes good physical control of who gets near the radiation and for how long."

In his own words, it's as though "you were to put up a fence and on one side permit certain individuals to get 40 hours a week of chronic, workaday exposure—maybe for 20 years. So far, for people on the other side of the fence (typical citizens not working directly with microwaves), we haven't seen any trouble to speak of. But because 10 percent of workers exposed to high levels of microwave radiation *do* develop cataracts, this is an operational risk that can't be overlooked."

Some people "on the other side of the fence"—housewives, restaurant employees, etc.—*are* being exposed to dangerous levels of radiation and in completely uncontrolled situations. You or one of your relatives may own one of the more than 100,000 microwave ovens in home and commercial use. If so, you can take little if any comfort in knowing that the U.S. Bureau of Radiological Health has set official government standards for these ovens. According to the latest directive, a new oven may leak 1 M.S.C. at the time of sale, older ovens, 5 M.S.C. This means that an oven can be delivered, according to Dr. Zaret, and "*a day later* be leaking 5 M.S.C. and still meet HEW (The Department of Health Education and Welfare) approval . . . And this is in the uncontrolled environment of the home, where you're not dealing with only healthy, young adults, but older people, infants, children and even pregnant women as well."

In its booklet, "Facts About Microwave Oven Radiation," HEW admits that oven safety is a very "iffy" proposition: "The only way to determine if a given oven is emitting microwave radiation is to have the oven tested with a specially-designed instrument . . . *it is impossible to state that a particular make and model of microwave oven is radiation safe unless it is surveyed.*" (our emphasis) While you're left wondering if your oven is too dangerous to use, the booklet closes with a "safety tip" recommending that you "stay at least a full arm's length away from the front of an operating oven."

And what good are oven "standards" anyhow if they exist only on paper? As a report by the U.S. Public Health Service indicates (*New York Times*, July 23, 1971), some ovens are sealed about as well as a sieve. They might as well be operated with open doors; the unsuspecting housewife is getting at least half as much dangerous radiation leakage as she would with the door wide open!

After testing 5,000 household ovens in 25 states, the HEW estimated that one oven out of every 10 is leaking radiation in excess of the industry's former voluntary limit of 10 M.S.C. Many ovens were found to be leaking up to 100 M.S.C. (Ovens tested with open doors registered only twice as much—up to 200 M.S.C.)

The agency blamed the widespread cases of leakage on faulty design (especially in pre-1968 models), shipping damage, and poorly adjusted safety interlocks (which *should* shut off the oven automatically when the door is opened). The consumer can also be at fault, however. If you allow food and dirt to build up in crevices along the seal, the safety door can't close properly.

Dr. Zaret was disturbed by these findings, especially since some industries—such as Bell Telephone Laboratories—have used a temperature/humidity index factor to come up with a permissible exposure limit of just 1 M.S.C. for their own workers using equipment that emits radiation. "I think it's ludicrous that the young healthy adult man who happens to work for Bell Labs is exposed to just 1 M.S.C.," he remarked, "while his family at home, assuming they own a microwave oven, can be exposed to 5 M.S.C. or more. It just doesn't make sense."

The Bureau of Radiological Health admits that "although researchers know that harmful health effects may be expected from exposure to certain microwave frequencies, they do not completely understand these effects."

But oven manufacturers aren't waiting for all the answers. Industry representatives expect that an increasing number of all cooking ovens sold in this country will be microwave ovens. As an official for Litton Industries stated, "It's now a product whose time has come" (*Wall Street Journal*, August 19, 1971). But is a potato baked in eight minutes or a 10-pound frozen turkey cooked in an hour worth the risk of exposure to damaging radiation?

145. New Hope For
The Glaucoma Patient*

Glaucoma, in its more common form, can destroy vision slowly and painlessly, sometimes without giving any warning signs or symptoms to its victim until most of the sight is gone. Although there are many types of glaucoma, one feature is common to all—increased pressure within the eyeball.

A healthy eye has an optimal or favorable pressure within it called the intraocular (within the eye) pressure. Without this force, the eye would collapse like a leaking balloon. Intraocular pressure varies somewhat in different persons and even from day to day in the same eye. This variation is similar to that of the blood pressure in that a fairly wide range is considered acceptable.

When the pressure increases to such a degree that damage to structures within the eye occurs, the condition is called *glaucoma* or hypertension of the eye (also commonly termed hardening of the eyeball). There is no direct relationship, however, between high blood pressure (arterial hypertension) and glaucoma (hypertension of the eye).

Although it is possible to become overly glaucoma-conscious, there are certain signs and symptoms which should induce one to be examined by an ophthalmologist (an eye doctor). Early detection is important because vision lost as a result of glaucoma is never regained (except to a very minor degree). It is a question of keeping what vision a patient has rather than any hope for appreciable improvement. While glaucoma can sneak up without warning, the following symptoms or danger signals can occur— *rainbow-colored rings (haloes) around lights, a narrowing of the visual field, frequent changes in eyeglass prescriptions without visual improvement, abnormally poor vision in dim light, fuzzy*

*Reprinted from *New Hope For Incurable Diseases*, copyright, 1971, by E. Cheraskin, M.D., D.M.D. and W. M. Ringsdorf, Jr., D.M.D., M.S., published by Exposition Press Inc., Hicksville, New York 11801.

or blurred vision which may come and go, vague headaches or eye aches, particularly after watching movies or television in darkened rooms, watering or discharge of the eye, any change in the eye color, clouding of the cornea and hardness of the eyeball. Another warning is a family history of glaucoma. Relatives of those with glaucoma have five or six times as much of this eye ailment as persons without glaucoma in the family.

What Causes It?

The front portion of the eye between the lens and the cornea holds a clear watery fluid called the aqueous humor. Throughout a person's life, this watery substance is constantly produced within this tiny chamber, flows through it to nourish the cornea, and then drains through a minute natural canal. For reasons not yet completely understood by science, this drainage canal may become blocked.

If this happens, the aqueous humor backs up and pressure within the eyeball builds up. This force is transmitted to the retina (on the back side of the eye). The retina contains sensitive nerve cells and fibers that relay light stimuli through the optic nerve to the brain. Increased intraocular pressure can cause destruction of these cells; and, with each cell destroyed, a portion of the field of vision is lost forever. Eventually all sight may be gone.

Glaucoma usually begins with the loss of peripheral or side vision, then slowly closes in until only straight-ahead vision is left, then none at all. A person may be unaware of the loss of side (lateral, peripheral) vision because he can see straight ahead with 20/20 central vision. It is generally concluded that an elevated pressure over a long period of time is necessary to produce visual field defects. While this may be correct for many patients who develop such loss of sight, it should be noted that there are also individuals with elevated pressure for long periods of time who do not develop visual field loss. Since so little is actually known concerning the cause of glaucoma, host resistance and susceptibility factors in the latter group might provide some clues. In fact, malnourishment of the disc (where the optic nerve attaches to the eyeball) because of impaired blood circulation has been suggested.

Basically, there are two divisions of glaucoma, *primary* and *secondary*. Although much is known about what happens in primary glaucoma, the fundamental cause or causes remain a mystery. Primary glaucoma occurs in both eyes and is called "primary" for the simple reason that it is apparently not "secondary" (or due) to some other disorder. The conditions which result in secondary glaucoma are almost too numerous to list. As the term implies, the high pressure within the eye is a result of some disease, tumor, inflammation, or injury. Secondary glaucoma is frequently limited to one eye.

Within the primary division there are three types of glaucoma. *Chronic* glaucoma is the most common and is the type usually referred to in this chapter. It is the classic sneak thief of vision and is an extremely deceptive disorder. *Acute* glaucoma is uncommon and attacks suddenly and painfully. The pressure must be reduced immediately or blindness will result. Although it presents a critical emergency, cure is more often achieved (medically and surgically) than with the other types. Finally, *infantile* glaucoma is a rare congenital type requiring surgery.

How Common Is It?

Numerous detection surveys have shown that the incidence of glaucoma (mostly undetected) is about 2 percent of the people over 40. This percentage increases progressively with age. It is estimated that approximately 2,000,000 American adults already have glaucoma and that half of them are not aware of it. The incidence and prevalence of glaucoma in blacks is almost twice as high as in white persons. In those with a positive family history of this affliction, screening surveys have shown that almost one out of every ten adults examined had glaucoma. This observation suggests a possible genetic influence. However, the mere fact that something runs in families does not preclude its being environmentally inspired.

Although glaucoma is primarily a disease of those over forty years of age, disturbances in sugar metabolism encourage its development much sooner. Generally, the duration of diabetes mellitus is directly related to the intraocular tension. In other words, the longer the duration, the higher the intraocular pressure. Thus, juvenile diabetes can produce high tensions in the first decades of life.

Next to cataracts, glaucoma is the leading cause of blindness. There are about 54,000 men and women in this country who are blind in both eyes and an additional 185,000 blind in one eye from this disease. According to health authorities, the blind population has been increasing at nearly twice the rate of the general public. Not only is this trend continuing, but it is believed that the increase will accelerate.

What Cures It?

Any mention of the treatment of glaucoma must be, for the most part, quite general, for no two cases are exactly alike. The therapy of one ophthalmologist may vary somewhat from that of another. Yet both may achieve similar results. However, it is of great importance that glaucoma treatment usually be looked upon as a control and not a cure! In other words, *glaucoma is controlled rather than cured!*

In acute (rather severe but of short duration) glaucoma, drug relief is usually followed by surgery. For chronic glaucoma (not severe and of a long duration), restoration of vision already lost due to nerve degeneration cannot occur. Thus, therapy is designed to preserve the remaining sight. Astute patient control is necessary in chronic glaucoma since treatment is lifelong and the disease is slowly progressive. Initially, miotic drugs (eyedrops) effectively increase the outflow of aqueous humor to keep the intraocular pressure down. Other eyedrop drugs may also be used to reduce the formation of this fluid and thus aid in suppressing the pressure. Failure to control the pressure with these agents may be followed by an oral drug designed to decrease the rate of aqueous humor formation. At some point in the progression of chronic glaucoma, a decision is usually made to improve the aqueous outflow by a surgical procedure. Where surgery does not control the intraocular pressure, progression to blindness is almost inevitable.

As additional aids in the control of glaucoma, the following instructions are applicable to most patients:

1. Follow the advice of your ophthalmologist to the letter. This is by far the most important thing to keep in mind. Return for checkups when advised.

2. Notify your ophthalmologist immediately if you should develop pain or redness of the eye or sudden blurring of vision. If intense itching accompanies swelling and redness of the eyelids and eyes, tell your ophthalmologist promptly. It may mean that you have developed an allergy to a medicine that you are using.

3. Avoid excessive use of stimulants such as coffee and tea. It is preferable that you give up all such stimulants. If you drink coffee, however, one-half to one cup a day should be your limit. You may have caffeine-free coffee.

4. Avoid excessive amounts of fluid intake at any one time. In hot weather, excessive perspiration may necessitate your drinking larger amounts of fluids than usual. Do not drink three or four glasses at any one time, however; spread them out.

5. Avoid excessive smoking. It is not known with certainty how much damage smoking causes in cases of glaucoma, but there is enough evidence to indicate that smoking does cause some harm.

6. You should attempt to lead as tranquil a life as possible. Avoid emotional upheavals as far as possible.

7. Avoid prolonged periods of darkness, such as several hours a week at motion pictures. Do not use sunglasses too much. In the very bright sun, however, shaded glasses do no harm.

8. Most ophthalmologists feel that the ordinary use of the eyes does no harm insofar as glaucoma is concerned. This means that you may read, sew, and watch television without fear of damage to your eyes.

9. When you consult your family physician or your surgeon, tell him that you have glaucoma. He will avoid giving you certain drugs that might adversely affect your glaucoma.

10. If you move or have any other reason to change your care to another ophthalmologist, request that your old records be sent to him.

11. Carry an identification card at all times. It is advisable to carry this card with information as to your condition, just as a patient with diabetes does. There are several reasons for this. If one is found unconscious from an accident or for some other reason, the examining physician, on seeing the card, will realize that the person's small pupils are due to the use of drugs in the eyes. Unless this information is known, the small pupils may be misinterpreted. On seeing the identification card, the physician will be on guard, too, about administering drugs that might adversely affect the glaucoma. Your ophthalmologist can secure these cards from the National Foundation for Eye Care.

Remember that the most significant factor in the treatment of your glaucoma is to follow your ophthalmologist's advice to the letter.

Is There More Hope?

At a recent meeting of the Roman Ophthalmological Society in Rome, Italy, four Italian physicians gave evidence of an exciting breakthrough in glaucoma treatment. Doctor Michele Virno and coworkers cited human evidence that the intraocular pressure in glaucomatous eyes could be dramatically reduced by an oral dose of vitamin C (ascorbic acid)! The report was immediately published in the United States by the *Eye, Ear, Nose and Throat Monthly*.

The initial approach by these investigators was to evaluate the effect of a single oral dose of vitamin C (0.5 grams of ascorbic acid per kilogram [2.2 pounds] of body weight) upon the intraocular pressure in patients with different kinds of glaucoma. For example, a person weighing 150 pounds would receive 35 grams of vitamin C. This megadose is over 500-fold the amount generally held to be an optimal daily intake. Doctor Virno and his associates observed a highly significant drop in pressure for all patients. This table is a summary of their findings (eye pressure is expressed in millimeters of mercury):

Type of glaucoma	No. of eyes	Average maximum eye pressure reduction (expressed in millimeters of mercury)
Chronic simple glaucoma		
initial pressure 50-69	7	25.0
initial pressure 32-49	7	19.0
initial pressure 20-31	11	6.5
Acute glaucoma		
partial angle closure	3	28.5
complete angle closure	4	10.5
Hemorrhagic glaucoma	2	17.0
Secondary glaucoma	5	11.5

It was noted that the intraocular pressure reached its lowest point about four to five hours after taking the single dose of vitamin C. This low point was maintained for more than eight hours. It was also observed that the blood vitamin C level, which was very low in the beginning, reached its highest point as the pressure reached its lowest level. This blood level was about eight to ten times greater than initially. After five hours, the blood vitamin C level began to decrease.

Since most patients treated with the single load of vitamin C developed disorders of the stomach and diarrhea, Doctor Virno decided to divide the single dose into several smaller ones. Thus, amounts of 0.10 to 0.15 grams per kilogram of the body weight were given three to five times a day. Thus, the 150 pound person mentioned earlier would be given seven grams five times each day. Although this produced mild stomach discomfort and diarrhea at the beginning, these symptoms disappeared after three to four days.

With these smaller doses, which were administered daily for periods up to forty-five days, it was possible to obtain acceptable intraocular pressure in many patients. This happened in some individuals whose pressure could not be controlled with oral drugs (such as Diamox) or eyedrops (miotics such as 2 percent pilocarpine).

Doctor Virno and his team expressed hope that others will use vitamin C in the treatment of glaucoma. Although the mechanisms are not completely understood, the administration of ascorbic acid in the smaller doses three to five times a day is very effective and perfectly safe.

Summary

Professor G. B. Bietti, Director of the Eye Clinic of the University of Rome, where this research has been conducted, recently offered these conclusions concerning the vitamin C treatment:

1. Vitamin C at high dosage is a very effective hypotonic agent for intraocular pressure, not only when administered by intravenous injection (sodium ascorbate: from 0.4 grams to 1 gram per kilogram of body weight), but also when given by mouth (ascorbic acid: 0.12 to 0.5 grams per kilogram of body weight).

2. The hypotonic effect on the eye of ascorbic acid by mouth lasts longer than other agents which have an osmotic action when given by both oral and intravenous routes (including sodium ascorbate), although the action of ascorbate lasts longer than that of urea, mannitol and glycerol given by mouth.

3. Ascorbic acid given by mouth has various intensities of action depending on the individual patients and the types of glaucoma and seems more effective in cases of chronic open-angle glaucoma.

4. Ascorbic acid has proven equally active whether given in a single dose of 0.5 grams per kilogram of body weight or in fractional doses during the day.

5. It has also been proved that the hypotonic action of ascorbic acid on the eye can be prolonged practically indefinitely, at least for the period observed in patients so treated (seven months) by the daily administration of divided doses of 125 mg. per kilogram of body weight two, three or four times a day. Normal intraocular

tension could be obtained by treatment with ascorbic acid by itself, or in association with topical antiglaucomatous medication (miotics), on occasions when miotics by themselves were unable to control the tension.

In some cases the lowering of the intraocular tension caused by prolonged treatment with ascorbic acid persisted for several weeks after the treatment had been stopped. Sodium ascorbate given by intravenous injection acts predominantly by osmotic dehydration of the eyeball, although it is possible that there is a different additional action of the ascorbate itself or of the ascorbic acid liberated from it in the body.

The other possible mechanism of action of ascorbic acid on intraocular tension, as proven by tonographic investigations and those with a suction cup (modified by Bucci), seems to be a chemical one causing a diminished production of aqueous by the ciliary epithelium.

An additional hypotonic mechanism, acting very possibly through a decreased production of aqueous, could be the shift of blood pH towards the acid side.

The medical profession emphasizes that the medical and surgical treatment of glaucoma should be looked upon as a control and not a cure. In many people, however, the control is not adequate to prevent the disease from progressing. Since the oral administration of vitamin C has been reported to be highly effective in reducing high intraocular pressures to a normal or near normal level, there are many good reasons for trying it:

1. Vitamin C is nontoxic (safe) in the dosage recommended.

2. Vitamin C is a cheap and convenient way to treat glaucoma.

3. Vitamin C, taken orally, does not produce the degeneration of eye and body tissues that occurs with the strong eyedrops and oral medications used in treating glaucoma.

4. The preservation of sight may be accomplished with vitamin C even after all drugs and surgery have failed.

Based on the earlier definitions and the evidence presented here, vitamin C must be regarded as a resistance agent in glaucoma.

The sensible course for the patient with glaucoma is to consult an eye doctor regarding the possible use of this treatment.

146. Therapy For Crossed Eyes

A person with crossed eyes sees two objects when he's looking at one, because each eye views the same object from a widely different angle. He squints or tilts his head, unconsciously trying to combine the two images or ignore one of them. Neither attempt fully succeeds. Eventually a strabismus (cross-eyed) victim stops trying to see with both the eyes. When he looks at things with only one eye, he sees only one image. Using one eye gets to be a convenient habit and soon the other eye becomes incapable of focusing on anything. Functionally, it is blind.

The basic cause of crossed eyes is the unequal pull of eye muscles. If the muscle on one side of the eye pulls harder than the muscle on the other side, the eye "looks" toward the side with the stronger muscle. An eye doctor works to equalize the pull of the muscles until the eye in repose is directed straight ahead. Sometimes glasses alone can force better direction, but rarely.

Another familiar device used to treat crossed eyes is an eye patch. The stronger eye is covered, forcing the weaker one to do all the sight work. The confusion of the double image is immediately resolved, and the idea is that increased work will restore muscular control of the weaker eye. Unfortunately, once the patch is removed, the eye usually goes right back to the old position.

Failure with these measures used to leave surgery as the last resort. The surgeon shortens the weaker eye muscle and equalizes the pull on both sides of the eye to make it look straight ahead. Sometimes several operations are required before the proper alignment is achieved.

Surgery Unsatisfactory

Sometimes eyes apparently respond to the operation, but still lack the versatility necessary for good vision. Peripheral vision may be obscured; distant focus might be fine, but not close up; the ability to follow moving objects or adjust focus rapidly to near and far away just isn't there.

The results are so unpredictable that one successful operation out of four is considered a pretty good average. In a child born with strabismus, chances that surgery will get the two eyes to work together perfectly are less than that. A good result depends largely on very early operations; some patients are no more than 18 months old. The recognized uncertainty and risks of surgery are so great that conservative Johns Hopkins University Hospital has established an Orthoptic Center that concentrates on treatments other than surgery for correcting eye problems.

Important among these treatments is exercise therapy, a technique deserving wider knowledge and application than it has yet received. Exercise therapy is simple, safe and, according to Dr. William M. Ludlam of New York City, successful in about 70 percent of the cases. The clincher: in most cases, even persons who have surgery need eye exercises later to round out the results. Parents are certainly sensible to try the exercises first.

The child in visual training works at machines that stimulate a variety of visual situations and help him adjust his sight to them. He repeats sighting patterns that force his eyes into proper positioning and coordination. Eventually the eyes can do the work with minimal assistance from glasses—sometimes without glasses.

The theory of eye exercise for improved vision is not a new one. The Bates System, evolved several generations ago, prescribed general exercises for eye strengthening and more specific ones for individual eye disability. Modern visual training has greatly refined the approaches and predictability of eye exercise. New equipment makes things easier and helps to maintain interest long enough to get results.

Most physicians agree that a tendency toward visual problems is inborn. This means that prenatal care can have some influence in preventing weaknesses. A healthful diet, high in protein and other vitamin-rich foods in pregnancy, will help to insure strong muscle tissue and healthful nerves that will work toward proper eye control in the expected baby.

147. Effective Eye Treatment For Diabetics

One of the most depressing statistical projections ever made about American health went relatively unnoticed when it was issued in 1971. At that time, it was estimated by the Harvard School of Public Health that by the year 2000, more people will be blind or severely visually impaired just by the complications of diabetes than are now blind from all causes put together.

Diabetic retinopathy, which is degeneration of the retina, the single most important part of the eye structure, afflicts 154,700 persons, the study estimated. By the year 2000, this number will rise to a staggering 573,000, the Harvard team reported in *Views* (Spring, 1972), the publication of the Wisconsin Society for the Prevention of Blindness, Inc., an affiliate of the National Society for the Prevention of Blindness.

The National Society estimates that 50 percent of diabetics who have had diabetes for 20 years will develop retinopathy. Ninety-five percent of those who have lived with diabetes for 30 years can expect to develop the disease.

Basically, diabetic retinopathy is atherosclerosis of the blood vessels in the eye's retina, similar to the better known form of atherosclerosis which causes arteries in other parts of the body to become clogged with fatty deposits. Frequently, because advanced diabetes is often accompanied by complications, the victim of diabetic retinopathy may have other eye problems, too. High blood pressure can cause vessels to hemorrhage within the eye, and cause fluids to ooze through membranes and accumulate in the eye, further reducing vision.

The prediction made by the Harvard School of Public Health is based on two assumptions. One is that the incidence of diabetes will continue to rise as steeply as it has in recent years. The other is that no cure will be found for this progressively disabling condition.

But there may be some very good news in store for the nation's six million diabetics. Simultaneously with release of the Harvard

667

projection in the publications of the National Society for the Prevention of Blindness, came a report by a southern California physician and his colleagues in the *Journal of Applied Nutrition* (Spring, 1972). The report was entitled "An Effective Thyroid-Vitamin Treatment for the Atherosclerotic Component in Diabetic Retinopathy," and it was written by Dr. Michael Walczak of Studio City, California, along with Dr. M. Israel of New York and Dr. I. R. Ross of Maryland.

As the title of the article suggested, their treatment consisted of oral doses of thyroid hormone extract, along with generous amounts of B complex vitamins. Vitamin C, enzymes, and diuretics were also given.

Using this regimen on 45 patients, 25 of whom were legally blind, for an average of 13 months, the authors reported that 40 were improved, two unimproved, while three became worse. For a disease which is considered incurable, and with which even stopgap measures are relatively ineffective, this record of clinical success, confirmed by eye specialists is extraordinary indeed! One patient had lost all sight in his left eye two years before seeing the physicians, and was rapidly losing vision in his remaining eye. He sat around the house all day, sinking into a great depression. His blood pressure, high cholesterol count, and other metabolic abnormalities made his prognosis far from favorable. During this time, the vision in his right eye was 20/200, which means that he perceived objects that were 20 feet away as if they were 200 feet away. After five months of treatment, the vision in his right eye dramatically improved to 20/60. His cholesterol count dropped from 294 to 215, his blood pressure was reduced, and his total health and attitude improved to the point where he was able to return to work.

A 57-year-old woman, the authors reported, "presented a pathetic picture" when they first saw her. He had lost virtually all the vision in her right eye ten years before and her left eye was only slightly better. All she could perceive were vague images. Complicating her general condition was the fact that at five feet two inches in height, she weighed 242 pounds. After 11 months of treatment, the vision in her right eye, which had been 4/200, meaning that at four feet she could perceive objects only with the clarity that normally sighted people can perceive them at 200 feet, improved to 20/200. The vision in her left eye improved from 6/200 to 20/100, the latter representing an astonishing improvement.

Long Experience With Thyroid Extract

The formulation of the thyroid-vitamin treatment was not something that Dr. Walczak and his colleagues stumbled upon. He and other physicians associated with the Vascular Research Foundation had been using thyroid and vitamins to attack atherosclerotic problems in the blood vessels of the heart, kidneys, brain, and other tissues for 20 years. They explained that atherosclerosis, in their view, is in part a gradually advancing thyroid deficiency. In the course of aging, both the production and utilization of thyroid secretion decreases. Whether this is "normal" or not is not the main issue. What's important is that by administering supplemental thyroid extract, processes associated with the decline of this hormone can be arrested, and in some cases, even reversed.

Thyroid hormone affects oxygen consumption and heat production throughout the body and stimulates the metabolism of certain isolated organs, such as the liver and muscles. It is believed, although it is not certain, that abnormal oxygen consumption by the retina is a major factor in diabetic retinopathy, and this may be the point at which thyroid hormone interferes with the progress of retinopathy. The action seems to take place at a very basic level, involving the transfer of enzyme electrons within the cell.

Knowledge of the beneficial effect of thyroid in patients with atherosclerosis is not new, but reports dating back many years indicate that there can be troublesome side effects. However, Dr. Walczak and his colleagues found that when the full B complex and vitamin C were given along with the thyroid, these unfavorable reactions were completely blocked. The B vitamins, he explained, achieve this by increasing the efficiency of electron transfer to the point where this accelerated process does not create side effects.

A Severe Case Responds Well

All this may sound rather complicated, but the important part is that the treatment appears to work. Consider the case of a 47-year-old woman with severe diabetic retinopathy, impending gangrene, marked fluid retention and high blood pressure. When first seen by Dr. Walczak, the main question was, as he described it, "Would the patient live long enough to become totally blind?"

Following treatment with the thyroid extract, vitamins, and diuretics, it was reported that her arms and legs felt warmer, pains diminished, her strength greatly increased and albumin stopped appearing in her urine. Most impressive, the examining clinician said, was that her improvement of vision in both eyes was "almost unbelievable." Dr. Walczak noted that this particular patient had received virtually every other treatment for retinopathy known, prior to being treated with hormones and vitamins, all without success. "Thus," he said "proof of the efficacy of the treatment does not require the inhuman procedure of administering placebos to 50 percent of such hopelessly ill patients."

Dr. Walczak said that this treatment is not useful merely as a last-ditch attempt to save failing eyesight. Rather, he said, it is most effective in cases where the disease has not yet caused deterioration of sight. Eye examinations showed that there was a definite improvement in 11 out of 12 patients whose vision had not yet begun to deteriorate at the time of treatment. This demonstrates, the authors said, *the truly preventive aspect of the treatment.*

Dr. Walczak, who is a specialist in preventive medicine and nutrition as they relate to chronic diseases associated with aging, had each of his patients carefully examined by an opthalmologist before and after treatment. Assessment of improvement, then, was not left solely to his judgment. The fact that 40 out of 45 people with an "incurable" disease improved was demonstrated by the most sophisticated medical techniques available. The researchers added, "From our experiences in the long-term treatment of this condition, *a large majority of these patients will retain their improved vision.*"

The work of Dr. Walczak and his colleagues remains in the "experimental" stage. That is to say, their results are not universally accepted by other physicians. This, of course, does not in the least diminish their importance. Nor should it deter anyone who has diabetic retinopathy from seeking similar treatment.

Greatly in favor of this new treatment is that it is primarily natural. Along with the thyroid extract, which patients take orally three times a day with their meals in custom-tailored doses ranging from 10 mg. to 60 mg., Dr. Walczak also administers vitamin B_1 and B_2, niacinamide, calcium pantothenate, and vitamin C. Vitamin B_{12} and calcium in the form of calcium gluconate are administered by injection, along with laevo-thyroxine to supplement the oral hormone. An enzyme (Varidase) is also given. Diuretics are administered to help the patient shed excessive fluid from the body.

148. How Nine-Out-Of-Ten Patients Conquered Conjunctivitis

Conjunctivitis is the general name given to a number of painful inflammations of the delicate mucous membranes, or conjunctiva, in the immediate vicinity of the eyes. Palpebral conjunctiva is an inflammation of the conjunctiva which line the eyelids, while burbular conjunctiva is an inflammation of the outer surface of the eyeballs, giving them a milky or blue sheen appearance. "Pink eye" is the common name for a more contagious and graver form of this condition, which physicians usually refer to as acute conjunctivitis. Another form, vernal conjunctivitis, which will start in the spring and normally last through to autumn, causes an aggravating itching and tearing condition of the eyes which is known to recur among sufferers every spring for a period of five to seven years.

The first symptom of conjunctivitis is the mistaken feeling that there is a foreign object in the eye. The next symptom is usually a discharge of a fluid that is rubbery or stringy in consistency. This specific symptom always occurs with vernal conjunctivitis. Other general symptoms include pain and swelling of the eye region and a nagging urge to rub an incessant itch, especially during hot, humid weather. The unyielding burning sensation is aggravated by an abnormal sensitivity to light (photophobia).

Vitamin D And Calcium For Conjunctivitis
Of all the treatments used in treating this most irritating of eye disorders, none has had such a dramatic effect as the combination of vitamin D and calcium supplements. Dr. Alexander Knapp, an ophthalmologists, has reported remarkable success in treating sundry types of conjunctivitis with these natural substances. In a paper presented to the *International Academy of Preventive Medicine* in March of 1974, Dr. Knapp reported, "For years vitamin D and calcium have been prescribed, and over 90 percent of the patients have improved."

671

The Eyes

Dr. Knapp's 40 years of research into the treatment of conjunctivitis with vitamin D and calcium was paralleled by his research in using these compounds to treat myopia successfully. In his first attempts to treat conjunctivitis, he used traditional methods of treatment with little success. He then turned to a method of conjunctivitis therapy never before tried in the annals of medicine. Noticing that vernal conjunctivitis has been associated with other eye disorders that seem to be allergies, he recalled research done at Columbia's College of Physicians and Surgeons. There, animals fed on diets deficient in vitamin D soon developed similar eye disorders. Furthermore, Dr. Knapp himself had previously treated humans with these related anomalies. The patients had responded well to vitamin D and calcium. In addition, the doctor found that some investigators had claimed that there is an underlying calcium deficiency in certain forms of conjunctivitis. He, therefore, began treatments with vitamin D and calcium in the form of mineral mixture tablets given to 41 of his conjunctivitis patients.

Vitamin D functions to aid calcium's absorption and transportation throughout the body once foods containing calcium have been digested. The vitamin helps in the assimilation of calcium through the walls of the intestines into the serum of the blood which feeds the various body regions including that of the eye. Hence, vitamin D is essential for proper calcium metabolism. In order to regulate this metabolism even better, calcium should be accompanied by phosphorus and magnesium. It is then understandable that the mineral mixture tablets prescribed by Dr. Knapp contained not only calcium but significant quantities of phosphorus and magnesium as well. (They were nearly identical to bone meal.)

After approximately four months, 20 of the 41 patients treated experienced complete relief while 11 others showed tremendous improvement with vitamin D therapy. Photophobia and excessive tearing had just about disappeared.

Later Dr. Knapp obtained further evidence linking vitamin deficiency to vernal conjunctivitis. A number of sailors serving during World War II returned to the States complaining of inflamed eyes, itching, burning sensations, and photophobia. It was unusual for any such patient to have had similar complaints prior to being at sea on restricted rations for long periods of time. Dr. Knapp diagnosed the sailors' malady as being conjunctivitis. Upon questioning them, he learned that they had subsisted on diets deficient in vitamin D, and their conjunctivitis responded to vitamin D therapy.

Another doctor followed Dr. Knapp's lead. Success with large dosages of vitamin D in treating vernal conjunctivitis was also gained by Dr. Saleh Ali Ibrahim and reported in a monograph entitled "Vitamin D in the Treatment of Certain Ophthalmic Cases." Vitamin D was directly instilled in the conjunctivae of 54 patients three times a day for one month. This was supplemented by oral doses of the vitamin. Sixty percent of the cases of spring conjunctivitis showed improvement. Most important, the most common and most annoying complication of conjunctivitis—eosinophilia—completely disappeared. Eosinophilia is the formation and accumulation of an unusually large number of a type of white blood corpuscles which form a sticky, stringy discharge. Dr. Ibrahim was pleased to find that eosinophilia was absent from the films examined of patients given the vitamin therapy. He further noted a rapid disappearance of the sticky discharge as well as a renewed sense of comfort and relief in his patients.

Dr. Knapp warns that very often the potential for conjunctivitis lurks within us without exhibiting overt symptoms. And while conjunctivitis is not a fatal disease, it is so miserably uncomfortable that anyone who can prevent its occurrence but still permits it to develop is very foolish indeed. It is so simple to prevent, by preventing vitamin D deficiency. The best and most reliable source known for a measured daily intake of vitamin D is natural fish liver oil. The vitamin is also found in egg yolk and fish.

Vitamin A, as well as vitamin D, is effective against conjunctivitis. An important secretion of the mucous membranes is lysozyme, which has an antiseptic action. But if there is a shortage of vitamin A, the outer cells of the membranes become scaly, preventing the effective secretion of lysozyme. Vitamin A then works directly to prevent drying and hardening of the mucous membranes.

A general rule of thumb is that green and yellow colored foods are good sources of vitamin A, as are animal and fish livers.

With proper nutrition, conjunctivitis need not be a problem. But if it should occur, the advances made by Dr. Knapp offer encouragement for a speedy and lasting recovery.

149. Nearsightedness In Children Can Be Cured

When rays of light enter the normal eye through the lens, they are bent to converge on a single point on the retina, the inside coating of the eyeball. Although it is only the thickness of a newspaper page, the retina contains ten distinct layers and between 125 and 150 million sensing rods. In the individual with myopia (nearsightedness), the light rays, instead of converging on a single point on the retina, are pinpointed in front of it, making distant objects appear blurred. Traditionally this problem has been treated by fitting the patient with negative (minus) lenses which make an adjustment to the light rays, resulting in their being properly focused on the retina.

The condition opposite to myopia is farsightedness, or hyperopia. This condition makes close images, such as the print on this page, appear blurred, though distant objects remain in focus. This problem is caused by light rays converging behind the retina. This problem has been corrected by fitting the patient with positive (or plus) lenses which also bend the light rays so that they focus on a single point of the retina.

However, a growing number of optometrists believe that the plus lenses traditionally used to lessen the aggravation of farsightedness may actually be employed to *cure* nearsightedness.

The eye functions by "accommodation," which is the term used to describe how the focusing apparatus of the eye adjusts to objects at different distances. "Accommodation" takes place by increasing the convex shape of the eye's lens through contraction of the ciliary muscles. In man, according to these optometrists, the eye's normal function is programmed to distant objects. But children start school at an earlier age and television plays a larger part in the child's daily routine, so the eye must "accommodate" to close up vision, which is unnatural for it at an early age. To perform such an adjustment, the curvature is altered, blurring distance vision.

Treatment Starts When Squinting Begins

The positive lens advocates believe that when a child starts squinting in school—one sign that myopia may be imminent—the child should be fitted with weak positive lenses. The positive lens, which is a magnifying glass, minimizes the need for major accommodation. For example, when a child wears a pair of plus glasses, it's impossible for him to read with comfort anything brought close to the eyes because the print appears to be blurred. So the child must hold the paper or book farther away from his eyes. This means the eye does not have to work as hard to "accommodate" if the child stops reading to look at something in the distance.

And, to minimize the number of times a child might have to put on and take off his glasses, those who advocate the use of positive lenses recommend a half-lens or "granny" glasses, so the child can gaze over the positive lenses when looking at distant objects.

But what happens if the child who develops a case of myopia is fitted with a pair of negative lenses? The negative lens corrects the blurred image and distant objects literally leap into focus. But, the negative lenses *do not* correct the overall problem of accommodation. The basic problem of adjusting to close-up work still exists. And what's worse is that the eye will continue on the same path, developing a worsening case of myopia. This means that until the individual is around 25, he will continue to need stronger and stronger negative lenses until the myopia gradually grinds to a halt. Even then, there is no guarantee it will stop.

On the other hand, according to the positive lens advocates, there is a good chance that if a child is fitted with positive lenses, he can slowly work his way out of a myopic state to the point where he will never have to wear glasses. By this theory, the use of plus lenses compels the child to use his distance vision all the time. This keeps the myopia from developing any further, and may, in many cases, eliminate it.

But is the positive lens treatment for myopia practical? "Yes, definitely," said Dr. William M. Ludlam, an optometrist and former Director of the Laboratory for Myopia Research in New York. "I've used that method for the past 20 years and have had good success with it."

Dr. Ludlam said that myopia can be cured and, what's more important, can actually be prevented through development of good reading and other eyesight habits such as holding books farther away from the eyes during reading and frequently looking at distant objects during and after long periods of reading. "But once they (optometrists or ophthalmologists) fit negative lenses, that's it. The child has myopia," he said.

On one occasion an accountant brought his young son to Dr. Ludlam for treatment of headaches associated with long periods of reading. After fitting the son with positive reading glasses and prescribing a series of visual exercises, Dr. Ludlam was asked if he could cure or at least help the accountant's myopia. "The accountant had normal vision up until he was about 23 or 24. In fact he had served in the Air Force. But by the time he came to me, he had 20/400," Dr. Ludlam said. 20/400 means that the accountant, who was in his early 30's, could see at 20 feet what people with perfect vision could see at 400 feet. In practical terms, he could read only the largest letter on an eye chart.

Dr. Ludlam treated the accountant with a series of exercises and positive lenses which increased the eye's flexibility. "I brought him down from 20/400 to 20/80 and 20/40 where he is now and I've held him there," Dr. Ludlam said. "He still wears glasses to drive, for the theater and to watch television, but other than that, he doesn't need them especially for his close-up work."

Dr. Ludlam has done the same for children, bringing them from extremely poor distant vision right down to 20/40 through exercises and positive lenses and "held them there for 10 years. I reported on 30 cases that I treated for over a 10 year period of time, so I know it can be done," he said.

Not All Myopia Responds

Dr. Ludlam has studied two different forms of myopia. One is caused by pressure of the eye growing too fast, causing the eye to become elongated. "It literally grows right out of focus." Its treatment calls for fitting the eye with contact lenses which press the eye into focus, acting like a pressure bandage. If a 10, 11 or 12-year-old child is fitted with contact lenses, there is a good chance that the myopia will be caught and not progress further, he noted.

But the other type of myopia can be reversed. It's caused by a spasm of the ciliary muscles. For example, a person is reading and then looks up. If the eye fails to focus on a distant object, the ciliary muscles are believed to be undergoing spasms. "If a child comes in and tells me that he has trouble trying to focus on a blackboard or a clock until he blinks a couple of times, he's accurately describing a ciliary spasm," Dr. Ludlam said.

The ciliary spasm form of myopia is controlled by use of positive lenses which tend to take the close-up environment and push it outwards, increasing the reading distance. "The nearer you hold something like a book, the greater the problem, because the more the ciliary muscles must contract," Dr. Ludlam said. "Reading at eight inches or less is murder on eyes and someone who does this continually will become nearsighted very quickly."

Dr. Ludlam pointed out, however, that other factors might play a role in myopia as well. "There are indications that nearsightedness is caused by a number of things such as the environment, nutrition and function (i.e. reading)," Dr. Ludlam said. "There are cases where one aspect of the problem is more important than the other. For example, if a child eats a well balanced diet and lives in a good home, but all of a sudden becomes a bookworm and develops myopia, it's pretty obvious what the cause is."

Dr. Ludlam cited a study done on Eskimos in which it was discovered that myopia had reached near-epidemic proportions among the current school-age generation. The study of 204 children in elementary grades in Alaska showed that the proportion of myopes in grade five approximated that found in grade 12 among Caucasians, or 26 percent. However, the proportion of myopes in grade six (59 percent) usually is never reached in any school population among Caucasians according to an article in the *American Journal of Optometry and Archives of the American Academy of Optometry*, (May, 1970).

Dr. Ludlam pointed out that the grandparents of these children had no myopia while the parents of these school children had less than a five percent incidence. "This near-epidemic of myopia may be a combination of many different factors," he said. "This is the first generation to read. It's the first to use electrical lights and it's the first generation to eat a non-protein diet. They're eating everything from popcorn to Coke. Who can say what is causing their nearsightedness?"

Dr. Ludlam said that heredity can pretty well be discounted as a cause of myopia simply because of the fact that it is growing much faster than if it were a genetic defect. Although the positive lens theory works and can possibly lead to a life free from the anchor of glasses, it is extremely difficult to convince many patients that it will work for them.

A Bucks County, Pa., optometrist, Dr. Carl Cordova, has stated that many patients are reluctant to try the therapy because it doesn't work right away. "They believe in making a distant picture clear and they'll go from doctor to doctor in order to hear the answers they want," he said.

But the onset of myopia is a gradual one. It can happen over a period of a year or two, and a person might first be conscious of it after being examined. And, as Dr. Cordova pointed out, most patients want the blurred vision eliminated immediately. They will not take the time to effect a cure but will settle for having their distant vision cleared. A cure, however, can take almost as long as the disease took to reach the point at which correction started.

Fitting the patient with bifocals containing a reading (positive) lens and a negative lens of a lower power than needed is a variation of the positive lens cure, said Dr. Cordova. He was eventually able to almost completely correct myopia in patients who were willing to use this treatment.

Childhood Prevention Of Myopia

Most parents are very concerned with how they can prevent their children from becoming nearsighted. There are several ways, the first of which begins in the crib. Mothers, according to Dr. Amiel Franke, of Washington, D.C., should keep a child out of the playpen as much as possible. By stimulating the baby's eyes, they are given more of a chance to develop. "When a child's activities, even in infancy, are limited, his vision growth and development is limited too," he said during a meeting of the Southeastern Congress of Optometry.

Along with close eye strain during adolescence, diet has been blamed for the near-epidemic incidence of myopia. Dr. Jin Otsuka, a leading Japanese authority on nearsightedness and professor of the Department of Ophthalmology, Tokyo Medical and Dental University, believes that diet as well as the environment plays a major role in myopia.

In his soon to be published book, *The Cause and Treatment of Myopia*, Dr. Otsuka attributes the rise in myopia to the extensive use of sugar and refined foods in place of a more traditional Japanese diet which was heavy on natural foods.

Myopia seems to be a disease which can often be corrected, if the proper steps are taken. For many, it's too late. The die is cast. But it would be wise for parents to:

- Make sure their infants get plenty of eye exercise;
- Insure that their children eat a balanced menu including plenty of vitamin D and calcium;
- Guard against excessive close eye work and long hours of reading, especially at distances of less than eight inches;
- Watch for signs of squinting, headaches and tiredness;
- Train their children to take breaks in reading and look at far-off objects; and
- Have a child's eyes checked regularly.

150. Reinforce Children's Vision With Sound Nutrition

Sound vision and proper nutrition are inextricably linked together. These findings are borne out by vision-nutrition researchers wherever they wander—Asia, Africa, Latin America, and the United States.

A 50-country survey conducted by Dr. Donald S. McLaren of the American University in Beirut and World Health Organization representatives established this startling fact: "More than one percent of the poorer children had visual defects traceable to faulty nutrition." Studies indicated that at least 100,000 children throughout the world develop corneal defects linked to poor nutrition (*Nutrition Today,* March, 1968).

According to Dr. McLaren, 80,000 children go blind annually because of faulty nutrition; one of every two of these children die; and many more children suffer vision defects at home and abroad because of what their mothers ate during pregnancy or what they were fed during early childhood.

Affluent America may also be displaying its own singular lack of vision by succumbing to a false sense of security about its accomplishments in the field of nutrition. It is claimed that there is no starvation here, everybody is well fed. Deteriorating eyesight is considered a normal phenomenon, an easily corrected deficiency.

"More careful consideration reveals that many of the defects are traceable to faulty nutrition—and could have been prevented," Dr. McLaren said. "Prevented" is the key word, for prevention of visual defects in children is often directly related to adequate maternal nutrition during pregnancy.

What the mother passes on to the developing fetus in the form of nutrients has been shown to be the difference between healthy, clear-eyed children and children who must suffer some form of optic degeneration.

The Essential Nutrients
Researchers have correlated eye health with the broad spectrum of nutrients ranging from vitamins A through E to protein, calcium and rutin.

Vitamin A is considered one of the most vital of these nutrients in relation to ocular pathology. The "fish liver oil vitamin"— also abundant in butter, milk, eggs and liver—prevents xerophthalmia, a major cause of blindness in malnourished children.

These vitamin A-starved youngsters suffer drying and hardening of their conjunctivas (inner linings of the eyelids). These conjunctival lesions may be followed by similar changes in the cornea, resulting in a condition known as keratomalacia. At this stage, ulceration and irreversible blindness may occur.

The importance of vitamin A to the eye is underlined by the fact that about one percent of a person's daily intake of the substance is used directly by the retina.

The retina is composed of cones, sensitive to bright lights and colors, and rods, sensitive to dim light and black and white. The rods contain rhodopsin ("visual purple") which is made of the protein opsin, and retinene, a form of vitamin A.

When light strikes rhodopsin, retinene and opsin split, joining again in the dark to allow detection of images. The drawback is that some of the retinene is destroyed in the splitting process and, unless vitamin A is continually replaced in the body, vision becomes impossible in darkness. It's a condition we all know as night blindness.

Symptoms of eye disease appear rapidly in the very young, whose requirements of vitamin A during early growth exceed their ability to store it in the liver. A proper supply of vitamin A to newborn infants is, therefore, of prime importance to visual health. Again, maternal nutrition during pregnancy and while nursing, is the key.

The B complex vitamins, available in such food supplements as brewer's yeast, desiccated liver, wheat germ and sunflower seeds, help prevent a host of ocular problems: a conjunctivitis which occurs with bloodshot eyes; watering of the eyes; itching and burning; and sensitivity to light.

Riboflavin plays the pivotal role in the B group, being necessary for the cornea to breathe. In the absence of riboflavin, tiny blood vessels are formed in an effort by the body to bring oxygenated blood into closer contact with the cornea. Bloodshot eyes, of course, are characteristic of many other eye disturbances as well as lack of riboflavin.

Vitamin C, well known for its intra-cellular tissue strengthening ability, is little known for its importance to the eye. This nutrient is vital to the oxygen uptake of the lens, helping prevent tissue hemorrhaging associated with the extreme cases of nutritional deficiency.

Glaucoma and cataract are usually accompanied by extreme vitamin C deficiencies. One rich natural source of this vitamin, is rose hips. The fruit of the rose plant, rose hips are 40 times richer in vitamin C than grapefruit or oranges. Other excellent sources are green peppers, broccoli, cauliflower, watercress, raw cabbage, strawberries, cantaloupe, tomatoes and fresh peas.

The dramatic effects of vitamin D upon the eye have been observed by researchers in ocular pathology. Keratoconus, a bulging of the cornea, has responded well to vitamin D treatments. Since vitamin D regulates the deposition of calcium in bone formation, a lack of it can result in bone deformity or disorder that can affect the eyes. Strong skull and orbital bones protect eyes from injury; bone inflammation in Paget's Disease has been observed to induce symptoms of double vision (diplopia); poor upper and lower jawbone formation is associated with squinting and bulging eyeballs, and decaying nasal bone hinders tear drainage.

Vitamin D is found mainly in fish livers—which are also rich in vitamin A—and eggs. The action of sunlight on the skin enables us to synthesize this vitamin.

Rutin, a bioflavonoid extracted from buckwheat leaves, has been used to cure capillary fragility of the eye. Its contribution to bodily health is found in its ability to strengthen artery walls, thus preventing strokes and hemorrhages.

Enough Protein Is Vital

Children at Guy's Hospital in London whose diets were enriched by protein showed definite progress in arresting the development of myopia, while children whose diets were unaltered suffered continuing visual deterioration.

Dr. J. J. Stern of Utica State Hospital, New York, writing in the book *Modern Nutrition in Health and Disease,* points out that amino acids are essential for the health of the eye's lens.

Dr. Stern found that a high proportion of laboratory animals deficient in amino acids developed cataracts. The cataracts disappeared if amino acids were fed before the condition progressed too far.

Recognition of the urgent need for vitamin-balanced diets administered in the earliest stages of a developing infant's life has not, however, been accompanied by an effective course of action in this nation and throughout the world.

More people are going blind each year in the United States than have ever gone blind before. A well known U.S. Public Health Service inquiry into eye disorders revealed that: "In the two decades between 1940 and 1960 the general population of the United States increased by 36 percent, while the blind population rose by some 67 percent." Today, 90 million Americans have some form of eye trouble and much of it could have been nipped in infancy.

In Dr. McLaren's own words: "The question that needs to be asked is 'How long is it going to take parents . . . to become actively desirous of incorporating foods into the diets of their infants which they have hitherto regarded as unnecessary or positively harmful?'"

151. What Tobacco Smoke Does To The Eyes

It has long been known that tobacco smoking can be irritating to the eyes of smokers and nonsmokers alike. The 1972 Surgeon General's report indicated that 70 percent of those people queried concerning their antismoking complaints listed ordinary eye redness and the tear inducing menace of cigarette smoke as two of the most aggravating factors. However, the irritation of cigarette smoke is far more dangerous to the internal structure of the eyes than commonly believed.

In 1974 research conducted by Smoking Research of San Diego, California, and the United States Department of Health, Education and Welfare, showed that both carbon monoxide and nicotene, two of the most harmful ingredients in cigarette smoke, were involved in cutting the oxygen supply to the eyes, causing a marked inability of the eyes to adapt to darkness. The studies proved that nicotene causes the blood vessels in the eye to become smaller, while the carbon monoxide diminishes the blood's ability to supply and regulate oxygen.

Other research showed that the oxygen limiting menace caused by the tobacco smoke also severely limits a person's field of vision, diminishing periphereal vision at night and creating a condition known as *tunnel vision*. Consider the danger in a smoke filled car at night where the driver has to be aware of vehicles or persons on either side of the road.

The California studies also confirmed the existence of a cigarette smoke induced disorder known as *tobacco amblyopia*. The disorder, although rare and often misdiagnosed, lessens visual acuity and the perception of colors. The initial symptom is presbyopia, the decreased ability of the eye to focus on near objects because of a loss of elasticity in the eye's lens. This is accompanied by the inability to perceive the colors red or green, or simply a case of incipient color blindness. These symptoms are paralleled by a general decline in circulation, the most obvious symptom of this being a "freezing feeling" in the tips of the fingers. *Tobacco amblyopia* is linked to a combination of smoking, poor diet, and abuse of alcohol. The condition begins to improve as soon as the sufferer gives up smoking, moderates his drinking habits and develops sound eating habits.

152. Tension Causes Eyestrain

Nervous tension may affect the eyes in many strange ways because anxiety and nervousness stimulate excessive eye muscle activity. This in turn gives rise to symptoms of eyestrain.

Take the case of Mrs. G., a storekeeper. She suffered with many signs of eye trouble: blurred vision, headaches, and burning and itching sensations in her eyes and eyelids. However, a thorough eye examination showed conclusively that she did not need eyeglasses.

"I have this eye trouble mostly at the end of the day," she said. "Usually after figuring my daily business and going over the bills."

Further investigation revealed that she found bookkeeping a complicated and distasteful chore. She also was having difficulty in meeting her bills, which further agitated an already tense situation. After assigning her book work to someone else and making more convenient arrangements with her suppliers, these symptoms disappeared. Eyestrain commonly is experienced by those who live in a state of nervous tension. This is because slight defects of the eyes, normally tolerated by calmer persons, become aggravated in nervous people.

If you are nervously inclined, and suffer the symptoms of eyestrain because of tension, you may be able to overcome these symptoms by simply relaxing. The first step is to plan a daily relaxation period. Seek quiet, comfortable surroundings, preferably at the same place and the same hour every day. Close your eyes lightly and allow your mind to relax completely. If your eyes sting or itch you can help them relax by applying hot compresses. A daily relaxation period will not only aid your eyes, but the rest of your body as well, because anxiety and tension adversely affect all body organs.

153. Eye Trouble?
Check Your Teeth

When it comes to dental work, many people search high and low to find the cheapest, quickest, and most painless treatment. This usually occurs because the dentist's chair has the terrifying and discouraging reputation of being a painful, time-consuming and expensive place to be.

Incomplete dental work may get done fast, but it can later return to plague you as visual problems. On the other hand, those extra few minutes in the dentist's chair could save you months of eye trouble later. The few more dollars could keep you from paying a full ophthalmologist's fee. And the little bit of discomfort now could help you avoid an agony of temporary loss in visual acuity, inflammation of the eye or, worse, a permanent visual impairment caused by a serious eye disease later.

And it's a two-way street. Not only can your dentist help prevent eye impairments by careful work on your teeth, but if you find yourself in the eye doctor's chair too often with an eye condition that just won't clear up, you might do well to see your dentist about it.

Eye problems can often begin in the mouth, and are sometimes solved by dental treatment. Cases of blurred vision or even complete blindness have been reported to be cured by the extraction of irritating teeth, as have incidents of "tics," or involuntary contractions, of eyelid or facial muscles.

Tooth Roots Cause Eye Problems

A Swiss dentist, J. L. Dephilippe, studied four patients with sight problems and eye inflammation ranging from mild to severe who found their cures in the dentist's office. Each was found to have small starting points of infection at the points where root canal work on an upper lacteral incisor, usually called an eyetooth, had been incompletely finished. This is understandable: Root canal work is a painful process undertaken in cases of advanced dental caries, involving the removal of the tooth's nerve, when properly performed, up to the jaw bone. In these four cases, repeating the root canal work and completely obliterating the root canal system resulted in an immediate improvement of symptoms and a restoration of full sight.

In other cases, part of the root may remain after extraction—especially in the case of teeth with curved roots, where a dentist may feel the time involved and the pain to the patient doesn't warrant reentering with a probe and picking out those pieces remaining in the bone. In one example, a man experienced persistent pain over his left eye, which could not be explained by normal eye or ear, nose and throat findings. A slight broadening of the site of a removed molar tipped his dentist off to the possibility of remaining root fragments; a dental X-ray showed this to be the case. The pain was caused by reflex process, stimulation of the common nerve between the teeth and the eyes; when the root fragments were removed, the pain disappeared.

Mouth Infection Can Lead To Blindness

But tooth-related eye problems are not always as simple as pain or inflammation: dental troubles are suspected of causing more serious diseases.

Uveitis is an inflammation of the front part of the eye which can cause scarring of the cornea and, in severe cases, blindness.

Studies by the Uveitis Clinic of the Philippine General Hospital showed the teeth and gums were responsible in about 60 percent of cases studied as a focus of infection for the disease (*Philippine Journal of Surgery and Surgical Specialties,* July-August, 1966). And Dr. M. E. Alvaro of Sao Paulo, Brazil, has reported that 52.27 percent of his cases were caused by foci of infection in infected teeth. Although it is difficult to demonstrate the technical mechanism, it would be hard to deny the causal relationship between diseases of the eyes and the teeth.

Another disease, endophthalmitis, is transmitted through blood vessels or lymph channels from the teeth to the eyes. This is characterized by negative vision, a whitish opacity seen through the pupil, and congestion of the eye. Usually, even if the infection is controlled the eye remains totally blind and atrophies.

In the viral disease Herpes Zoster Ophthalmicus (shingles), vesicles, or fluid-filled sacs, form on the terminal endings of the fifth cranial nerve, the common nerve between the eyes, causing severe pain and visual problems. This disease has been reported to develop after a tooth extraction or even a simple crowning.

Allergy Is Involved

According to Dr. Liborio Mangubat, assistant professor of ophthalmology at the University of the Philippines College of Medicine, there are two ways infections can travel from your dental area to your eye area. Transmission of the disease through the jaw bone, veins or lymph channels leads to what he calls direct extension or metastatic spread. But more often, he said, eye infections are caused by antibodies formed by the system to fight bacterial antigens produced by dental troubles. Researchers are still trying to discover the manner by which this phenomenon occurs (*Pakistan Dental Review*, October, 1970).

The connection between your teeth and your eyes is shown even more forcefully through the congenital defects relating them. The Oculo-Dento-Digital Syndrome, documented by three scientists in 1966, is characterized by deformation of the fingers and nostrils, abnormally small eyes and defective and yellowed tooth enamel. There have been only 10 cases reported in world medical literature, and no one has explained how the syndrome is caused—but the connection is there, and it is strong. Even more astonishing is the case of a five-year-old girl with abnormally placed teeth—in her eyelid. "This is a very unusual condition, and the explanation for its presence on the lid is just conjectural," said Dr. Mangubat. "But could you think of a better way of showing how close the eyes and teeth can be?"

But incomplete dental work cannot be blamed for causing all your vision troubles—lack of dental care can be just as debilitating. If you don't protect your teeth and keep them strong and healthy, you may find yourself with eye impairments caused by dental infection, pulp exposed by caries, degenerated or injured pulp or pulp stones. And putting off the removal of that neglected or impacted wisdom tooth that's giving you dental agony can put pressure on the nerves leading to your eyes, causing them pain and problems too.

Nutrition For Teeth Will Help The Eyes

Good nutrition and eating habits can help you prevent eye problems caused by tooth troubles, as well as improve your whole health outlook. Vitamin A helps build the enamel of your teeth while preventing pulp tumors, said Dr. James H. Shaw, Ph.D., of the Harvard School of Dental Medicine; these tumors, reported Dr. Mangubat, can travel from the pulp through the upper jaw bone and into the orbit of the eye. According to Dr.

The Eyes

Karl Rinne in *Zahnarztl Rundschau*, a German dental journal, vitamin A can also enable you to avoid gum diseases such as gingivitis, which causes gums to shrink away from the teeth, forming pockets and inviting collection of food debris to stimulate infection. Fish liver oils are especially good sources of valuable vitamin A. And fish liver oil also is a rich provider of vitamin D, which scientific studies have shown to reduce the incidence of new cavities and slow the development of old ones.

The B complex vitamins also aid the health of the mouth, lips and tongue, and therefore are important for full dental health, noted Dr. Rinne. Vitamin B_6 was reported at the first meeting of the American Society for Clinical Nutrition (*Drug Trade News*, May 15, 1961) as particularly useful in the full utilization of calcium and has been reported to lessen the incidence of dental caries. Wheat germ, desiccated liver and brewer's yeast are all excellent sources of the whole vitamin B complex.

Rose hips, green peppers and cabbage are providers of vitamin C, which Dr. Shaw stressed is a must for healthy gums. Without sufficient quantities of vitamin C, gums can be inflamed and spongy, and more susceptible to damage. And this weakening of the gums can lead to a loosening of the teeth.

Another tip: avoid simple sugars and refined foods, which are recognized worldwide as the major cause of tooth decay. They lack the important "protective" factor, which some doctors suspect to be phosphorus. You can find phosphorus, all-important calcium and other minerals needed for strong teeth and bones in bone meal, helping your teeth to resist damage and decay. Your best bets for good dental health are foods as close as possible to their natural state, without excessive refining, and a diet with a minimum of high carbohydrate foods.

Good saliva flow, important for the natural cleaning action of your teeth, should be aided by sufficient quantities of water, proteins, niacin, folic acid, iron and vitamin A. Citrus juices, although a good source of vitamin C, should be avoided—they can promote tooth erosion, reported Douglas N. Allan, M.D.S., D.D.S., in the *British Dental Journal* (April 4, 1967). Also, stay away from abrasive toothpastes; they can damage tooth enamel. Instead, eat plenty of raw fruits and vegetables.

154. If You Wear
Contact Lenses . . .

Contact lenses, now worn by millions of people in the United States, are chosen not only for their cosmetic value. Eyeglasses can be an impediment in certain sports and in certain areas of work. Contact lenses correct highly myopic conditions and aphakic conditions (having no lens in the eye), and are helpful in correcting certain eye defects in children.

But, according to P. Thomas Manchester, M.D., an Atlanta ophthalmologist, wearers of contact lenses often develop inadequate eye warning systems and can sometimes do harm to their eyes without experiencing pain (*Journal of the American Medical Association*, October 5, 1970). This is because the contact lens exerts pressure on nerve endings, so the sensitivity of the cornea is reduced. Dr. Manchester maintains that greater pressure exerted by a contact lens can also cause objects to be buried deep in the cornea, making them extremely difficult to detect or find. "Foreign bodies . . . and various chemicals and pollutants from the atmosphere cannot be flushed away so easily as was possible without the lens," he said. "Smoke, mascara, hair spray, detergents for cleaning the lenses—all may accumulate beneath the lenses. Even food particles and spirochetes are likely to be found if the patient cleans the lenses in his mouth."

Dr. Manchester discouraged any one over the age of 20 from wearing contact lenses. Youngsters adjust quickly and without as much discomfort as adults, he said, "but I can't recommend contact lenses to anyone, because his eyes are better off without them and health must come first."

Dr. Manchester conceded, however, that contact lenses are generally believed to retard myopia so that some young patients can wear the same prescription for five or even ten years without a change. If these patients had been wearing eyeglasses, they would probably have required several adjustments in prescription. Why is this so? Dr. Manchester said that an alteration in the refractive index of the cornea, possibly influenced by a change in water content, often accounts for the longevity in lens prescriptions.

In March, 1966, six ophthalmologists reported in the *Journal of the American Medical Association* the results of a nationwide survey covering almost 50,000 contact lens wearers. While the great majority had no complications, there were 7,600 who showed some temporary changes in their eyes. These were readily treatable. But, there were 157 cases in which patients suffered permanent, though minor, damage. In 14 persons, however, the damage was not minor. They lost the sight of one eye. The authors of the report concluded that "the popularity of contact lenses has exceeded the public knowledge of potential hazards associated with their use."

Permanent damage occurred only when contact lens wearers wore their lenses for days or weeks without interruption in the presence of corneal infection or in the presence of "overwear" or poor fit.

Tips For Lens Wearers

Millions of lens wearers suffer disappointment with their lenses and risk eye damage, according to Jeffrey Baker, author of *The Truth about Contact Lenses* (Putnam, 1970). Contact lenses have their dangers, he points out, but when the wearer is deeply motivated and exercises care and proper hygiene, the lenses serve him well, and in special circumstances eliminate some of the handicaps of spectacles.

Here are some pointers suggested by Mr. Baker which might help contact lens wearers avoid trouble:

Always carry wetting solution with you. If the hands can't be washed before inserting a lens, wet both lens and fingertips with solution. But don't use saliva. Bacteria from the mouth can be dangerous to the eye.

When holding a lens by the edge, do not squeeze; lenses warp easily and then cause abrasions.

When reading, doing close work, or while at concentrated physical work, a person should consciously relax now and then, look away from his work and gaze about, blinking normally. This will relieve the burning and itching which sometimes is the result of concentrated hard wear with insufficient blinking. The same problems that cause eye burning and itching during concentrated work may also cause tiredness and headaches.

Be careful about using wetting and soaking solutions that may cause hazing of lenses. Use solutions produced by the same company to avoid this incompatibility.

Wearers who use cosmetics should insert the lenses before contaminating the hands.

Never use hair spray while wearing lenses. Hair spray can permanently alter lens plastic since it remains in the air long after use.

Men should insert their lenses before handling hair oils or shaving lotions.

If there is any eye infection or allergic discomfort, don't wear contacts.

When traveling with contact lenses, do not use local water for lens rinsing and cleaning if there is doubt about its purity. Changes in altitude and water content can cause lens irritation.

Do not accept discomfort or disturbed vision as routine to contact lens wear.

Carry a pair of eyeglasses at all times. Wear the eyeglasses periodically during the day even if contacts feel perfectly comfortable.

Drugs, such as diuretics or birth control pills, may cause difficulty. Avoid them if you use lenses.

155. The Pill Can Affect Your Vision

Despite the discomforts experienced by many users of the pill, despite the disadvantages of weight gain which often accompanies the use of the drug, and even in spite of possible serious, long-term side effects reported by some authorities, oral contraceptives are taken by more women today than any other medication alone.

Disturbing reports of serious, immediate side effects also are heard from time to time, effects that are mainly concerned with the vascular system of the body. Among those that are seldom mentioned, however, are side effects that frequently manifest themselves in ocular and general circulatory disturbances, changes in vision, and in interference with the general health and well being of the eyes.

The eye is a highly vascular organ, richly supplied with blood vessels which extend to and nourish all its parts, especially the light-sensitive retina that is responsible for vision. Any interference with blood circulation to or from the retina for even a brief period will cause rapid loss of sight in the affected area, resulting in a scotoma, or blind area, in the visual field. If the involved retinal area is large, loss of sight in the entire eye may result. The loss is a permanent one, in most cases, and sight will not return even if blood circulation is restored.

One of the more serious side effects of oral contraceptives is the possible formation of a venous thrombus, or blood clot of the vein. This can occur anywhere in the body, of course, but far from the common belief that it concentrates in the legs, it will most frequently occur in small vessels such as those found in the eye and surrounding the brain. Dr. Frank Walsh and associates at Johns Hopkins Hospital reported that they had tabulated the more common ocular and cranial side effects of the pill. Of 59 cases of undesirable effects possibly related to oral contraceptives, Dr. Walsh listed 33 percent from either vascular thromboses of the retina or optic neuritis (inflammation of the retinal nerves), 29 percent had stroke-like symptoms, suggesting involvement of the cranial blood supply, and 37 percent with migraine headache, a head pain often associated with vascular dysfunction.

Edema Of The Eye

The cornea, that clear transparent window in the front of the eye, is completely without blood supply. It derives its nourishment from soaking up fluids from the blood supply furnished to the adjacent white of the eye, the tears which bathe its front surface, and the interior fluid contents of the eye. Since the cornea is surrounded by and completely dependent on body fluids, any imbalance producing a retention of fluids by the body tissues, a condition sometimes caused by using oral contraceptives, will be marked by pronounced swelling of the corneal tissue.

Subjective effects of corneal swelling from oral contraceptive use include blurred vision, dizziness, headache, and difficulty in depth perception. These can be disturbing enough for the woman who normally has good eyesight, or who habitually wears glasses to correct a vision defect. They can be many times more troublesome for the lady who wears contact lenses.

Success in contact lens wearing depends, to a large degree, on maintaining a stable corneal curvature, and consequently a constant physical relationship between contact lens and corneal surface. When well fitted, a contact lens will match the radius of curvature of the cornea to within a few hundredths of a millimeter. Change of even one tenth of a millimeter in this relationship may blur the wearer's vision and in many cases will make the lens extremely uncomfortable to wear.

Corneal edema from use of the pill is not a stable entity, but may fluctuate from day to day, or hour to hour. Once this condition begins, not only will the vision be blurred from corneal swelling, but also from changes in the lens-corneal relationship. In addition the eyes may burn, sting, and water as they do from exposure to smoke or wind. A hot, dry feeling often accompanies corneal swelling behind a contact lens, and if wearing persists in spite of the symptoms, severe pain and possible permanent eye damage may result.

In most cases the edema is easily reversed upon discontinuation of the pill, and occasionally upon adjustment of the diet to restrict the intake of sodium. Under no circumstances, however, should self-diagnosis and do-it-yourself therapy be attempted. All symptoms noted above can result from causes other than contraceptive therapy, and any disturbances of this nature should be reported to your doctor immediately.

156. Beware The Sunburned Eye

Each summer millions of Americans expose their eyes to large concentrations of solar radiation, unaware that this action could lead to severe ocular irritation and/or loss of vision. While some solar radiation may be beneficial, excessive doses are harmful and potentially dangerous.

Sunlight is composed of many different kinds of radiation. The sun's rays range from long infrared to short ultraviolet radiation, and that which creates sight, the visible spectrum, is actually a very small portion of the total energy striking the eyes. Ordinarily, moderately bright light from the visible spectrum cannot and does not harm the eyes. Long exposure to visible light rays may cause eyestrain, particularly when the eye is not properly corrected, but no physical harm will result from such use. However, when the eyes are bombarded by mixed infrared and ultraviolet as well as visible radiation, which always occurs in direct sunlight, the physical effects can be pronounced.

Almost everyone is familiar with ordinary sunburn. Too much exposure to summer sun will cause skin to redden and become painful to the touch. The burn comes from the action of ultraviolet radiation on surface skin cells and is not unlike a mild burn from a hot iron.

Sunburn does not require the presence of direct sunlight. Serious burns can occur to someone sitting in open shade, as under a beach umbrella, and even on a cloudy day when there is no sunshine at all. Ultraviolet rays are extremely short, and being so, are easily scattered and reflected into areas where longer, visible rays, do not travel. Similarly, ultraviolet radiation is not obstructed by clouds, as is direct sun, but filters through overcast to cause harm when least expected. The eyes, too, can be sunburned.

Effects Of Ultraviolet
The effect of ultraviolet on the visual system varies with the areas affected and the intensity and duration of the exposure.

Symptoms familiar to most people are the redness, irritation, and dry sandy feeling in the eyes experienced after a day at the beach or on the open road. The condition is known to doctors as actinic conjunctivitis, and it results from exposure of the conjunctiva (the fragile covering membrane of the eye) to ultraviolet radiation. Usually transient, the irritation most often disappears after a good night's sleep. Deeper irritations from repeated or prolonged exposure may develop into chronic conjunctivitis, which is much more difficult to relieve.

The iris diaphragm, which regulates the amount of light entering the eye, and the crystalline focusing lens, whose action permits us to see clearly both far and near, may also be affected by excessive exposure to ultraviolet radiation. In the latter case a form of cataract, appropriately called "radiation cataract," can develop as a result of extreme and prolonged exposure to ultraviolet energy.

Ultraviolet radiation is usually stopped at the lens of the eye and seldom penetrates to harm the light-sensitive retina. However, infrared rays, constant companions of ultraviolet, easily penetrate into the deep parts of the eye and can cause temporary or permanent harm from retinal burns. Retinal damage from infrared energy usually results from looking at or near the sun, or its reflection in water or snow. Astronomers, life guards, airplane spotters, and the like, are especially subject to the hazard and must take special precautions to avoid harmful exposure. In greater danger are the curious, who may be tempted to view an eclipse or other solar phenomenon through the ill-advised protection of colored glass or plastic. Many cases of permanent eye injury have resulted from such practices.

Danger Of Night Blindness

There is yet another disability resulting from ocular overexposure to the sun: night blindness.

The eye can adjust its sensitivity to nearly any level of light, dim or brilliant, and it functions more efficiently because of this adaptation. The familiar experience of entering a movie theater and being temporarily blinded until the eyes "get used to the dark" is a common example. The normal eye will become 90 percent accustomed to the dark in seven to ten minutes, and vision in the dark markedly improves during this period.

Not so with the sunburned eye. Dark adaptation is severely restricted in the sun saturated eye, and the inability to see in dim illumination can be great enough to deserve the title "night blindness."

What does all this mean in a practical sense? Imagine the end of a hot summer weekend at the beach, in the mountains, or on the highway. You and thousands of others are eager to get home. Your mind and body are tired. You speed up a little in your desire to get some rest before Monday morning rolls around. Darkness falls, but you are unaware that your sun jaded eyes have failed to adapt. It's a situation that invites an accident.

The only solution to night blindness is prevention. The diet must contain adequate amounts of vitamin A, the nutritional tool for eye adaptation to light variations. Since few of us are certain to get the vitamin A we need, and in fact more than one-third of the population is deficient in this vitamin, a daily supplement of halibut or cod liver oil is recommended. In circumstances where exposure to much sunlight is expected, a vitamin A supplement becomes imperative.

Eye protection from ultraviolet and infrared radiation, as well as overbright visible rays, is also needed, and such protection can be found in good quality sunglasses. Sunglasses act as optical screens, filtering out all of the harmful and excessively bright radiation, and allowing only that which is good for your eyes to pass through. Today's sunglasses are durable, comfortable, and attractive, and should be part of every sun lover's outdoor equipment.

Sunglasses come in varied colors and, assuming good quality lenses, the filtering capacity is nearly equal for each. Choice can be made largely on an aesthetic basis alone. But note the term "good quality." Pits, waves, and optical distortions are common in the cheaper glasses and often create eyestrain and headache for even the normal sighted individual.

157. Are Eyeglasses Always The Answer?

When Marilyn B. Rosanes-Berrett, Ph.D., was a young woman of 27, her eye problems were such that there was never any doubt in anyone's mind that she'd wear glasses for the rest of her life. She had hyperopia, commonly called farsightedness, an eye dysfunction in which rays of light entering the eye converge behind the retina rather than on it. Those who suffer from hyperopia see things at a distance more clearly than they do close objects. Another problem from which she suffered was astigmatism. This is a slightly flattened cornea, causing such symptoms as eye fatigue and difficulty in focusing. She also suffered from strabismus, or crossed eyes.

In spite of getting successively stronger glasses from her eye doctor, her eyes continued getting worse. On the advise of a friend, she went to a clinic where, after several training sessions, she threw away her glasses and found a new profession. For more than 25 years since then, she has been helping people see better without the eyeglasses prescribed by conventional eye doctors. Those she's helped range from the very young who would have been consigned to a lifetime of wearing glasses, to the very old whose vision had faded to the point where they could recognize nothing but shadows.

The techniques she uses are controversial. In a sense, they are based on the theory that if a weak, flabby body with stiff joints can be gradually whipped into shape through proper conditioning, so can the eyes. But does the theory actually work? "Definitely yes," declares Dr. Rosanes-Berrett, Director of the Gestalt Center for Psychotherapy and Training in New York City, "I've proved it. I know it can be done. I also think that there is a psychological aspect to good sight. We've got to have a readiness and willingness to see the world. This is a big factor. You must want to see well if my program is going to do you any good at all."

Some of the people she's helped seemed hopeless. For example, one of her first patients was an 84-year-old woman who had been virtually immobilized by obesity and arthritis. She was almost totally blind. In addition, she had undergone five operations, three for glaucoma and two for cataracts. She could distinguish only between light and darkness.

Dr. Rosanes-Berrett said that she visited the woman once each week for 90 minutes. Three months after her first visit, the woman could distinguish the table and chairs in her kitchen. After six months of practice, she could read headlines in the newspaper. A few weeks later, she was enjoying photographs in a magazine and reading the large captions. Shortly after that, she began to play solitaire, then to write letters with large crayons. Five years later, the woman was able to read newspapers for brief periods with the help of strong glasses.

Let The Light Shine Through

One of the basic techniques she uses and describes in her book, *Do You Really Need Eyeglasses?* (Hart Publishing Company, Inc., 1974), is a process called sunning, which consists of simply bathing the *closed* eyes in light, either natural or artificial. She says the process stimulates the retina, which grows dim and insensitive if it is deprived of light over a long period of time. Concurrently, she noted, there is a theory that sunning, because it stimulates the retina, slows the aging of the brain because the retina transmits images to the brain and is actually an outpocketing of the brain. And if the brain is stimulated, the theory goes, it will age more slowly.

To practice sunning, get a comfortable, straight-backed chair and an ordinary, incandescent light of almost any strength. Eventually, she says, you should progress up to a 150-watt bulb mounted on a reflector. The lamp should be placed about three feet in front of the chair. Seat yourself comfortably but erectly in the chair with your nose pointed straight ahead. Take off your glasses and close your eyes gently. Then, turn your head slowly, smoothly and rhythmically from side to side, midway to each shoulder but no farther.

Dr. Rosanes-Berrett said the light should soak into your closed eyes as your head passes through the glow. Sunning should be restricted to one or two minutes but gradually increased over several weeks to a total of ten minutes a day.

"When you feel like an old hand at it," she says, "move the lamp closer—to within two feet of your chair—and sun several times a day if you can. Many short periods are better than a few long ones. In case of serious eye problems," she says, "sunning for a minute or two every hour is advisable."

Ease Eyestrain With Palming

Another technique which she teaches is called palming. This can be done utilizing a pillow, a briefcase or small suitcase, or even the kitchen table. Begin with warm hands to increase blood flow. You can rub your hands together to warm them. Sit erect in a comfortable but straight-backed chair. Put a pillow or your briefcase on your lap, and rest your elbows to support your upper arms. Then, close your eyes gently. Next, relax your hands and cup your palms lightly over your eyes with the sides of your hands against the sides of your nose. The overlapping fingers should be on your forehead. Although there isn't any pressure on the eyeballs, no light should reach your eyes if you palm correctly. Dr. Rosanes-Berrett says that you should palm as often as you can, as long as you can. Even five minutes a day during a busy day at the office will refresh you and your eyes, she says.

Give Your Eyes The Grand Tour

Another of the techniques that Dr. Rosanes-Berrett recommends is the long standing swing, which should be performed three times a day. With soft music playing and your glasses off, stand in the middle of a room facing a window. Keep your feet parallel and comfortably apart. Let your arms hang loosely and keep your nose pointed straight ahead. Swing your body—head, trunk and all—to the right putting your weight on your right foot and letting your left heel rise from the floor. When your shoulders are parallel to the wall that was on your right as you started, swing back to the center and, without pausing, swing on to the left. Your weight will transfer to your left foot and your right heel will rise. She warns not to swing too far since you are attempting to relax and not to exercise.

While you are swinging, she recommends letting your eyes drift along the lines where the walls meet the ceiling. But, after a few swings you should lower your eyes to a level just beneath the top of the window and follow an imaginary line along the wall, keeping the line straight, flowing smoothly. When your eyes pass the window, she says, let them gaze out as far as the vista permits—the change of focus will loosen the eye muscles. This exercise, as she points out, should be done three times a day for about a minute each time.

Dominoes For Myopia

Dr. Rosanes-Berrett explained that anyone can do these exercises if he or she wants to have healthier eyes and wants to see better. However, she recommends specific programs for specific diseases. Consider myopia or nearsightedness, as just one example.

Dr. Rosanes-Berrett's exercises are similar to those of Dr. William H. Bates, a distinguished New York ophthalmologist who became a rather controversial figure in modern ophthalmology more than three-quarters of a century ago when he announced that the main reason behind poor eyesight is the fact that people work too hard at seeing. Poor vision and even glaucoma, according to Dr. Bates, could be caused by strain and emotional stress.

Therefore, the key word to the regimen of exercises Dr. Bates developed, known as the Bates Method, was "relaxation." For example, the muscle that will cause an eye to be "crossed" by pulling the eye off center is simply pulling too hard. It is not relaxed, and unfortunately the patient does not know how to relax it. To relieve this tension, Dr. Bates suggested sunning, palming and swinging, the same methods suggested by Dr. Rosanes-Berrett.

Myopia affects many sometime between the ages of six and ten. It is the result of an elongation of the eyeballs from the front to the back. First, Dr. Rosanes-Berrett recommends sunning and palming for several short periods and then palming for one longer period.

Then come the specific steps. Stand 14 ordinary dominoes, each having no more than 12 dots, approximately an inch apart at face level. You can put them on a stack of books on a table or on a desk or on a bookshelf or even on the top of your television set. Then, she directs you to sit just far enough away so that the dominoes appear slightly blurred. Close your eyes and inhale deeply and slowly. Exhale slowly and deeply. Then, open your eyes and let them gently wander around the sides, top and bottom of the domino farthest to the left.

She says that you should not try to focus on the dots. Just look around the domino's boundaries. Follow this procedure at least six times before moving on to the next one. Dr. Rosanes-Berrett says that by the time you reach the sixth domino, the slight blur with which you began should have disappeared and the domino should stand out vividly. She notes that if the domino's dots are not bright, sharp, and white, you should close your eyes and visualize the first domino, mentally intensifying its image sharper and brighter than what you actually saw. With this imprinted image on your memory, open your eyes and let them move around the side of the first domino. No matter how you actually see the domino, the visualized image will snap into focus.

Repeat the procedure with the other dominoes. Once they all stand out, move your chair back six inches and start the game again. It shouldn't take as long as you think, Dr. Rosanes-Berrett says. A half hour should be sufficient. On the second day, use regular playing cards, but only the spades with numbers. Tape the cards with clear tape to the wall at eye level, an inch apart. Then sit where they appear slightly blurred and use them as you did the dominoes. On the third day, substitute a calendar with numerals big enough to be read at ten feet or closer, if necessary, without glasses and only slight blurring.

After eight days of alternating near and far work, take the dominoes and place some of them where you can see them perfectly and another group where they appear slightly blurred. Look back and forth between them for ten minutes or so, pausing frequently and concentrating on their peripheries rather than on their patterns.

She says the routine should be kept up for at least a month, alternating the dominoes, playing cards and the calendar. She also recommends playing solitaire whenever you can because that particular card game induces muscular mobility and is devoid of many of the tensions that exist in competitive card games. She predicts that by the end of one month, anyone with no worse than average myopia should note a considerable improvement in vision. In more serious cases, she adds, it will take longer.

"The whole idea of this program is relaxation and enjoyment. You should be doing it with a good feeling, to give yourself a treat," Dr. Rosanes-Berrett stresses. "After a while these exercises will become a part of you and you'll have a good feeling. Let your vision come to you."

158. You Can Learn To See Better

According to a leader in the field of visual training, Dr. Robert Kraskin, O.D., F.A.A.O., we all have it in our power to help ourselves toward better vision and when we do, we will not only see more, we will learn more, and remember more.

Better vision can mean greater ability in every aspect of life—better reading skill, better school and work performance, a higher I.Q. score and greater success in sports, Dr. Kraskin maintains in his book *You Can Improve Your Vision* (Doubleday, 1968).

The vision system plays a vital role in everything we do. Eyesight—movement of hand to eye—movement of the entire body—these are the practical ways a person turns his thoughts into acts. Trying to do this with an erratic visual system is like a good airline pilot trying to land in the fog with a badly adjusted radar and a set of inaccurate instruments. Good vision is learned, Dr. Kraskin maintains, just as truly fine diction or superb athletic form is learned.

You Can Learn To See Better

Visual training is a process of learning to see better. It involves a whole series of visual abilities. Vision is not like snapping a still picture. It is an ongoing, unending process of coping with movement. The eyes must be controlled to stay on target, they must change focus instantly, their signals must be integrated and interpreted and used as the basis for the new eye movements.

When he gives visual training, Dr. Kraskin sets up a great many devices to stimulate the visual challenges of ordinary life. Some are as simple as rotating disks and a swinging ball suspended from the ceiling; others are sophisticated and complex instruments. All are aimed at heightening the many skills that combine into the process of seeing.

To tone and improve the visual system, Dr. Kraskin suggests certain exercises that can be done at home, whether or not you have a specific visual problem. These exercises benefit every member of the family because they increase the smooth coordination of muscles that affect the eyes.

All procedures are done in a relaxed, well balanced posture—standing with feet slightly separated and weight distributed equally. One way to achieve this posture is to stand with feet about eight inches apart. Then go up on your toes and reach stiffly for the ceiling so hard that you feel the tension in the back of your legs; then drop down flat on your feet.

Deep Breathing—Stand in your relaxed posture. Inhale through the nose, raising your head, and pause for three seconds. Then exhale through your mouth, lowering your head, and pause again. The goal is to do ten deep breaths in this way but you may be able to do only two or three at first.

Neck Rotations—Standing with your eyes gently closed, rotate your head around your shoulders three times in a clockwise direction, then three times counterclockwise. Open your eyes and look. If there is no dizziness, repeat this whole procedure three times. Make the movement as full and smooth as you can, but do as much as possible with the neck, trying not to sway the whole body.

Alternate Wink—Make a target by drawing a letter in crayon on a plain white three by five card. Place this at eye level and stand back five feet from it. Looking steadily at the target, wink your eyes alternately, up to a total of 40 winks. The goal is to keep the target clear throughout the procedure and keep it stable—that is, it should not appear to jump.

Concentration—Here is an old card game that the whole family will enjoy. From a deck, take eight pairs of cards and four single cards. Shuffle these 20 cards and deal them face down in four rows of five cards each. The goal is to match pairs. As each player takes his turn he selects a card, turns it over exposing it to his opponent, then selects another card to see if it matches. If it does, the pair becomes his property and he gets another turn. If not, both cards are turned back face down. Remembering the positions of these cards is the key to succeeding on future turns so the game is a fine exercise in memory control of visualized objects.

While these visual training exercises suggested for home use won't cure any major problem all by themselves, they will, Dr. Kraskin says, invigorate and smooth your visual system in much the same way that simple physical exercises can turn a flabby body into a hard-muscled one. The only reason that such results seem rare is that few persons stick to simple exercises long and hard enough to carry through their dramatic possibilities. Dr. Kraskin says he has seen their effects on hundreds of patients— seen them mirrored in the form of better school grades, easier reading, disappearance of headaches, superior sports performance and more graceful bearing.

But basic seeing habits are practiced so constantly that they far outweigh the few hours of special work in or out of the optometrist's office. This makes it vitally important to be sure your living and working arrangements tend to be good influences— not only for people who already have visual problems, but as a means of preventing them.

Ways To Help Your Eyes

Dr. Kraskin suggests some practical arrangements that will minimize stress on your eyes, the greatest enemy of good vision.

Avoid sharp contrasts in light. Working with just a desk lamp is unwise. The whole room should be illuminated. If a desk lamp is used in addition, be sure the bulb is shaded. When contrast is reduced, stress is reduced. For this reason, you should avoid writing on white paper that rests on a dark mahogany desk.

Other room lights should be turned on when watching TV. Looking at a TV screen is identical to staring into a low power light bulb. The contrast must be reduced by having light all around, with lamps carefully placed to avoid any direct reflection on the screen.

Don't become glued to the TV. While adults normally move away from the set frequently enough to break excessive concentration, children have to be watched more carefully. If you speak to someone who is watching TV and get no response, it's likely that he is too deeply engrossed and should be interrupted.

Furniture used for close work should enable a person to maintain proper posture. The desk or table should be at waist level when you are seated. Whenever possible, the work surface should be tilted to about a 20 degree angle. When this is done, and the head is bent slightly forward toward the work, the face will be parallel to the book or paper. The ideal distance from eyes to reading matter can be gauged by making a fist and measuring the distance from the middle knuckle to the elbow—which is about 14 inches for the adult.

Reading in bed, although pleasurable, is usually harmful. This is especially true when one is ill with a high fever. At such times both reading and TV should be avoided. Try the radio.

Generally speaking, Dr. Kraskin recommends avoiding sunglasses for children, to maintain the widest possible range of freedom to adapt to different light conditions, especially in the formative years. Use of sunglasses in moderate light, when there is no real need for them, has nothing to recommend it.

While indirect sunlight is never harmful, a real glare is another matter. People who do a lot of boating, fishing, or winter sports and who notice glare should wear protective glasses—usually Polaroid, since the nature of the glass cuts out direct reflection.

Two Nervous Systems

If you are over 40 and have trouble threading a needle or reading the phone book, you have lots of company. Age affects vision because your eyes are governed by two nervous systems—the only part of your body that is. The voluntary nervous system moves the entire eyeball so that you can consciously aim your eyes wherever you wish. The involuntary nervous system controls the focusing without you realizing it.

It is the difference in the aging of the two systems that eventually creates a problem. The voluntary system declines very slowly, but the involuntary system drops off more steeply in its activity—beginning in the early teen years. The gap goes on growing for about 25 years without being noticeable, Dr. Kraskin points out. But, at a certain point—usually in the mid-thirties—it begins to cause troubles: discomfort, lower efficiency, reduced reading speed, errors in typing or addition, poorer golf scores.

Why does this happen? When the two systems are not working in partnership, a stress is set up in the mind and body. The brain gets conflicting information that it translates as a blur. It signals the whole system to try harder, thus racing the engine and the stress in itself does further damage to the involuntary nervous system. Now your visual acuity really takes a nose dive that drives you to an eye doctor for reading glasses.

While this process cannot be prevented, Dr. Kraskin says, it can be minimized. What it takes is careful observation to anticipate the time when the divergence of the two systems will become a threat—before it is noticeable to the patient. If the optometrist can identify this early presbyopia before it begins to put stress on the seeing system, he prescribes reading lenses that can really be called preventive glasses. We cannot stop the normal physiological changes, Dr. Kraskin says, but we can prevent the maladaptations that multiply the ills.

Many adults, persons whose eye measurements seem all right

but who cannot enjoy or profit from their reading can be helped by visual training. Dr. Kraskin describes one retired admiral who came to him feeling quite low because the dream he had nurtured for years while waiting to retire had gone sour. He had accumulated a great library of books that he had never had time to read. His big wish was to spend days quietly reading all these works. "I find I can't really read for long," he told the doctor. "I get headaches, or I become very sleepy—no matter how interesting the subject is. The job of reading just seems to spoil all my pleasure in the contents of the book." This man, Dr. Kraskin explains, had perfectly good "eyesight" but his visual system was tuned to the reading of short memos. It just wasn't keyed to long reading. He took visual training directed straight at his particular goals, and in a very few months he was completely happy.

"Your visual system is not a finished product just because you are grown," the doctor says. "It is flexible, dynamic, ever evolving. While part of its future is rooted in the past, a big part is still up to you."

Section 28
Feet

159. When Your Feet Hurt, You Hurt All Over

Human hands appear to be marvels of fine workmanship and design. What miracles may not be accomplished by a human hand, trained in some delicate skill or made powerful by practice for anything from violin playing to carpentry! But it seems that our hands are mere slabs of insensitive flesh compared to our feet. Dr. Frederick Wood Jones of the University of Manchester says that man's hand is a "ridiculously simple and primitive appendage . . . (but) man's foot is all his own. It is the most distinctive human part of his whole anatomical makeup." He adds that the foot is man's crowning achievement, his finest piece of adaptation.

The 52 bones and 214 ligaments composing our two feet are small, delicate and finely balanced. Yet they carry our weight over the eight miles or so that most of us walk in a day, and they endure, for the most part uncomplainingly, hours of standing on hard floors or walking on hard sidewalks. No human engineer could construct so efficient a machine for weight bearing and motion.

Yet we esteem our feet so little, treat them so badly and neglect them in such a wholesale fashion that something like 75 percent of us suffer from some foot disorder, of which we may or may not be conscious. For evidence of foot troubles does not necessarily appear first in the feet. Pain in your legs, your back, your neck or your head may be coming from your feet. Poor posture may be the result of faulty foot function and likewise, painful feet may result from poor posture. Your weight is important, too, for it goes without saying that every extra pound adds to the work your feet must do.

Consider for a moment how feet were made to be used. Primitive man walked barefoot. His feet were adjusted to soft earth, which he could grasp with his toes as he walked. Today even those of us who live in the country spend much of our time walking on hard level floors. City-dwellers pound the hard sidewalks every time they step outdoors. Practically none of us who are adult ever go barefoot, preferring to wear slippers even for that short walk from our evening bath to the bedroom. From the time we are toddlers our feet have been shod in shoes—usually badly fitted shoes. The women of modern times have earned countless foot disorders because they tend to select shoes that look small and flattering regardless of what they do to feet.

The way we stand and walk has more to do with the health of our feet than any other single factor. The weight of the body should be borne on the outside arch of the foot, which is made of bone for the express purpose of bearing weight. The inside arch is made mostly of ligaments and muscles. When we walk incorrectly and stand with an incorrect posture, the weight is thrown instead on the inside arch. Muscles and ligaments endure all they can and then give way, resulting in fallen arches, one of the most painful conditions known, which may involve all kinds of apparatus necessary to take the place of the muscles that have collapsed. Exercise is important, too, in relieving fallen arches, as well as specially designed shoes.

Good Posture Helps Prevent Foot Trouble

What can we do to prevent foot trouble? As you might expect, we should concentrate our preventive efforts in childhood, and much of the literature dealing with foot health concerns training and proper shoeing of children. We must be aware of the fact that foot disorders are very often not apparent for years, and a child's foot may become deformed so gradually that he experiences no pain and his parents may not suspect that anything is wrong. Posture is of the utmost importance. One's feet should at all times be straight—that is, parallel to one another, rather than turned out or turned in. Pigeon-toes suggest immediately that something is wrong and the pigeon-toed child will usually be taken to the doctor. But until recent times, it was considered genteel to turn the toes out in walking and many of us suffer today as a result of this fad. When the toes turn out in walking or standing, the weight of the body is thrown on the inner arch, which sooner or later is bound to give way. Therefore, the first and most important exercise for healthy feet is learning to walk and stand with feet parallel. When we take a step the weight should be first on the heel, then as we go forward, it is transferred to the outer arch, across the ball of the foot and finally to the great toe.

But it is impossible to walk correctly unless you have comfortable shoes. There is considerable controversy as to what constitutes correct shoes. They should, of course, be big enough. Many foot troubles have their start in childhood when little feet are growing rapidly, getting too big for shoes long before the shoes wear out. A survey of the feet of 8,995 children was conducted in the District of Columbia from 1967 to 1969. Of the more than 5,000 children surveyed who were less than six years old, 3,363—over a third—had abnormal foot posture.

Children Outgrow Shoes Rapidly

An active youngster takes 30,000 steps in one day. If his shoes do not fit properly, is it any wonder that his feet soon suffer from all kinds of ailments? Unfortunately, children's shoes are designed primarily to follow adult shoe fashions. Children should begin to wear shoes only when they start to walk on harsh surfaces like cold ground, concrete, tile and pavement. Shoes for young children should serve to protect the feet, rather than to act as a stylish accessory.

Children's shoes should be replaced as soon as there is any indication that they are too small. The fitting should be carefully made, with the child standing, so that the full weight is on the feet. There should be the width of an adult's thumb between the toes and the end of the shoe. And since you never know how fast your child may be growing during any given time, you should make frequent examinations between shopping trips, just to make sure that junior's feet still have enough room inside his shoes. In general, shoes should be firm enough to give support, yet should not be made of stiff, unyielding leather which might be appealing because of its durability.

Until the age of 16 or so, children's shoes should be renewed every three or four months, if you want to be certain their shoes are not too small. Hand-me-downs are an acceptable way to save money on clothes, but poor economy in shoes. No one, child or adult, should ever wear shoes that someone else has been wearing. Heels should be straightened whenever they seem to be run over. And, incidentally, heels worn down either on the outside or the inside are an indication that posture is poor and feet are not functioning as they should.

Flat-soled oxfords that tie on securely still seem to be the best shoes for young, active feet. Proper fit is most crucial to a child's growing foot. Shoes must not hinder the development of young feet, or the child will suffer deformities that will cause him many painful foot problems as an adult. A shoe that is too short or long, too wide or narrow, or made from too heavy or too flimsy a material can deform a child's foot.

The first evidence of badly fitted shoes appears on the skin—redness or blisters anywhere on the foot indicate friction or pressure, which mean poor fit. Corns and calluses may develop in a person with foot deformity who wears perfectly fitting shoes and also in a person with perfect feet who wears badly fitting shoes. One of the major causes of foot trouble in housewives is wearing old shoes to do housework and saving the comfortable good ones for going out. Any housewife knows that she walks miles during the average work day and uses her feet constantly. She should make certain that her everyday shoes are the most comfortable ones she has—of course, with low heels. And always remember that properly fitting stockings and socks are just as important as properly fitting shoes.

Form Doesn't Always Follow Function

The platform and wedge shoes so popular in the past few years illustrate the impracticality of most shoe styles. They are noisy, and the rounded shape of many of the platforms makes the shoes unstable. To walk on them successfully, one must develop a stiff-legged, awkward-looking gait.

To allow comfortable, graceful walking, a shoe must be flexible at the ball of the foot. The rigid, heavy platform shoes make correct walking impossible, because to take a step, the entire foot must be lifted and put down at once, and cannot bend naturally.

Despite the difficulties in walking created by platform shoes, many of them have only thin straps to hold the foot in the shoe. Such flimsy straps increase the hazards of the shoe even more, for the foot can slip in the shoe, resulting in sprained or even broken ankles.

An American Medical Association release on platform shoes cautioned wearers to "be prepared to fall down, hard." Wearers of platform styles can expect sprained ankles, broken bones, and skinned knees and elbows. "When stepping down from a curb, or into a small chuck hole in the pavement, it is easy for the ankle to turn away from the shoe, resulting in a crashing fall."

Today's high-heeled shoes are less harmful than the spike heels of the 1960's, because the heels are broader and more stable. But, as in any type of high heel, the toes are pushed toward the front of the shoe, and the chances of developing corns, calluses and bunions are great.

The Earth Shoe

A revolutionary and widely popular idea in modern footwear is the so-called Earth Shoe. The shoe was designed by Mrs. Ann Kalsø of Denmark, and it is one of the first shoe styles designed for the foot instead of the eye.

The shoe is wide and deep across the front to allow plenty of room for the toes. Instead of the conventional raised heel, the Earth Shoe has a raised sole, which makes the wearer's heel lower than his sole when standing in the shoe. The sole is made of a thick, inflexible, ridged rubber material, and uppers are of leather.

A study completed at the California Podiatric Medical Center late in 1974 concluded that Earth Shoes could help about 70 percent of the population to walk better. The other 30 percent—people with flat feet, high arches or shortened calf muscles—will find the shoes uncomfortable.

Most of the patients participating in the study found that wearing Earth Shoes relieved the pain of bunions, corns and calluses. Because the shoes are so wide, they relieve most disorders caused by pressure on the foot for patients with normal feet.

However, not all the experts agree on the value of the Earth Shoe. Proponents of the Mensendieck system of body alignment do not favor these shoes. The Mensendieck system is a method of learning to use all muscles according to the laws of body mechanics in order to achieve correct posture and freedom from pain. Jennifer Yoels, noted Mensendieck instructor and author of the book, *Re-Shape Your Body, Re-Vitalize Your Life* (Prentice-Hall, 1972), states that negative heel shoes make for poor posture. When body weight is shifted from the balls of the feet onto the heels, the body is thrown into a backward, out-of-alignment position which makes correct posture impossible.

Moulded Shoes

A forerunner of sorts to the Earth Shoe is the moulded, or "Space" shoe. These shoes were created by Alan E. Murray, a professional ice skater who was unable to find shoes that didn't hurt his feet.

The moulded shoe is made from a plaster cast of the individual foot, and must be prescribed by a doctor. The shoes fit almost as tightly as a second skin; each toe is outlined. The inner sole is a soft platform into which the toes can sink, just as they do when a person is walking on sand.

As might be expected, these custom-made shoes are expensive and they do not look like ordinary shoes. One observer compared them to a catcher's mitt. But the moulded shoe does seem to be helpful in relieving painful feet. They are supposed to gradually remold the foot into their original perfect shape which sidewalks and hard floors have so cruelly deformed.

Your Feet Require Special Care

If there is a comforting thought about foot trouble, it is that no one who has it is suffering alone. Experts estimate that 80 percent of the women in the United States and 60 percent of the men suffer from disorders of the feet. Most of them are painful enough to keep corn plasters and bunion pads moving off drug store counters at a very fast pace. Many victims are driven to more drastic attempts at self-help, and risk serious infection by razor-blade surgery. When foot problems reach those proportions, it is safer and more helpful to consult a podiatrist, a doctor who specializes in diseases of the feet.

Podiatrists are supported and recognized by the American Medical Association. They have one or two years of college required before entry into one of several approved schools, and the courses require four years for completion. In these four years the student attends 4200 to 4400 hours of classes in the usual medical school courses such as bacteriology, pathology, dermatology, plus special courses in foot gear, foot orthopedics, etc. The podiatrist works side by side with a medical doctor, in the same way that a dentist does.

Shoes Create Need For Podiatrists

If there is one factor in modern life, one single thing which has made the doctor who specializes in foot disease indispensable, it is shoes. Not only are fit and style to blame for many foot problems, the materials of which a shoe is made can also have a great deal to do with foot health. Many synthetics are being used, and they have one basic fault. They don't "breathe" with the foot. In leather there are many minute air holes which permit some circulation for air around the foot. Many synthetics do not allow for this, and the climate is ripe for infection in a foot that is so confined.

The construction of the shoe usually varies with the price. In well-made shoes, inner seams are finished so that the welting is at a minimum. Protrusions, such as nails from the heels, are never felt. The lining is securely anchored and not likely to fray. All of these things conspire to make a shoe comfortable and to spare you trouble with your feet.

Even if the material of the shoe is the finest, individual peculiarities often enter into the problem. Sensitizing and irritating chemicals such as monobenzyl ether of hydroquinine, used to prevent rubber oxidation, have a bad effect on some feet. The dyes and resins can cause sensitive feet to burn intolerably. If such problems beset you, and you can see no visible reason for the trouble, change the brand of shoes you wear. Different manufacturers use different chemicals and formulae for dyes, and a change of maker could solve the problem.

Must We Wear Shoes?

Why don't we just go without shoes, as nature obviously intended? The hard floors and sidewalks of civilization have just about eliminated that possibility. Bare feet would be ruined by these hard surfaces. When man was walking on resilient earth and grass, bare feet were able to hold their own without damage. Now, life without some foot protection and support would lead to serious breakdowns of foot comfort and health. It is significant, though, that foot disorders seen among shoe-wearing societies are not known among those that go barefoot.

The American Podiatry Association has made some worthwhile comments on the most common foot problems we run into as shoe-wearing Americans: Corns and calluses are symptoms of ill-fitting shoes, or malformations of the foot bones. They should never be cut with a razor blade or any other non-sterile instrument. Foot infections can easily result and force long periods of inactivity. If such a condition becomes painful enough to cause you to contemplate cutting it out, see a podiatrist who is trained to care for such conditions properly.

Athlete's Foot And Other Ailments

Athlete's foot, a type of ringworm, is a skin disease caused by a fungus. Fungus thrives best in a warm, moist, dark environment—just the kind provided by the inside of a shoe. Athlete's foot is uncomfortable in itself, and can also provide a breeding ground for other, more serious, foot infections.

Wear shoes or sandals which are well ventilated to avoid

excessive perspiration, and change shoes and socks (or stockings) every day. Wash the feet at least once a day, and make sure to dry thoroughly between the toes. A dusting with powder or cornstarch will help keep the feet dry. Don't walk barefoot in public showers, or on any heavily traveled floor.

Ingrown nails are caused by pressure from tight shoes, or by cutting the nails improperly. Many people seem to believe that trimming the toenails without rounding the corners is not neat, so they clip off the corners. When growth begins again, instead of growing straight out, the tapered nail takes a new path—inward—and begins to cut into the flesh of the toe. Ingrown nails cause excruciating pain, inflammation and if severe enough, infection and other complications result.

To avoid this painful problem, wear shoes with rounded toes, and trim your nails straight across with a toenail clipper or emery board. If you do develop an ingrown nail, have it treated by a doctor.

A bunion, a severe swelling and tenderness of the joint of the great toe, is sometimes caused by an inherited weakness of the ligaments, muscles or bone structure of the foot. Usually, though, bunions result from crowding the big toe into pointed or tapered shoes.

Corns and calluses make life miserable for millions of Americans. A corn is a cone-shaped growth of horny skin on the toes, usually caused by badly fitted shoes. If your toes slip forward against the front of your shoes as you walk, you are likely to develop corns. To relieve the pain of a corn, you must ease the pressure from your shoe. Place a corn pad cut into the shape of a horseshoe behind the corn, or use a piece of moleskin (separated from the corn with a bit of cotton or gauze). Stay away from chemically treated corn pads or over-the-counter "remedies." If your corns persist, see your doctor.

A callus is similar to a corn, but the hard tissue is shallow and spread over a broader area. Friction from shoes and improper weight distribution across the sole of the foot are usually to blame for calluses. To get rid of calluses, find a pair of shoes in which your feet are held securely, and which don't rub against the feet in walking.

Plantar warts, found on the bottom of the foot, are warts that the weight of the body has forced to grow into the foot. A plantar wart may have a hard surface like a corn, but unlike a corn, the wart is composed of living tissue—it has blood vessels and nerve endings. Some plantar warts may go away by themselves, but most require medical treatment. Never try to remove them yourself. Bathroom surgery is quite dangerous and generally unsuccessful.

Flatfeet may be present from birth or developed at some point in life. Congenital flatfoot, the kind many people are born with, is as serviceable and pain-free as a normal, healthy foot. In fact, a congenital flatfoot has been found ideal for military service, as the arch cannot break down under the strain of prolonged marching.

The acquired flatfoot, in which a normal arch has "fallen," brings great agony. Acquired flatfoot may result from obesity, excessive walking or standing, or wearing poorly fitting shoes in childhood. There is no cure for fallen arches; a doctor can only redistribute the stress on the feet with special supports built into shoes.

Foot odor is a cause of acute embarrassment, but it causes no physical pain. This disorder is generally due to excessive perspiration, and can often be controlled by wearing loosely woven cotton hose and shoes of a porous material, applying powder to the feet and inside shoes, frequently cleansing the feet and changing footwear often.

Tired, Aching Feet

When the feet tire quickly and ache at the end of the day, and no noticeable disorder is present, the problem may be a simple lack of exercise. After being confined all day in shoes, feet need a chance to spread out. Walk barefoot or in stocking feet as much as possible around the house. Hard surfaces such as asphalt and concrete are rough on bare feet, but when you have the opportunity to walk on soft grass or sand, by all means take off those shoes! Walking on these resilient surfaces is excellent therapy for tired feet—the muscles of the foot are strengthened as the toes grasp the soft earth, and tension is relieved because the toes can flex naturally and relax.

Overweight Adds Problems

The obese person is far more likely to develop painful foot problems than a person of normal weight. The added strain that excess poundage puts on the bones and joints of the feet can bring on degenerative arthritis at an early age. Overweight people get more corns and calluses, and the extra pressure put on the ligaments in their feet causes arch problems for many.

Dr. H. Darrel Darby, a member of the Board of Trustees of the American Podiatry Association, warned that, "The obese person often suffers from ingrown toenails, caused by excess flesh about the nails, and athlete's foot, brought on by the greater perspiration that results from tight-fitting shoes."

Dr. Darby advised that while an overweight person is trying to reduce, he also should trim his toenails carefully and often, and pay special attention to foot hygiene (*Evening Chronicle,* Allentown, Pennsylvania, October 15, 1973).

Sports Can Lead To Sore Feet

Sports have always been responsible for many foot injuries. And now that such activities as tennis and jogging are gaining more and more popularity, the ranks of footsore folk continue to grow.

"Tennis toe," a throbbing pain and purplish discoloration under the toenails, is sending many racqueteers limping off the court and into the podiatrist's office. The disorder is caused by new kinds of tennis shoes which provide so much traction that when a player stops suddenly, his toes are jammed against the front of the shoe, and the nail is injured. Damage from "tennis toe" is increased by hard playing surfaces such as wood or concrete. Playing on a clay or grass court decreases the likelihood of injuring the feet.

Overzealous joggers suffer much needless foot distress. The tissues of the feet and ankles take quite a pounding from the blacktop and concrete traveled by the jogger, and the feet must be conditioned gradually to take such a beating. When the jogger does not allow his feet time to accustom themselves to hard pavements before embarking on a full scale program, the tissues in his feet simply break down. He experiences pain similar to that of traumatic arthritis, and may injure his Achilles tendon. And his jogging days are over before they've really begun.

Section 29
Flu

160. One Of The Most Infectious Diseases!

Influenza, also known as the flu or the grippe, is one of the most common of the infectious diseases. The symptoms of the flu encompass cold symptoms as well as the chills, prostration, muscle aches and general malaise. Although weather conditions have nothing to do with the causes of flu, outbreaks generally occur in the winter months. Flu epidemics usually begin in February, which is considered the kick-off month for the virus season.

There are numerous viruses which are known to cause the flu. Since the first viruses were isolated in 1933, new viruses, including additional types of the groups already known, have been discovered every year. Prior to 1974, 38 major flu outbreaks had been recorded, including the disasterous pandemic in 1918 which "attacked an estimated 500 million people, leaving 20 million dead," according to *Science Digest* (March, 1975). The severity of the 1918 pandemic was due largely to the fact that it lasted for more than 14 months; ordinary virus epidemics in the average community often last no more than six weeks before running their course.

Although common influenza is decidedly more aggravating than it is serious, it may be hazardous for older people who could suffer severe complications of the upper respiratory tract. Influenza viruses are airborne and highly contagious, infecting susceptible individuals who inhale the infectious droplets in the air. It becomes extremely dangerous when the virus invades the mucous membrane cells in the lungs, inducing cases of pneumonia which can lead to death. This complication accounts for the majority of influenza deaths of people over 55.

Vaccines have been developed to combat some strains of the flu virus, but they only work for certain strains of virus which are not continually mutating. Despite the containment of other classic plagues such as typhus, small pox and yellow fever, the volatile nature of the flu viruses is the primary reason doctors have been unsuccessful in eradicating flu epidemics, which appear to run in cycles every two to three years.

Flu Shots More Effective With Vitamin C

A Czechoslovakian doctor told an International Nutrition Conference in London that vitamin C extends a helping hand to preventive inoculations. Roger Lewin, writing in the *New Scientist* (April 18, 1974) reported that Dr. Smola determined that when people get a flu shot along with vitamin C, the protection they get from respiratory infection is greater than what one would expect from the sum total of protection from either an inoculation or vitamin C alone.

One explanation for this curious effect, observed Lewin, "is that, because the cells of the immune system—the lymphocytes—appear to require vitamin C, an underlying deficiency of the vitamin might blunt the teeth of the immune system; conversely, boosting the vitamin C intake may boost the immune response."

Moral: If you have just taken a shot of flu vaccine, as many physicians are now recommending for their older patients, increase your vitamin C and you will enjoy far better protection, not only against the flu virus, but bacterial bugs as well.

These two important clinical trials we've reported on here are hopefully just the first steps toward a true understanding of which infectious diseases can be subdued by vitamin C, and how much is necessary to do the job. A great deal of the basic research has already been done. Back in 1937, Jungeblut reported in the *Journal of Immunology* (32:203) that, "ascorbic acid is capable of bringing about inactivation of tetanus toxin *in vitro*" (in the test tube).

In 1939, it was shown that bacteria that cause whooping cough are neutralized in the test tube by vitamin C. In 1942, it was *Proteus vulgaris*, another nasty germ that weak patients pick up in the hospital, that was brought under control by vitamin C—in a test tube. The year 1950 saw vitamin C bring about this same bacteriostatic activity on Group A hemolytic streptococci.

Dr. Frederick R. Klenner of Reidsville, North Carolina, who has been using vitamin C on his patients for many years, has reported that it is capable of rendering harmless a wide variety of viruses and bacteria. While small amounts can bring a degree of immunity, huge doses are what Dr. Klenner uses to beat down an actual infection (*Journal of Applied Nutrition*, Winter, 1971).

Dr. Klenner has used massive doses of vitamin C to treat such serious illnesses as encephalitis, meningitis, poliomyelitis, viral pneumonia, tetanus and other infections. He has administered it by injection in amounts ranging from two to four grams approximately every two to four hours around the clock. "Ascorbic acid is a powerful-oxidizer when given in massive amounts; that is, 50 grams to 150 grams intravenously," Dr. Klenner points out. "In serious pathological conditions, this amount is 'run in' as fast as a 20 gauge needle will allow. Then it acts as a 'flash oxidizer,' often correcting the pathology within minutes."

To interested practitioners, Dr. Klenner cautions that with continuous intravenous injections of large amounts of ascorbic acid, at least one gram of calcium gluconate must be added to the fluids each day. This is done because massive doses of ascorbic acid pull free calcium ions from the vicinity of the blood platelets. The first sign of calcium ion loss, he says, is nosebleeding.

While all this exciting research into better and more natural means of combating infections goes on, millions of Americans are being told by high-pressure commercials—and maybe even their own doctors—that when the flu or another infection is on them, the appropriate behavior is to start gobbling aspirin. Aside from the fact that aspirin, even in small amounts, causes bleeding from the lining of the stomach, in large amounts it seriously limits the availability of vitamin C to the immune system. This was recently proven by Drs. Loh, Watters and Wilson of the University of Dublin, Ireland (*Journal of Clinical Pharmacology,* November-December, 1973).

By seriously inhibiting the uptake of ascorbic acid by the leukocytes, those circulating bodies which play a crucial role in policing germs which get into the body, aspirin can impede recovery from serious infections, the Dublin researchers point out. To the extent that you're taking aspirin, you're crippling your vitamin C! Even when 500 mg. of vitamin C were given to normal adults, the Irish doctors found, simultaneous administration of 600 mg. of aspirin (about two tablets) "completely arrested uptake of ascorbic acid into the leukocytes. It is concluded," the doctors said, "that supplementary ascorbic acid should be administered to individuals receiving aspirin therapy."

Put Iron In Your Flu Resistance

New research suggests that a major role in our defense system against infection such as flu viruses is played by a nutrient that few people had previously suspected of doing battle on this front. It turns out to be iron.

But even more important than the identification of this mineral as an infection-fighter is the discovery that the body's defense lines are weakened long before the appearance of outright anemia or gross iron deficiency.

Slight Iron Deficiency Is The Worst Kind

This was dramatically shown by work conducted at the Massachusetts Institute of Technology, reported by Dr. Raymond B. Baggs and Dr. Sanford A. Miller at the 1972 meeting of the Federation of American Societies for Experimental Biology in Atlantic City, N.J.

The researchers divided rats into five groups and fed them diets with an iron content ranging from 0 to 35 parts per million a day. A daily intake of 25 ppm is considered the minimum amount necessary for satisfactory growth.

All the animals were then infected with *salmonella typhimurium,* a bacterial strain which can also infect man. The animals with the least iron intake had least resistance to infection, Dr. Baggs said. But curiously, the animals that got sick first and died the earliest were not those getting the least iron, but those receiving a dose of 15 ppm, which is in the range of a moderate iron deficiency. The next most vulnerable group fared somewhat better, while the animals receiving the highest dose of dietary iron, which was greater than the minimum required amount, fared best of all. Only one of these animals even became sick, and none of them died.

"This unexpected finding is important in that marginal iron deficiency is much more common in man than severe deficiency," the researchers declared. (In fact, marginal iron deficiency is *epidemic* among millions of Americans, particularly women and children.)

Babies Left Vulnerable By Mothers' Diets

In case anyone should have doubts about the relevance of laboratory experiments to human beings, another researcher told the same meeting that babies born to iron-deficient women developed fewer white blood cells. Dr. L. G. O'Connell of the Coombe Lying-In Hospital in Dublin said that these white blood cells are, of course, one of the body's chief lines of resistance to all infections.

It happens often in science that researchers in different laboratories make remarkably similar discoveries almost simultaneously, and this is the case with iron nutrition and resistance. In the same year, 1972, Dr. B. N. Nalder and colleagues published in the *Journal of Nutrition* (102:535) their own remarkable findings.

They began their extensive experiments armed with the knowledge that malnutrition is known to increase susceptibility to infection. But Dr. Nalder and his associates set out to identify specific dietary components which would prove to be most closely linked to the production of antibodies. Antibodies are those custom-produced physiological soldiers which specialize in turning invasive germs into immobilized prisoners of war.

One of their findings was that as the diet fed to their test animals was diluted with sucrose, or table sugar, there was a steady fall in antibody production. But the blockbuster was the entirely unexpected discovery that iron deficiency has a tremendous effect upon antibody production. A summary of their work in *Nutrition Reviews* (April, 1973) puts it this way: "In fact, antibody production was found to be more sensitive to the decreases in dietary iron than levels of hemoglobin, serum iron, serum protein, liver iron, or body weight."

First Effect Is Lowered Resistance

That is really a fantastic discovery. It had always been assumed that if hemoglobin and other measurements of body iron, such as the amount stored in the liver, are "normal," then the person is not deficient in iron.

Dr. Nalder's work tells us that the *first effect* of less than optimum levels of dietary iron is a reduction in antibody synthesis, which means, of course, a weakening of resistance to flu and infections of every kind.

The practical significance of all this, which is to say, its relevance to your health, is that a so-called "normal" level of iron as measured by a hemoglobin or serum iron-test, is absolutely no guarantee that our iron levels are all they should be to keep production of critical antibodies at the greatest possible level.

You can easily see why it is a very tricky matter to determine if you or your children are enjoying the protection afforded by optimum iron nutrition. Yet, this is a question of vital importance to all of us. Short of having your level of antibody production monitored before and after a period of nutritional supplementation, the only way to answer this question is statistical. And statistics tell us that your chances of not getting enough iron every day are dangerously high.

The comprehensive Ten-State Nutrition Survey of 1968-1970, conducted by the Center for Disease Control in Atlanta, Georgia, concluded that iron deficiency is the number one nutritional problem in the U.S. This is true for men and women, children and adults, black people and white people. It is doubly true of pregnant women and nursing mothers.

Getting Iron From Food

So much for the bad news. Let's get on to the good news. First of all, whole grain bread is a fine source of iron (as well as many other nutrients). And if you want to get some of the considerable amount of iron which is in eggs, but which is not ordinarily absorbable, you can get it by drinking orange juice along with your breakfast, because it is well known that vitamin C greatly enhances the absorption of iron. There are several studies which show that approximately 500 mg. of vitamin C is the optimal amount for increasing iron absorption regardless of where the iron comes from.

In general, meat is the best source of iron, not only because it contains a generous amount of this mineral, but because protein is vital to the whole process of iron absorption and utilization. Liver and other organ meats are the best sources of iron.

Beans and wheat germ are two other excellent sources of iron although they don't come up to the efficiency of liver. But in a healthy, mixed diet, they have an important contribution to your iron nutrition.

Although the importance of adequate iron in the body's defense system is now known to be enormous, it is not the only nutrient which you need to build the most powerful resistance. Vitamin C has been shown in many carefully controlled studies to be of great help both in preventing colds and flu.

Vitamin A is another infection-fighter, helping to keep all the epithelial tissues, including those in the nose, throat and lungs in a healthy, elastic condition.

Plenty of sleep is a resistance-booster that too often is neglected. Many people have been amazed at how much better they feel by getting just one more hour sleep every night, or taking a nap during the day.

Flu

With the combination of nutritional insurance and personal health practices, you can give your total resistance just the boost it may need to get you safely through the miserable season of the flu.

161. The Soviets' "Secret Weapon" Against Flu

You more than likely will not find garlic in your doctor's little black bag. But in Russia, pharmacologists are making an antibiotic drug from a substance in garlic called allicin, according to a report in *Today's Health*, November, 1971. Russian scientists claim that unlike other so-called antibiotic "wonder drugs" which have powerful side effects, allicin destroys only specific harmful germs and leaves the body's natural bacteria untouched.

During a flu epidemic in 1965, the Soviets had a 500-ton emergency supply of garlic flown in. Public notices in the *Evening Moscow Journal* advised more garlic consumption because of its "prophylactic qualities for preventing flu." When a *New York Times* reporter asked a U.S. specialist in internal medicine about it, he got nothing but a laugh and the old saw to the effect that garlic's strength lies in its ability to keep people more than a breath away.

Actually, there's much more to garlic's reputation as a powerful infection fighter than that.

For centuries it was a European remedy for many types of infectious disease, including clogged and running nose, cough and sore throat. Nobody who used it then could say just why it was effective, but they knew that a good dose of garlic held the cure for many an illness that would respond to few other things.

Until the Soviets isolated the active protective agent in garlic's essential oil, the remedy had long been discarded as a product of an old fashioned era. How could those ignorant peasants find a cure for diseases which the modern laboratories have not been able to conquer? And how could a common and odorous bulb hold the answer?

Curiosity Led To The Answer

Someone did get curious enough to find out if garlic really could do what antibiotics and sulfa drugs had been unable to do. The man was Dr. J. Klosa, and he reported his findings in the March, 1950, issue of a German magazine entitled *Medical Monthly*.

Dr. Klosa found that garlic oil had that elusive ability to kill dangerous organisms without attacking organisms vital to the body's health. It is this danger to bodily health that rules out (or should rule out) the use of many proposed compounds as medications, even though they are effective germ killers. For example, formaldehyde inactivates all viruses—including flu "bugs"—but it also reacts unfavorably with the body's own protein, and is, therefore, a deadly poison to the body. (Unfortunately, many of the drugs actually being used today have shown themselves to be antagonistic to body processes, but because the reaction is not as immediate nor obviously violent as with formaldehyde, they continue to be used.)

Dr. Klosa experimented with a solution of garlic oil and water, and he administered this preparation in doses of 10 to 25 drops every four hours. It was found that the desired effect was enhanced by the inclusion of fresh extract of onion juice in the dosage.

Results Of Treating Grippe And Sore Throat With Garlic

Dr. Klosa reported results of patients suffering from grippe (a feverish, flu-like disease), sore throat and rhinitis (clogged and running nose). Of 13 cases of grippe treated with this garlic oil solution, fever and catarrhal symptoms were cut short in every case. All patients showed a distinct lessening of the period of convalescence required. No patient suffered from any of the common post-grippe complaints such as chronic inflammation of the lungs, swelling of the lymph glands, jaundice, or pains in muscles and joints. Even the cough that often accompanies grippe was considerably suppressed.

In 28 cases of sore throat, the garlic oil had a prompt and salutary effect. The burning and tickling abated to the point of disappearance in 24 hours. Dr. Klosa found that, if caught in its first stages, the further development of sore throat could be completely stopped by about 30 drops—or about two doses—of the garlic oil solution.

There were 71 cases of clogged and running nose treated in this manner. The oil was taken partly by mouth and partly directly into the nostrils. The congestion of the nostrils was completely cleared up in 13 to 20 minutes in all cases. There were no further complications.

Dr. Klosa demonstrated that garlic is indeed effective against viruses like the flu. Later, the identification of allicin, the natural antibiotic in garlic, explained *why* it is effective.

So instead of using aspirins and other over-the-counter drugs that sell by the millions during the "flu season," why not give garlic a chance? You will be using a natural remedy whose properties have been proven to affect favorably many unhealthful conditions, and a remedy you can be sure will do you no harm.

The offensive odor of garlic on the breath, it is true, is one good reason for not using it in the quantities in which it is most beneficial. The problem, though, is one that is easily overcome.

If you want to add garlic to your diet the unoffending way, try garlic perles. These are tiny capsules of garlic oil which you swallow whole. The garlic does not get on your breath, but it does get into your stomach and digestive system, where you need it.

Garlic, it seems, is always good for a laugh. New research is proving that those who use it liberally may instead have the last laugh.

162. Pneumonia And Pleurisy

One of the most serious of the infectious diseases is pneumonia, a severe inflammation of the lungs which is usually accompanied by chills and a high fever. Earlier in this century, pneumonia was among the leading causes of death, but now pneumonia is quite successfully treated with modern antibiotics cautiously used by a physician, sharply reducing the mortality rate.

In treating pneumonia, the physician's first task is to identify the specific microorganism causing the infection. Then an appropriate antibiotic is prescribed. For example, one of the most common types of pneumonia which strikes people of all ages is caused by tiny organisms called *pneumococci*. Penicillin is the remedy of choice in such cases. Often the patient is up and around again in less than two weeks.

Mycoplasma pneumonia or "walking pneumonia" often goes undiagnosed because its symptoms are relatively mild and mimic influenza. Victims are usually adolescents and young adults. Penicillin is ineffective against mycoplasma pneumonia; tetracycline or erythromycin are the drugs of choice.

In some cases of pneumonia, pleurisy may also develop. This is a painful inflammation of the pleura, a thin membrane attached to the outer surface of the lungs and the inner surface of the chest wall. A knifelike pain in the side, chills and fever followed by dry cough are typical symptoms of pleurisy. The pain is intensified by breathing and coughing.

Although antibiotics prove extremely effective in treating such infectious diseases as pneumonia and pleurisy, a steady diet of these powerful drugs will deplete the body of such essential nutrients as vitamins C and K, and the entire B complex. This is especially true in the cases of adolescents and the elderly, where careful monitoring of the nutrient levels in the blood is most advisable.

Section 30
Food Poisoning

163. Food Poisoning— As Dangerous As Ever

Many of us can remember the time when food poisoning was an ever-present household fear. Unregulated butchers used to restore the redness of spoiling meats with benzoate of soda. Egg salads and fish would quickly spoil in the old fashioned icebox. The ice itself, sometimes made of untreated water, could communicate salmonella infections when used in cold drinks.

We now have better refrigeration and most of our food is processed in enormous plants that represent the height of modern sterile technology. Food poisoning should have become a thing of the past. But has it?

Today, poisoning yourself and your family has become as simple as opening a can or thawing a freezer package.

Food poisoning is caused by living bacteria which can infest foods. These minute organisms, once inside the body, may cause illness ranging from mild gastrointestinal distress to death.

Drs. Bob Park and Wilkie Harrigan reported in the July 29, 1971, *New Scientist and Science Journal* that despite mounting concern about limits for toxic chemical pollutants, "probably far more suffering is caused by readily controllable bacterial food poisoning than by chemical pollutants. Moreover, changes in food processing and kitchen practice may be increasing the risk of food poisoning." News reports from the past year alone testify that now only one mistake or omission in a food processing plant may directly affect the lives of thousands upon thousands of people.

It has become apparent that the latest increase in food poisoning is directly due to the greater sophistication of food handling methods. That is, more processing steps are being taken in order to make possible longer storage time and shelf life for the products involved. At each step of the way there is another opportunity for food contamination to take place. Of course, no food industrialist *wants* his product to be a carrier for a food-borne poison, and there is no doubt that many brilliant people are working hard and singlemindedly to prevent it. But as long as the objective in preparing foods for the market place remains longer shelf life, then periodic episodes of food contamination will be inescapable.

Not all contaminated food is discovered even after it is eaten, and many cases of mild food poisoning are mistaken for minor gastrointestinal upsets. "Food poisoning," says the August, 1970 *Consumer Bulletin*, ". . . quite often is not correctly diagnosed, but written off as the virus, stomach flu, or the 24-hour bug."

There Are Several Kinds Of Food Poisoning

Salmonella is among the most common causes of food poisoning in developed countries. Authorities believe more than two million cases of salmonella poisoning occur each year in the United States.

Very young and very old people are affected most severely by salmonellosis. From eight to 72 hours after the contaminated food has been eaten, the victim suffers pain, diarrhea, nausea and vomiting, chills or fever. Salmonella poisoning is not often fatal, but if another infection is already present, the additional contamination can result in a critical situation.

Salmonella bacteria are most often found in raw meat, poultry, fish, eggs and milk products. Foil-wrapped chocolates have been another noted offender in recent years. "The most vulnerable foods," says *Consumer Bulletin*, "are, of course, those that are handled or processed in excess or those that are used after only light cooking or none at all. Once a food is contaminated, bacteria may grow at an alarming rate. . . Careful food handling is the only way to avoid salmonellosis, as the presence of the bacteria does not affect the appearance, smell, or taste of the food within which they grow."

Many of the latest convenience foods are processed in ways which make them particularly vulnerable to salmonella contamination. Several factors contribute to the problem. First, introduction of salmonella organisms into the processing chain is frustratingly easy, especially when foods of animal origin are being handled. Second, food batches in modern processing plants are so large that one or two infected lots of incoming food can contaminate tons of the finished product. Third, processors have relied increasingly on chemical additives and low-heat dehydration to preserve food. Neither technique is effective in controlling the growth of salmonella organisms.

Salmonellae do not die, but cannot reproduce in cold temperatures. It is their rapid increase that makes it hard, or impossible, for the body to fight them. This makes it important to keep meats refrigerated right up to the time they are prepared. Cooking will destroy these bacteria provided that the temperature reaches 160° throughout the meat, down to the very middle of the portion. Use a meat thermometer to be sure meats are thoroughly cooked. Also, heat all leftovers completely. Gravy or broth should be brought to a rolling boil for several minutes when reheated.

Clostridium perfringens is another widespread cause of food poisoning. Although its name is unfamiliar to many people, this bacterium is found in many places—it occurs in soil and dust, clings to food, and inhabits the intestinal tract of man and other warm blooded animals.

Illness from perfringens bacteria usually occurs when large quantities of food are kept too cool or too warm for several hours or overnight. The worst culprits are restaurants, cafeterias and similar establishments where foods are kept in warming devices for hours on end.

Symptoms of perfringens poisoning appear four to 22 hours after the contaminated food is eaten. They include diarrhea and abdominal pain.

To destroy perfringens bacteria, meats must be cooked thoroughly and kept at temperatures above 140°F until serving. When meat is cooked for later use, it must be refrigerated immediately and kept cold until it is used.

Staphylococcus bacteria, known as staph, produce a toxin in food unless they are destroyed in time by high heat. The toxin, if already present, will not be destroyed along with the bacteria. Staph can grow in all meats, poultry, eggs and egg products, cream-filled pasteries and potato, macaroni, tuna or chicken salads.

About two or three hours after the tainted food is consumed, the person becomes violently ill, with vomiting, nausea and cramps, while the body tries to remove the toxin. Recovery is likely within 24 hours, and death is rare. But the grueling interval before recovery is enough to make anyone take all possible steps to avoid such a fate.

Botulism
Botulism is the least common type of food poisoning, but by far the most dangerous. Although rare, botulism is often fatal. It

differs from other food poisons in that it affects the central nervous system rather than just the digestive tract.

The hazard lies in the nature of the botulism microbe, *clostridium botulinum.* In the natural world, botulinum is widely distributed in soil, and also in some lakes and bays. It would seem, then, that botulinum-caused disease would be more widespread. The explanation of the paradox is that the microbe itself is harmless—you probably ingest millions in your lifetime. It is not the microbe but the poison it produces that causes illness and death—and the poison is produced only under special conditions.

The toxin (a protein) is a by-product of the microbe's process of growth, and it grows only under airless conditions. It is one of the anaerobes—a class of microorganisms that cannot multiply in the presence of oxygen.

To protect itself when food and growing conditions are lacking, botulinum changes its form. From a rod-like organism it becomes a round, tough spore, highly resistant to destruction. It can survive indefinitely, lying in wait until the right conditions exist for it to grow.

There are a number of types of botulinum, types A, B and E being the varieties that cause poisoning in man. Of these, type E (usually associated with poisoning from seafood) is distinctive in that it can grow and form toxin at temperatures below 40°F. In other words, it can do its damage at temperatures below the level of ordinary household refrigeration.

For decades, botulism had been considered under control in this country, with the handful of cases occurring annually almost always attributable to inexpertness or carelessness of home canners in preserving their own foods. Then, in 1963, this nearly extinct form of food poisoning began to stage a comeback.

There was a great uproar in the popular press at the time. The 1963 outbreaks suggested that in this age of nationwide mass distribution, relaxed standards in guarding against botulism at a single plant could lead to catastrophe of immense proportions.

New processes of food treatment, packaging, storage and marketing pose different problems in botulism control. The danger signal points to the many "mildly processed" foods, prepared and packaged to retard spoilage, but not subjected to treatment that would destroy botulinum spores. Particularly when these foods are vacuum packed, thus providing the airless environment required for the production of botulism toxin, they could carry death if at any time during storage or shipment refrigeration became weak and the temperature rose enough to enable the bacteria to start growing.

The problem of refrigeration, however, is more complex than merely educating food stores and consumers. Education does not guarantee compliance, especially in the face of the constantly rising cost of electricity needed for refrigeration. And we still do not have all the facts we need to determine what level of cold is necessary if the food is to be kept for a long time.

The types of foods responsible for botulism vary according to methods of preservation and regional eating habits. In 1974, the Institute of Food Technologists' Expert Panel on Food Safety and Nutrition reported that botulinum toxin has been found in many different foods, including canned corn, peppers, green beans, beets, asparagus, mushrooms, ripe olives, spinach, tuna, chicken, chicken livers and liver pate. The deadly bacteria have also been discovered in luncheon meats, ham, sausage, stuffed eggplant, lobster and smoked fish.

The publicity afforded to outbreaks of botulism caused by commercially processed foods tends to obscure the fact that the danger of botulism may also be present in foods canned at home. If you turn to the canning pages of your cookbook, you will notice the warnings.

Low-acid foods such as vegetables and meats can support the botulinum microbe. These foods must be processed in a pressure cooker to insure that they will reach a temperature high enough to destroy any botulinum spores that might be present.

Foods with a high acid content, such as pickles, jams, tomatoes and all fruits may be processed in a boiling water bath. Unless sauces or similar substances are added, which is unlikely, the botulinum microbe cannot survive in these foods. If you are uncertain whether some newly developed strains, such as the low-acid tomato, contain enough acid to kill the bacteria, add a teaspoon of vinegar or lemon juice to each pint you process.

When there is any question about the safety of canned foods, boiling the food in an open pot for 15 minutes before serving it will destroy any botulism toxin that may have developed. The toxin, unlike the spores, cannot survive this level of temperature.

Botulism toxin causes paralysis of the muscles by interfering with the myoneural junctions in body tissues. The paralysis usually begins in the face, then progresses downward to the throat, chest, arms and legs. If enough toxin is in the bloodstream, the muscles of the diaphragm and respiratory system will also become paralyzed, and the victim may die from asphyxiation.

The symptoms of botulism generally appear from eight to 72 hours after the contaminated food is eaten. The first signs to appear are weakness, fatigue and dizziness, followed by blurred vision. Speaking and swallowing become difficult. Labored breathing, weakness of the muscles, abdominal pain and distension, and constipation frequently develop. The type of botulism caused by seafood also produces nausea, vomiting and inflammation of the throat. Botulism can be difficult to diagnose, and is sometimes mistaken for other disorders of the central nervous system.

Since government control of botulism is practically impossible, we must protect ourselves from this deadly illness. Canned foods must be discarded when the ends of the cans bulge or show any other evidence of spoilage such as leaks, discoloration, souring or gas formation. Dispose of such containers where children and pets cannot get at them. Do not even taste the contents—throw them out immediately.

Certain commercial foods are especially susceptible to contamination with the botulinum toxin and should be routinely avoided: mildly processed meats (ham slices, cold cuts, chicken and turkey slices, frankfurters, etc.) and smoked fish.

Frozen foods are less suspect, since botulinum cannot multiply and produce toxin at sub-freezing temperatures. But to be absolutely safe, in case the package has been allowed to thaw at any time during storage, you might wish to boil the product 10 to 15 minutes.

By far the best guideline is to stick to fresh foods whenever possible. Unprocessed meats, fish and vegetables, when kept unspoiled, are also kept free of the lethal botulism toxin. Whether eaten raw or cooked, fresh foods have never caused an outbreak of botulism, so why not play it safe?

Illness From Seafood

Contaminated seafood can be responsible for two types of illness, paralytic shellfish poisoning (PSP) and infectious hepatitis.

Paralytic poisoning may be carried by mussels, clams, oysters, shrimp, crabs and lobsters. The PSP toxin is present in the type of algae whose coastal invasion cause what is known as the "red tide." Fish and shellfish eat the algae, which are harmless to them, but poisonous to man when he consumes the shellfish that ate the algae. Lobsters, shrimp, crabs and scaled fish don't concentrate as much of the toxin in their bodies as do mussels and clams, so they are not as likely to cause PSP.

Seafood which carries the toxin has no telltale appearance, and no off-taste to warn you of danger. There is no way to tell if you are eating infected seafood until the disease attacks.

The symptoms of paralytic shellfish poisoning are fast and frightening. In a severe case, the victim notices a slight tingling and numbness of the lips and fingertips within five to 30 minutes, then loss of strength in the muscles. After four to six hours, he is able to raise his head or move his arms only with great difficulty. Breathing also becomes difficult, and the victim must often be put in a respirator or he will die within hours.

Because the poison acts so swiftly, if you should happen to encounter it, remember that action must be taken at once. The usual practice is to induce vomiting with an emetic, or purge with a strong laxative. But doctors agree that these measures cannot always be relied upon to intercept a fatal dose of poison. As soon as difficult breathing develops, artificial respiration should be applied, sometimes for several hours. In severe cases, this procedure may save a life.

Shellfish that live in polluted water can become tainted and cause infectious hepatitis. Symptoms of infectious hepatitis include yellowed eyes, dark urine, nausea and severe abdominal discomfort. Although a person may not die from hepatitis, he can be incapacitated for weeks or even months.

The only way to eliminate any chance of contracting hepatitis from clams, oysters and other shellfish is to cook them long and properly. Clams must be steamed from four to six minutes to destroy hepatitis organisms. Frying clams and oysters will also eliminate the hepatitis virus, but milder cooking methods such as preparation of chowders or stews may not be effective. For additional information on infectious hepatitis, refer to the Liver section.

Trichinosis

Trichinosis is the painful and often fatal disease contracted from contaminated meat, usually pork. Most people believe that government inspection guarantees that meat will be free of disease-causing organisms. But the trichina larvae which cause trichinosis may be present even in inspected meat.

The United States has yet to develop a program for detecting trichina in meat. The inspection required by the federal government does not include a test for trichina larvae. Other countries have been able to work out criteria for condemning meat infected by the parasite, and as a result of our lack of effort, Americans suffer more cases of trichinosis than the rest of the world put together.

The disease is named for the parasitic worm that causes it, *Trichina spiralis*. In its larval stage, the worm embeds itself in the muscles of animals, particularly pigs. Humans acquire the disease by eating raw or undercooked meat that is infected. Once in the human body, the digestive processes liberate the larvae from the meat, and they attach themselves to the lining of the lower intestine. As they mature, they are carried to the lymph nodes, heart, lungs and brain, and throughout the rest of the body.

At each stage of their progress, the parasites produce some symptom of invasion. When they attack the intestine, the victim experiences nausea, diarrhea, abdominal pain and/or fever. In the lungs, symptoms may suggest pneumonia; if the larvae reach the heart, they can coil themselves around it and interfere with its function; they produce inflammation in the brain. Eventually the trichina seek out their natural haven, the skeletal muscles. There they coil up and work cysts around themselves which cause stiffness, pain and swelling in the muscles. The patient develops fever, sweating and insomnia. Many victims carry encysted trichina larvae in their muscles throughout life, mistaking their symptoms for those of other illnesses. The clinical symptoms of trichinosis often resemble a viral infection and it is believed that many acute cases of trichinosis are misdiagnosed as "flu" or "a virus."

When hospitalization is necessary, it is the symptoms, not the disease itself that must be treated. In two or three weeks, the symptoms subside; after this time the patient may never have any further difficulty with the disease, or the condition could cause aches and pains for the rest of his life.

It is up to the individual to protect himself from trichinosis, and the best way to do that is to cook meat, especially pork and all pork products, thoroughly. Cooking temperature must be high enough to kill any trichina larvae which might be present—350°

for pork roasts, for 35 minutes per pound. The temperature of the meat itself, measured with a meat thermometer, should be at least 185°. For fresh pork, a good rule is to cook the meat until it is gray in color, or at least white. Never eat pink pork. Pork products, such as frankfurters, also should never be eaten raw.

How To Avoid Food Poisoning

Sensible shopping habits can go a long way to help protect your family from food poisoning. A book entitled *Evaluation of Public Health Hazards from Microbiological Contamination of Foods*, published in 1964 by the Food Protection Committee of the Food and Nutrition Board, National Academy of Sciences and National Research Council, made these points:

1. Since mild processing (usually low heat) eliminates low-temperature spoilage microorganisms, the consumer is not warned of contamination because there is no visible spoilage; furthermore, with these competing microbes eliminated, "conditions are probably made more favorable for growth and, perhaps, toxin production by potentially pathogenic organisms."

2. Vacuum-packing adds to the hazard—not only because anaerobic conditions are "suitable for the development of botulism," but also because this airless condition inhibits the growth of any surviving spoilage bacteria, so that the chance of the consumer's being warned is further diminished.

A publication on food poisoning released jointly by the USDA and FDA in 1974 offers other tips on careful shopping and cooking practices to prevent the growth of bacteria that cause food poisoning.

Plan your shopping so the grocery store is the last stop on your way home. Buy meat, poultry and frozen foods last so they don't defrost or warm up in the cart while you finish your shopping.

When you get home, put any frozen foods in the freezer, and meats and poultry in the refrigerator right away. The temperature in your freezer should be 0°F, and refrigerator temperature should not exceed 40°F.

Never allow frozen foods to thaw at room temperature. Thaw them in the refrigerator or cook the food frozen. If you must thaw something quickly, put it in a watertight plastic bag and submerge it in cold water.

Don't keep prepared dishes at room temperature for more than two hours before serving them and always refrigerate leftovers as soon as the meal is over.

The best way to avoid food poisoning, of course, is to avoid processed and packaged foods altogether. Prepare and serve only fresh foods, carefully and thoroughly washed. When cooking, be sure to heat foods through and through to a temperature high enough to kill any dangerous bacteria.

And don't neglect to keep up your defenses—naturally—against harmful bacteria that enter your body. Vitamin C, or ascorbic acid, has for more than thirty years been known to function as an antibiotic, that is, a bacteria-killer. Keep an abundant amount of fresh, raw fruits and vegetables in your diet, especially such vitamin C-rich foods as bell peppers, cabbage and black currants.

Another food that will help to keep your gastrointestinal tract in good health is yogurt. This wonderful food product contains millions of harmless bacteria which produce lactic acid, a powerful deterrent against the development of toxin-producing bacteria. People who have begun to eat yogurt regularly after not having done so, soon notice that many of their gastrointestinal disturbances disappear within days of when the new food makes its appearance. Buttermilk produces similar effects. Besides aiding digestion, yogurt also favors the production of the valuable, water-soluble B vitamins, which, like vitamin C, cannot be stored for very long and must be constantly replenished.

Possessing an abundance of the right, friendly bacteria will help, and so will tissue saturation with vitamin C. Yet the only complete answer is fresh, healthy food that has never had a chance to get contaminated.

Section 31
Gallstones

164.   Is Surgery The Only Answer?

164. Is Surgery The Only Answer?

An estimated 16 million Americans are afflicted with gallstones. This condition is fifth among causes of hospital admissions, and the third most common surgical procedure. Although surgery, in which the entire gallbladder is removed, is ordinarily successful, older people and heart patients can undergo such an operation only at a very high risk.

Cut a gallstone in half and you will see that it is made up of glistening crystals of a white, wax-like solid material. This is cholesterol, a word formed from the Greek *chole*, meaning gall or bile, and *stereos*, meaning solid. Cholesterol is a vital ingredient in the bile which is secreted by the liver and stored and concentrated in the gallbladder. From the gallbladder, bile pours into the intestines to help digest fatty foods. The trouble begins when, for reasons which are not clear, cholesterol begins to crystallize out of solution and form stones. Sometimes these stones can pass harmlessly into the intestine, but they can also block up the ducts of the gallbladder. When this happens, the duct contracts in an effort to dislodge the blockage, and the result is a pain said to be worse than childbirth. To make matters worse, the pain is frequently accompanied by vomiting. Only the most powerful analgesics give even a measure of relief.

When the stone obstructs the common bile duct completely, bile is diverted into the bloodstream, resulting in jaundice. If the cystic duct is blocked, bile trapped in the gallbladder becomes so highly concentrated that the organ becomes inflamed.

Adding to the general confusion about the cause of gallstones is the uncertainty as to why people have gallbladders at all. The surgical removal of this organ doesn't seem to cause any metabolic disturbance—at least any that can be observed. A fairly fatty meal can still be adequately digested. Many animals, in fact, do not have gallbladders. The horse, elephant, camel, and whale, as well as many birds, are among this group. So is the rat, but not, for some strange reason, the mouse.

No one has been able to explain why, but if a woman is fair (it is true; blondes do have more gallstones), fat and over 40—and especially if she has had several pregnancies—she is a typical candidate for a battle with her gallbladder. This is not to say that she's alone; gallstones are open to anybody. You can be fat or thin, young or old, male or female, brunette or bald and still be a victim. If you suffer with indigestion and constipation, if you are jaundiced or pass clay-colored stools frequently, and if you get occasional, but severe attacks of colic with pain and vomiting, especially after eating fatty meals, you ought to be suspicious enough to consult a doctor about the state of your gallbladder.

Unsaturated Diet Linked To Stones

Now it turns out that your chances of developing gallstones are more than doubled if you are eating a "prudent," low-cholesterol diet designed to prevent heart disease.

This unsettling discovery was reported by three medical researchers in Los Angeles, who carefully reviewed autopsy protocols from a large group of patients at a Veterans Administration Hospital. During the years 1959 to 1969, 422 of these patients (all male) were put on a diet high in polyunsaturated fats and low in saturated fats, such as cholesterol. Another 424 patients ate the "standard American diet." This long-term experiment, which received considerable publicity, had several interesting results. One was that the heart attack rate among the polyunsaturated group was considerably lower—48 as compared to 70. But although spared from heart attacks, the experimental group suffered a strikingly high incidence of gallstones.

An analysis of the experiment was reported by Drs. Sturdevant, Pearce, and Dayton in the *New England Journal of Medicine* (January 4, 1973). What these doctors found is that while only 14 percent of the patients eating the usual American diet developed gallstones, 34 percent of those on the polyunsaturated diet were found to have gallstones upon autopsy. Suggesting a very definite cause-and-effect relationship was the further finding that there was a direct correlation between the incidence of gallstones and the total number of polyunsaturated meals consumed.

Earlier studies have pointed to the fact that people who are overweight tend to develop gallstones more frequently than others, and this same trend was found in the Los Angeles study. However, there were more overweight men in the control group than in the experimental group, so this could not be used to explain the vast difference in gallstone formation.

These findings are startling not only because they are entirely unexpected, but also because gallstones are composed chiefly of cholesterol. And if you eat a diet very low in cholesterol, and tests show that your serum cholesterol is dropping, why should you develop cholesterol stones in your gallbladder? Dr. Sturdevant and his colleagues admit that the solution to this mystery eludes them.

Lecithin Balances Bile Composition

What then do you do to protect against gallstones if you are on a polyunsaturated diet? The answer is surprisingly simple. Take lecithin every day in generous amounts. What is lecithin? Ironically, it consists largely of polyunsaturated fatty acids, the foundation of any diet designed to reduce cholesterol levels. But more important, it is extremely rich in phospholipids, which prevent fats from clumping together. And of all the theories as to what causes gallstones, the one with the most circumstantial evidence backing it up is that they are precipitated by a decrease in the ratio of phospholipids to cholesterol in the bile.

Dogs have a very high amount of phospholipids, or lecithin, in their bile in relation to their cholesterol, and almost never develop gallstones. Human gallstones dissolve rapidly in dog bile. The most promising pharmaceutical approach to the gallstone plague is an experimental drug called chenodeoxycholic acid, which is thought to be effective largely because "it increases the lecithin content of the bile, augmenting the capacity of the bile to solubilize cholesterol . . ." (*New Scientist*, December 28, 1972).

Does eating lecithin, which is usually extracted from soybeans, instead of a drug, accomplish the same goal? Yes! This was discovered and reported in 1968 by a team of investigators at Ohio State University, which included specialists in physiological chemistry and surgery. Dr. Ronald K. Tompkins told the annual meeting of the Federation of American Societies for Experimental Biology at Atlantic City in that year that he and his colleagues first confirmed the fact that patients with gallstones do indeed have an abnormally low phospholipid-cholesterol ratio in their bile. Patients who had healthy gallbladders had six times as much phospholipid as cholesterol, while those with gallstones had only twice as much of the emulsifier, a very significant three-fold difference.

For their experiment, the researchers gave 10 grams of lecithin a day to each of six patients. The patients had a choice of swallowing 20 half-gram (500 mg.) lecithin capsules daily or eating 5 cookies into which the lecithin had been baked. This succeeded in doubling the bile concentration of phospholipids, Dr. Tompkins reported.

How Vitamin C Can Help

Another important study by Dr. Emil Ginter of the Institute of Human Nutrition in Bratislava, Czechoslovakia, revealed that vitamin C is an important link in the conversion of cholesterol into bile acids, a necessary step if cholesterol is to be rendered harmless in the bile. (*Science*, February 16, 1973.)

Dr. Ginter induced a state of vitamin C deficiency in guinea pigs which, like humans, do not synthesize this vitamin. He did not induce outright scurvy because acute scurvy in developed countries occurs rarely as compared to latent vitamin C deficiency, which is quite common.

He gave 26 control animals 10 mg. of ascorbic acid every 24 hours. To induce a vitamin C deficiency in another 26 animals, he fed them a scurvy diet for 14 days and then gave them a maintenance dose of 0.5 mg. of ascorbic acid every 24 hours. After three months, the animals were all given an injection of cholesterol. Then they were sacrificed and autopsied. What did Dr. Ginter find? Enough to make anyone who has ever been told to watch his cholesterol reach for more vitamin C instead of cutting down on eggs.

The control animals, or those who got the vitamin C supplement from the beginning, had almost eight times as much vitamin C in their livers, four times as much in their spleens and just half as much cholesterol in their blood. They also showed less cholesterol in their livers, about 25 percent less than those animals deficient in vitamin C. *But the most amazing finding was the decreased levels of bile acids in those animals who were deficient in vitamin C.* The lower the level of these acids in the bile, the more likely it is that gallstones will eventually form.

A Doctor's Advice: Eat More Bran

Extra fiber-rich bran in the diet may also help prevent or treat gallstones. That was reported by Dr. E. W. Pomare, of the Bristol Royal Infirmary in England.

When patients with radiographically-detected gallstones were fed additional bran every day (as much as they could tolerate) in a short-term study, the cholesterol saturation of the bile was significantly lowered, Dr. Pomare told The Canadian Society for Clinical Investigation's annual meeting in Winnipeg (*Internal Medicine News*, March 1, 1975).

Dr. Pomare recommended completely unprocessed bran—the kind available in health food stores. The larger particle size of unprocessed bran is believed more effective than the smaller particles found in packaged dry cereals, he said.

Dr. Pomare suspects long-term treatment using bran might possibly reduce the size of existing gallstones. In less-developed countries—where levels of dietary fiber are extremely high because foods are not refined—gallstones are very rare.

Section 32
Goiter

165. Metabolic Impairment
Of The Thyroid Gland

165. Metabolic Impairment Of The Thyroid Gland

To understand the condition we call goiter, we must first know something about the thyroid gland and its function in the human body. Located at the base of the neck, over the Adam's apple, the thyroid is a ductless gland. That means it is an organ of the body which secretes a fluid, but it has no "duct," or opening, through which this fluid passes to some other part of the body. So the fluid manufactured by the thyroid gland passes directly into the blood stream. This fluid, or hormone, thyroxine, is made by the thyroid gland out of iodine and the amino acid, tyrosine.

The thyroid, through the hormone thyroxine, determines growth, controls body temperature, regulates the metabolism or the burning of food in the body and influences, to a great extent, mental and emotional balance. Also, it is of special importance for a proper functioning of the reproductive system. The interrelationship between reproductive functions and thyroid functions is very complex and not entirely understood, but it is known that various changes, especially in girls and women, are apt to cause changes in thyroid function. For instance, a slight enlargement of the thyroid gland is common at puberty, during pregnancy and menopause.

When the thyroid gland is functioning properly, we are hardly aware of its existence. It stores practically all of the body's supply of iodine, releases thyroxine into the blood stream at intervals and regulates all the bodily functions we have mentioned above. Disorders of the thyroid gland are apparently caused by two conditions: (1) lack of sufficient iodine in the diet, so that the thyroid cannot obtain enough to manufacture thyroxine; or (2) some disorder of the body which creates a demand for far more thyroxine than the gland can manufacture.

Goiter, generally speaking, refers to any abnormal enlargement of the thyroid gland. *Simple* goiter, called also *endemic* goiter, is an enlargement of the thyroid caused, apparently, by increased need for the thyroid secretion. The gland becomes larger in an effort to produce more and more thyroxine. This condition is not accompanied by other symptoms, except possibly a feeling of fatigue. *Toxic* goiter, called also *exophthalmic* goiter, is marked by the suddenness of its appearance, and its accompanying symptoms of extreme nervousness, emaciation, irritability, sweating and rapid heart beat. We do not know what causes toxic goiter.

Myxedema occurs in complete atrophy of the thyroid gland. That is, this gland does not function at all, and all the other body operations which it regulates are affected, with resulting headache, lassitude, obesity, depression, subnormal temperature and mental dullness. Children whose thyroid glands are atrophied at birth, are said to have "cretinism." Such children are mentally defective, lethargic and dull, with scanty hair and pasty, thick skins. Many do not survive to adulthood. Adult cretinism is the result of thyroid deficiency over many generations. It frequently results in heart trouble, deafness and deaf-mutism.

What Part Does Iodine Play?

J. F. McClendon, Professor of Physiological Chemistry at the University of Minnesota, was one of the leading authorities in the branch of thyroid study that has concentrated on iodine deficiency in the diet. His classic book, *Iodine and the Incidence of Goiter*, (University of Minnesota Press, 1939) was one of the first works to contain a full discussion of the world distribution of the ailment, as compared with the distribution of iodine in food, water, soil and rocks. In 1910, Professor McClendon noted that a woman who had lived in a region where goiters were common was relieved of this illness when she began to eat quantities of seafood, which contains a lot of iodine. This observation convinced him that iodine is an essential food constituent and that lack of it may lead to a deficiency, just as lack of a vitamin may. The deficiency disease in the case of iodine would be goiter.

Though Dr. McClendon admitted that many of the more complicated phases of thyroid function needed much more investigation to be adequately understood, he believed that enough was known about goiter for us to relate it purely and simply to the iodine content of the diet.

Kelp Protects Against Goiter

There are whole sections of the world where iodine is completely lacking in the soil. These iodine-poor areas are well plotted in every country; in fact, probably no other single nutrient has been pin-pointed around the globe so comprehensively. Regions of endemic goiter—that is, areas where goiter is prevalent because of iodine lacking in the soil and food—have been identified for many years. Many parts of the middle inland sections of our country, especially the Great Lakes regions, are deficient in iodine content in the soils. These localities are called "The Goiter Belt."

For a long time public health authorities have promoted the use of iodized salt to prevent goiter. This is plain table salt to which potassium iodide has been added by chemists. Most of us get far too much salt. Why not get the iodine from kelp?

Borden's *Review of Nutrition Research* states that to get 100 micrograms of iodine (estimated as the normal daily requirement for human beings) one would have to eat

10 pounds of fresh vegetables and fruits, or
8 pounds of cereals, grains and nuts, or
6 pounds of meat, freshwater fish, fowl, or
2 pounds of eggs, or
.3 pounds of marine fish, or
.2 pounds of shellfish.

It goes on, "The problem of obtaining sufficient iodine from food of non-marine origin may be seen from values shown in this table. Iodine-rich seaweed is an abundant source on a limited scale for some peoples. Kelp contains about 200,000 micrograms per kilogram and the dried kelp meal nearly ten times as much, or .1 percent to .2 percent of iodine. Used as a condiment this would provide ten times as much iodine as American iodized salt."

Kelp has long seemed to many the perfect answer for a dietary mineral supplement. It is practically the only reliable food source of iodine, aside from seafood. It is rich in potassium and magnesium. It contains, in addition, all of the trace minerals that have been shown to be important for human nutrition and many more whose purposes we have not yet discovered. It grows without commercial fertilizers and is never sprayed with pesticides.

Water Pollution And Goiter

Sir Robert McCarrison, a famous British physician, devoted his life to the study of the causes of goiter. Starting off in his search with no preconceived ideas of what might or might not be the cause, he traveled widely, to obscure corners of the world looking for clues.

He visited the country of Hunza and found that, in nations in the territory surrounding the Hunzas, goiters were common. The terrain, the amount of iodine in soil and water, and the climate of these nations were similar to that of Hunza. Yet, among the Hunza people, goiter is unknown. Sir Robert studied the water supply of Hunza and found that it was carefully guarded against pollution. Aside from the fact that the Hunzas themselves are meticulously clean in their way of life, they know that water for drinking must be pure. They keep their drinking water in roofed tanks or closed cisterns inaccessible to animals and well protected from any kind of contamination.

"In nine villages about 60 miles from Hunza," said Sir Robert, "the water comes from a single source and is conveyed to the different villages in open kuls or channels . . . it will be observed that there are two main channels on the banks of which the villages are situated, one below the other. Each village in this way receives the drainage of the village or villages above it, till at the last village, Kashrote, the drinking water has been polluted by the eight villages above.

"The water in these open channels not only supplies the inhabitants with drinking water, but it irrigates their extensive crops, serves as an open sewer, is used for the cleansing of their bodies, household utensils and wearing apparel. The drainings from cultivated and manured fields flow into it. It can readily be imagined, therefore, that considerable organic impurities find their way down to the lower villages."

Sir Robert then gave the goiter statistics for each village. "From this table, it is seen that the percentage of infected houses, of infected individuals in these houses and of the total population suffering from goiter, goes on increasing from the highest to the lowest village on the water-channels."

Vitamin A Deficiency And Goiter

"In articles, and even in books, on the possible influence of the soil (and the water that springs from it) on man, it is generally stated that the only known example of such an influence is that exerted by iodine on the thyroid." These words are from a book, *Soil, Grass and Cancer,* By André Voisin (published by the Philosophical Press, New York). Dr. Voisin noted that iodine has been used to treat goiter for about 140 years.

Goiter

Goiter is a reaction on the part of the thyroid to a disturbance in the metabolism of iodine—that is, the way the body uses iodine, said Dr. Voisin. One extremely important clue to the way the body uses iodine is the amount of vitamin A present in the diet. For the last 20 years, we have known that lack of vitamin A is one cause of goiter. A thyroid gland already goitrous contains about one-tenth of the normal amount of vitamin A. If the epithelial cells present in the thyroid are deficient in vitamin A, then enough thyroxine will not be made, for it is apparently in these cells of the thyroid gland that the hormone is manufactured.

It is true, too, that a lack of vitamin A disorders the function of the pituitary gland. The pituitary gland secretes a substance which regulates the thyroid. Lacking vitamin A, this entire process goes awry. Night blindness is one of the first symptoms of vitamin A deficiency. It has been observed that people who suffer from night blindness also suffer from goiter, another indication that lack of vitamin A is involved. Dr. Voisin quoted a Dr. Rhein of Strasbourg, who believed that an original lack of vitamin A probably is responsible for setting in motion both these two disorders. He thinks perhaps the vitamin lack may sensitize the thyroid to some goiter-causing element in the environment.

Section 33
Hair and Scalp Problems

166. What Keeps Hair Healthy?

What we call hair is actually a hardened, hollow, pigmented shaft that grows from the hair follicle, a tubular pit in the outer layer of the scalp. The scalp has more of these hair follicles than any other surface part of the body. Each follicle is a cluster of cells, called the matrix, from which the hair grows as it receives nourishment. The nourishment comes from the papilla, a microscopic, nipple-shaped nodule, often erroneously referred to as the "root" of the hair follicle. The papilla is actually a part of the bulb-shaped skin membrane which surrounds the matrix, and it is directly supplied with nutrients by blood vessels and capillaries. This matrix in the human scalp will produce a little more than 1/100th of an inch of hair every day. And each hair is unique in its thickness, varying from 1/140th to 1/1500th of an inch in diameter.

The energy the body uses to produce this amount of hair is extremely large compared with what it takes to produce other body tissues. If the products brought to the follicle via the blood vessels and capillaries are missing anything vital the hair will not grow, or if it does manage some growth, it will not have a healthy and glossy appearance—it will, in fact, be weak and brittle.

It is obvious that the quality of hair cannot depend solely on applications of external conditioners but depends upon the circulation and quality of the blood brought to it, which in turn depends on the quality of nutrition. "Hair flourishes when the body prospers, weakens when the body languishes, not as a parasitical attachment but as an integral functioning organ does," according to Dr. Irwin I. Lubowe in his book *New Hope for Your Hair* (E. P. Dutton and Co., Inc. 1960).

The importance of sound nutrition and healthy hair growth is by no means a new discovery. Back in 1913, Dr. Richard Muller, who studied at leading institutions in London, Vienna, and Berlin wrote a book entitled *Hair, Its Nature, Growth and Most Common Affections*. "The growth of hair," he said, "depends entirely on the blood supply. Anemic, sclerotic, ill-nourished people will grow no hair while their condition is below normal."

Dr. Muller's diet for promoting the growth of hair was interesting. He advised raw eggs, carrots, oatmeal, toasted bread, raw milk, gelatin and a soup made of two parts of meat and one part bones. In other words, he included in his diet those foods that contained nutrients similar to those contained in the hair.

Diseases directly caused by malnutrition—such as marasmus and kwashiorkor—often manifest their first symptoms in the make-up and appearance of the hair. Many researchers use hair analysis to gauge the degree of malnutrition. Dr. Robert B. Bradfield, reporting in the *American Journal of Clinical Nutrition* (April 1971), noted a change in hair follicles due to protein and calorie malnutrition. During a three-month study of six male volunteers between the ages of 21 and 45, Dr. Bradfield and his colleagues studied the effects on the hair of nutritionally sound liquid diets which excluded all protein. The volunteers, who were in good health throughout the study, showed significant changes in their hair follicles after only 11 days: atrophy, dyspigmentation, bulb-diameter reduction and sheath absence. But when protein was readmitted to the diet, the hair follicle changes reversed themselves.

167. What Can You Do About Baldness?

Hair loss and baldness come in different forms, some permanent, others only temporary. Hair loss, an affliction which affects 90 percent of the male population and 20 percent (or more) of the female population of all ages, is a traumatic blow to the psyche. The essential questions in matters of hair loss are: Is the hair loss inevitable? And, if not, what can be done about it?

Whether lost hair can grow back does not depend on the damage to the hair itself, but on the condition of the follicles involved. "When there is hair loss," reported Dr. Norman Orentreich in the *Journal of the American Medical Women's Association* (June, 1969), "either the living hair follicle or the keratinized hair shaft may be involved. When the dead hair shaft involved is affected, hair loss is temporary since the follicle continues to produce normal hair. If the living follicle is damaged or diseased, the hair coming from it may cease to grow and finally fall out. This may be followed by (1) the immediate regrowth of new hair; (2) the temporary failure to regrow a hair, or (3) the persistent inability to regrow a hair from that follicle. If the follicle is destroyed, the resultant *alopecia* (baldness) is of course always permanent. . ."

Baldness In Men

The most common form of baldness is *male pattern baldness,* which accounts for approximately 90 percent of all male baldness. Its symptoms are easily recognizable. It usually begins with a uniformly receding hair line, or an expanding circle of baldness on the crown of the head, or hair may gradually disappear on the back of the head and the balding area may gradually work its way forward. Each of these forms results in a horseshoe pattern leaving a swath or fringe of hair around the ears. (Actually, there is hair on top of the head, but it is colorless, very fine, and averages only about three millimeters in length.)

The medical consensus is that most male pattern baldness is based upon hereditary influences and is irreversible. The only success in regrowing hair, according to many medical researchers, is found in the technique of the surgical hair transplant. First developed by Dr. Norman Orentreich in the 1950's, the transplant technique involves the following procedure:

Using a rotary biopsy punch, the physician cuts a small round segment from the area where there is hair, the back or side fringes. This is implanted in a segment already prepared in the bald area. The receiving area must be exactly the same size as the circle of scalp being inserted. These circles are called "plugs." Each one contains from 10 to 15 hairs with their follicles, and, as a rule, 10 to 25 plugs are transplanted in a single session. Some doctors will transplant an increased number if the patient is in a hurry. On the average, it takes from 10 to 20 sessions to achieve a good growth. At this point, the patient may have a bad case of nerves, because the transplanted hairs fall out after a few weeks. This is because hair that is transplanted immediately goes into a resting phase (*telogen*). In about three months, however, new hair growth will become apparent in the transplanted sections.

Medical World News (July 19, 1974) reported that well over a million persons have had transplants in the 20 years since the procedure was developed. When the operation is done by a trained surgeon skilled in its intricacies, the rate of graft survival is close to 100 percent.

The cause of hereditary male pattern baldness is still a mystery to medical researchers, but it is known that the production of androgen, the male hormone, is a prime factor. A hereditary tendency to over-produce this hormone will cause baldness (even in women). Baldness does not occur in men who do not reach full sexual maturity, which is why it happens after adolescence, usually after the age of twenty.

Some of the most hopeful research being done to prevent male pattern baldness is in the area of manufacturing an anti-androgen which can be directed to the hair follicles without tampering with the rest of the body. This would require considerable modification of the anti-androgen substance, but it is a procedure that still remains in its formative stages. But *how* and *why* is male pattern baldness connected with androgens? Dr. Lubowe suggests that excessive male hormones may reduce the thickness of the fatty subcutaneous tissue of the scalp, thus making it more susceptible to impaired blood circulation, which, in turn, causes baldness.

But, according to Dr. Lubowe, there must be more responsible for male baldness than androgens alone. The fact that brothers, who share the same family inheritance, do not necessarily go bald at the same rate suggests a matter more complex than the simple diagnosis of *heredity—nothing can be done to prevent it.* Dr. Lubowe believes that there are other causes which contribute to baldness which must be investigated. "While it is always possible that in the end, all functional tests will check negatively, the least feeling of despair should be resisted until the investigation is complete. There are now too many known reasons for baldness, and too many known means of coping with it, to warrant any other initial assumption than marked optimism."

Female Pattern Baldness
Female pattern baldness, though it afflicts a low percentage of women, is on the increase at a significant rate. This form of baldness will rarely assume the degree experienced by males— that is, nothing left but a halo of hair around the sides and back of the head. Naturally, a woman becomes alarmed at the first signs of hair loss, but a dermatologist will assure her that there is much that can be done to alleviate the problem.

Until the mid-1950's the number of balding women in the United States was not spectacular and it appeared unchanging. Then, suddenly, the number of women losing their hair doubled, then tripled, and soon even the new number tripled again. A report from 170 members of the American Dermatological Association in 1962 confirmed the trend. The Association noted a 122 percent increase in women losing their hair dating from 1956. Statistics worldwide showed a similar increase.

Some doctors speculate that the changing social position of women may have something to do with this increase of hair loss. As more women enjoy equal job opportunities, it appears that they encounter more stress and anxiety in the positions they achieve. Stress can trigger a hormone imbalance in women, which may take the form of increased androgen production. All women produce androgen naturally, but much less of it than men do. It only takes a minute upset of the hormone balance to cause symptoms of "masculinization" in females, of which pattern hair loss may be one. Other symptoms of such hormonal imbalance include hirsutism (increased body and facial hair), disturbances in the menstrual cycle, and difficulty in becoming pregnant. Another source of this imbalance could be an ovarian tumor, which interferes with the proper hormone balance.

Female hair loss not associated with masculinization symptoms is sometimes referred to as *diffuse cyclic hair loss*. This is an "overall" rather than "patterned" loss, a diffuse hair loss without disease of the scalp. "This condition is by definition cyclic and reversible," reported Drs. William B. Guy and Walter F. Edmundson (*A.M.A. Archives of Dermatology* (February, 1960), "... it occurs in transitory episodes, lasting for several weeks only. It is the source of much perplexity because there is no apparent cause. Those afflicted would invariably seem to be women."

Diffuse cyclic hair loss appears to be the result of systemic stresses, disease, excessive anxiety or physiologic situations (such as recent major surgery). Leading major doctors in their field note that it is difficult to tell in the emotionally-charged atmosphere of excessive hair loss, whether anxiety is the cause or result of hair thinning. But it's been noted that some cases can be clearly seen to have originated in emotional strain.

Even normal male pattern baldness, which most authorities agree is strictly a result of the genetic "throw of the dice," has been linked by other researchers to personality factors. Tension, stress, and anxiety can "tighten up" the scalp, causing impaired circulation that promotes hair loss. In her book, *Hair: Sex, Society, Symbolism* (Stein and Day, Co., 1971) Wendy Cooper observed, "that primitive races are usually exempt from baldness is offered in support of this idea, as is the increased tendency to hair loss in women, who, happily emancipated, now bear their fair share of stresses."

Ms. Cooper also cites the amazing theory of two psychiatrists from the University of Chicago, Drs. Thomas A. Szasz and Alan M. Robertson, who claim that smiles and laughter can be a cause of baldness. "The facial nerve, which allows fluidity of facial expression, has branches that activate the muscles of the scalp and ears. Broad smiles and hearty laughter cause this muscle to pull on the scalp and tighten it, and, worse still, the suddenly tautened muscles themselves constrict the blood vessels supplying the hair."

Other Causes Of Excessive Hair Loss In Women

Speaking at the Symposium on Biopathology, Disorders and Treatment of the Pilosebaceous System, at Crans, Switzerland, Dr. Irwin Lubowe reported that "... hormonal disturbances with genetic susceptibility have been documented as prime factors. . ." in the "startling" increase in hair loss among women, as well as many external causes (*Clinical Medicine*, March 1972). He said that some hair loss was due to the indiscriminate use of certain cosmetics; "hair appliances" which caused "temporary hair breakage and damage;" such coiffures as the ponytail, which required tight braiding of the hair, using rollers and bobbypins (he noted that in some of these "severe" cases of hair strain the loss could be permanent); and hair waving or straightening preparations which contain triglycolates, which are also used in certain depilatory creams, in the manufacture of industrial iron and as a stabilizing agent in the production of plastics.

Dr. Lubowe noted that among the deficiencies seen in patients suffering from hair loss was vitamin deficiency. "In the majority of patients, deficiency of vitamins because of poor diet is known to exist," he said. For treatment of female pattern baldness he said that he had used a "sustained-release vitamin tablet" made up of the following: thiamine, riboflavin, pyridoxine HC1, vitamin B_{12}, nicotinic acid, pantothenic acid, ascorbic acid, alpha tocopherol, cysteine HC1; and the minerals: potassium iodide, manganese, copper, zinc, as well as inositol and folic acid, the last added as a metabolite which may favorably affect hair growth.

Pregnancy, The Pill And Hair Loss

There are other causes of hair loss which are much more specific and easily diagnosed. Temporary hair loss, or *post partem alopecia*, can occur in a woman after she has given birth or after an abortion. Since a woman's body produces a large amount of estrogen during pregnancy, the sudden decrease of this estrogen production at the termination of a pregnancy, whether natural or artificial, will shift the hormone balance abruptly. In some women the hair loss will barely be noticeable and in others it will be quite noticeable, usually lasting for three months. Repeated pregnancies, however, may extend the duration of this form of *alopecia*.

Women taking oral contraceptives also risk excessive hair loss. Since the Pill convinces the body that it is pregnant, the same hormonal changes take place. The hair loss is often experienced after the Pill is discontinued. Dr. Lubowe reports that hair fall may sometimes not occur until three or four months after the birth control dosage is stopped, but the hair, he notes, is restored within six months.

Medicines That Harm Your Hair

There are several antibiotics that may cause temporary baldness or hair loss, including penicillin, the sulfanomides and mycin drugs.

The anticoagulant drug, heparin, which is now being widely used as a heart treatment, is another drug which is an often unsuspected villain when an uncommon amount of hair shedding takes place. Ordinarily, about ten percent of the hairs on a normal scalp are in what is known as the "resting phase." When this "resting phase" ends, a new hair starts to grow, and as it does, the old hair falls from the scalp. Heparin, heparinoid and coumarin cause vast numbers of the hairs to go into the "resting phase" long before they should. Of course, the result is a drastic thinning of the hair. Occasionally, people who are taking carbimazole, a drug used in the treatment of hyperthyroidism, find to their surprise that they are suffering a loss of hair. The cause often goes undetected and everything from hair spray to hat bands is blamed, while the patient goes on taking the drug, unaware that this is the bandit which is destroying his hair.

168. Dandruff Can Be Defeated By Diet

Dandruff is the most common disorder of the scalp. Basically there are two types of dandruff: (1) simple dandruff which forms when the scalp is dry and flakes off as the hair is brushed or combed; and (2) the more severe form of dandruff, *seborrheic dermatitis*, which forms when the sebaceous glands become overactive. Ordinarily, these glands are useful in providing a lubricant for the skin and hair, but over-production and blockage of the glands by normal accumulations of dandruff can bring on this most irritating form of dandruff. Dr. Albert M. Kligman and colleagues at the Department of Dermatology, University of Pennsylvania School of Medicine, in distinguishing between ordinary dandruff and seborrheic dermatitis, have stated that sudden exacerbations of the latter are a common occurrence following emotional traumas and illnesses of various kinds, whereas ordinary dandruff is more stable. An upset in hormonal balance, which can be triggered by the emotions, can also cause excessive oil production by the sebaceous glands.

The body malfunctions related to dandruff are similar to those related to acne, according to Dr. Irwin Lubowe in his book *The Modern Guide to Skin Care and Beauty* (E. P. Dutton and Company, 1973). However, while one might expect that they would occur simultaneously, they don't. Dandruff usually begins to show at about 20, when acne has become a painful memory, and it is not seen much after the age of 40. That does not mean that you can't have dandruff after 40. If you do, Dr. Lubowe noted, it is not necessarily evidence of prolonged youth. However, within the age range of 20 to 40, dandruff affects 80 percent of the population.

Excessive Starch And Dandruff

Dandruff itself is not a disease, but only a symptom of one that is less visible. Far more serious than the snowflakes on your shoulders is the fact that dandruff can lead to hair loss and even to baldness. But there are steps that you can take at your very next meal that will help you overcome your dandruff problem and, at the same time, overcome some other problems. One of the most important is to reduce your consumption of starchy foods and also reduce, or better still, eliminate sugar completely. Sugar and starch are two of the dietary excesses which Dr. Lubowe scores as triggers of the internal difficulties which can lead to dandruff. There are external influences, too. Some cosmetics and medications can cause inflammations and chemical changes of the scalp surface with resulting dandruff. An increased volume and activity of the bacteria and fungi normally residing on a human scalp is another cause. But sugar particularly, could well be the substance that triggers the conditions that cause dandruff.

When Dr. John Yudkin, internationally famous nutritionist and researcher affiliated with Queen Elizabeth College, University of London in Great Britain, investigated the relationship between sugar and various forms of disease, he discovered that people who suffer with seborrheic dermatitis are more often than not heavy sugar users. In fact, those with the flaky stuff on their shoulders were eating more than half again as much sugar as those who did not suffer the embarrassment and annoyance of dandruff (*Nature*, September 22, 1972).

In order to double-check these conclusions, Dr. Yudkin told half his patients to abstain from sugar; not the natural form found in fruits and vegetables, but the refined form found in processed foods. When Dr. Yudkin followed up a year later, he found that of 11 patients who were not instructed to cut out refined sugar, two were cured, but nine had experienced no improvement at all. Of eight patients who abstained from sugar, all but one were cured of seborrheic dermatitis at the end of the year.

Vitamin B$_{12}$ Involved

Dr. Wolfgang Caspar of St. Vincent's Medical Center in New York City, reporting new findings regarding seborrhea of the scalp at the International Conference of Dermatology in Venice in 1972, said that improper diet leads to seborrhea. Also, seborrhea patients suffer from an easily disturbed carbohydrate metabolism with malabsorption or malutilization of vitamin B$_{12}$. He did not say which came first. But he did suggest that it would be advisable in cases of such seborrhea to supplement the diet with vitamin B$_{12}$ orally or by injections from a physician.

Hair And Scalp Problems

It would be logical to assume that the malabsorption or disturbed metabolism came first, resulting in the disturbed pH of the skin, rendering it more alkaline than acid, thus favoring the growth of the bacteria always present on the scalp. "Where dandruff is present, the acid mantle has been temporarily changed because the balance has shifted toward the alkaline side," says Dr. Lubowe. If you go to a dermatologist or a physician with a bad case of dandruff, he will very likely prescribe an acid buffered cortisone liquid and shampoo for external application.

A do-it-yourself measure which would involve less expense and perhaps fewer consequences, would be to add lemon or vinegar to your final rinse water after shampooing. This is a measure you would be wise to take whether you have dandruff or not, simply to restore the acid balance on your head which tends to become alkaline immediately after shampooing. Be sure to dilute your lemon juice or your vinegar as full strength would be much too acidic.

Reporting in the *Journal of the Canadian Medical Association* (July 15, 1968), Dr. A. P. Caspers notes that "Many patients with *pityriasis capitatis* (common dandruff) or frank seborrheic dermatitis have low basal metabolic rates, who admit to consuming an excess of carbohydrates, fats or alcohol." In some instances, Dr. Caspers noted a deficiency of vitamin B was present. It is therefore his practice to supplement local treatment with nutritional measures. He forbids alcohol, chocolate, and excessive amounts of cream, butter, milk and sweets. Any suspected vitamin B deficiency is rectified. Sugar needs the B vitamins in order to be metabolized. When you eat natural carbohydrates like fruits, vegetables and whole grains, the vitamin B you need is supplied by the food itself. But when you eat refined sugar or white flour products, your body must steal vitamin B from your muscles, nerves and organs in order to metabolize that sugar. Obviously, if you eat large quantities of refined sugars and starches, you may suffer from a vitamin B deficiency that can cause fatigue, nervousness, constipation, and other symptoms like dandruff.

Which of the B vitamins have particular relevance to the health of your scalp and hair? "Riboflavin, niacin, pyridoxine, and possibly pantothenic acid are the members of the B complex group that have clinical dermatological significance for man," says Dr. W. A. Krehl in *Modern Nutrition In Health and Disease* edited by Drs. Robert S. Goodhart and Michael G. Wohl, Lea and Febiger Co., 1968.

Besides, says Dr. Krehl, "The dermatitis of riboflavin deficiency is primarily a seborrheic dermatitis with many fine greasy scales on an erythematous (reddish skin) base."

169. Retaining Hair Color

Artificial Hair Dyes And Cancer

There has been growing evidence of a causal relationship between the use of commercial hair dyes and cancer. According to Dr. Bruce N. Ames, a member of the National Academy of Sciences and a biochemist at the University of California, tests indicated that 150 of 169 different hair dyes genetically changed the characteristics of Salmonella bacteria (*Proceedings Of The National Academy Of Science*, May 15, 1975). The ominous fear that these dyes may in some way be carcinogenic (cancer-causing) was raised because Dr. Ames had estimated from past experience that 70 to 75 percent of known carcinogenic substances are also mutagenic. The California studies began in 1970 following earlier reports of other scientists who found that certain chemicals in hair dyes could be absorbed through the skin and were found in routine urine analysis.

The 250 million dollar hair dye industry, which services 20 million Americans every year, attacked the findings of Dr. Ames as "inconclusive." Because of early commercial pressures in the 1930's, hair dyes were deemed exempt from regulations pertaining to dyes in the original Food, Drug and Cosmetic Act of 1938. Commercial pressure has retained this exemption status even under the stronger Kefauver amendments of 1962.

The National Cancer Institute (NCI) began its own investigations into the carcinogenic properties of hair dyes in 1970 after a Japanese scientist, Nobuyuki Ito of Nara Medical University, discovered that small amounts of a hair dye ingredient, known as toluenediamine, induced liver cancer in rats. The 1970 NCI test on the hair dye ingredient proved inconclusive in the first round trials, even though the chemical produced a varied number of tumors in the control rats. Shortly after the commencement of the NCI investigations started, the hair dye industry dropped toluenediamine as an ingredient in its products. According to Clyde Burnett, manager of toxicology at the Clairol plant in Stamford, Connecticut, "It played only a small part in the manufacturing of hair coloring; we decided to withdraw it because of publicity" (*Medical World News*, May 5, 1975).

Though tests into the carcinogenicity of hair dyes on higher level organisms are still officially inconclusive, and probably will remain so for quite some time, a specter of doubt surrounds the safety of the use of these preparations, according to some researchers. Dr. Nathaniel Shafer, an internist in Manhattan, reported in April, 1975 (*Medical World News*) that 87 of 100 breast cancer patients he examined had "been long-term users of permanent (oxidative) hair coloring."

Fortunately, artificial hair dyes are not the only means available for retaining or heightening the color of your hair.

Graying And Good Nutrition

Good nutrition and retaining one's natural hair color seem inextricably bound together. Although there is no one formula that will guarantee the return of one's original hair color once it has faded, there are breakthroughs in the field of nutrition giving us hope that eventually we can avoid fading and complete loss of color merely by consuming enough of the right foods.

Actually, many persons have experienced a complete reversal of the graying syndrome by changing their diets. But since food requirements are highly individual, there is no known formula that will invariably restore lost hair color.

There are so very many facets to each function of one part of the body, and each part is so interdependent on the others, that it would be difficult to separate the causes of any one condition. According to nutritionists in the field, loss of hair color indicates losses or deficiencies in other parts of the body also.

It would seem that the wisest approach to rejuvenation of any one part of the body, then, is an overall plan of improvement to the whole body. That way one is assured of the best performance of any and every part.

Foods that some people have found helpful in restoring original hair color include brewer's yeast, liver, wheat germ, blackstrap molasses, sunflower seeds, whole grain cereals, rice polishings, sea food, kelp, yogurt, and cold pressed vegetable and nut oils.

These foods would have to be included in a regular diet to be most effective. This would mean adding them to a daily diet consisting of fresh fruits, vegetables, and protein dishes such as cheese, nutmeats, animal meats, and fish.

Natural Hair Colorings

Another method of combating the onslaught of fading color is to use *natural* colorings on the hair. With some of these, a measure of an original shade can be restored. Others will at least darken hair that is graying. One can even prepare a rinse from golden headed flowers that will lighten blonde hair and another herbal rinse to remove drabness.

While these colorings from herbs and flowers can have some positive effect on the hair in returning it to its original shade, they are seldom as concealing as a chemical dye. They are also more inclined to wash out or lighten with successive shampoos. So herbal treatments must be used on a frequent basis. This is a general rule, though of course there will be exceptions.

Some women find that a monthly rinse with a sage shampoo keeps their hair a soft brown. Other women use camomile rinse instead of a bleach on their blond hair, and though they may be in their forties, there is no darkening or fading of highlights as is usually the case with blond hair after the earlier years.

Because of their more gentle qualities, these herbal rinses are not as powerful or long lasting as the chemical ones, but they are certainly much safer.

Section 34
Hay Fever

170. A Safer Way To Treat The Wheezes And Sneezes

For all too many people, the sunshine-filled days of late summer mean watering eyes and a runny nose, sneezing and sniffling, itching and scratching in the throat, choking and gasping. In a word, hay fever. Hay fever is an allergy specifically to pollen. It is just like any other type of allergy except that it is seasonal. Once the pollen is gone, so is the allergy until next year. But when the pollen is in the air, it cannot be avoided, and high concentrations bring exquisite suffering.

Almost one out of every ten Americans—or approximately 20 million—suffer from one allergy or another, according to the Allergy Foundation of America. And somewhere between seven and eight million suffer from hay fever.

In all, the problem is essentially the same. The body over-reacts to the pollen, producing inordinately large numbers of antibodies which, when they are actively battling an allergen, somehow induce the tissues to produce histamine. The histamine makes the capillaries more permeable, which results in edema, swelling and irritation of the nerves in the region.

There is no "one-shot" cure for allergies such as hay fever, although almost everything from injections of urine to keeping a chihuahua in the house has been tried to alleviate the symptoms. The 1618 edition of the London *Pharmacopedia* recommended a diet of fox's lungs. Until the 1800's, leeches were used to suck out the evil humors. And, in 1831 the British physician, John Elliotson, recommended hypnotism. Unfortunately, none of them has worked. Nor is the score much better for today's desensitizing injections of small amounts of pollen. They do reduce the intensity of some people's attacks, but most sufferers are helped little, if at all.

Drugs Have Nasty Side Effects
It's at this point a person starts reaching for the popular drugstore remedies containing antihistamines to counteract the histamine which is causing all the distress.

774

But the antihistamines have dangerous side effects. One of those is sedation. In fact, some antihistamines are actually sold as sedatives.

This sedative effect makes driving cars or operating machinery a dangerous proposition. Reaction time is slowed, and it becomes all too easy to fall asleep at the wheel or otherwise endanger life and limb under influence of the drug. Antihistamines have also been known to dry up the mucus in the nose to the point where severe nosebleeds occur.

In children, large doses of antihistamines have reportedly caused cerebral edema and convulsions. In adults, convulsions are less common and overdosage is more likely to cause depression of the central nervous system. Other side effects include the inability to concentrate, dizziness, and disturbance of coordination. Dryness of the mouth, pharynx and bronchial mucosa with an irritating dry cough may occur (*British Medical Journal*, December 28, 1963).

So even though the neutralizing of histamine can be expected to relieve an attack of hay fever, the antihistamine drugs are actually too dangerous to be used regularly by a sensible person.

Vitamin E: A Natural Antihistamine?

Vitamin E may be a better answer, at least for some. A Japanese researcher, Dr. Mitsuo Kamimura of the Department of Dermatology at the Sapporo Medical College in Japan, believes that vitamin E has effective antihistamine properties which might help hay fever sufferers through their misery, while avoiding the torpor, raised blood pressure, and other side effects that render pharmaceutical antihistamines undesirable (*Journal of Vitaminology*; 18, 204-209, 1972).

Dr. Kamimura decided to investigate the anti-allergic potency of vitamin E in his own tests for two reasons that make good sense. One, several other Japanese researchers reported significant results using vitamin E. And two, he pointed out that: "It is a well-known fact that vitamin E is often effective in the treatment of various inflammatory skin diseases."

In his own work, Dr. Kamimura used both animals and humans. In every test carried out, *vitamin E suppressed symptoms of allergy* and the kind of fluid accumulation that characterizes an allergic reaction.

First, the animal studies: Dr. Kamimura injected a group of rats with a chemical (dextran) to produce typically allergic swelling and puffiness such as occur around the eyes and nasal passages of the hay fever sufferer. Some of the animals were then immediately injected with 20 I.U. of alpha tocopherol (vitamin E), some with just 10 I.U., and some with only sesame oil, to serve as controls. Twenty-four hours later, the animals that had received no vitamin E developed "severe" edema, or swelling. Those which had been given the smaller dose of vitamin E developed much less swelling, while those receiving 20 I. U. of vitamin E developed no swelling whatsoever!

The dermatologist also tried painting the shaved backs of rabbits with an irritating chemical. On some areas of the skin, Dr. Kamimura also applied either vitamin E ointment or sesame oil ointment, along with the irritant.

Although in this case the vitamin E was applied topically instead of by injection, the results were similar. It was apparent that in the areas treated with alpha tocopherol ointment, "the inflammation was suppressed and the duration of lesion was shortened." The total area of inflammation was only about one-third of that which occurred when no vitamin E was applied, and the degree of hemorrhage and wound infiltration was much less.

What about human beings? The Japanese researcher injected a group of people with histamine, the substance which when released in the body in reaction to an allergen is directly responsible for the swelling and puffiness associated with allergic reactions. Some of the subjects had long suffered from chronic hives (an allergic skin condition), while the others had not.

After taking 300 I. U. of oral vitamin E a day for five to seven days, the allergic reactions in those not susceptible to hives decreased by 37 percent, while in those who were very susceptible, the area of the reaction was reduced by up to 33 percent.

In another test, Dr. Kamimura applied preparations containing irritating plaster to various portions of the backs of 100 people. In some areas, only the irritants were used. Other areas contained, in addition to the irritants, either vitamin E or a substance known as glycyrrhetinic acid, which Dr. Kamimura says is "claimed to have antihistaminic action." The results were that without either ointment 37 persons developed either redness or itching. With the glycyrrhetinic acid, 23 persons developed symptoms. But with vitamin E, only 19 developed symptoms.

Dr. Kamimura, who has been studying vitamin E for a number

of years, admits that he is not certain exactly how vitamin E works to reduce inflammation. But it works. He believes it does so in *two* ways: first, by decreasing the permeability of capillaries, which would prevent the accumulation of fluid outside blood vessels, and second, by directly suppressing the release of histamine. Although vitamin E is not usually recognized as possessing antihistamine activity, Dr. Kamimura feels confident that it does, and points out that this is consistent with his finding that vitamin E is more effective if given *before* irritation than when administered after the fact.

Food Allergy And Vitamin E

In an indirect way, vitamin E also plays a role in allergic reactions to food that affect children, particularly, much as hay fever does. Such reactions are often misdiagnosed as hay fever, according to Howard Rapaport, M.D. and Shirley M. Linde in their book, *The Complete Allergy Guide* (Simon and Schuster, 1970).

They report that Dr. Joseph H. Fries, a pediatrician at the State University of New York Downstate Medical Center, believes the evidence is strong to show that chocolate candy is a major cause of allergy, especially in children. And the effects of chocolate can intensify the effects of other allergies already present. As little as half a chocolate bar can set off an acute attack of wheezing, sneezing, skin rashes and abdominal upset in children with allergy to other substances.

Dr. Fries says that many children are slightly sensitive to chocolate, and do not always have clinical reactions to it. But if chocolate is taken, for example, during some other particularly sensitive period such as the pollen season, there is a reaction.

Other children have very severe reactions to chocolate. In tests of children from age three upwards, one-half to three chocolate bars caused symptoms that varied from rashes and hives to itching, redness around the mouth, weeping lesions, clogged-up noses, sneezing, coughing, wheezing, abdominal pains or vomiting. When chocolate was taken away, the symptoms were dramatically reduced.

Rapaport and Linde warn that if your child craves chocolate, you would be better off giving him vitamin E. Removing chocolate and replacing it with vitamin E will not only eliminate allergies arising from chocolate, but may also help reduce the severity of hay fever or any other allergies the child may be suffering from.

Hay Fever

Remember that vitamin E has been shown to have a natural antihistamine effect. It will not make you tired or sleepy. It will not dry up your mucous membranes. It will not do you any harm at all, in fact. But it may help your hay fever symptoms. Those who suffer from the allergy know what such help can mean.

171. Vitamin C Eases Breathing In Allergy Season

Early in 1974, a doctor from the Yale University Lung Research Center in New Haven, Connecticut, published a brief medical report that offers new hope of relief to the millions of Americans who suffer in the throes of annual hay fever attacks.

Dr. Arend Bouhuys wrote a short letter to the *New England Journal of Medicine* (March 14, 1974) in which he suggested that the well-known beneficial effects of vitamin C in respiratory disease might be linked to its natural antihistamine properties.

Dr. Bouhuys referred to a very carefully controlled study by Dr. John L. Coulehan and others which had earlier been published in the same medical journal. This study showed that school children taking one or two grams a day of vitamin C didn't have any fewer colds, but the actual number of days in which they had symptoms were reduced by nearly one-third. The children receiving vitamin C also did less coughing and sniffling than other children. From this and other studies, many people have concluded that vitamin C helps protect the body against invading viruses. But Dr. Bouhuys suggests that this may not be the whole story.

He puts it this way: "If histamine plays a part in promoting mucosal inflammation in acute respiratory illness, the antihistamine action of vitamin C might explain, in part, the reduced symptoms and duration of these illnesses."

But where did Dr. Bouhuys get the idea that vitamin C has "an antihistamine action"?

The answer is simple: he proved it in his own experiments. Along with colleagues Eugenija Zuskin, M. D., and Alan J. Lewis, Ph.D., he published the results of these trials in the *Journal of Allergy and Clinical Immunology* (April, 1973).

Breathing Easier With Vitamin C

In the first set of experiments, 17 healthy people inhaled identical histamine mixtures. Histamine is a substance which reacts dramatically with the walls of the capillaries, making them more permeable and allowing more waste material from the blood to enter the cells. This, in large part, causes that uncomfortable swelling in the nose and around the eyes which is associated with hay fever. Although the release of histamine by the body in response to an allergen is thought to be a protective reaction, in the case of sensitized individuals the reaction is so exaggerated that breathing can become sheer torture. Statistics tell us that all too many people know exactly what this feeling is, and how terrifying it can be.

After the histamine was taken by the 17 subjects, the doctors measured their breathing ability immediately afterwards, then at three hours, and finally at six hours. Later, they measured breathing ability at each of these times after the subjects had been given either 500 mg. of vitamin C, a placebo, or nothing at all.

They discovered a "significant" increase in the ease of breathing after the subjects received vitamin C. They said that a "single oral dose of 500 mg. of ascorbic acid (vitamin C) inhibits the constrictor effect on airways of human subjects." The beneficial effects lasted for up to six hours, they added.

The doctors point out that large doses of ascorbic acid are excreted for the most part in about four to five hours. To maintain the antihistamine effect, they speculated that it might be a good idea to give smaller doses—they mention 250 mg.—at three-hour intervals throughout the day.

They emphasize, though, that the doses of histamine that the research subjects received were relatively mild: "We have not investigated the action of ascorbic acid against more severe degrees of histamine-induced airway constriction."

Vitamin C Better Than Drugs

The same year that saw publication of this fascinating study from Yale also brought another clinical study published in the *British Journal of Industrial Medicine* (30; 1973). This study, by Drs. F. Valic and E. Zuskin, of Zagreb University in Yugoslavia, showed that supplemental vitamin C is of great benefit to people who must work in environments polluted with dust.

Twenty female textile workers were the subjects. As a result of chronically breathing large quantities of flax, 13 of the women were diagnosed as byssinotic, meaning that their lungs and breathing function had been adversely affected over the years from the constant breathing of dust. The other seven were considered non-byssinotic.

The object of the study was to determine which would help these women most—vitamin C, a chemical antihistamine, or a bronchodilator. Traditionally, the workers showed a significant decrease in breathing efficiency as exposure to their polluted environment continued through the week. To evaluate the comparative effect of the different medications and the ascorbic acid on the loss of breathing ability, the study was conducted on four consecutive Mondays.

The first week, their breathing capacity was measured without any treatment at all. On the following Monday, orciprenaline, a bronchodilator, was administered by inhalation before the work-shift. On the third Monday, the women were given an antihistamine orally before they started work. Finally, on the fourth Monday, one tablet of a placebo was given prior to work and then, beginning the following day and continuing through the remainder of the week, 500 mg. of ascorbic acid were given daily, including the following Monday before the shift began.

Everyone who received some form of medication or the vitamin C showed a better rate of breathing when tested. In addition, those who suffered from byssinosis were helped more than those who did not. But when the doctors looked closer at how the women responded to each treatment, it became clear that vitamin C had won the contest hands down.

After taking the antihistamine or bronchodilator treatment, eight of the byssinotic workers said they felt better, with less difficulty in breathing and less tightness of the chest. But after vitamin C, 12 of the women reported that they felt much better. The vitamin C was 50 percent more effective.

Of the seven workers who did not have byssinosis, none felt better after the placebo, three felt better after the antihistamine, and four felt better after either ascorbic acid or the bronchodilator. It seems, then, that those who need help the most get the most help from vitamin C, while those who aren't so bad off get as much help from vitamin C as they do from medication.

The authors note that the mechanism of the preventive effect of ascorbic acid is not quite clear. Previous studies in textile workers showed that the reduced lung capacity resulted from the bronchial constricting action of histamine and/or some other active substances. However, other factors such as swelling of the mucous membrane or other changes narrowing the respiratory airways may play an additional role, they speculated.

It has also been reported that ascorbic acid decreases the

permeability of small blood vessels. It is possible that ascorbic acid, by decreasing capillary permeability (opposing the effect of histamine), prevents edema or fluid formation and consequent narrowing of the bronchial tubes. The researchers suggest that more study is needed to clarify the exact mechanisms of the working of ascorbic acid. However, the only question is *how* it works—they are positive that it *does* work.

More Vitamin C, Less Suffering

In fact, the discovery that vitamin C is effective in alleviating allergy symptoms is not really new. As long ago as 1942, for example, H. W. Holmes, M.D., wrote in *Science* (96, 1942) that he gave 200 to 500 mg. of vitamin C every day for a week to his patients and succeeded in relieving not only the hay fever and asthma, but food allergies as well.

A quarter of a century later, the *Eye, Ear, Nose and Throat Monthly* (July, 1968) described results of a study that measured ascorbic acid levels in the plasma and urine during the active stages of allergy. It was found that vitamin C values were considerably lower than normal, indicating the unsaturated state of the tissues. According to this medical journal: *Heavy medication with vitamin C produced a rise in the blood and urinary ascorbic acid levels which coincided with the subjective and objective improvement of the allergic disorder"* (emphasis ours).

Success in medical studies done on large groups means that the majority of the people are helped. Whether or not the treatment is going to work—or to what extent—in the case of any particular person is more difficult to predict. In a letter, Mrs. Susan Thyer McCormick of Toronto, Canada, describes her personal experience with taking vitamin C for hay fever.

After a visit to her allergist, she discovered that she was allergic to almost every plant, including trees, grass, and ragweed—even common dust.

"So I started taking shots—every week I would have three needles in one arm, and every week my arm would be swollen and painful for at least four days afterwards." But, she says, she had "good results" with the treatment so she continued it.

"However," she wrote, "after a while, the shots themselves began to bother me so much I began to start missing treatments, because always one of my arms was hot, swollen and red due to the severe reaction of the allergens I was receiving."

'Prayed For The First Frost'

So she gave up the shots altogether and hoped she would get better. She was wrong. The next summer she suffered with hay fever "worse than ever, and prayed for the first frost that would kill the miserable ragweed."

After reading of earlier studies that showed the benefits of vitamin C in allergy and respiratory cases, she began to take 1,000 mg. of vitamin C or more every day, "just to see what would happen."

The outcome? "I am happy to say that now hay fever season is half over, and I have only sneezed a few times! I'm not completely cured. I know that. But the relief is so great, especially when I remember the misery I went through before, both with the allergy itself and then those painful shots."

She added this P.S.: "Vitamins are a *lot cheaper* than allergy drugs!"

If every hay fever sufferer could be helped to the extent that Mrs. McCormick was, it would be wonderful. But that would probably be too much to hope for. No one can say exactly what the chances are that you will be helped, if you have an allergy, but all the evidence we've seen indicates that vitamin C is certainly worth trying.

Keep in mind that, as the Yale physicians suggest, it is better to take vitamin C every three or four hours throughout the day, rather than all at once. This translates to a total of about 1,000 mg. to 1,500 mg. a day during the allergy season. This much vitamin C is perfectly safe, the Yale doctors say. It can only do you good.

172. The Honey Treatment For Hay Fever

From time to time there have been reported seemingly miraculous cures of hay fever in connection with honey. Usually a particular kind of honey that is unstrained and rich with pollen is mentioned. When people have speculated on why such honey should restore the defenses of chronic hay fever sufferers, the results have always been attributed to the pollen that the honey contains.

There is one big question that must immediately arise in the minds of many readers. Isn't pollen the stuff that causes hay fever and won't eating it cause an allergic reaction, especially if it is the type of pollen to which a person is already sensitive?

Apparently not.

One resident of Tucson, Arizona, after 16 years of suffering, was freed of hay fever after taking honey for a few weeks. Another Tucson resident reported his lifelong hay fever finally disappeared when he began eating honey at the age of 70.

An article by Wayne Amos ("The Honey Hassle," *Arizona Days and Ways Magazine,* July 3, 1966) reported that many people in Tucson are being relieved of sneezes, itches, and swelling of the eyes and nose by taking merely one or two teaspoons of honey.

There is a limitation, however. The honey must be locally made by bees in the areas near where the hay fever is occurring. Before we can examine these "cures," we must see what causes thousands of people to suffer embarrassing runny noses in late summer and early fall.

Hay fever is an allergy. We inherit the tendency to develop an allergy, but not the allergy itself. In hay fever, the irritant is usually pollen from ragweed, although tree and grass pollen can affect some people all year. Pollen is the yellow powdery dust we see in great concentrations on flowers. The pollen grains stick to the furry legs of bees collecting nectar. Carried back to the hive, pollen becomes mixed with honey, usually accumulating at the bottom, where dark residues called honey-scraps fall. Ironically, "pure" honey is devoid of the valuable honey scraps.

Honey is a natural sugar, used as a food and flavoring, a food preservative, a mild laxative and sedative, an antiseptic, and a quick source of energy. Easy to digest, it is the only unrefined sweetener available commercially. Honey contains some vitamins (B complex, C, E, K) and minerals (calcium, magnesium, iron and others). If filtered and heated to 150 degrees, honey loses its cloudy appearance and becomes clear because certain elements, including pollen, have been removed.

Immune Mechanism Stimulated
Interestingly enough, the people of Arizona ate honey that was neither too finely filtered nor heated above 140 degrees. Such honey still retains its pollen. What becomes difficult for many to comprehend is why people would eat substances to which they are known to be allergic. The concept behind such a seemingly harmful act is that by putting some amounts of the irritants into the body, one induces the system to build defense or immunities against the foreign substance. Thus, honey, with its bits of pollen, is thought to build up immunity to hay fever and to relieve victims of the symptoms.

Although literature on allergies in general is relatively abundant, the question of honey as a cure for hay fever is almost ignored. Some information comes from D. S. Jarvis, M.D., author of the popular book, *Folk Medicine*. He writes, "If honey comb cappings (which, again, are rich in pollen) are chewed once each day for one month before the expected hay fever date, the hay fever will either not appear or will be mild in character." In *The American Bee Journal* (December, 1950) he mentions the value of propolis, or bee glue, a constituent of comb honey. It is supposed to have "a special action on the breathing tract . . . It opens the nose, produces a drying effect . . . lessens catarrhal discharge and . . . cough. It is for this . . . effect and the sedative effect on the body as a whole that comb honey with its propolis is used."

P. M. Winter, Ph.D., of Kingston, Pa. considers "honey to be the best cure." Replacing sugar with honey, he found that the first year his hay fever declined and was not serious, and in the succeeding years, the hay fever left him completely.

Some doctors take a dim view of this remedy. In "The Honey Hassle" Mr. Amos summarizes in his own words the attitude of

Hay Fever

Arizona doctors who label the whole idea as nonsense: "It is a specific protein in the pollen that sensitive people are allergic to and once this protein hits the acids in the stomach and certain enzymes in the upper intestine . . . it is no longer the same protein. Thus . . . the eating of honey cannot relieve hay fever symptoms." Doctors say the pollens must be injected, not swallowed. They see the "miracle cures" as faith healings.

Impossible—But It Works

Yet, an increasing number of people in Tucson disregard the medical argument, take local honey, and find themselves considerably relieved of symptoms. Many residents are putting their own bee colonies in their backyards to make sure they can obtain local honey containing the precise pollen to which they are sensitive. The question remains: do the curative powers of pollen have validity? Handicapped by limited information, we can only speculate about why pollen might help.

The strongest possibility, we would guess, is that some of the pollen protein does not go through the digestive process but is assimilated unchanged into the bloodstream. This is likely in view of the sheer toughness of the membrane enclosing each pollen grain. It is the membrane alone that protects the pollen and keeps it alive for weeks or months until the pollen comes into contact with a flower stamen and begins its development into a seed. Grains of pollen have been known to survive snow, rain, wind and sunshine for decades, protected only by their thin but hardy membranes.

The membranes will succumb to digestive acids and enzymes, but perhaps they are sufficiently resistant so that in any given amount of pollen swallowed, a portion of the grains will remain unaltered as the absorptive processes go on.

In conventional treatments for allergies, the patient is told to avoid the irritant altogether, take drugs, or go to the doctor for injections containing small amounts of the offending allergen to build up immunities. Taking a trip across country is often inconvenient; drugs can have bad side-effects; and even injections, the major form of therapy, have not always proved effective.

Shots Might Also Be Called "Faith Healing"

Results from allergy tests, supervised by Dr. L. Emmett Holt, showed that both ragweed and placebo substitute injections affected 68 children similarly. The conclusions, revealed at a meeting of the American Pediatric Society, (June, 1955), were that "by and large the comparison between placebo and ragweed therapy failed to show any difference . . ." For as many people helped by shots, just as many are not helped.

Presently, there is not enough evidence to prove that either pollen or honey actually cures and prevents hay fever. If you are suffering from this allergy, and your doctor has not been able to help you after testing and treatment, you might want to try small amounts of unclarified honey, made nearby where the offending pollens are. Or, if your doctor has succeeded in isolating the precise pollen to which you are allergic, ask your doctor if under his supervision you can try taking by mouth small amounts every day of the allergenic material. He will probably laugh at the idea. The fundamental fact of allergy seems to be that it is stirred up by the body's recognition of a foreign protein and production of antibodies to fight it. And there is no doubt that proteins taken by mouth, including the protein of pollen grains, will largely be broken down into their constituent amino acids before they are assimilated into the bloodstream. No amino acids are in themselves foreign to the human body. It is only a strange molecular arrangement of them that the body recognizes as an enemy. So the amino acids, in theory, should have no more effect on the system than the amino acids from eggs or a T-bone steak.

We cannot dispute the theory nor are we in any position to say that the pollen is going to help your condition. However, hay fever is a nasty and sometimes unbearable affliction. Your doctor will be happy to give you injections of the same pollen with no assurance whatsoever that they are going to improve your reactions. He certainly ought to be willing to let you experiment with another way of attempting to desensitize yourself.

Section 35
Headache

173. What Is A Headache?

At least two million headaches are in progress at any given moment in the United States alone, and probably many more if we include the twelve million migraine sufferers, some of whom might be going through some phase of an attack. Some headaches are as excruciatingly painful as a difficult childbirth without anesthetics and some are no more than pounding reminders that a body cannot take too many cocktail parties. For their headaches Americans combine to swallow a total of more than 500 pills for head pain relief *every second*. Clearly, we are willing to spend many more millions to dull pain than we are to eliminate its causes.

The brain can interpret pain from other parts of the body, but is totally incapable of feeling pain itself. So the ache of a headache results not from pain directly involving the inner cerebral matter but from pain affecting the highly sensitive nerve filaments (or nerve plexus) within the arteries supplying blood to the brain. These fibers are found in the membranes comprising the inner and outer covering of the brain and are extremely sensitive to any stretch movement.

Headaches may be clinical symptoms of other medical problems such as eyestrain, glaucoma, sinus condition or brain tumor. But the overwhelming number of headaches fall into two categories: (1) tension headaches which result from an involuntary contraction of muscles on the neck, scalp and forehead in response to stress-provoking situations; and (2) arterial or vascular headaches which result when the large and small blood vessels in the membrane covering of the brain are unable to dilate at uniform rates. This latter group includes the infamous migraine. In headaches of a vascular character, as some vessels become larger, the velocity of the blood passing through the smaller vessels is increased as well, causing painful displacement and dilation of the smaller vessels as they stretch to accommodate the increased arterial flow. As the entire artery undergoes this general distension, the pain of headache is registered by the nerve cells.

174. Tension Headaches Explained—Some Do-It-Yourself Techniques For Relief

What do you do when you or someone in your family suffers a severe throbbing tension headache? Do you throw up your hands in distress and resort to pain-killing drugs such as aspirin?

It is now well known that repeated use of aspirin can cause gastric bleeding which could lead to anemia or ulcers. In some cases aspirin ingestion may even cause headache. But most of us know less about the way our bodies work or what causes our pounding headaches than we do about the mechanics of our cars, lawn mowers and washing machines. And when we are hit by a blinding headache, we feel utterly useless and, in desperation, either take a couple of aspirin or, fearing the worst, make an appointment with the doctor, ophthalmologist, dentist, neurologist, or psychiatrist. If the headache is painful and persistent, it would, of course, be wise to keep that appointment.

But medical researchers seeking an understanding of the basic ailments that may hide behind headache have found that in 90 percent of all cases, headaches are *not* connected with brain tumors, brain infections, hardening of the cerebral arteries, trouble in the eyes, sinuses, ears, teeth or even the frequently-blamed stomach upset.

"Nine times out of ten," said Dr. Arnold P. Friedman, chief of the headache unit at New York's Montefiore Hospital, "headaches are totally unrelated to any specific organic disease condition. Most are tension headaches—a mild form of torture that almost everyone is familiar with. They are triggered usually by emotional tension or occupational situations in which the head or neck have been held in an awkward or fixed position for long periods of time such as driving in the rain at night" (*Business Week*, June 20, 1964).

"Why some people react to stress with their muscles (tension headache) while others get ulcers, skin troubles, or asthma and a favored few escape any such symptoms, is a mystery," Dr. Friedman said.

Seventy-five percent of the people suffering from tension headaches are women, according to Dr. James W. Lance in his book, *HEADACHE: Alleviation and Understanding* (Charles Scribner's Sons, 1975). "Why women should be more susceptible to tension headache than men remains a mystery. Women traditionally have shown their feelings more than men, but their emotional tone fluctuates more widely and they are generally more sensitive to minor frustrations or disappointments." Dr. Lance suggests that this may be due to the variances of hormonal changes in the menstrual cycle, because women also comprise 75 percent of migraine sufferers and it has been shown that their migraine, which is vascular in nature, can be influenced by their hormonal changes. But it is still perplexing, according to Dr. Lance, because, although the statistical correlation is high, there is little evidence yet that tension headaches may be influenced by the same vascular reactivity.

However there are ways of relieving the pain of tension headaches that are no mystery.

A Doctor's Prescription For Tension Headaches

Several do-it-yourself techniques for relieving a tension headache are described in detail in *A Chiropractor's Treasury of Health Secrets*, by Samuel Hamola, D.C. (Parker Publishing Co., 1970).

Dr. Hamola's therapies are based on a chiropractor's knowledge of the integrated functions of all systems of the body and on the importance of good nutrition for prevention as well as correction. His tips may help you understand what it is that triggers the headache in the first place. Why, for instance, does a headache usually clobber us when we are anticipating a big event, facing finals, a Cub Scout picnic, or a deadline?

According to Dr. Friedman, you brought it on yourself. Because you were operating under pressure, you became tense and contracted the muscles on the back of your neck.

A Pain In The Neck

There is a relationship between emotion, neck muscles and cranial blood vessels. Such common remarks as "He gives me a pain in the neck" are more than figures of speech. They are literally medical truths in the case of tension headaches.

"Little is known," Dr. Hamola reports, "about how tight neck muscles actually cause a headache, but we do know that the pain usually stems from reflex dilatation (expansion) of the blood vessels around the brain. This causes a throbbing pain that pounds in rhythm with the heart beat."

While brain tissue itself feels no pain, the walls of the blood vessels near the brain have many sensitive pain fibers. When these vessels dilate and stretch the vessel walls, each beat of the heart transmits an acute hammer-like pain to the head.

Most tension headaches, Dr. Hamola points out, can be relieved with such simple remedies as moist heat, cold packs, massage or traction. Whenever a muscle becomes too tight from nervous tension, some of its fibers contract. This kind of involuntary contraction can usually be relieved by placing pressure on the muscle or by stretching the fibers which have shortened. There are several procedures by which you can apply traction to the muscles of your neck and nip that tension before it goes to your head. For instance, you can apply traction with your hands whenever you feel the need of a stretch.

Place both hands on the back of your neck with fingertips overlapping. Then let your head fall back. Your hands will act as a wedge to pry your neck vertebrae apart while the base of your skull is resting on the edge of your hands. Try this exercise whenever possible. It's particularly effective if done when you're leaning back in a reclining chair. This effect is heightened by the pull of gravity.

After you have tilted your head backward, drop it forward and stretch the muscles on the back of your neck by pressing the base of your skull forward and upward with your fingertips.

If you work over a desk, typewriter, a sewing machine or in any occupation that necessitates a downward tilt of your head for long hours, you should straighten up and drop your head back several times each day. This reverse bend will serve two purposes. First, when the neck muscles are forced to remain contracted for a long period of time, there is an accumulation of lactic acid and other waste products which irritate the muscles and cause inflammation and spasm. Second, there is a danger of reversing the normal curve of the spine in the neck region. Once this happens, the muscles of the neck must work even harder to hold the head up. This can give you a pain in the neck as well as a headache.

A stronger form of traction can be applied by using the partner method—"You stretch my neck and I'll stretch yours." For partner traction, you sit erect on the edge of a low stool, or "side saddle" in a straight chair. Your partner stands behind you with his foot on the edge of the chair seat. He cups his hands around the base of your skull and jaws, his right elbow supported by his right knee and simply raises the heel of the foot that's on the stool. His wrists should be held rigid so that movement of the supporting knee will lift your head. By raising his heel and then lowering it he can apply "intermittent traction" which will relieve neck tension by alternately stretching and releasing the neck muscles.

Heat And Massage

As soon as you feel the slightest tension building up in the muscles of your neck or shoulders, you can head off bigger troubles if you apply moist heat right away. Try standing under a shower and letting a thick stream of hot water ripple over your neck and shoulders. If this is inconvenient, try wringing out a towel in hot water and drape it over the back of your neck. An infra-red heat lamp or an insulated heating pad will help to keep the towel nice and hot.

Massage is another technique that can help relieve tightness and soreness. Every household should have at least one member skilled in the art of giving a pain-relieving massage. Dr. Hamola's detailed instructions provide an excellent guide. Try this method on a friend, then let him return the favor. Seat your friend on a low stool or chair. Now place your left hand (if you're right handed) on his forehead and encourage him to let his head rest against your hand so that the muscles on the back of his neck will be completely relaxed. Now circle the back of his neck with the thumb and forefinger of your other hand. Massage his neck by moving your hand in a circular motion making sure to press the hand firmly against the neck so that it stays in contact with the skin and does not ride over the muscles.

Other Headache Treatments

If, after trying these measures you still have a headache, you may obtain relief from an ice pack. Your headache may be due to dilated blood vessels around the brain. A cold pack may relieve the symptoms because cold will constrict the swollen vessels. Try the ice pack on your forehead or on the top of your head, or place it on the front of your neck like a turtleneck collar for several minutes.

Sometimes a cold foot bath will relieve a headache. But, if your headache is caused by a cold or congestion, take a hot foot bath while you keep an ice bag on your head.

Remember that impure air can cause a headache. Excessive carbon monoxide in the air can invade your bloodstream and deprive your brain of oxygen. Keep a few growing plants in your home. They convert carbon dioxide to oxygen.

Use a thin feather pillow under your head, Dr. Hamola suggests, but fluff up the bottom edge so that it will fit into the hollow of your neck. This will relieve strain on the joints and ligaments and permit you to relax. Avoid the use of foam rubber pillows which do not offer enough support and cause excessive neck tension and headaches.

Low Blood Sugar

Another frequent cause of headache is low blood sugar. Your brain cannot function without glucose. When there is insufficient sugar in your blood, the resulting condition is similar to that of oxygen starvation. To meet the demands of the brain more blood is needed; hence, the blood goes pounding through your head at a faster clip and the result is a throbbing headache. Also, if you are excited or nervous or under pressure, your adrenal glands go into high gear and consume sugar at a faster rate, thus further depriving your blood of the sugar and causing headache discomfort.

If you get hungry between meals and develop a headache, try a snack of fresh fruit or protein-rich food like nuts or sunflower seeds to boost your energy stores. Because the end result of eating sugar is a depletion of sugar in your blood, persons who are constantly eating candy for "energy" may feel more tired and headachy at the end of the day than those who eat nothing at all between meals.

Eat and live in such a way as to keep a normal blood sugar level and you should be able to solve your low blood sugar problems. The first step would be a good high-protein breakfast.

If you have a chronic headache that does not respond to improved nutrition and self-help techniques, then you should certainly seek medical investigation of the underlying cause.

Temporal Arteritis: A Headache Warning To Senior Citizens

One type of headache that medical science now knows how to deal with, fortunately, is *temporal arteritis*. This disease attacks older people almost exclusively, causing excruciating headache pain and if not treated, often blindness. Dr. Bayard Horton, who discovered the disease, urges doctors to "think first, not last, of *temporal arteritis* in diagnosing the cause of headache in senior citizens."

Early diagnosis of the disease assures treatment before permanent blindness strikes. Sight does not come back once lost. "It is my impression," says Dr. Horton, "that *temporal arteritis* frequently goes unrecognized and that there are hundreds of older people in America today who could have had their vision preserved if the medical profession had been alerted and educated in this special field." Two telltale signs of *temporal arteritis* are pain when chewing and a marked bulging of the temporal artery in front of and above the ear.

175. Migraine Misery: There May Be A Way Out For You

Of the headaches which are vascular in character, none is more aggravating than the sinister migraine, or *Hemicrania*. The incessant throbbing pain, which usually affects only one side of the brain, may be accompanied by any or all of these disturbing symptoms: vomiting; nausea; altered hearing and visual distortions, such as light flashes or dark spots; speech difficulties; and a general clamminess of the skin. If the pounding pain is accompanied by these symptoms, it is known as "classic" migraine; if not, then it is known as "nonclassic."

The unique feature of "classic" migraine, according to Dr. James W. Lance, is that the "large arteries and veins dilate while the network of smaller vessels, which normally carry the blood from the arteries to the veins, is shut off by constriction (so that blood bypasses areas of the cerebral cortex). The cells, deprived of their normal blood supply, first become excited so that the person sees stars, flashes or zigzags of light or feels other extraordinary sensations." After this reaction, and as the nerve cells become inactive, the "classic" migraine sufferer has visual and speech problems, partial paralysis on one side of the body, and enlarged pulsating veins on the outside of the skull which become clearly visible beneath the scalp, according to Dr. Lance.

Migraine is known to run in families and is considered by many researchers to be genetic in origin. If you are one of the many Americans periodically coping with migraine headaches and the accompanying symptoms, you are in exalted company. It may not ease the pain of the white hot spikes that pierce your skull, but it might comfort you a little to know that the same kind of pain afflicted Sigmund Freud, Ulysses S. Grant, Thomas Jefferson, Napoleon, musicians Frederic Chopin and Peter Tchaikovsky, writers Heinrich Heine, Leo Tolstoy and Lewis Carroll, whose Alice in Wonderland expresses some of the distortions in size and perception that migraine sufferers know so well. Anyone who periodically faces the prospect of uninvited imps pounding in his head should have some understanding of what it is that invites these imps in the first place. Is it allergy to specific foods, odors, or inhalants? Or is it a vitamin deficiency? There is evidence that all of these phenomena are involved.

The Nutritional Aspects Of Migraine Headaches

In a study published in the *Archives of Otolaryngology* (Vol. 75, p. 220, 1962), Dr. Miles Atkinson, an otologist who was at the time of the study on the faculty of New York University, considered migraine and its accompanying problems a matter of nutrition, ruling out the possibility that it could in some way be psychosomatic in origin. He postulated that vasoplasms (spasms of a blood vessel) produced the visual disturbances and other symptoms of the syndrome while it was vasodilation (dilation or stretching of the blood vessels) which produced the major symptom, the intense throbbing headache.

Dr. Atkinson believed that B complex vitamins, especially B_3, were essential to the maintenance of normal vasodilation. In fact, he often noted a severe vitamin B deficiency in his patients suffering from migraine. However, he did not blame migraines on a lack of B vitamins in the average American diet but rather on the internal factors which inhibit utilization of the vitamins. "What about absorption? This may be interfered with by gastrointestinal disease, for example, and by many drugs. Of the drugs, antibiotics are at the present time the most significant offenders because of their widespread use . . . Always when antibiotics are given," Dr. Atkinson warned, "vitamins should be given at the same time. How often is this done?"

Some doctors now recognize the necessity for reestablishing the colonies of bacteria (demolished by antibiotics) which help your body to manufacture the B vitamins. When Dr. Eric Ask-Upmark, a distinguished Swedish surgeon, prescribed a preparation containing lactobacillus acidophilus, he found that not only did his female patient's intestinal condition greatly improve, but, unexpectedly, her migraine disappeared almost completely (*The Lancet*, August 20, 1966). Dr. Ask-Upmark tried the same treatment on 10 migraine patients who had failed to respond to the ordinary regimen and he reported that there was substantial improvement in eight patients—who incidentally had some degree of gastrointestinal disturbance.

Some migraine sufferers may find relief by replenishing their intestinal flora through the addition of yogurt or buttermilk to their diets—a simple expedient well worth trying. Others may not. Each one of us has a different metabolism. Some of us do not manufacture any B vitamins in the intestine. Those with liver disease do not utilize or store vitamins sufficiently. This suggests something more than inadequate dietary intake such as a defect in the utilization of the B vitamins, due perhaps to a metabolic fault. Dr. Atkinson did not overlook the fact that there are other possible causes for this neurovascular dysfunction. He suggested that allergy, eyestrain, alcohol, tobacco, stress and emotional strain are factors which serve as triggers in particular cases.

While such factors may trigger an attack for certain individuals, they provide no explanation of the basic cause of the neurovascular instability which is the crux of the matter. The acid test is, does the theory work in practice? Does the administration of vitamins overcome the deficiency which is assumed to be responsible for the dysfunction and, consequently, does it abolish the attacks?

Vitamin Therapy For Other Causes

The answer, according to Dr. Atkinson, was a resounding "Yes." One patient treated by Dr. Atkinson had suffered severe migraine headaches since girlhood and at the age of 45 was almost bedridden. She suffered constant headache, and all sorts of accessory symptoms. Neither ergot (a drug derived from fungus growth) nor any other drug was of avail. It took two years of vitamin therapy to show any improvement and even at that time she was far from recovered. "That was 15 years ago," Dr. Atkinson recalled. "Today she is a fit and energetic person even though she still has a very occasional mild migraine, insufficient to put her to bed. Presumably some irreversible damage has taken place, but she regards herself as cured."

Another of Dr. Atkinson's patients was a lab technician of 35 who had to support her mother and feared she would have to give up her job because of the severity of her migraine attacks. "Again, ergot had ceased to help and," the doctor said, "was producing side effects—so usual a story. When finally she persuaded someone to give her the vitamin injections, for she lived too far away to come to see me, there was profound skepticism in the hospital where she worked. In six months her headaches were under control and it was only with great difficulty that she could be persuaded to stop injections. In 12 months, she was a new woman."

Dr. Atkinson's therapy included both injection and oral administration, in order to gain control as rapidly as possible. Injections, he points out, must be intravenous because the solutions used in the dosage necessary are painful if given intramuscularly or subcutaneously. Injections are given daily for the first one or two weeks, then three times weekly until a large measure of control has been established, usually as many as 100 injections may be necessary in migraine. Oral therapy is given together with injections, again to the maximum dose compatible with response and tolerance. This is continued thereafter for several years.

Diet Is Important

What about diet? "It would be illogical to treat a condition along nutritional lines and not give attention to eating habits," Dr. Atkinson said. "Investigation of such habits will also produce surprising results, as people who can well afford a good diet might be expected to know one but are often the worst delinquents. Perhaps the two most common faults are inadequate breakfasts and an excess, often a gross excess, of carbohydrates. Diets should be high protein, low fat, medium carbohydrate and consideration should be paid to the possibility of allergenic foods such as chocolate and cheese as etiological factors in migraine."

It has been known for centuries that certain foods caused headaches in some people. Long before the phenomenon of allergy was discovered, it was known that milk was likely to cause headache. Burton, writing in the 17th century, quoted Pythagoras as saying that members of the pea family would also cause headache. Both milk and the pea family are now recognized as common offenders.

Even though the official position of many doctors, including the National Migraine Foundation, is that diet plays only a minor role in headache problems, many physicians expressed concern about certain foods as a causal factor in the onset of migraine at a conference of the American Association for the Study of Headache and the National Migraine Foundation in June, 1974. "I don't like to push the diet-migraine connection very far," said Dr. Seymour Diamond, a past president of the Foundation, "but some foods do seem to initiate migraine attacks in some patients."

Chocolate, red wine, aged cheese and citrus fruit head the list of foods that dietary migraine sufferers think precipitate their attacks. Some researchers have theorized that certain enzymes which influence the body's metabolic processes may be the culprits, and for a number of years tyramine, one of these substances, was thought to be public enemy number one. However, the problem is that chocolate contains little or no tyramine. What's more, Robert Ryan, M.D., St. Louis, conducted tests which seemed to show that dietary migraine sufferers reacted with a headache more often when they *thought* they were getting tyramine than when they were actually getting it! At any rate, if you have headaches that you've tried "every way to get rid of" it won't hurt to skip chocolate, alcohol, citrus, and cheese for awhile. Allergists might add wheat products, onions, pork, fried fatty food, and seafood, as foods that cause migraine headaches.

Other Causes Of Migraine

Inhalants and even odors can trigger a migraine, too, according to Dr. Seymour Speer of the University of Missouri (*Modern Medicine*, February 8, 1971). Molds and house dust are the most common of the inhalants. Patients allergic to molds usually notice that either nasal symptoms or headache are caused by exposure to musty basements, farm contacts, and grass cuttings. Patients sensitive to house dust may feel worse after housecleaning or during remodeling.

Not many migraine sufferers realize it, but certain odors, too, can start off the cycle which culminates in a blinding migraine. Tobacco smoke is the most common of the odors that may bring on an attack, Dr. Speer reported. Other offenders are perfumes, motor exhausts (especially from buses), smog, paint, paint thinner, aerosols, frying odors, flowers, formaldehyde (present in some stay-press garments), chlorine and ammonia.

Nervous, perfectionist people possess what doctors call a "migraine personality." When one woman who was suffering with a blinding migraine visited her doctor, he said, "You can't possibly have a migraine. Your hair is messy." One of Dr. Speer's patients remarked that she had had only two attacks of migraine in her life. The first was when she got married, and the second was when her daughter got married. Other typical sources of psychic stress which can bring on a migraine are death in the family, disputes with husbands, wives, or children, and a severe scolding by teacher or boss.

A Greater Incidence Of Migraine Among Women

The causal connection between hormonal estrogens and migraine in women has been firmly established. Dr. Lee Kudrow, director of the California Medical Clinic For Headache, reported fresh evidence in support of the connection at the June, 1974 meeting of the National Migraine Foundation.

In his study of 300 patients with migraine headaches, Dr. Kudrow discovered that oral contraceptives and other estrogenic preparations significantly increased headache frequency. And when the hormones were withdrawn, headaches decreased significantly. Dr. Kudrow's research also lends more evidence to the idea that estrogenic hormones can start migraine headaches in women who never had them before.

In an addenda to his study, Dr. Kudrow observed, "It is my impression that in some cases where supplemental or replacement hormones were being given to women, the need for therapy was questionable and, in many cases, the dosage prescribed was greater than necessary. This could be due to the practice of determining estrogen deficiency by vaginal smear examination. Estrogen concentrations adequate for tissue of reproductive organs may be excessive for other tissue, particularly the vascular system." By lowering the dosage, Dr. Kudrow believed the hormonal therapy might be just as effective without causing headaches.

Intelligence Myth Out Of Date

For years, the only consolation sufferers of migraine received for their misery was the satisfaction of thinking that migraine was an affliction of the intelligent. But that is no longer the case, according to Dr. Craig Burrell, a vice president of Sandoz Pharmaceuticals. "Migraine occurs in patients at every level of intelligence, in every ethnic group and in all types of genetic and environmental backgrounds. There's no proof that neurotic and mentally active individuals are more apt to be afflicted with migraine than phlegmatic and dull ones."

Dr. Burrell claims the myth arose because only well-educated and prosperous patients with migraine were coming to the attention of medical practitioners. For a full half century statistics related to migraine were distorted.

Successful Treatment Is Hard Work For Both Patient And Doctor

Oftentimes physicians find it much easier to ameliorate the pain of migraine rather than to get at the core of the problem. In order to accomplish this with as little reliance on dangerous drugs as possible, it will take understanding and diligence by both the patient and doctor.

Successful treatment of the migraine will be no easy matter, according to Dr. Donald J. Dalessio, head of the Division of Neurology, Scripps Clinic and Research Foundation, La Jolla, California. "Patience and perseverence on the part of both physician and patients may be necessary," reported Dr. Dalessio. "The art of medical practice may be more important here than scientific pharmacology. The physician must first remember to do no harm (*primum non nocere*), since headache complications associated with analgesic abuse are always more dangerous than the headaches themselves. Nonetheless, with careful attention to the whole patient, some resolution of the problem can be achieved in the majority of patients who complain of migraine." (*Medical Tribune*, October 16, 1974.)

Migraine Headaches And Acupuncture

At the 1974 World Acupuncture Congress held at the University of Pennsylvania in Philadelphia, Pa., hundreds of practitioners from all over the world met to discuss the state of the 2,000-year-old art of acupuncture in relation to a number of diseases ranging from the common toothache to cancer. One of the health problems in which attending doctors reported tremendous success with acupuncture treatment was migraine headaches. As those who are prone to migraine attacks know only too well, the usual medical treatments for these severe headaches leave much to be desired. And all the drugs now in general use are designed to be taken only after an attack has actually begun. In contrast, acupuncture treatment seems to be very effective in preventing the attacks from ever occurring, or rendering them much less severe when they do hit.

Dr. Howard D. Kurland of the Northwestern University Medical School and senior attending psychiatrist at the Evanston Hospital in Evanston, Illinois, reportd that he and his associates completed a two-year study of headache treatment with acupuncture techniques. Their patients had a variety of headaches, including migraine, histamine cephalalgia (cluster headaches), whiplash and tension headaches.

Dr. Kurland said he usually administers needle acupuncture in the head area. Following this, the patient is often taught how to treat himself with acupressure on certain points on the ear. These points are massaged and pinched when the patient feels an attack of migraine coming on. "My treatment for headache is either acupuncture or acupressure," Dr. Kurland said. "I do not give any prescription medicine for migraine headaches."

Far Fewer Drugs Needed

Using these new techniques, Dr. Kurland reported achieving great success, with a reasonable degree of relief in *all cases* where the patient adequately participated. The efficacy of acupuncture and self-administered acupressure treatment was verified, he noted, by the fact that prescriptions for narcotics, painkillers and other drugs were eliminated entirely in most cases.

Some of Dr. Kurland's most gratifying success has come in treating cluster headaches, which many people consider to be the very worst kind. The headaches usually come in "clusters" of from five to seven and may last for several days. Ordinarily, a person affected with these headaches can do absolutely nothing for himself except lie down in a dark room with shades drawn and wait until the agony goes away. With acupuncture, followed up by acupressure at the first hint of an attack, some patients with a history of very severe headaches—who had been on some of the strongest pain-killing drugs known—have had to resort to drugs only on a few occasions over the two years.

Another benefit in using acupuncture treatment for headaches, Dr. Kurland said, is that it is nontoxic and non-habit forming, which makes it a welcome addition to the physician's therapeutic arsenal. Dr. Ralph M. Coan, who is not an acupuncturist, but is the Medical Director of the Acupuncture Center of Washington in Washington, D.C., reported that practitioners at his clinic had also achieved impressive results.

One patient was a 55-year-old woman who had been suffering from headaches for more than 40 years, including two to three migraine headaches every month. These headaches lasted from two to five days. In early 1973, she had four acupuncture treatments and has not had a migraine headache since then, Dr. Coan said. She does, however, still have mild tension headaches and takes one over-the-counter analgesic every other day, instead of the three or four she used to take daily.

Another patient was a 68-year-old man who had almost constant pain for over seven years. He had three operations in which nerves in his head were cut to try to deaden the pain, but the results were not what he had hoped for. The pain continued and forced him to retire from his job earlier than normal. When he sought acupuncture treatment, he was taking at least seven very strong pain-killing pills as well as codeine every single day. Acupuncture treatment began in January, 1973. In this case, Dr. Coan said, the pain returned after an initial remission, and the patient underwent 15 more treatments. The patient then reported that the headaches he had were only half as bad as they had previously been.

In some cases the headaches are completely vanquished. A 41-year-old man who had a 20-year problem with migraine headaches reported that the headaches hit him four or five times a week, each lasting four or five hours. When medically evaluated at the clinic, he was taking 50 Darvon capsules every month. Following six treatments administered between January and March of 1973, the man became free of pain for the first time in 20 years.

Average Remission Is 10 Months

Dr. Coan said that when he looked at the results obtained from treating 40 consecutive patients with migraine headaches, he discovered that 23—or 58 percent—reported substantial improvement. The average length of the remission of pain after a single series of five to six acupuncture treatments was 10.2 months, Dr. Coan said. In 11 patients there was no relapse at the time of the Philadelphia meeting, an average of 15 months. In the majority of cases, Dr. Coan added, there is usually a marked reduction in medication.

"If the remarkable cure of acupuncture is related to a placebo effect, autosuggestion or hypnosis, as some have speculated," Dr. Coan said, "this ancient form of therapy would have to be rated as an outstanding psychosomatic therapeutic adjunct. Acupuncture cannot be dismissed as something that only works on Chinese."

A relatively new form of acupuncture, new in this country at least, is auriculotherapy, in which areas of the external part of the ear are stimulated. Two researchers using energized needles which impart microcurrents of electricity to various acupuncture points of the ear, are Dr. Sae-il Chun, M.D., of the University of Pennsylvania School of Medicine, and Dr. Arthur J. Heather, M.D., of the Delaware Curative Workshop. The doctors, who used this technique for many conditions, said that so far they had only treated two cases of headache. One was migraine headache and the other a tension headache. But in both cases, they said, excellent success was achieved with energized needles.

Help May Be Related To Blood Flow

Two researchers from the Departments of Anesthesiology and Biophysics at the Indiana University of Medicine believe that acupuncture may be connected with the blood flow to the head. In an article in *The American Journal of Chinese Medicine* (October, 1974), Drs. K. C. Kim and R. A. Yount reported on a series of acupuncture treatments they gave to 25 patients, 21 of whom were female, for migraine headaches. After six months of treatment, the pair reported that the frequency of headaches was reduced 68 percent and the duration 60 percent. Their results showed that 68 percent of the patients were able to completely halt their use of pain-killing medications. Twelve of the patients were considered completely cured. Another impressive statistic reported by the pair was an 82 percent reduction of such common migraine problems as vomiting, absence from work and the need to lie in bed.

In a discussion of their findings, they noted that other studies show that blood flow to the head is increased during the headaches. The blood flow is increased even more to the side of the head in which the migraine occurs. The speculation of other researchers is that this increased flow is connected to the migraine. They hypothesize that acupuncture—in some way—affects the blood circulation in the head by balancing this "improper" blood flow to the head.

Although acupuncture seems, at this point, to be a very potent weapon in the fight against migraine headaches, it takes an expert acupuncturist to get the desired results. Even though patients may be taught acupressure massage points at home, the person who suffers from this malady has to be taught the correct procedures to follow.

Just as all surgeons are not equal to their skills, not all doctors who practice acupuncture are equally skilled. Those who seem to be leaders in the field, however, do agree that the most reliable acupuncturists are either medical doctors who have been intensively trained, or Oriental practitioners who usually work in cooperation with M.D.'s . By making some phone calls to hospitals in your area, particularly teaching hospitals, you may find a convenient acupuncture clinic.

BioFeedback: A Treatment Of The Future

Acupuncture is by no means the only answer to migraine. Many people have been helped with psychological counseling. An increasing number of headache sufferers are now learning to abort migraines in the early stages by undergoing special training at biofeedback clinics. This is a technique which teaches a person how to actually control the flow of blood in his head so that headaches never reach the stage of serious pain. The theory is that headache pain caused by the abnormal constriction of blood vessels in the head might be preventable by controlling the tone of the sympathetic nervous system. Relaxation causes blood vessels in the head to dilate, get warm, increasing the flow of blood, triggering the same reaction throughout the sympathetic system. But the actual practice is still in its early stages and, despite several successful studies, is still in the experimental stage.

Section 36
The Heart

176. A Glossary Of Heart Terms

What does your doctor mean when he says you have a cardiac infarction? Or angina pectoris? Or endocarditis?

Here are the explanations of some of the terms used in referring to heart and circulatory disorders.

Acrocyanosis. A bluish discoloration of the skin (usually fingertips) which indicates lack of blood. It may be the beginning of Buerger's disease.

Acroparesthesia. A feeling of pins and needles in the fingertips.

Acrosclerosis. Raynaud's disease—see the later definition of this.

Adrenalin. A secretion of the adrenal glands, which constricts the small blood vessels (arterioles), increases the rate of the heart beat and raises blood pressure.

Aneurysm. A blood-containing tumor in the wall of a blood vessel. The wall is weakened but does not burst.

Angina pectoris. Severe attacks of pain over the heart or in the mid-chest region. Easily confused with gas pains stemming from indigestion.

Angiocardiography. An X-ray examination of the heart and great blood vessels after an opaque fluid, or dye, is injected into the bloodstream.

Angioma. A tumor formed of a blood vessel. These are seldom dangerous unless they are exposed to injury.

Anoxia. A lack of oxygen for an area of heart muscle caused by a blood clot cutting off the blood supply. The affected tissue dies.

Anticoagulant. A drug capable of slowing the clotting of blood.

Aorta. The main trunk artery of the body. From the aorta many arteries branch off transporting blood to all parts of the body except the lungs.

Aortic insufficiency. Improper closing of the valve between the aorta and the heart, permitting some backflow of blood from the aorta into the heart.

Apoplexy. Stroke. A hemorrhage in the brain. The term may be used also for hemorrhages in other parts of the body.

Arrhythmia. An increase in the rate of heart beat when you breathe in, a decrease when you breathe out, caused by interference with breathing out. Usually this condition has no adverse significance, but it may be aggravated by rheumatic heart.

Arterioles. The smallest arterial vessels. They conduct blood from the arteries to the capillaries.

Arteriosclerosis. Commonly called "hardening of the arteries," in which the arteries become thickened and lose elasticity.

Artery. A blood vessel which transports blood away from the heart to some part of the body.

Atherosclerosis. A form of arteriosclerosis, characterized by clogging of the arteries with fatty deposits on the walls.

Athrombia. Insufficient clotting of the blood.

Atrium. One of the two upper chambers of the heart. The right atrium receives "used" or unoxygenated blood from the body; the left atrium receives oxygenated blood from the lungs.

Auricle. Another name for the upper chamber in each side of the heart. See *Atrium.*

Auricular fibrillation. The rapid and irregular quivering of the auricles (or upper chambers) of the heart. The pulse becomes completely irregular with a beat as high as 150 to 160 per minute. Causes may be rheumatism, hyperthyroidism, acute infections like flu or pneumonia, poisons like tobacco, or emotional strain. If one does not have heart disease, there is probably no danger. The condition may go on for many years without harm.

Auricular flutter. Much the same as auricular fibrillation except that the contractions are regular. This condition is rare.

Blood count. A measurement of the number and kinds of red and white cells.

Blood pressure. Refers to both systolic pressure (when the heart contracts) and diastolic pressure (when the heart is fully relaxed). Measured by the pressure of the blood against the walls of the vessels.

Blue babies. Babies whose skin has a bluish look because of insufficient oxygen in the arterial blood. This is often the result of a heart defect but may have other causes, such as impaired respiration or premature birth.

Bradycardia. Slow heart beat. Any pulse rate under 60 per minute is classed as bradycardia. If one's heart normally beats slowly this is an extremely healthful condition. But slow heart beat resulting from interference with the nerves to the heart is quite serious. Present in a fairly young person and causing fainting spells and epileptic-like convulsions, this is called Stokes-Adams syndrome.

Buerger's disease. Also called *thromboangiitis obliterans.* This is the inflammation of the inner lining of small blood vessels with constriction and clogging due to blood clots. Because of impaired circulation, the feet or hands become cold and tender. More than any other reason, tobacco appears to play a large part in causing this disease.

Capillary. A narrow vessel through which oxygen and nutritive materials pass into the tissues and carbon dioxide and waste products move from the tissues into the bloodstream.

Cardiac. Pertaining to the heart. Sometimes used to refer to anyone who has heart disease.

Cardiovascular. Pertaining to the heart and blood system.

Carditis. An inflammation of the heart.

Cerebral vascular accident. Also called *cerebrovascular accident,* or stroke. It denotes impeded blood supply to the brain. It may be caused by (1) formation of a blood clot in a vessel supplying the brain (*cerebral thrombosis*); (2) rupture of a blood vessel wall (*cerebral hemorrhage*); (3) blockage of a brain blood vessel by a clot or other material formed elsewhere which moves to the cerebral vessel (*cerebral embolism*); (4) pressure on a blood vessel—by a tumor, for example.

Claudication, intermittent. A spasm in the artery, causing muscle cramping in the legs, with pain and limping. There is a diminished blood supply to the legs.

Congestive heart failure. The heart cannot effectively pump out all the blood that returns to it, and blood backs up in veins leading to the heart. Congestion, or fluid accumulation, may occur in various parts of the body, such as lungs, legs or abdomen.

Constrictive pericarditis. A shrinking and thickening of the heart's outer sac which interferes with normal expansion and contraction of the heart.

Coronary disease. A number of different disorders. *Coronary sclerosis* is the hardening of the arteries that lead to the heart. This may cause *coronary occlusion* which is the obstruction of the coronary artery by a blood clot or embolism. Occlusion occurs suddenly and is accompanied by severe pain and shock. *Coronary insufficiency* is a partial blockage of the coronary artery so that some blood gets through but not enough to nourish the pericardium (the sac in which the heart is enclosed). This then becomes diseased—and the name of this condition is *coronary infarction.*

Coronary thrombosis. The formation of a blood clot in the coronary artery leading to the heart.

Cyanosis. Blueness of the skin caused by insufficient oxygen in the blood.

Decompensation. A person is said to be decompensated when the heart fails to maintain normal circulation. See *Congestive heart failure.*

Dextrocardia. The heart is on the right rather than the left side of the chest. Apparently this causes no impairment to health.

Diastole. The period of relaxation of the heart in each heartbeat.

Digitalis. A drug made from leaves of foxglove that strengthens heart-muscle contraction, slows the contraction rate and improves efficiency of the heart so that fluid may be eliminated from body tissues.

Dropsy or edema. The abnormal accumulation in the tissues of fluid that has escaped from blood vessels. It usually indicates heart disease or circulatory obstruction of some kind. When it occurs in the abdomen it is called *ascites;* in the brain—*hydrocephalus;* in the chest—*hydrothorax.*

Effort syndrome. Simple weakness of the circulatory system. Breathlessness, heart palpitations and rapid heartbeat are symptoms. Individuals with this condition become exhausted when ordinary persons are merely tired.

Electric cardiac pacemaker. An electric device that discharges rhythmic electrical impulses to control beating of the heart.

Electrocardiogram. Also called EKG and ECG. A record of the electrical currents produced by the heart.

Embolism. A small clot or other substance which has been detached from the wall of a blood vessel and is floating in the blood stream. A *pulmonary embolism* is a blood clot that lodges in the lung, causing a pulmonary insufficiency and sometimes death.

Endocarditis, acute. Acute inflammation of the lining of any membrane of the heart. Usually it is present in cases of rheumatic fever.

Endocarditis, bacterial. Inflammation caused by some bacteria. It may be streptococcus. The acute form involves chills and fever. The chronic form may simply show fatigue, loss of weight, breathlessness.

Endocarditis, chronic. Sometimes called chronic valvular heart disease. The valves in the heart become warped or shrunken and let the blood flow backward. The most common cause of this is rheumatic fever.

814

Extrasystole. A heart contraction which occurs prematurely and interrupts normal rhythm.

Fibrillation. Uncoordinated contractions, virtually mere twitchings, of the heart muscle.

Heart enlargement. A condition which might occur when one is doing extremely hard physical work (an athlete for instance) for which the heart increases in size to accommodate the extra work. Usually it is from other causes, however—to compensate for such conditions as valvular disease, kidney disease and so forth, where the load on the heart is greatly increased. *Fatty heart* is an enlargement of the heart, usually of those who are sedentary and obese.

Heart murmur. An abnormal sound of the heart heard through the chest wall indicating a functional abnormality or the site of a structural abnormality.

Hemangiectasis. Enlargement of the blood vessels.

Hypertension. High blood pressure.

Hypotension. Low blood pressure.

Infarction. Blockage of a blood vessel.

Myocarditis. Inflammation of the myocardium or heart envelope. It is usually due to rheumatic fever. *Chronic myocarditis* and *myocardosis* are in much the same category as heart disease with great enlargement.

Neurosis, cardiac. Symptoms may be dizziness, nervousness, weakness, sleeplessness, palpitation—all these without any apparent cause. The assumption is that such symptoms may be imaginary or neurotic.

Open-heart surgery. Surgery carried out on the opened heart while blood is diverted through a heart-lung machine.

Palpitation. An inordinately strong, rapid, or irregular heartbeat. Most are completely normal, the result of fatigue, emotional stress, or overexertion, but some forms might be clues to more serious heart problems.

Periarteritis nodosa. Inflammatory condition of medium-sized arteries. This results in the formation of a series of nodules in the middle and outer coats of arteries.

Pericarditis. This is the inflammation of the pericardium or heart envelope.

Phlebitis. Inflammation of a vein. *Thrombophlebitis* is phlebitis with blood clots. Frequent causes are injury, infection, childbirth and varicose veins.

Plasma. The liquid, cell-free portion of uncoagulated blood.

Pulmonary. Pertaining to blood circulation between the heart and lungs. The *pulmonary artery* is the large artery that carries unoxygenated blood from the lower right chamber of the heart to the lungs. The *pulmonary valve* is located at the junction of the pulmonary artery and the lower right heart chamber. The *pulmonary veins* are four veins (two from each lung) which carry oxygenated blood from the lungs to the left upper chamber of the heart.

Pulse, alternating. Strong and then weak beats. The heart is trying to rest with every other beat. *Asymmetrical*—strong one side of the body, weak on the other side. *Bigeminal*—two regular beats, a pause, two regular beats, a pause, etc. *Dicrotic*—this means a double beat. *Intermittent*—sometimes called *extrasystoles.* This means dropped or skipped beats, or pauses instead of beats. Often this is not associated with heart disease, but may result from fatigue, emotion, worry, coffee or tobacco. If heart action is speeded up with exercise, extrasystoles may disappear. If they do not, myocardial heart trouble may be present. *Irregular*—loss of rhythm of pulse. If this is chronic it may denote something quite serious.

Raynaud's disease. Constriction of the blood vessels causing impaired circulation in the hands, feet, ears and nose. The hands are affected most often. They may become pallid, numb and purplish.

Rheumatic fever. A disease most frequent in childhood, which can cause serious heart damage. The valves of the heart may be scarred so they no longer open and close properly. Rheumatic fever may develop a few weeks after a streptococcal infection. Its symptoms include fever, sore, swollen joints, skin rash, and involuntary twitching of muscles.

Serum. The clear fluid that separates from blood when it clots. *Serum cholesterol* is the term used in measuring the cholesterol level in the blood.

Stenosis. A narrowing of an opening. Aortic stenosis, pulmonary stenosis, etc., mean that the indicated valve has narrowed so that it doesn't function properly. This is often caused by rheumatic fever.

Stroke. See *Cerebral vascular accident.*

Systole. The period of contraction of the heart in each heartbeat. *Atrial* systole is the contraction of the upper chambers of the heart; *ventricular* systole is the contraction of the lower chambers.

Tachycardia. Rapid heart action. Fast pulse. A beat of 90 or higher per minute. The heart must work faster to do the work done by other hearts with 70 beats a minute. It may be a symptom of infections, or may be emotional or neurotic.

Thrombosis. Formation of a clot. If the *thrombus,* or blood clot, tears loose from the blood vessel wall and arrives eventually at a blood vessel too small for it to pass through, there will be an embolism at this point.

Varicose veins. Dilated and swollen veins. May come from an infection. Fat persons are more susceptible than thin ones. Standing for long hours is undoubtedly one of the causes.

Vein. A blood vessel which carries blood from some part of the body back to the heart.

Ventricle. One of the two lower chambers of the heart. The left ventricle pumps oxygenated blood through the arteries to the body. The right ventricle pumps unoxygenated blood through the pulmonary artery to the lungs.

177. Your Personality And Your Heart

Some people have unhealthy personalities, particularly from the point of view of heart disease. They are hard driving, aggressive, and overly conscious of the need to save time. Those coronary-prone people tend to run, not walk, pound their fists when talking or use other vigorous gestures. When they talk they spout out words in an explosive stream. They are competitive people, having an inner urge to show superiority.

Although we have all read a great deal about the pattern of life that makes people susceptible to coronary disease, the personality factor has not been in the forefront of the news. There are several reasons. First, personality is not a clear-cut, black and white thing. Not everyone can be classified as having a coronary prone or coronary immune personality. Some are in the middle ground, and for them the idea of personality has no significance to heart health. Also, many doctors are hesitant to use the personality test procedure, because they don't think they can be objective in testing a subjective thing like personality.

Also, personality is only one of many factors in the heart health equation. If you are overweight, have high blood pressure, and smoke cigarettes, your chances of having a heart attack are high even if you have a "good" personality. Likewise, lack of exercise and hereditary factors are important, as are vitamin and mineral nutrition. Even a person with the most high-pressure type of personality can continue pounding his fist with a certain degree of safety if he will nourish himself properly, exercise, avoid smoking, and do the other things that tend to insulate us against heart attack. Still, personality is something we should learn about, because we have to use every tool at our command to try to achieve health in this artificial and unhealthful world.

Two doctors have been in the forefront of the study of personality and heart health. They are Dr. Meyer Friedman and Dr. Ray H. Rosenman, both of the Harold Brunn Institute of Mount Zion Hospital in San Francisco. Back in 1959 they reported that people with a dangerous heart personality—which they call type

A people—had seven times more coronary heart disease than a group who were similar in all characteristics except personality. The "good" personality people are categorized as type B.

A later study of 3,000 men aged 39 to 59, showed that occurrence of coronary heart disease was about three times greater in the type A (aggressive, hard-driving) group than in the type B people (slower, more calm). But when the doctors considered only the younger men, between ages 39 and 49, the difference was more marked. Six times as many type A men in that group got coronary disease. Those are impressive figures, and indicate that knowledge of personality factors is essential to a well-rounded heart attack prevention campaign.

How is your personality type determined? Doctors use an interview method. They talk to the subject and ask a series of special questions designed to get people to expose the complex of characteristics that make one person different from another. Interestingly, the interviewer is less interested in the answers given to the questions than in the style with which they are delivered. The interviewer is on the lookout for loud and explosive statements, vigorous gestures, and other physical signs that match an aggressive, competitive personality. A person who just sits calmly through the interview and answers in a quiet voice will no doubt be placed in the type B category, unless it is suspected that he or she is trying to hide normal characteristics. Of course, it is important to realize that there is aggressiveness and competitiveness in almost everyone, but the type A people have more in their makeup than is perhaps normal, and the type B people have less.

Drs. Friedman and Rosenman say that this interview method is about 75 percent to 85 percent accurate, when the test is given by an interviewer who is oriented to detect subtle personality differences and is himself the type of person who is perceptive of people's emotions. That leaves considerable room for error. If even the best interviewers could let 25 percent of people slip through with the wrong personality brand, the average result is likely to be considerably less accurate. So the team that pioneered personality investigations of heart attack risk has also been looking hard and long for a better way to separate people into the different personality groups.

A voice analysis test could be the answer, Drs. Friedman and Rosenman and Alvin E. Brown, M.A., reported in the May 5, 1969 *Journal of the American Medical Association*. They were led to investigate a voice test by their observation that type A people have a characteristic way of talking, using semi-violent accents, an aggressive timbre and similar styles. The type B person, on the other hand, speaks in a rather smooth, unruffled manner. Using that information, they have found that the way people read a standard test passage can provide enough information to separate them into type A and type B personality groups with almost as much accuracy as the best interviewer.

Of course, the paragraphs to be read are not something from *Little Women*. They are literally blood and guts stuff designed to stir the emotions. The people to be tested are asked to read this speech, modeled after what a military commander might say to his troops before they go into battle:

"This is the way that you and me, every God damned one of us, are going to lick the hell out of whoever stands in our way. And I don't give a damn whether you like what I'm telling you or not. This is the way I say it's got to be done. First, we're going to smack them hard with mortar fire, understand? I want you to pour it on them! Let the bastards feel it get hot, really hot around them. Singe the hell out of them! Scorch the bastards, fry them, burn their guts out. Make ashes out of them.

"After the mortars, I'll tell you when to advance. And when I give the signal, don't crawl, you run forward! Remember, it's your skin or theirs! All right, enough talk, now let's get the lead out of our pants and get going. Hey! One more thing, good luck!"

The readings took place with only the subject and an investigator present. First, the subject was told to read the paragraphs as if he were alone in his own home, having read them in a novel and then decided to read them out loud to himself. Interestingly, more than half the type A people then asked, "Do you want me to read them with expression?" None of the type B people asked that.

During the tests, vocal recordings were made which showed the intensity and loudness of the speech used. The type A people being tested read the passage louder than the type B people. But even more revealing was a second reading, in which these instructions were given to the test group:

"Now we would like you to reread these same two paragraphs, but this time we would like you to pretend or imagine that you are not here but are on a battleground and that you are the commanding captain or sergeant of about a half dozen, tough, hard-bitten soldiers who are just about ready to attack an enemy force a few miles ahead of you. These soldiers are huddled about you. You and they too are in a hurry to begin the attack. The seconds are ticking off as you talk. You want them to do a good job. Now read the paragraphs with these things in mind."

On that second reading, the difference in style between the coronary-prone and type B really became apparent. The average type A person rushed through the little speech in 38 seconds, in a tone of voice with many "vocal oscillations," quite loudly at times. The type B people took an average of 44 seconds, and used a more quiet style of talking.

The hope of the voice test researchers is that they have now developed a method of personality testing that can be widely used, because it doesn't depend on the availability of extremely skilled interviewers. They feel that personality typing is extremely important to the prevention of coronary heart disease, and that many lives can be saved if vulnerable people will be identified and warned of the hazard their own personalities create.

Can people change their personalities? Drs. Friedman and Rosenman and Alvin E. Brown say that they have seen a number of type A people who appeared to alter their behavior patterns after having suffered a heart attack. Before being struck down, they refused to do anything to change their ways, trusting to "luck" to protect them. But after having an attack, the lesson was hammered home and some of those type A's were able to start living differently.

The big question remains, though, whether accurate testing for personality can bring home to type A people the hazard of their way of life without the dramatic lesson of a heart attack. People are notorious for thinking that they live charmed lives, and that the bad things only happen to others. Perhaps that is a good human trait, for otherwise we would be dragged down by all the possibilities for harm that surround us. The smartest people, though, realize that luck comes more often to those who plan ahead and try to smooth out the road on which they travel through life.

By this time you have thought some about your own personality and have wondered if you are type A or type B. Probably we can take a pretty good guess at our own personality type by thinking of the way we talk and especially what our personal attitudes are toward time and deadlines. But we can't really be accurate in assessing ourselves, and that is why a good test of personality is needed.

Whatever your personality type, though, be sure not to confuse the calm, good type B personality with laziness or a life of ease and self-indulgence. To be really healthy you must sometimes drive your body hard physically, work up a sweat, breathe hard, and even tire yourself. The type A person is said to walk fast, it is true, but how far does he walk? Chances are it is just to the nearest garage or bus stop. The truly healthy person walks an hour or more a day at a steady pace.

In the past doctors crippled untold thousands of heart attack victims by telling them to take it easy physically for the rest of their lives. That is a prescription for invalidism. True, a person with a heart attack must rest for a while, but today he is often told by his doctor to start a gradual program of exercise and to keep it up. Doctors now know that vigorous use of the body is in some ways a prescription for heart health, when it is done carefully.

The personality theory of heart health is valid as a means to identify those people who are more likely than others to have heart attacks. However, a type A person probably has to do far more than change personality to gain protection from coronary heart disease. Evidence that personality changing alone can prevent coronary disease is sketchy at best. There is, on the other hand, a growing and impressive body of evidence that good diet, exercise, avoidance of smoking, and other generally sensible routines of life can protect against coronary disease. More than anyone else, the type A person needs to learn how to use those proven techniques of prevention.

178. Heart Disease Symptoms In Patients With Normal Hearts

"There is no evidence that stresses cause heart disease," wrote Kurt Aaron, M.D., of East Brisbane, in the November 14, 1959, issue of the *Medical Journal of Australia*. However, he went on to demonstrate that stress of certain kinds can cause certain heart symptoms in patients whose hearts are perfectly normal.

From time immemorial we have associated the heart with our emotions. Language is full of phrases like "heartfelt," "lion-hearted," "broken-hearted." We know, too, that the heart is actually associated very closely with the emotion of fear and its natural accompanying physical preparedness. Physical response to danger requires increased blood supply to the muscles, dilation of the small arteries that lead to the muscles, the release of the gland secretion, adrenalin, and an increase in the "output" of the heart—that is, the heart must beat harder, faster or both.

In earlier days, of course, danger meant the same thing it means to animals—one had to fight or run. So these body preparations took place to give strength for fighting or swiftness for escape. It is true that the clotting time of the blood is shortened when one feels fear, anger or hostility. This means the blood tends to become thicker—apparently as an adaptation to protect a person if he is wounded, so that he will not bleed to death. Today most of us are far removed from danger of actual physical wounds, yet fear and anger still produce this same reaction—a thickening of the blood. One can easily see, therefore, that chronic fear or anger may lead to dangerous blood clots.

It is true, too, wrote Dr. Aaron, that recalling an event that made one fearful or angry will produce the same body reactions as if the event were taking place in the present. One's heart beats faster, or harder, one feels the rush of blood into the muscles and the stimulation given by adrenalin as it moves swiftly to all parts of the body to ready it for an emergency. Undoubtedly, people with very vivid imaginations must go through almost the same sensations of fright when they are telling or re-living some fearful event.

However, the perfectly normal patients who come to doctors with complaints of heart symptoms are suffering from something else, in Dr. Aaron's opinion. They have a neurosis. This does not mean that their difficulty is imaginary. It's real enough, all right, but it is the result of something in their personalities—nothing in their heart physiology.

Some of the symptoms of this type of patient are heart palpitations, difficulty in breathing, pain in the chest and fatigue. Any one of these singly or in conjunction with some other symptom like frequent urination, indigestion or headache constitute the major complaints of patients who have nothing wrong with their hearts.

Dr. Aaron then described these symptoms. His description of heart palpitations is particularly good: heart palpitation is "the consciousness of the heart beating." It is usually painless and may be felt in the chest or over the heart. The heart may seem to be pounding very hard; it may seem to be beating in places removed from it or the tissues directly around it. Beats may occur that are out of step with the preceding beat or following beats, or the heart may beat very rapidly.

Palpitations may not be felt in times of real stress or crisis. Usually patients feel the palpitations while lying in bed recalling difficult situations.

Breathlessness or labored breathing is another symptom: "The patient calls it shortness of breath and means two varieties. The first is an increase in respiratory rate and the second is the feeling of inability to take a deep breath, as if he could not get enough air into the lungs. Yet this particular type of breathing is associated with deep sighing respiration. It is a feeling of oppression as if something was stopping the thoracic (chest) cage from expanding. I find it a particularly useful symptom in favor of the diagnosis of neurosis, of which it is characteristic. It occurs at any time, has no relation to effort, and is particularly prone to happen in association with recall of fearful and unpleasant situations. It often occurs at night, waking the patient in a panic."

Chest pain, another symptom, can cause a lot of diagnostic trouble for both patient and doctor, for how can you tell it from the pain of angina pectoris? The kind of pain Dr. Aaron referred to does not occur as a result of effort on the patient's part. It may go on for days. It may yield to rest, but it may be necessary to rest for several hours. One patient told Dr. Aaron that he would have to go to bed for the rest of the day to get relief from his pain caused by visiting the doctor in the morning. It is hard to describe pain. Patients may have read accounts of the pain experienced by angina patients and may confuse their own pain with this.

What causes such heart symptoms, if there is nothing organically wrong with one's heart? Dr. Aaron said that emotional happenings in one's past life are responsible. Recalling situations that caused fright or anger stimulates the same physical reaction throughout the body as if one were frightened or angered.

Dr. Aaron wrote, "I have no doubt that most, if not all, patients suffering from anxiety states have gone through prolonged periods of fear without relief in action. An insecure childhood is the most common factor, particularly mother-deprivation, a violent alcoholic father or over-strictness of well-meaning parents. These features are almost always found in the history of these unfortunate persons . . . My conception of the etiology (cause) of these disabilities is, then, conditioning of prolonged anxiety and insecurity as a rule in childhood up to the age of 18 years, resulting in unduly violent emotional reactions to later stresses. These may be everyday stresses of life, recall of difficult life situations, dreams or new severe emotional upsets. The reaction remains the same—stimulation of the automatic nervous system. If the fear of heart disease is superimposed on this, the threat to life is added and a vicious circle is established."

It is also possible for people with organic heart disease to have heart symptoms that arise from anxiety neuroses. In such cases the doctor must first treat the organic heart trouble, then, if the symptoms persist after the actual working of the heart has been corrected, the patient must work to correct the emotional background that is causing them.

Do emotional stresses cause heart disease? Not according to Dr. Aaron. He takes up the commonly held notion that executives have more heart attacks because they "worry more." He asks, "What about the executives in Japan and other countries where heart attacks are comparatively low? Do their executives worry less?"

Are mental symptoms the result of heart disease? So far as neurosis is concerned, Dr. Aaron stated that people who have heart disease and know that it may get worse and eventually cause a heart attack usually become adjusted to this idea and do not worry greatly about themselves. "The patient with advanced heart disease has reason to worry about his state of health and the eventual outcome; yet it is surprising how well adjusted most of these patients are, and how infrequently they show neurotic traits."

However, mental symptoms are frequent in association with *advanced* heart disease, especially in the elderly. Difficulties in sleeping, nightmares, disturbing dreams—all these may contribute to the distress felt by these patients.

Finally, Dr. Aaron considered the patient who has been made fearful about his heart by a doctor. "It is stated that some doctors, through ignorance, carelessness or failure to recognize the mental state of the patient, diagnose organic heart disease where no such disease exists, and cause severe disability in these patients who consequently believe themselves to be suffering from serious heart disease. There is no doubt that this occurs. Of 631 persons referred to a work classification unit for assessment because of the presence of heart disease, 175 had no heart disease at all. . .

"I recall a number of patients requesting examination of their hearts who, when told that I could not find any evidence of heart disease, informed me that they had been told that they had heart disease but did not believe it." He noted that many people are made ill by a doctor through misinterpretation of what he tells them about symptoms.

Dr. Aaron concluded that neurosis is a common cause of certain symptoms which appear to be symptoms of heart disease. Adjusting to life situations rather than taking medicine is the cure for such symptoms.

179. How's Your Blood Pressure Doing? (Why Not Find Out For Yourself!)

Here is one person's experience with blood pressure readings. The story is valuable because it shows why blood pressure readings need to be double-checked and analyzed.

"I was first informed I had high blood pressure while I was in the Navy and trying for an ROTC scholarship—I wanted to go to college when I got out of the service. I flunked the physical, of course, and was ruled out for the scholarship. But that disappointment was nothing compared to my shock and fright on learning I had high blood pressure. I was only 20! I couldn't believe what they told me. It really bothered me. I was panicked for days if I was scheduled for a physical—and, sure enough, at college and again when I wanted insurance, that high blood pressure showed up each time.

"Then I applied for the Peace Corps. This time, for my physical, I went to an elderly doctor attached to a nearby VA hospital. He had all the time in the world, and when I told him my story he just said, 'Well now, let's see.' And we sat there together in his office for close to an hour while he took my blood pressure over and over and over again, now on the right arm, now on the left. The pressure showed high at first, but by the end of the visit it was right down where it belonged. And stayed that way. I was accepted by the Peace Corps, met my future wife while we were fellow corpsmen—or should it be corpspersons?—and now I'm 35 and have never since shown up with high blood pressure in any examination.

"All along, you see, when I wasn't tensed up, *normally* I was *normal*. But it took that blessed old-fashioned VA doc to set the matter straight."

This story illustrates a fact widely acknowledged in the medical profession: doctors often get a reading of hypertension (high blood pressure) in perfectly normal people, especially on initial visits. Anxiety can temporarily shoot the pressure up. Usually doctors want a series of visits and repeated pressure measurements before they will diagnose high blood pressure.

The truth is, your physician probably *never* gets a wholly accurate picture of your normal basal blood pressure—that is, pressure when all distorting factors have been eliminated. Even when hypertensive patients are hospitalized, kept quiet and relaxed over a period of days, and have their pressures taken repeatedly, Dr. Walter Kirkendall and associates report in *Circulation* (December, 1967), "Blood pressures recorded by the nurse tend to be lower than those taken by the doctor because of the emotional response generated by the presence of the physician."

The authors then suggest: "Nearly all basal blood pressures also can be taken in the home, preferably by a member of the family. Daily recordings taken in the home usually trend downward during the first week to a lower, more constant level."

It would seem, then, that you and the familiar members of your own household are, for *you*, the very best blood pressure measurers in the world—or would be once they learned the quite simple (but initially awkward) technique of using the blood pressure measuring apparatus, the sphygmomanometer. (If your tongue twists on this tongue twister, think of it as two words and it'll come out easier; *sphyg*mo, pertaining to pulse, plus ma-*nom*eter, pertaining to measurement, as in the thermometer.) The apparatus indirectly measures the pressure of blood against artery walls at the height of its force when the heart muscles contract (systolic pressure), and again in between beats when the heart is at rest (diastolic pressure).

There are sound reasons for having a household sphygmomanometer and using it regularly. "Blood pressure measurements should become a common household practice to aid in early detection of hypertension," says Dr. George Burch, of the Tulane University School of Medicine, according to *Internal Medicine News* (April 15, 1972).

It Pays To Know

Of the estimated 23 million Americans with high blood pressure, 85 to 90 percent have what is known as "primary" or "essential" hypertension. That means they have the typical form of disease, whose cause is still unknown. Certain specific and often correctable causes, however—for example, a non-malignant kidney tumor—are responsible for high blood pressure in the small proportion of patients said to have "secondary" hypertension. The doctor may want to conduct various tests to eliminate other possibilities before primary hypertension is diagnosed.

Of all the people with high blood pressure, detection surveys indicate that half are unaware of their condition. This disease has no symptoms in its early stages, but damage to the vascular system, which can eventually affect heart and kidneys and accelerate the risk of heart attack and stroke, continues unnoticed. Controlling high blood pressure—that is, keeping it down to reasonable levels, preferably by natural means (diet, exercise, rest), but by medication if need be—substantially reduces the risk of these grave complications. In 1971, Dr. Edward Freis of the Veterans Administration won medicine's coveted Lasker award for his clinical studies establishing that patients with an elevated diastolic pressure of 105 or more can triple their chances for escaping hypertension-related disease and death when their blood pressures are controlled (*Medical World News*, August 24, 1973).

So you can see why "early detection" is very important indeed. If someone in your family is developing high blood pressure, you should want to know it.

As for the hypertensive patient who already is under a doctor's care, here again the household sphygmomanometer can be of great value. "One cannot manage hypertension without checking the patient's blood pressure regularly any more than one can manage a diabetic without checking his urine sugar at home," Dr. Burch points out, arguing that a carefully kept home record of blood pressure readings is a doctor's best guide in managing this very common disorder.

Here's the word from the High Blood Pressure National Task Force (appointed by the U.S. Department of Health, Education and Welfare) as reported by *Medical Opinion* (April, 1974): "Both patients and physicians are increasingly accepting the use of home blood pressure readings taken by the patient or his family as an important adjunct to therapy. This is especially true for patients who need frequent monitoring to check on the effectiveness of therapy."

We still have with us, of course, the Doctor who won't even reveal blood pressure readings to his patients—let alone trust them with taking their own pressures and keeping accurate records. But let's hope this type will soon be educated out of existence. We might recall that the thermometer, too, was once considered a highly scientific instrument to be entrusted only to physicians.

Making The Purchase

For taking blood pressure you need both the sphygmomanometer and a stethoscope—the latter is the instrument with which to listen to the pulse beat as the sphygmomanometer registers the pressure. Both instruments can be purchased in medical supply houses which serve doctors and hospitals. However, quite satisfactory instruments for home use are now available from many mail order houses and pharmacies.

If you are living alone and plan to take your own blood pressure, Dr. Kirkendall (whom we quoted earlier) recommends a home instrument in which the stethoscope "head"—the disk or cone that is placed on the arm and catches and magnifies the sound—is built right into the sphygmomanometer. This combination device is probably not quite as accurate as the two separate instruments used in partnership, he acknowledges, but having just one instrument to handle instead of two will make things a lot easier for you.

Examining The Instruments

Your purchase arrives, along with the merchant's brief description of the instruments and how to use them. Unless you've ordered the combination instrument, mentioned above, you'll find yourself with what you've often seen in the doctor's office. Here's the stethoscope, with its buttons to place in both ears and tubes from the ear-buttons leading down to the instrument's head. And here's the sphygmomanometer: an inflatable rectangular bag, known as the cuff, which wraps around your upper arm; an attached bulb which you press to pump up the cuff; and an attached dial from which you will read your pressures as the pumped-up cuff is deflating. (Instead of the dial found on the aneroid sphygmomanometer, the mercurial sphygmomanometer—which is slightly more expensive—has a glassed-in column of mercury from which you read your pressure on a graduated scale. Pressure readings are actually a measure of the height of mercury (Hg) in millimeters (mm)—hence the formal reading of a pressure such as 105 diastolic is written 105 mm Hg. Either type of sphygmomanometer—aneroid or mercurial—is satisfactory.)

Now then. You're ready to begin.

Taking Blood Pressures

Let's start with a caution. True, taking blood pressure is a simple operation. Youngsters still in high school perform this job in some hospital summer programs. "People who can hardly read or write can take a blood pressure," says Tulane University's Dr. Burch. But first attempts are often fumbling and frustrating. It takes practice to handle the instruments with ease. So be patient. Play around with the gadgets for a few days before keeping any records at all—and before putting any credence in the readings you get. These will probably shift all over the place until you become experienced.

Say you're going to take your wife's blood pressure. Have her sit with her arm (slightly flexed) resting on a table. The arm should be at about heart-level; so if the table is too low, provide a platform with a box or a couple of big books.

Step No. 1 is to wrap the cuff around the upper arm. This used to be quite a task. But nowadays cuffs come with self-adhesive surfaces, so that one end sticks to the other without any fastenings necessary. The cuff should fit snugly around the arm but not bind tightly—the tightness will come when the cuff is inflated.

A tip if you're taking your own blood pressure: you'll find it absurdly difficult to fasten the cuff around your arm using only your one free hand, so don't try. Instead, fasten the cuff together while it's still on the table before you. Now you have an oversized bracelet, which you can quite easily slip up your arm to the proper position. Now rest your arm on a table, palm up.

Step No. 2: Place the stethoscope buttons in your ears. Gently touch the face of the stethoscope head and you'll hear how the soft sound of your finger's touch is magnified. Place the instrument's head just below the arm's bend, towards the inside of the arm (towards your body). Here it will be resting on a major artery. Don't allow the head to touch your clothing. Hold it firmly but without undue pressure.

Now sit back for a few minutes and just listen. You'll hear various muted cracklings and rumblings, and you want to get used to these vague noises so you won't confuse them with the pulse-beat sounds. The pulse you won't hear yet—not while the cuff is still uninflated and applying no pressure on that main artery carrying blood down the length of the arm.

Step No. 3: Straighten out the arm wearing the cuff—this will give you a sharper sound. Now, with dial clipped or propped so you can easily watch the moving hand, begin to press on the bulb to inflate the cuff. There is a fastener on the bulb which you must tighten in order to pump air—and loosen when it's time to let the air escape.

Inflate the cuff until the pressure gauge registers around 160 (or higher if you know your top pressure tops this figure); then loosen the fastener slightly so that the air gradually escapes. (If your one hand is holding the stethoscope head over the artery of the arm and the other hand has been pumping on the bulb, this final operation—loosening the fastener—can sometimes be tricky. You will soon learn to reach out with your thumb and forefinger and manipulate the fastener while the rest of your hand is on the bulb. To make things easier, you can get a combination "stetho/sphyg," with the stethoscope head built right into the cuff, which is suggested for people taking their own pressures.)

Step No. 4 is the reading of blood pressure levels as the cuff deflates. Here, perhaps, we should go into a little background. When the cuff is inflated, its pressure stops the flow of blood through the arm's arteries. In effect, it's a tourniquet. At the point when the pressure in the deflating cuff has lowered enough to let through the first surge of renewed blood flow, you hear the first sounds of the pulse in your stethoscope. That's your systolic pressure, reflecting the force exerted on artery walls when the heart beats. As the cuff continues to deflate and circulation returns to the lower arm, the diastolic pressure is gauged by the pressure in the cuff when your stethoscope picks up no more pulse sounds.

To translate all this into practical instructions: As the cuff deflates, keep your eyes on the dial, or manometer, as you listen for sounds. At the first noise—faint clear tapping sounds—note the pressure level. Let's say it's 130. Keep your eyes peeled and your ears alert. The sounds will increase in intensity, change in quality, then (usually) there's a muffling, then silence. Note the cuff's pressure reading at the point when sounds disappear. Let's say it's 85. Now you have your blood pressure reading: 130/85. (The most accurate readings are obtained when pressure in the cuff drops at the rate of two to three mm per second. When you become practiced in the art of blood pressure taking, you'll know just how quickly to let air out of the cuff to achieve this perfection.)

Step No. 5: Quickly deflate the cuff completely. If you want to take a second reading right away, switch to the other arm. You don't want to block circulation again till the arm has had a chance to recover from its first cut-off. If for some reason you must use the same arm, you will find that if you don't wait at least two minutes, the second reading will be abnormally high.

More Whats And Whys About Blood Pressure

Do without food (and smoking!) for half an hour before you take your blood pressure: just prior to a reading, both can influence the results. So can exertion, pain, cold, climate changes, emotional turmoil, a distended bladder—and even the time of day. Try to stick to a particular time (or times) when you regularly measure your blood pressure and, as best you can, eliminate other factors that might affect pressure readings. (Note to obese persons: your reading may be artificially high; discuss this with your doctor.)

Not everyone can use the common equipment for measuring blood pressure. If your hearing's poor, you won't catch the pulse sounds. If your vision's poor you won't see the gradations of the manometer. There is, on the market, a transistorized electronic apparatus that many such incapacitated people might find usable. However, it is quite expensive.

The adult size of the sphygmomanometer (which properly should be 5 to 5½ inches wide) is unsuitable for use with children. Pediatricians have a special size for their small patients.

The old notion that rising blood pressure is a normal and inevitable accompaniment of old age has been discredited by many investigators of primitive people not yet hooked on the "Western Way." In a study of six tribal societies in the Solomon Islands, led by Dr. Lot Page of Tufts University, it was found that people in the three isolated tribes, who still followed a primitive way of eating and living, did not develop high blood pressure with aging—whereas hypertension showed up increasingly with age in the three more Westernized tribes. Dr. Page concludes as quoted by *Medical Tribune* (March 7, 1973): "Failure of blood pressure to rise with age is normal in human beings." Hypertension is a "civilized" disease.

Thus it is not normal (though it may be average) for an 80-year-old man to have a high systolic pressure of 180—despite that old saw that the "top" pressure "should be" 100-plus-your-age.

What's Normal Blood Pressure?

Just what *is* normal pressure? And when should you be concerned because it's "too high"?

Generally, adults are considered within the normal range if the higher, or systolic, pressure falls between 100 and 140 and the lower, diastolic, pressure readings are in the range of 60 to 90. A reading of 120/80 is considered a normal blood pressure for a healthy young adult.

Though some authorities dispute the emphasis, it's the diastolic pressure that most physicians consider the key to the diagnosis and management of hypertension. In classifying groups of hypertensive patients and recommending appropriate treatments, the High Blood Pressure National Task Force goes by the diastolic pressure only. Here are the four groups they identify: (1) from about 90 to 105 mm Hg. diastolic pressure; (2) between 105 and 120; (3) between 120 and 140; and (4) greater than 140. We might dub these classifications mild, moderate, severe, and very severe.

Patients in Group Four—the very severe—should be hospitalized for individualized therapy, the Task Force says. For those in Groups Two and Three, medication is recommended—and in escalating amounts if smaller doses prove ineffective. But for the mild cases—those with a diastolic pressure of less than 105—the Task Force recommends "observation and management," preferably *without* the use of drug therapy. To date, at least, there is no evidence that antihypertensive drugs cut down the risk of future complications in patients with mild high blood pressure.

This is not to say that the mild form of the disease is harmless. On the contrary, as insurance statistics have long indicated, elevated blood pressure—even when mild—increases the risk of future complications. Even within normal ranges, you're better off at the lower end, as insurance figures also show. But for those patients in Group One, drugs have not yet been shown to be helpful.

When it comes to patients in Groups Two and Three, the recommended initial drug (the one with the fewest bad side effects) is a diuretic. Diuretics promote the excretion of water and salt and thereby cut down on fluid retention. This (it is thought) reduces the volume of blood the heart must pump, and so lowers the pressure (like reducing the pressure in a garden hose by turning down the water faucet).

As a side effect, most diuretics also promote the excretion of two important minerals—potassium and magnesium. If the doctor ever puts you on a diuretic ("water pill"), be sure to take the supplement dolomite for its magnesium, and eat plenty of potassium-rich foods, which include bananas, oranges, and dried peaches and apricots. (Some diuretics are chemically engineered not to cause potassium loss; be sure to find out which kind has been prescribed.)

More than 50 antihypertensive drugs swamp the market, all falling into one of three broad classes. Besides the diuretics, there are compounds that relax the tiniest arterial vessels (the arterioles) so that peripheral resistance to blood flow is reduced. A third class of drugs acts upon the sympathetic nervous system. Doctors often add one or another of these medications to diuretic therapy.

Is There A Cure Without Drugs?

If you can help it, you don't want to take drugs—any drugs! If you find you have mild hypertension (or even a diastolic pressure slightly over 105), stop the doctor when he reaches for the old prescription pad. Tell him you'd like to bring your pressure down by natural means if at all possible. Chances are he'll work with you on this; "change in life style" is one of the medically recognized treatments for hypertension. The National Task Force recommends the following: regular exercise, adequate rest, low-salt diet, abstinence from tobacco, minimizing all types of life stress or anxiety-provoking situations, and keeping the cholesterol level normal by diet or other means.

Without expanding on the above, here are a few more tips on natural methods for lowering pressure. There's scattered evidence that both onions and garlic are antihypertensive. Eat these vegetables plentifully or take daily concentrated garlic supplements, and see what happens.

Yoga exercise, which produces mental and physical relaxation, significantly reduces blood pressure in hypertensive patients, writes Dr. C. H. Patel in *The Lancet* (November 10, 1973). So join a class in yoga and see what happens.

Regular exercise, authorities agree, decreases blood pressure. But some people with the best of intentions lack resolution when it comes to scheduled trips to the gym, the pool, or the great outdoors; there's always some reason why *this* time it's inconvenient. If you're this type, a stationary bicycle (or a regular bike on a stand) could be your answer. Put in an hour's workout four or five times a week (regularly!) and see what happens to your blood pressure. With your own sphygmomanometer you can see what happens any time you want.

180. Hypertension, Nitrites And Nitrates

While food additives account for a large share of man's exposure to nitrites and nitrates, the agricultural pollution of lands and water sources with nitrous substances is at least of equal importance. An epidemiological study in Colorado links hypertension to high nitrate levels in the water supply.

Dr. William E. Morton, professor of public health and preventive medicine at the University of Oregon Medical School, reported on the study at the annual meeting of the American Public Health Association, meeting in Houston in October, 1970. This is a rural area in Colorado's eastern plains, Dr. Morton said, that showed (in a 1960 survey) a surprisingly high incidence of hypertension and death from that disease. In an attempt to find an explanation for Colorado's 1960 geographic pattern of hypertension distribution, the research team analyzed the hypertension figures in conjunction with a U.S. geological survey of Colorado water supplies in 1959-1960.

They found that only one constituent in the water supply showed marked similarity to the hypertension pattern—namely, the concentration of nitrate. Water hardness or softness, levels of chlorine, levels of sodium—none of these varied in relationship to the incidence of hypertension. The researchers even checked out socio-economic conditions and the availability of physicians as possible factors in the different incidence of hypertension. But no relationship could be inferred from these statistics. However, where hypertension rates were significantly high, there the water showed significantly high nitrate pollution.

Clearly, a cause-and-effect relationship is suggested in this epidemiological picture.

Adding strength to the case is the fact that workers exposed to nitrates in plants that manufacture explosives tend to develop hypertension. Dr. Morton calls attention to findings to this effect in Europe, Japan, and the U.S.: "Chronic cardiovascular toxic effects among workers exposed to organic nitrates in the explosives industry include elevated diastolic blood pressure, lowered pulse pressure, and increased risk of angina pectoris and/or sudden death. In Pennsylvania, male explosive workers aged 20-54 years have been reported to have a coronary artery disease mortality rate about 15 times greater than that of the general male population in that age group."

Most physicians, Dr. Morton noted, are not familiar with the findings on hypertension incidence in the explosives industry. Rather, they think of nitrates in terms of medication for the relief of angina pectoris. However, Dr. Morton cited evidence from a number of research laboratories which "raise the possibility that therapy with long-acting organic nitrates might hasten the progress of coronary artery disease rather than alleviate it. Clearly, this possibility must be investigated."

181. What About Low Blood Pressure?

Some doctors believe that low blood pressure is a blessing, for if you have it, chances are that you won't be afflicted with high blood pressure. Some physicians believe that a systolic (upper reading) blood pressure of 90 is so low that something should be done about it. Others feel that a systolic pressure of 100 to 110 is an indication that something is wrong. The insurance companies hold that a pressure as low as 100 or even 80 is perfectly compatible with good health, if that has always been your blood pressure. But if your average pressure is 120 and suddenly it goes down to 90 or 80, then probably there is something wrong.

Edward P. Jordan, M.D., expressed the feeling of the medical fraternity in his book, *You and Your Health:* "... most of those with low blood pressure are well off and can expect a long life. There are few exceptions; there is a condition known as Addison's disease which, among other symptoms, is characterized by low blood pressure, but this is rare and there are only a few other things which have any serious significance ... In most cases of below-normal blood pressure the cause seems to be exceptionally elastic arteries and this is a good thing. This generally means that hardening of the arteries will be slow to develop and this in turn has much to do with the expectation for a longer life."

Other medical books warn that low blood pressure may be simply an indication of poor nutrition and it is often accompanied by low blood sugar, low basal metabolism, sub-normal temperature, anemia, or hypothyroidism (that is, a thyroid gland which does not secrete normal amounts). In general, low blood pressure seems to go with people who do less of everything than other people do. That is, they may not eat enough or exercise enough which causes their glands to slow down and decrease their secretions. In cases of outright starvation, of course, the blood pressure is always low.

One kind of low blood pressure has been dignified with a medical name—postural hypotension. Hypotension is, of course, low blood pressure, the opposite of hypertension or high blood pressure. Many of us are inclined to feel dizzy or lightheaded when we stand up or sit up from a lying-down position. But the individual with postural hypotension is quite likely to have these symptoms to a serious degree. Any sudden change in posture necessitates a change in blood pressure all over the body. In some people the mechanism which adjusts this change is disordered. So, when they rise suddenly from a prostrate position, the blood does not reach the brain rapidly enough, and they may faint.

Improved Nutrition Can Help Low Blood Pressure

Suppose you are one of those people who feel weak and tired all the time, and suppose your blood pressure is low. The doctor may tell you that there is nothing to worry about. But do you want to go on feeling "all dragged out"? If there is indeed no disorder that is causing your low blood pressure, it's possible that improved nutrition can raise it to the point where you will no longer feel tired.

One study showed that lack of a B vitamin (thiamine) can cause low blood pressure. In this experiment, reported in the *Archives of Internal Medicine*, Vol. 69, a number of volunteers agreed to live on a diet in which there was no thiamine. They ate white bread, canned fruits and vegetables, meat, potatoes, sugar, coffee and so forth. The doctors who conducted the experiment even gave them brewer's yeast so that they would not be deficient in the other B vitamins. But they destroyed the thiamine in the brewer's yeast. In addition, the volunteers got supplements containing vitamins A and D, iron, calcium and phosphorus.

Without exception the volunteers suffered from personality changes as well as physical symptoms. They became tired, grouchy, inefficient, forgetful. Physically, they became constipated and sleepless; they developed neuritis. Their hearts beat abnormally and became enlarged. Their digestive tracts developed all kinds of disorders. They all developed low blood pressure. The experiment had to be stopped in less than six months for it would perhaps have been fatal had it been carried on longer. As soon as the subjects took some thiamine, the symptoms began to disappear and before long they all felt fine once again.

Another diet that can lead to low blood pressure is one lacking in first-class protein. The blood vessels are made of protein as are the other parts of the body and if enough protein is not available they get flabby and gradually waste away, just as muscles do.

If you are worried that your blood pressure is too low, make certain you have no underlying disorder that is responsible. If there seems to be no good reason for your hypotension, then concentrate on making your diet a good one. From the Superintendent of Documents in Washington, D.C., you can secure Agriculture Handbook Number 8 (Composition of Foods) which lists all the common foods according to protein content, giving as well their content of starch, fat, vitamins and minerals. With this book at hand you can easily figure out just how good your nutrition is and what foods to eat to improve it.

182. Stroke!

What is a "stroke"? Why should the aftereffects of this sudden "striking down" kill about 200,000 Americans a year and incapacitate hundreds of thousands of others? Because a stroke does the worst of its damage within a matter of moments or hours, it seems that prevention is the only sure answer. The many warning signals which generally precede the actual stroke provide the perfect means for prevention of a serious stroke. What are these warning signals and what can be done when they occur?

A "stroke" (we used to call it apoplexy) is an insufficiency or complete stoppage of blood to a part of the brain. It may be the result of several different malfunctions or disorders in the blood vessels. One kind of stroke is caused by blood vessels in the brain breaking or giving way so that there is a hemorrhage throughout the brain's tissues. A stroke may be caused, too, by a thickening or a clot in a brain blood vessel which prevents the blood supply from entering the brain. It may also come about as a result of a floating blood clot which lodges in a brain capillary or artery shutting off the supply of blood, hence the supply of oxygen. The brain requires enormous amounts of oxygen for proper functioning—about 20 percent of all the oxygen required by the body. Shutting off this supply of oxygen for even a very short time results in damage.

Each part of the brain is involved with a different part of human activity; one section controls speech, another the movement of the arms or the legs on one side of the body, another controls the muscles of the mouth or the eyes and so forth. Therefore, damage from a non-fatal stroke is immediately reflected in some other part of the body.

There may be extensive paralysis of a limb or limbs. There may be paralysis of a facial muscle, or lasting sensations of numbness in certain parts of the body. There may be difficulty with speech, sometimes involving frightening complexities—for instance, the afflicted person may not be able to associate words with objects so that he calls a table a tree, or a chair a house; he may not be able to write sentences in proper order or may omit important words; there may be "thickness" of speech.

During the months or perhaps years that are sometimes necessary to rehabilitate a victim of stroke, it may appear that his mind is permanently afflicted; whereas the sufferer thinks as clearly as ever, but simply cannot communicate well. Crippling of an arm or a leg may follow a stroke if the affected part of the body is not immediately given good, intensive physiotherapy to keep muscles from deteriorating.

Many of us have warnings of the possibility of major strokes by the occurrence of "little strokes" which indicate that all is not well inside the blood vessels that feed oxygen to the brain. If we act wisely and promptly, we might prevent the "big stroke" which paralyzes or permanently injuries.

What Are The Symptoms Of Little Strokes?

The late Dr. Walter Alvarez, an authority on "little strokes," once stated, "One of the commonest diseases of man is that in which, over the course of 10 or 20 years, a person is gradually pulled down by dozens or scores of thromboses (clots) of little arteries in the brain." Although these little strokes are so common, many physicians never think of diagnosing them as such, partly because patients just don't give their doctors all the symptoms or because the physician is not familiar with all the bizarre, peculiar things that can happen to an individual as the result of a little stroke.

Dr. Alvarez told of a friend who had been incapacitated by a pain in the abdomen (no ulcer was present) and by a slowing down both mentally and physically. The man's wife remembered that the trouble had begun one morning when, for 20 minutes, her husband had been confused and unable to talk. Since then he, who had always been kind and understanding, had become unreasonable and irascible. He was so changed his wife hardly knew him. Dr. Alvarez believes that on that morning the man suffered a little stroke which was responsible for the symptoms that followed. "Often when a suspicious episode is seen, if only the physician would ask the relatives to remember some peculiar spell followed by changes in character and ability, they will tell him that the disease must have started many years before." Physicians rarely see more than one episode in the illness.

Here are some of the many known symptoms of the little stroke: acute indigestion which does not seem to be related to any overindulgence in food or eating any food that disagrees; temporary weakness in one leg which occurs suddenly when one awakes in the morning; sudden unexplained clumsiness of one hand; mental or nervous disability that is all out of proportion to the little stomach or chest pain that may be there; a nervous breakdown or queer group of symptoms that come on suddenly—on one day; a sudden dizzy spell, a blackout or a fall after which the patient shows changes in character or ability to work; sudden drops in a formerly high blood pressure; sudden spells of crying unaccompanied by any feeling of sadness; sudden changes in handwriting or composing sentences in a letter; difficulty in finding words to express oneself; sometimes difficulty in swallowing so that food will go down "the wrong way" and cause choking; the saliva may be thick and ropy, some may drool out of the corner of the mouth; burning of the tongue or mouth, bad taste in the mouth, especially if it occurs only on one side; a burning of the skin or scalp or a feeling of extreme heat or cold on skin or scalp; in rare cases sudden blindness in one or both eyes, or even seeing double for a day or two.

A sudden pain shooting down through the chest is surely cause to suspect a stroke, if there is no evidence of shortness of breath or heart difficulty when walking. However, it is perfectly true that the same disordered vascular system that results in strokes may produce heart emergencies, too. Pain shooting into the abdomen may indicate a little stroke, if it comes on suddenly and if no stomach or digestive symptoms are present. Sudden brief attacks of nausea and vomiting may be little strokes. Most elderly people with supposed Meniere's disease (a disorder involving the organs of balance of the inner ear) may have no trouble at all with their ears so that the dizziness they experience comes from the brain instead—a little stroke.

After a little stroke there may be a sudden burning pain in the hand, wrist or forearm. There may seem to be sudden arthritic changes in a hip or wrist. A fall which the patient says was caused by blacking out may be the result of a little stroke.

An old case of migraine headache may be reactivated by a little stroke. A stroke can bring a psychosis. Tendencies toward depressive feelings or suspicions of others, no longer closely controlled, can completely overtake an individual after a little stroke and change him into someone unfamiliar to his family.

These are some of the symptoms that may indicate that a little stroke has taken place. Undoubtedly there are many more. There seems to be one circumstance common to all—the change comes about suddenly. Symptoms can be traced to the happenings of one day when the stroke took place even though at that time it was not recognized as such.

However the little stroke is merely one part of a long-term disease. The unhealthy condition of the arteries and capillaries which prevails when the little stroke occurs almost always involves hardening of the arteries and may involve high blood pressure.

183. Quick Action In Case Of A Heart Attack

It's the first few minutes of a heart attack that count in terms of "doing something" to help the victim. Dr. Herman Hellerstein, heart specialist in Cleveland, Ohio's University Hospital advises anyone who might be faced with such an emergency to take prompt action because what you do can be a life-saver.

If a person suddenly complains of pains in the chest, loses color, sweats, contorts his face and collapses, do this before doing *anything* else—even before calling the doctor or an ambulance:

Lay the victim flat on the floor—don't let him remain in a heap.

See if you can detect any breathing or a pulse by feeling the artery in the neck. If not, pinch the nostrils and tilt the head back with one hand. With the other hand, hold the neck up and begin breathing into the victim's mouth—two breaths, then rest. During the rest, put the head down, release the nostrils and place one hand on top of the other on the center of the victim's breast bone and press down firmly. Do this 15 times, about once a second, then go back to breathing two breathes into the mouth as before.

Dr. Hellerstein directs, "Repeat this procedure until you can detect a pulse or until the patient has resumed breathing on his own . . . then rush to a telephone and call an ambulance. Scream for help or have someone else phone, but don't ever leave the victim until you see that he is breathing on his own."

Estimates have it that such measures taken regularly could save 50,000 lives a year.

184. Heart Patients Need A Nutrition Program

Victims of congestive heart failure have one overriding concern—to get better and to never, never let it happen again. They follow doctor's orders; they avoid stress and they exercise moderately, according to directions; they don't permit themselves to get excited; they take whatever drugs are prescribed. But one serious problem that chronic congestive heart failure patients have in common is often ignored by their doctors, hence by the sick. They are malnourished.

Joseph G. Pittman, M.D. and Phin Cohen, M.D., writing in the *New England Journal of Medicine* (August 20, 1964) warned that malnutrition is the usual aftermath of heart failure. It might be due to any of three problems: poor appetite, a mixed-up metabolism that mishandles the foods the victims do eat, or excessive nutrient loss through the urine or feces.

A lack of interest in food is common to all wasting diseases, but especially congestive heart failure. Drs. Pittman and Cohen say loss of appetite is so common that there may be some self-protective mechanism behind it, perhaps the body's unconscious effort to avoid the strain a large meal puts on a bad heart. Further, physicians must often impose necessary dietary restrictions that cut out foods that the patient likes best, thereby reducing even more his desire to eat.

Intensifying the problem, the cardiac patient frequently suffers from vague abdominal pains and abdominal swelling along with a frightening difficulty in breathing. Sometimes eating intensifies abdominal distress. Slow digestion and delayed gastric emptying add to the patient's woes. In the presence of congestive heart failure, normal hunger contractions are diminished or replaced by a premature sensation of fullness and satisfaction because of reduced stomach capacity and retarded emptying.

Ordinarily, a sick person with a poor appetite, if he rests quietly, reduces his total energy requirements. By contrast, a patient with heart failure usually burns more energy than before, because he develops a fast heart beat, a rise in body temperature, excessive sweating and other heightened sympathetic nervous system activities. Even with a bed-chair type of existence, the cardiac patient expends abnormal amounts of energy.

Heart failure makes abnormal demands on the breathing muscles, the heart muscle and the blood manufacturing system—all contributing to increased oxygen consumption. The energy expended in labored breathing is clearly more than average, and probably accounts for much of the excessive oxygen consumption in cardiac patients. There is a greater resistance to breathing, attributed to congested lungs, reduced total lung capacity and enlargement of the heart.

Fever is common in congestive heart patients, and fever costs the body valuable nutrients. A rise in body temperature of even one degree increases the body's energy consumption by about seven percent. One study of 172 patients with congestive heart failure showed elevations to 100 degrees F. or greater in 89 percent of the patients. In another study of 200 hospitalized patients with varying degrees of heart failure, researchers found only four who were entirely free of fever. In general, researchers agree that the cardiac patient is highly susceptible to fever-inducing infections.

Some type of increased nutrition seems to be essential to the full recovery of a patient with heart failure. Because he cannot eat more, a daily ration of all of the natural food supplements, especially the B vitamins and vitamin E, must have a high place in any therapeutic program—vitamin E to maintain the extra oxygen he needs, and B vitamins because they are essential to digestion and use of the food he does eat.

The cardiac patient has every reason to be concerned about his chances of recovery, and to guard diligently against another attack. But any plan that does not include good nutrition is incomplete and shortsighted.

185. Statistics Show It— Heart Health Requires Vitamin E

Paralleling the growing recognition of vitamin E's essential role in human physiology is a mounting concern about the widespread—in fact, *prevailing*—deficiency of this nutrient in the American diet.

It is Dr. Wilfrid Shute's theory that deficiency in vitamin E is causally linked to this country's staggering rise in cardiovascular deaths. He points out that a major dietary source of the vitamin, the wheat germ, was removed from the American diet 70 years ago with the widespread practice of milling wheat into refined white flour; it is in the past half century that mortality rates from heart disease (particularly coronary thrombosis) have climbed so steeply as to take on plague dimensions (*Vitamin E for Ailing and Healthy Hearts*, Wilfrid E. Shute, M.D. with Harold J. Taub, Pyramid House, 1969).

Two Alabama professors checked this theory through statistical analysis of heart symptoms in relation to daily vitamin E intake. The study was limited in the number of subjects involved (299); nevertheless, in a given presumably healthy population, low vitamin E intake correlated with a high incidence of cardiovascular symptoms in the older years. Furthermore, correction of the diet over a one-year period led to a reduction of the symptoms.

Dr. E. Cheraskin and his colleague Dr. W. M. Ringsdorf, Jr., of the University of Alabama's Department of Oral Medicine, reported their findings in "Daily Vitamin E Consumption and Reported Cardiovascular Findings," (*Nutrition Report International*, August, 1970). The subjects who were studied in the investigation of vitamin E and cardiovascular symptoms came from Ohio and California. They included 171 dentists and 128 wives. The vast majority were between the ages of 30 and 60.

Each individual in the study was given a dietary analysis. Through a questionnaire based on "food frequencies," the daily average intake of foods and their specific nutrient content was arrived at through computer analysis—a technique of dietary survey (offered by a California firm) which Dr. Cheraskin described as simplified yet broadly accurate and as reliable as any food-intake study "short of putting a patient for a week's stay in a metabolic ward." Because it is inexpensive, convenient, and speedy, this technique could be of enormous value as a routine tool of the medical practitioner, Dr. Cheraskin suggested.

In the Cheraskin-Ringsdorf study, subjects were divided between those whose diet analyses showed they received less than the National Research Council's daily recommended allowance of vitamin E (30 I.U. for men and 25 for women) and those who received the minimum or more. It turned out that, in this population of educated, health-oriented, well-to-do individuals, a full 80 percent were getting less vitamin E than they needed as a bare minimum! Dr. Cheraskin comments that this proportion is consistent with that found in other studies—in other words, typical of Americans, rich and poor.

In addition to the dietary analysis, the patients' cardiovascular health was established in terms of their reported symptoms. For this inventory, the investigators used the subjects' answers to the cardiovascular section of a standard medical form—the Cornell Medical Index Health Questionnaire. The participants answered questions, for example, about chest or heart pains, breathing difficulty, tendency to get out of breath, swollen ankles, cold hands or feet, and leg cramps; they also reported if a physician had ever diagnosed high or low blood pressure or heart trouble.

When the answers to these questions were analyzed in terms of age groups, the investigators found (as expected) that "the data confirms the well-established fact that, with advancing age, there are progressively more cardiovascular symptoms and signs."

However, when the cardiovascular data was studied in relation to vitamin E intake, this startling discovery was made: there was *no* increase with age in the incidence of heart symptoms among the group consuming vitamin E in the minimum recommended amount (or more). As Drs. Cheraskin and Ringsdorf put it: "Cardiovascular findings do indeed increase with age but only in those subjects consuming sub-optimal amounts of vitamin E."

Heart Symptoms Removed With Vitamin E Increase

A still more striking finding was made in a follow-up study conducted one year later. After the original dietary and cardiovascular surveys were completed, the participants convened for a lecture on what the investigators had found out and what they recommended in the way of dietary reform. Some of the dentists and their wives apparently took the lecture most seriously and added vitamin E to their diets either through supplementation or improved eating habits. When, a year later, both the dietary analysis and the cardiovascular questionnaire were repeated (among 95 of the original participants), those individuals who had improved their diets found themselves answering "no" instead of "yes" to a string of questions about suffering heart disease symptoms. Those who had not profited by the lecture experienced no such "luck."

Summarizing the findings, Drs. Cheraskin and Ringsdorf stated: "During this (one year) interval, those who increased vitamin E intake were paralleled by a decrease in cardiovascular symptoms and signs. Those who did not increase vitamin E consumption did not improve with regard to the clinical picture."

As the authors pointed out, theirs is not a "controlled experiment" in the usual sense and "hence the results must be viewed with caution." It also should be recognized that a certain amount of subjectivity could enter the individual's answers to the cardiac questions. Nevertheless, to Drs. Cheraskin and Ringsdorf, the evidence they uncovered "suggests that vitamin E may play a more significant role than heretofore recognized," and they expressed the hope that their observations "will catalyze interest in this apparently new area and generate additional study."

A large-scale controlled study on vitamin E and heart disease, comparable in scope to the massive research on heart disease and dietary fats, would be a dramatic step toward reversing the tragic pattern of mounting heart deaths in this country.

But we do not have to wait for that day to benefit individually from the research of the Alabama professors. Bring vitamin E-rich foods to the table. Among the richest sources are seed and germ oils, alfalfa (tablets or alfalfa tea) and lettuce. It's advisable, too, to take a natural vitamin E supplement as well.

As the Cheraskin-Ringsdorf study shows in the case of the dentists and their wives, vitamin E may forestall cardiovascular symptoms—and even reverse them if brought to the rescue in time. Even more important, a daily intake of several hundred units (build up to this slowly, starting with 100) may be the nearest you will ever come to insurance against coronary thrombosis.

Vitamin E In Heart Surgery

In open-heart surgery, there's evidence that a high vitamin E level in the patient's blood protects against some of the damage to red blood cells that normally occurs during this lengthy and complicated surgical procedure. However, Max K. Horwitt, Ph.D., of the Chemistry Department at St. Louis University School of Medicine, established—"conclusively," he thought— that giving the patient an extra boost of vitamin E prior to surgery did not result in sustained higher vitamin E levels in the blood.

But he had based these findings on what happens when vitamin E is given in an intramuscular *injection*. More recently, he discovered that when adequate doses are given by mouth (the way people normally *do* take vitamin E supplements), high levels of serum tocopherol (vitamin E) were maintained. A gram or two of vitamin E given orally a day or so before surgery is scheduled, Dr. Horwitt said, provides levels of serum vitamin E that should allow the antioxidant effect of the nutrient to reduce oxidative damage to red cells during the operation. Data gathered by Dr. Horwitt and his colleagues (J. D. Marco and J. F. Schweiss) at the St. Louis School of Medicine, indicated that raising the patient's plasma alpha-tocopherol level should be considered before open-heart surgery is performed.

At the April, 1975, meeting of the Federation of American Societies for Experimental Biology, Atlantic City, Dr. Horwitt presented a paper on "Use of Alpha-Tocopherol to Decrease Oxidative Hemolysis During Cardiac Surgery."

186. Anti-Cholesterol Drugs Deplete Vitamin E

Vitamin E's major role in the prevention of heart disease is its antithrombotic (anti-clotting) function. Coronary thrombosis, which is caused by a clot blocking the coronary arteries, is the major cause of death from heart disease. Vitamin E, by preventing and dissolving clots, is a specific preventative of this catastrophe. In the words of Dr. Wilfrid E. Shute, pioneer clinical investigator in this field: "Not only will vitamin E dissolve clots, but circulating in the blood of a healthy individual (it) will prevent thrombi from forming." (*Vitamin E for Ailing and Healthy Hearts*, Pyramid House, 1969.)

Yet this natural protector of the heart and circulatory system is the victim of drugs taken for the purpose of avoiding heart disease!

Johns Hopkins Study

The discovery that hypolipidemic drugs (drugs used in reducing serum fat levels) have the side effect of lowering the patient's store of vitamin E was reported in the October, 1969, issue of *The American Journal of the Medical Sciences*. The authors of the article, Drs. Peter Weiss and J. R. Bianchine, of the Johns Hopkins School of Medicine, reported on a clinical study performed with 17 out-patients at the Johns Hopkins Hospital. All the patients had high serum levels of either cholesterol or triglycerides (another fatty substance also implicated in the formation of deposits on arterial walls). The drugs used were clofibrate and SU-13437.

Both drugs reduced the fats in the serum and also the vitamin E content. The total reduction of vitamin E amounted to as much as two-thirds in some patients. Vitamin E levels returned upward when the therapy was discontinued.

Just how the hypolipidemic drugs act to cut down the level of vitamin E is still a matter of speculation, Drs. Weiss and Bianchine indicate. "The drugs may impair the absorption or increase the metabolic breakdown of tocopherol," the authors suggest; or they may reduce the synthesis of substances in the blood carrier (lipoprotein) that provide carrier sites for fat soluble vitamins. In the present experiment, the authors note, vitamin E levels parallel serum lipid levels in the patients studied; and, they report, patients with hyperlipidemia (abnormally high concentration of lipids, or fats, in the blood) have higher than normal tocopherol levels. This, very likely, is how the body tries to protect itself against high lipid levels.

The Hopkins researchers conclude by pointing to some very suggestive findings that the drug, clofibrate, has on occasion caused side effects similar to diseased conditions noted in experimental animals made deficient in vitamin E. These involve liver damage and muscular degeneration.

Questions about diet and its relation to cholesterol level, atherosclerosis, and death from heart disease have been the subject of continual investigation since the late 1940's. Several dietary factors have been blamed in the course of research. The most familiar and widely accepted of these theories pertains to the ingestion of fats; a diet low in saturated fats (the hard fats such as animal fat, butter fat, and hydrogenated vegetable fats such as oleomargarine and shortening used in baking) and high in polyunsaturated fats (liquid vegetable oils) is often recommended as a preventive of atherosclerosis and heart disease.

However, results from research testing this and other diets are inconclusive and often contradictory. There is still no satisfactory direct evidence from controlled clinical trials.

Another major failing in the studies of diet and heart disease is that they do not take into consideration the role of vitamin E. Now, regardless of the cholesterol level and regardless even of the condition of the arteries, the most frequent cause of death through heart disease, coronary thrombosis, occurs *only* when a blood clot forms. Thus vitamin E, which is known for its anti-clotting properties, is surely a dietary factor that ought to be considered in assaying the relation of diet to the incidence of heart deaths.

187. B Vitamins Could Save Your Heart

Pyridoxine (vitamin B_6), along with potassium, was used regularly for five years by John Ellis, M.D., to treat emergency myocardial infarction. In *Vitamin B_6, the Doctor's Report*, (Harper & Row, Publishers Inc., 1973) he asserted, ". . . I believe that this routine treatment has reduced the mortality rate of my patients. The demonstrated difference in the cardiograms is sufficient to conclude that pyridoxine improves electrical conduction in the heart that has suffered a recent infarction. This seems sufficient reason for using B_6 in treating patients who have suffered myocardial infarctions."

A colleague at the same hospital, Dr. Vanis Pennington, a specialist in internal medicine, was asked if he thought it was the pyridoxine or the potassium that had led to improvement in the cardiograms of Dr. Ellis' patients. He acknowledged that although he often gave his own patients potassium, they did not enjoy the same degree of improvement in their electrocardiograms as those who also took pyridoxine.

Dr. Ellis stated, "On the basis of my studies I would suggest that there is a dietary relationship between myocardial infarction and advanced vitamin B_6 deficiency . . . somewhere between the early life of the fetus and the terminal gasps of the coronary thrombosis victim, an increased need for vitamin B_6 stands paramount as an associate in the cause of the deadly heart attack and myocardial infarction."

In *The Cholesterol Controversy* (Sherbourne Press, 1973) authors Edward R. Pinckney, M.D., and Cathey Pinckney state that vitamin B_3 (nicotinic acid) has long been used as a treatment for high blood cholesterol counts. The exact way this vitamin works is not known, nor is it successful with every patient. The Pinckneys suggest one explanation B_3 is used in treating certain mental and emotional problems. "It is possible that its reported anxiety-reducing action could have some effect in cholesterol lowering."

The B vitamin that has stirred the most investigative activity in its relation to heart health is thiamine. Some researchers link thiamine shortage to excessive carbohydrate consumption, particularly sugar.

When heart attacks strike down heavy consumers of carbohydrate foods, most laymen and many doctors attribute the calamity to too many calories. Most carbohydrate foods do have a heavy calorie count, but experiments are showing that the action of the sugar in the calorie-rich foods is probably the major trouble maker, not the calories. Thiamine, notably lacking in patients with heart trouble, is a known victim of excessive sugars in the body.

A convincing demonstration of the relationship between carbohydrate consumption, thiamine shortage and incipient heart trouble among relatively healthy individuals appeared in *The International Journal for Vitamin Research* (37, No. 4, 1967) by E. Cheraskin, M.D., D.M.D., professor and chairman of the Department of Oral Medicine at the University of Alabama Medical Center, and associates. Cheraskin recruited 74 dentists and their wives to answer the questions in the standard Cornell Medical Index Health Questionnaire dealing with cardiovascular symptoms and signs: ("Do you have pains in the heart or the chest?" "Are you often bothered by thumping of the heart?" "Does heart trouble run in your family?" "Do you get out of breath long before anyone else?" etc.) Twenty-six of the men and 15 of the woman (a total of 55.4 percent) had no cardiovascular complaints whatsoever, but 16 percent of the total group had at least one complaint, and 10.8 percent had two complaints. One woman said yes to seven out of 13 questions that might indicate cardiovascular problems.

The same group participated in a seven-day dietary survey through which the researchers calculated the daily thiamine intake. The subjects with the most heart problems, it turned out, were the older people in the study who consumed the least thiamine.

Less Thiamine, More Heart Trouble

In order to compare the cardiovascular complaints to dietary consumption, the dentists and their wives were divided into two equal subgroups: of these 74 individuals, 37 consumed .13 to .91 milligrams of thiamine a day (Group One); the remaining 37 consumed .92 to 2.95 milligrams of thiamine a day (Group Two).

The same division was done for consumption of non-processed carbohydrates and processed carbohydrates.

When all of these groups were compared, the two groups with the highest number of cardiovascular complaints were also found to have a higher consumption of processed carbohyrates and a lower consumption of thiamine than the rest. "Additionally," wrote Cheraskin, "the three groups with the highest mean cardiovascular scores (the most complaints) have a common denominator of smaller thiamine consumption." In other words, the paper was able to demonstrate that persons with heart complaints tend to be those who consume more carbohydrates and less thiamine. (It is important to note that, when carbohydrates are consumed, increased amounts of thiamine are necessary to process them in the system.) "It should be underlined that the relationships observed here do not, in themselves, prove cause-and-effect. However, it is noteworthy that the findings are consistent with other reports indicating the relationship of carbohydrate consumption to cardiovascular disease."

Plenty Of Support

Although Dr. Cheraskin is among the most renowned and influential of the research scientists who have delved into the problem of carbohydrates, thiamine and heart disease, he properly called attention to the many previous experiments that support this relationship. The major difference between Cheraskin's work and that of other scientists is that his has included living humans. Others have worked largely with laboratory animals or deceased humans.

Earl E. Aldinger, Ph.D., from the Department of Medicine, Tulane School of Medicine, put living rats on a thiamine-free diet for five weeks. During that time the tissues surrounding the heart showed a marked loss (69 percent) of tension and elasticity. The animals were also inclined toward an erratic heartbeat. As the weeks without thiamine went on, the irregularity was more and more pronounced. Many of the rats died during the experiment.

The role of thiamine in heart failure was touched on briefly in *Nutrition Reviews* (October, 1955). M. G. Wohl, *et al.* did their testing on human cadavers. Wohl measured the thiamine content of the heart muscle and of the liver and kidney tissues in 12 patients who died from heart failure with evidence of various kinds of severe organic heart disease.

These tissues were compared with similar tissues taken from ten patients who had no heart disease and who died of other causes. The doctors found a consistent decrease in the average thiamine content of the heart muscles in the cardiac patients as compared with the control subjects.

The total thiamine in the "non-cardiacs" was 1.37 micrograms per gram of tissue as compared to .60 micrograms for the cardiac subjects. *Nutrition Reviews* commented, "Because of the nature of the study, it was presumably impossible for the author to obtain histories of food intake on either the cardiacs or control individuals prior to death so that these could be compared. The assumption would seem valid that the patients dying of severe cardiac disease had not been well nourished for a considerable period of time prior to death. Whether the deficiencies found were sufficient to impair the metabolism of heart muscle was not known, although, as the authors indicate, these evidences of under-nutrition with respect to thiamine are certainly suggested."

The possible relationship between sugars and heart disease was clear in the 1950s, but at that time the medical world was primarily involved with the cholesterol-heart trouble theory. Generally speaking, it still is.

188. Vitamin C, A Natural Heart Medicine

Many people think of vitamin C in terms of protection against infection, but few are aware of its value as a tool for surviving a heart attack.

Although their work is not widely known in the United States, a Scottish medical research team has demonstrated that, following a myocardial infarction, the heart is in such dire need of vitamin C for healing itself that it snaps up the available supply to the extent that the rest of the body is reduced to outright deficiency levels.

Dr. R. Hume and his colleagues at Southern General Hospital, Glasgow, Scotland, reported in the *British Heart Journal* (1972, 34, 238-243) that their patients were 31 individuals (26 men and 5 women) who were admitted to the hospital very shortly after suffering a heart attack.

The first finding that they made was that within six to twelve hours after the attack, leukocyte ascorbic acid levels dropped precipitously all the way down to levels typical of people suffering from the vitamin C deficiency disease, scurvy. (Leukocytes are white blood cells, and their ascorbic acid levels are considered the best measure of the general ascorbic acid sufficiency of the body as a whole. Circulating in the bloodstream, the leukocytes' vitamin C load is always available to tissues in need.)

Continuing their measurements, the team of five Scottish physicians found that circulating levels of ascorbic acid rose very slightly after one day and continued rising gradually for several weeks, "eventually reaching normal levels one month after infarction."

But where did all the vitamin C go during the acute phase of the heart attack?

The immediate suspicion was that it went to the heart. Since the earliest days of ascorbic acid research, it has been known that the most obvious function of vitamin C is to participate in the formation of the body's connective tissue. This tissue is actually a variety of substances which are found everywhere in the body, and which literally hold all soft tissue together. If the skeleton is something like the beams in a house, the connective tissue is the mortar between the bricks (the cells)—only more so, because there are billions of times more cells in the body than there are bricks in the largest house. Without vitamin C, there can be no tissue repair, because the proliferation of new cells would be a meaningless jumble of mushy tissue, unable to hold its shape or perform any function.

In a heart attack, the blocking of a coronary artery has caused oxygen deprivation and consequent death or damage to portions of the heart muscle, and tissue repair is exactly what the heart must have following this injury.

Vitamin C Helps The Heart Heal Itself

To determine if the heart muscle had indeed picked up the ascorbic acid supply of the circulating leukocytes, the investigators undertook a second study. This time they compared 17 samples of heart muscle from patients who suffered a coronary death to 26 samples from patients who suffered non-coronary death.

Their suspicions proved correct. They found that the hearts of the coronary victims contained much greater concentrations of ascorbic acid. *The average level of the vitamin in the injured hearts was 25 percent higher than the presumably normal level found in the non-injured hearts.*

Dr. Hume and his colleagues concluded that: "The low leukocyte ascorbic acid for the two weeks after infarction is probably a reflection of (the) healing process, and is due to the deviation of ascorbic acid-laden leukocytes from the circulation to the heart muscle."

This period of healing with ascorbic acid, which lasts for about two weeks, is of special importance, because, as the physicians note, "Thereafter, healing by fibrous scar formation takes place."

Dr. Hume and his co-workers see profound implications in these findings, and many intriguing links to other recent research into vitamin C and the heart. They tell about a 1966 experiment by S. Gudbjarnason and others involving dogs in which myocardial infarction had been induced. Compared to unsupplemented animals, dogs given ascorbic acid showed a 122 percent increase in protein synthesis *in the very center of the infarcted area of the heart muscle.* Protein, of course, is the primary substance required for tissue repairs—more specifically, the fibrous protein called collagen, whose synthesis is dependent on vitamin C action.

Dr. Richard Bing of Wayne State University in Detroit, found ascorbic acid to be of great value in promoting healing in experimental animals after myocardial infarction.

Because heart failure causes not only vascular incapacity and restriction of capillary blood flow, but also changes in enzyme patterns, Dr. Bing did enzyme studies which showed that the process of repair in the damaged heart muscle can be accelerated by three different treatments: ascorbic acid, the anabolic steroids and a treatment called the Sodi-Pallares polarizing therapy.

Dr. Demetrio Sodi-Pallares of the National Institute of Cardiology in Mexico used the term 'polarizing therapy' to refer to an electrolyte therapy utilizing a combination of diet and a solution of glucose, insulin, and potassium chloride which contributes to repolarization (the orderly arrangement of nuclei and tissue permitting normal life activities, such as cell regeneration and rhythmic contraction and expansion) of myocardial fibers, the first step in the restoration of heart health. Dr. Sodi-Pallares told a meeting of the New York Academy of Sciences in January, 1967, that "digitalis compounds and diuretic drugs in heart failure, the vasodilator agents in angina and coronary insufficiency, the hypotensive drugs and diuretics in hypertension, have yielded their place of honor to this treatment."

Vitamin Avoids Drug Dangers

Supplementing the work of Dr. Sodi-Pallares, Dr. Bing of Detroit achieved the effect of the 'polarizing therapy' using ascorbic acid which plays a vital role in cellular metabolism. The insulin in the original polarizing solution, Dr. Bing said, acts like a growth hormone, stimulating the growth of new tissue. But insulin can promote dangerous complications, especially where there is diabetes or problems of renal function. Potassium is a valuable adjunct in this therapy because it helps restore the alkaline balance necessary for optimal regularity of the heart beat. Severe heart attack is usually accompanied by severe acidosis. However, potassium intake, too, must be carefully regulated. Over-dosage can produce weakness, confusion, paresthesia, and an irregular heartbeat.

Use of the anabolic steroids, while helpful in providing the adrenal hormone which triggers heart action and promotes the growth of new cells, is riddled with dangerous side-effects. Continued use of cortisone, for instance, tends to deplete the system of calcium, another element vital to the health of the heart. Patients on cortisone develop abnormally round faces and abnormal growths of hair. Steroids can also cause ulcers, high blood pressure and diabetes.

Of the three therapies found effective in promoting the regeneration of the heart muscle, the only one without any deleterious side-effects is vitamin C.

This is not surprising. What a vitamin helps to prevent, it often helps to cure, and the effect of vitamin C on cardiovascular health is well known. Vitamin C triggers the enzyme which breaks down cholesterol and triglycerides into free fatty acids, thus clearing the blood vessels for healthy circulation. When the tissues are well supplied with ascorbic acid, there is less chance for lipids to accumulate into the kind of fatty plaques that cling to artery walls, clog them and keep the arteries themselves from receiving an adequate blood supply, a condition which is a precursor of myocardial infarction or heart block.

Fights Stress Damage
Stress is another condition leading to the formation of blood clots. Stress triggers the adrenal glands to produce more of a substance which uses up vitamin C. It is felt that exposure to the stress of surgery is responsible for blood clots after operations, and some surgeons are prescribing massive doses of ascorbic acid before, after, and even during surgery.

A Natural, Miraculous Medicine
All of this presents a picture of vitamin C as a natural medicine for the ailing heart. It rushes to the precise scene of the injury, reaching maximum concentration in less than half a day. It immediately goes to work to spark the natural healing process—something which no drug claims to do. It has several weeks to complete the job. After that, whatever healing takes place is not in the form of new, viable tissue that can help the heart back to its normal function, but merely scar tissue.

These revelations in turn provide a double rationale for vitamin C supplementation as routine for heart patients.

First, it makes sense to insure that the absolute maximum amount of vitamin C is available to be carried to the heart by the circulating leukocytes.

Second, supplementation would bring the levels of vitamin C

in other parts of the body to normal levels, after they have been severely reduced by the migration of the vitamin to the heart. Being flat on your back in a hospital in a very weakened condition leaves you so vulnerable to infection that it would be foolish not to try to build up the body's natural defenses with large amounts of vitamin C.

Vitamin C is clearly an emergency first aid for the damaged heart. Of course, the main interest is in preventing an emergency from ever arising. Can vitamin C actually help in accomplishing this goal?

The Scottish doctors seem to think it can. They think it's a question that needs some very serious looking into. Here's why:

Atherosclerosis is said to develop in arteries "at sites of mechanical stress," Dr. Hume says. Referring to a study by Willis and Fishman which was published in 1955, he goes on to say that when these stressed areas of the arteries were examined at an autopsy, "localized depletion of ascorbic acid" was discovered. Adjacent, healthier segments of the arteries which were not stressed had a higher content of vitamin C. Further, "there was some evidence to suggest that it was possible to replenish the ascorbic acid in the arteries by ascorbic acid therapy."

It would be foolish, of course, to assume that adequate vitamin C is the sole nutrient required for arterial health. Many nutrients—other vitamins, fatty acids, protein, and minerals—are needed for the proper functioning of all body cells. Smoking, lack of exercise, and heredity also undoubtedly play an important role. But it does seem that, for many people, insufficient vitamin C is likely to be the decisive contributing cause when arteries begin to degenerate.

In this sense, atherosclerosis and its often fatal consequences to heart and brain could be described as a deficiency disease— marginal deficiency in ascorbic acid. Quite apart from research on animals and individual human patients, there's epidemiological evidence to support this concept. A British study showed that deaths from heart attacks and strokes were directly related to low dietary intake of vitamin C. In regions of England and Wales where the typical diet contained few vitamin C-rich foods such as fresh fruits and vegetables, the incidence of death from these diseases was high, researchers from the University of Birmingham discovered. And the reverse was also true: where dietary vitamin C intake was high, there was a low incidence of these fatal disorders stemming from atherosclerotic arteries.

We know from Dr. Hume's work that when a heart attack strikes, vitamin C is rushed to the scene by the body's natural and infinitely complex healing processes, so we know that vitamin C is of vital importance in restoring the injured heart to health.

How essential is vitamin C for *preventing* a heart attack? The evidence clearly suggests its great value.

189. Vitamin D And Your Heartbeat

Most of us are aware of the many roles played by calcium in our bodies. But not many of us realize that without another essential material—vitamin D—calcium is a lame duck. Most of the calcium in the body is used by the bones, the teeth, the nerves and muscles. Only one percent is present in the body fluids. Vitamin D helps to keep that calcium level strategically balanced.

Long known as the "sunshine vitamin," vitamin D has been recognized for 40 years as a preventive and cure for rickets— once a widespread threat to a baby's normal growth. Without vitamin D, calcium cannot be absorbed through the intestinal wall, and it cannot be deposited in the bones. These functions of vitamin D have been known for many years.

But research reported at the Second Drummond Memorial Lecture held at University College, London (October, 1970), demonstrated that vitamin D plays a far more critical role than was formerly believed. Not only is vitamin D necessary to make deposits of calcium to the bones, but vitamin D retains possession of the key that permits calcium to be withdrawn again, when needed. Dr. E. M. Lawson of the Dunn Nutritional Laboratory of the University of Cambridge pointed out at the Drummond Lecture, that "the function of vitamin D is two-fold, being required for the proper mobilization of bone, for example calcium acquisition and, in addition, for the mobilization of calcium into blood." Vitamin D is actually required for the body's proper regulation of calcium from the time it enters the body, through the various avenues through which it is utilized. As Dr. Lawson points out, "The balance of calcium between the plasma and bone is maintained by vitamin D, calcitonin, and parathyroid hormone, with the latter hormone only able to act in the presence of vitamin D."

Bone Regulating Hormones Need Vitamin D

Calcitonin, the thyroid hormone discovered by Peter Sanderon and his associates at the Peter Bent Brigham Hospital in Boston and Dr. Harold Copp at the University of British Columbia, controls the flow of calcium from the bones into the plasma. By inhibiting the breakdown of bone and keeping the calcium in the blood from reaching excessively high levels, it plays an important role in metabolism, Howard Rasmussen and Maurice M. Pechet reported in *Scientific American,* October, 1970.

A constant supply of calcium and phosphate is required in the circulating blood for the building of bone and the control of important functions of cells. If the concentration of calcium ions (electrically charged molecules) in the blood plasma falls below normal, the nerve and muscle cells begin to discharge spontaneously and the voluntary muscles go into continuous contraction. The heartbeat becomes irregular and weaker. To prevent such disturbances, the body endeavors to maintain a good supply of calcium in the blood, borrowing from the bones when necessary and returning it when possible. Vitamin D is essential to both functions and their proper control.

It is the parathyroid hormone that causes the release of calcium to the blood from bone and induces the kidney tubules to capture calcium that would otherwise be lost in the urine and return it to the circulating blood. Calcitonin exerts a control on the level of accumulation of calcium in the blood. It is a check on the activity of the parathyroid hormone. Both hormones are essential to the mobilization and positive control of calcium, and both need vitamin D in order to perform their functions.

The fact that vitamin D plays an indispensable role in both the deposit and withdrawal of calcium gives to this vitamin much more importance than was formerly recognized. Besides being necessary to bones, teeth, and nerves, calcium is absolutely essential to every beat of the heart.

If for some reason your calcium pool becomes dangerously low, your heart will flutter and fibrillate (twitch) and send out an SOS for more calcium. *Vitamin D must be on the job before this calcium can be withdrawn from the bones to come to the aid of your heart.*

This important bit of teamwork between vitamin D and calcium might provide a clue to the mystery of why perfectly healthy men with no history or evidence of any heart problems, when they undergo a strenuous exercise session, will sometimes develop cardiac arrhythmias (variation from the normal rhythm of the heartbeat). That is what happened when exercise tests were given to healthy male executives at NASA's Manned Spacecraft

The Heart

Center (*Medical Tribune,* June 7, 1972). Dr. Earl F. Beard told
the Ninth International Conference of Cardiology that "significant cardiac arrhythmias were encountered during exercise or
recovery" in 154 of 1,385 ergometric tests periodically administered to the study group.

On entry into the program, the men had no "clinically detectable cardiovascular disease" Dr. Beard emphasized. The fact that
34 percent of the subjects or 84 participants demonstrated some
irregularity in heartbeat during testing at some time during
participation was a puzzle to Dr. Beard, who commented that
previous studies, showing that arrhythmias may occur during
exercise, had suggested that these heart irregularities occur more
often in patients with organic heart disease. *But none of the men
in the NASA study had "detectable cardiovascular disease."*

Dr. Beard wondered if some of the subjects might have latent
ischemic heart disease (insufficient blood supply to the heart).
But none of them demonstrated ischemic ST segment depression
on the electrocardiograms performed during exercise and after
exercise. "This suggests that an impaired oxygen supply to the
heart muscle is unlikely," Dr. Beard noted.

What then could have been causing the irregular heart beat in
these healthy men? Dr. Beard was mystified. The mystery might
have been cleared up with the realization that increased heart
activity requires increased calcium, which will not be supplied
unless there is enough vitamin D in the system.

Remember that these NASA executives were subjected to
intensive monitoring of their vital signs—pulse, electrocardiogram and other ergometric tests of physical stamina. This is
certainly a wise precaution because these are good measurements of sensible limits to physical exertion. The executives also
underwent an annual physical examination in which their nutritional status was evaluated. But this examination was done in a
different department and whatever nutritional data was elicited
was not channeled into the "fitness" program which uncovered
the arrhythmias. And, in any event the nutritional evaluation did
not include a determination of serum calcium status.

Vitamin D Shortage Deprives The Heart Of Calcium

So vital is calcium to the heart, that when the heart is short of
calcium, the bloodstream withdraws calcium from the bones and
carries it to the heart. *But, if vitamin D is lacking, the blood is
unable to complete this lifesaving maneuver.* It is certainly a

probability that the strenuous exercise which the NASA executives were undergoing, by increasing the work of the heart, reduced their plasma calcium pools. Among those who had too little vitamin D in their systems, the body's normal adjustment process would be unable to work. The expected result would be variations in the heart beat.

Unlike other vitamins, vitamin D is not present in significant amounts in the normal diet. This "sunshine vitamin" is produced in the skin. W. Farnsworth Loomis of Brandeis University described the process in *Science*, August 4, 1967: solar rays from the far-ultraviolet region of the spectrum convert the pro-vitamin 7-dehydrocholesterol into natural vitamin D. Vitamin D also occurs in the liver oils of bony fishes and, in very small amounts, in a few foodstuffs in the summer. Almost none is present in foodstuffs in winter, Dr. Loomis says.

The term vitamin D, is, in fact, almost a misnomer, says Dr. Loomis, because this factor resembles the hormones more closely than it resembles the vitamins in that it is not eaten but is synthesized in the body by the skin and then distributed by the bloodstream for action elsewhere in the body.

As with hormones, but unlike most other vitamins, too much vitamin D is as bad as too little. Rickets, osteomalacia, and other disabilities relative to the use of calcium are the result of too little. When there is too much vitamin D, the blood carries high levels of calcium and phosphorus and lays it down in the soft tissues causing multiple calcifications.

Unlike other vitamins, this essential calcification factor which mediates the absorption of calcium from the intestine, the deposition of minerals as in growing bones, and the withdrawal of it in cases of emergency is not present in significant amounts in a normal diet.

More than 50 years ago we learned that the way to stop vitamin D deficiency is to make sure we get enough fish and especially fish liver oil. The same sources are available to us today.

Many physicians whose patients question them about vitamins will tell them, "Take them if you want—it's your money. But I must advise you to avoid vitamin D. You're getting plenty in your diet and too much can cause serious trouble."

True, too much can be toxic but the fear of toxicity has become so exaggerated that we are in serious danger of getting too little rather than too much. The National Research Council recommends 400 units daily. Yet when teenage girls were given 1,250 mg. of calcium daily—the amount supplied by five glasses of milk (containing 650 units of vitamin D) they excreted far more calcium than they retained. (*American Journal of Dis. of Children* 67, 265, 1944.) When the vitamin D was upped to 3,900 units daily, ten times more calcium was retained in the body.

Roger Williams points out in *Nutrition Against Disease* (*Pitman*, New York, 1971), "There is no vitamin that cannot be administered safely at a level ten times that of the usual supposed need."

When calculating your own needs, remember that stress, illness and aging bones increase the drain on vitamin D stores. R. W. Smith *et al* point out in the *American Journal of Clinical Nutrition* that 2,500 to 5,000 units daily is advantageous to adults.

190. Calcium For Heart Health

Exercise and good nutrition are allies in the good fight to keep your heart ticking away rhythmically year after healthy year.

One food element which is absolutely vital to the health of your heart is calcium. And, it is important to bear in mind, the more you exercise the more calcium your heart needs. Calcium has been termed "the prime instigator of vital activity." It is present in every single cell of the body.

Most of us realize that calcium is necessary to good teeth, good bones, and strong fingernails. But not many people realize that one of the most vital functions of calcium in the body is regulation of the very beat of your heart. And since every beat of the heart requires this important mineral, it stands to reason that every time you jog, bike, swim, ski, do push-ups, lift weights, push a lawnmower, swing a golf club, play ping-pong, tennis or badminton, you are quickening your heartbeat and therefore increasing your calcium requirements.

The fact that calcium is indispensable to the heart's ability to keep working was discovered by Dr. Winifrid Nayler of the Baker Medical Research Institute. He described what takes place in the *Heart Journal* for March, 1967. It involves an electro-chemical process which takes place within every cell in your heart with every beat. On the outer surface of each heart tissue cell there is a thin filament called actin. The actin reaches with a kind of magnetic attraction toward the center of the cell, thereby shortening its length. The result of many cells shortening at one time brings about contraction of the muscle, and it is calcium, fed to the actin by the bloodstream, that provides both the stimulus and the means by which the actin does its work. A shortage of calcium must inevitably result in a weakened heartbeat, which can be sped up by drug stimulants but cannot be strengthened, as long as the calcium is deficient.

Calcium is not a loner. No nutrient is. An important partner to calcium for cardiovascular health is magnesium.

It is vital that the actin absorb and release the calcium; absorb and release; push—pull; push—pull. If the heart muscle could not do both actions, your heart would contract and stay that way or else refuse to contract at all. What gives it the rhythmic push—pull? The mineral magnesium. In very small amounts it plays a heart saving role. It provides a tiny positive electrical charge that repels calcium, pushing it to the opposite side of the cell and thus reversing the contraction.

The older you get the more you need calcium because your ability to absorb it diminishes with advancing years. In the mature years, then, especially if you are exercising, it is important to make up for the poor absorption mechanism by insuring a higher level of intake. "In general," Dr. Carl J. Pfeiffer says in *Clinical Nutrition* (January, 1968), "the amount absorbed increases with the amount in the diet." In other words, the more calcium you consume, the more will be absorbed into your bloodstream and bones, and the more will be available for the activity of your heart muscle.

Bear in mind then, that even though you are consuming now just as much calcium as you did in your younger years, you may not be getting enough. How do you get more? By eating more high calcium foods. If you get your calcium from natural food sources you will also get more magnesium. Bone meal is an excellent natural supplement. Green, leafy vegetables help a lot. Nuts are good sources too.

191. Potassium: Protection For Your Heart

The L. Peter Cogan Foundation of New York, issued a report in 1967 suggesting that national heart disease rates are inversely tied to the amount of potassium in a nation's traditional foods. Where potassium-rich foods are frequently consumed (Japan, Scandinavia, Italy, France, Germany, Netherlands and Switzerland) the heart disease rates are low, compared with countries whose diets are not particularly rich in potassium (United States, Australia, Canada, New Zealand, United Kingdom). The Japanese eat plenty of potassium in seafood and seaweed (kelp), and the potassium-rich mushrooms that appear frequently in their national dishes. Italians are fond of seafood; olive oil and grape wine (both good potassium sources) are part of every meal.

Essential To Heart

The contributors to *Electrolytes and Cardiovascular Diseases*, edited by Eors Bajusz (Williams and Wilkins, 1966) detail the many ways in which this mineral plays a protective role in the heart's metabolism. Kenter and Falkenhahn describe an extensive experiment in which potassium and magnesium were administered to 97 just-hospitalized heart patients. Only five died, or slightly more than five percent, as compared to 12 percent mortality in an earlier group given all the standard treatments except potassium. Besides the 50 percent drop in mortality, the doctors reported that the patients given potassium and magnesium had much less pain, shock syndrome and irregular heart rhythms.

Dr. Samuel Bellet in his book *Potassium: Cardiac Aspects, The Role of Potassium in Health and Disease* wrote, "Animals fed diets low in potassium failed to grow at a normal rate. After several weeks the heart showed evidence of myocardial necrosis. . . . A heart lesion may be produced in four days by a diet low in potassium and high in sodium chloride, together with injections of desoxycorticosteroneacetate." A famous heart researcher, Dr. Hans Selye of the University of Montreal, performed experiments on rats, injecting them with potassium and magnesium to protect them against sudden extreme stress. Those not treated in this way developed damage in the heart muscle and died.

Investigators are still working to find out exactly what it could be in the potassium-rich foods that has such a beneficial influence against heart disease. One important consideration is potassium's effect on the skeletal muscles which contain about six times as much potassium as sodium. It influences the power of contraction of the smooth, skeletal and cardiac muscles and profoundly affects the nerve tissues. It could be that potassium's greatest contribution to heart health is its maintenance of the heart's muscle power.

Need Doesn't Have To Be Major

Major deficiencies of potassium, so serious that they are obvious upon examination, are rare. But it doesn't take a major deficiency to cause trouble. Even minor shortages of potassium can bring on vague weakness, impairment of neuromuscular function, poor reflexes and mental confusion. The muscles become soft and saggy and healthy cell growth is sluggish, when optimum potassium is missing.

While it is true that Americans don't eat as much seafood and mushrooms and drink as much wine as the people of many countries, there would be no problem in our getting enough potassium if our diet habits were pegged more to fresh, natural foods than the processed ones we favor.

There is plenty of potassium in meats, seeds, green leafy vegetables and fruits. But the popular choices are the highly processed items. Raw peaches contain 880 milligrams of potassium per 100 grams. Can them and the reading goes down to 450. Frozen peaches contain only 133 milligrams of potassium per 100 grams. Wheat germ contains 780 milligrams of potassium per 100 grams, while self-rising, enriched, fortified, all-purpose wheat flour has 90. The popular fig bar cookies contain absolutely no potassium, but dried figs have a reading of 780 milligrams per 100 grams.

Dr. W. A. Krehl, writing in *Nutrition in Clinical Medicine* (August 22, 1966) said, "If food habits had always been sound, the event of potassium deficiency and depletion would not have developed as a major medical problem." He affirms that poor dietary habits, restricted diet selection, misuse and inappropriate choice of foods are all to blame for any potassium deficiencies that exist.

Dr. Krehl emphasized the extreme importance of good stores of potassium when he said that "the mortality rate from all causes is much higher in potassium-depleted patients than in the undepleted. As a matter of fact, several studies have indicated that a potassium deficiency exists in perhaps as many as 20 percent of all hospitalized patients."

The fact that so many people are deficient in potassium may be one reason why the death toll from heart disease is so tragically high in our country. It is not a surprising fact when you consider the many millions of prescriptions written every year for diuretic drugs, one of the two classes of drugs which are particularly conducive to the problem of potassium deficiency. The other is the adrenocortical steroids (cortisone), so widely used in a variety of medical circumstances.

Dr. Krehl warned that the physician must always be alert to the fact that with every excellent result obtained with a drug there may be an accompanying adverse reaction or effect. "Potassium deficiency occurs in such a large variety of diseases and in so many therapeutic situations that the doctor must be particularly concerned with the possibility that loss of potassium can occur. Early clinical suspicion of undue potassium loss and prompt correction may prevent more serious difficulties."

Some signs of potassium depletion are: listlessness, fatigue, weakness, constipation, insomnia, slow and irregular heartbeat, absent reflexes, mental confusion and soft, flabby muscles. Sometimes neuromuscular function is impaired. There may be just a slight muscular weakness or frank paralysis.

Potassium Guards Cell Integrity

Potassium is vital to the life of the cell, while sodium is an intruder from the surrounding fluid. When potassium is low, it is as if there was a chink in the cell wall and sodium, always lurking at the gates in the extra-cellular fluid, barges in. The sodium changes the acid-alkaline balance of the cell, making for a toxic condition which fosters the formation of necrotic (dead or dying) tissue.

There are other spontaneous causes of potassium depletion such as tumors of the adrenal cortex, Cushing's syndrome (a disorder of the pituitary gland), and diabetes insipidus (which in addition to the disorder of glucose metabolism is marked by great thirst and excessive urination).

Gastric juices and intestinal secretions are rich in potassium. Therefore, any disease which produces vomiting or diarrhea may

873

be responsible for depletion of potassium. In fact, any circumstances that lead to a reduced intake of potassium-containing foods, such as has been reported in alcoholism and in cases where there is a loss of appetite, will lead to serious potassium depletion.

One cause of potassium depletion which has been largely overlooked, however, is stress. Stress invokes a mechanism that accelerates potassium loss. According to Dr. Krehl, it works pretty much the way the corticosteroid drugs work—by stimulating the pituitary with a subsequent release of ACTH which in turn stimulates the adrenal to produce hormones that induce potassium loss and consequent increased sodium retention.

Potassium is one of those minerals which are easy to deplete but hard to store. While the normal kidney functions well in removing excessive amounts of potassium in the plasma, it seems to have little capacity for conserving it in the face of deficiency. In fact, excretion of potassium continues even when the body's level is dangerously low.

But here is an important point: *Only if sodium intake is sharply restricted, does potassium conservation take place.*

Since sodium or table salt (sodium chloride) tends to drive the potassium out of the cell, one of the best ways to insure a good potassium balance is to throw away your salt shaker. While your body does need some sodium, there is so much of it in all processed foods, and in most natural foods, you cannot help getting more than you need. Any that you add at the table can only be excessive.

Potassium is also very important to the ability of the heart to pump blood with adequate force. When the level of potassium in the cardiac muscle is reduced, the myocardial tone is depressed. Furthermore, the body's ability to manufacture growth protein and repair damaged tissues is dependent on a good supply of nitrogen which is impossible to maintain in the face of a potassium deficit.

There are, of course, many gradations of potassium depletion. If very severe, death may occur. Potassium depletion produces an increase in the permeability of cellular membranes, leading to fluid saturation (edema) and consequent damage. Although the lesion may heal after potassium is administered, there is a resultant scarring of the tissue. In the heart, potassium deficiency leads to muscle degeneration, necrosis, connective tissue degeneration, and cellular edema, as in other tissue cells. In other words, the diuretics which are given to spare the heart by removing fluids from the body can, by causing a potassium depletion, actually encourage the retention of fluid in the cells of the heart.

Even minor shortages of potassium can bring on significant cardiovascular features such as poor pulse, and weak and distant heart sounds. Later on, falling blood pressure and evidence of heart block may appear.

Unfortunately, electrocardiographic findings of potassium depletion may not be present with moderate potassium loss. Even a normal electrocardiogram does not exclude intracellular potassium depletion.

In most instances potassium deficiency or depletion may be prevented by proper attention to the inclusion of potassium-containing foods in your diet. If for any reason you must be on a diuretic drug or on an adrenocortical hormone, the development of potassium deficiency may be very rapid, particularly if you are not getting enough of it in your diet. It is particularly interesting that a selection of foods that provides a favorable balance of potassium also provides the desired restriction of dietary sodium or salt.

Dr. Krehl pointed out that there is little need to prescribe costly drug preparations of potassium. It is far easier to invoke sound nutritional practices which include the appropriate potassium-containing foods. Pharmaceutical potassium preparations often have an irritating effect on the intestinal tract. Furthermore, some of them provide excessive levels of potassium that may produce undesirable side-effects.

Maintaining a good potassium supply is one of the prime requisites for good vital health. Among the best sources are sunflower seeds.

To put the sunflower seed into some kind of perspective as a source of potassium, sunflower seeds offer 920 milligrams per 100 grams (about a quarter of a pound), virtually the highest potassium value for any food analyzed in the *United States Department of Agriculture Handbook No. 8.*, while bananas and oranges, usually thought of as excellent potassium sources, contain respectively only 370 milligrams and 200 milligrams per 100 grams.

192. Magnesium—That Vital Spark For The Heart's Mechanism

Magnesium is a rather insignificant part of the body's bulk. It makes up only one-half of one percent of the body's mineral content, but it does a big job. Magnesium can prevent calcification or hardening of the coronary artery; protect the heart muscle during severe strain, even heart attack; strengthen weak bones; and infuse new energy and zest for life into fatigued housewives and burned-out athletes.

That small amount of magnesium triggers the necessary electrical activity within each cell which keeps the muscular action of the heart going.

With the turn towards preventive cardiology as the only answer to the growing problem of heart disease, there is renewed interest in the biological mechanism which keeps the heart pumping for 24 hours a day and magnesium's crucial role in that process.

Magnesium is an electrolyte. That is, its molecules carry a small electrical charge termed a magnesium ion. There are several different types of electrolytes (potassium ions are one) which interact with each other in vitally important activities, especially where the heart is concerned. For example, it is a reaction between two electrolytes which stimulates the contraction and relaxation of cardiac muscle fiber. Electrolytes stimulate enzyme reactions, eventually providing energy for the heart's work.

Without magnesium, these vitally important functions can't take place. But it's also important to keep these elements in balance. Otherwise, the whole mechanism of the heart can go haywire. For example, since magnesium—together with oxygen—has the job of providing the potential muscular strength for the heart to contract, while potassium is necessary to release this energy, any drastic shift in the magnesium-potassium-oxygen balance will disturb the cardiac muscle metabolism, causing heart problems, according to Dr. Eors Bajusz, M.D. (*Nutritional Aspects of Cardiovascular Disease*, J. B. Lippincott Company, 1965).

"Due to differences in structure and biological composition, as well as in metabolic and functional activities," Dr. Bajusz wrote, "the heart cells have nutritional needs that are distinct from those of many other types of cells in the body."

Essential To Enzymes

Besides its electrolytic quality, magnesium affects enzymes. Like the match to paper and the paper to wood, magnesium lights the fire that gives us energy. Essentially, it starts the enzymes working. The enzymes cause the food to be utilized. Therefore, without a sufficient supply of magnesium, the body cannot receive the proper amounts of energy-producing nutrients, even though they may be there for the taking! And, instead of being used, they're flushed out of the system, thereby weakening the whole body.

Though the question of enzymes, electrolytes and ion balance may sound complicated, the results aren't complicated at all.

In studies done with over 100 patients suffering from coronary heart disease—including one-third who were acute heart attack victims—Drs. H. A. Nieper and L. Blumberger reported that treatment with a magnesium compound saved all but one of the patients' lives. Compared to the record for the previous year when 60 out of 196 cases died after treatment with the traditional anticoagulants, magnesium was the life-saver (*Electrolytes and Cardiovascular Disease*, The Williams and Wilkins Company, 1966).

Dr. Bajusz was even more emphatic about the role of magnesium in protecting the myocardium. The myocardial cell is the primary site of injury in most common cardiac diseases, he pointed out in an article in *Lancet* (April 1, 1967).

His experiments along those lines showed that when magnesium and/or potassium deficiency was induced in laboratory animals, "severe disturbances in cardiac function, degeneration of myocardial fibers, and cardiac death" followed.

Translated into human terms, a lack of adequate magnesium—or potassium—in the myocardium may set the stage for the later development of a host of structural abnormalities in the heart. Mineral nutrition, therefore, may explain why one person is able to resist the devastating effects of stress while someone else can't, even though both are exposed to the same stresses!

In his experiments, Dr. Bajusz identified 18 different types of heart disease. He was able to prevent these diseases from developing in laboratory animals by administering doses of magnesium and potassium salts.

But magnesium doesn't simply protect the heart muscle from deteriorating. It works throughout the vascular system, keeping blood vessels open.

Dr. Hans Selye, M.D., found that, in rats, low-magnesium diets produced changes in the rhythm of the heart, calcification, fibrosis and inflammation (*The Chemical Prevention of Cardiac Necroses*, Ronald Press, 1958). In humans, he found that magnesium prevented cholesterol accumulation which can obstruct the blood flow. Magnesium prevented arteriosclerotic degeneration and atherosclerosis, the formation of plaques in the arteries.

Dr. Bajusz agrees with Dr. Selye and identifies magnesium as the most important element in stopping experimentally-induced atherosclerosis. When rats are fed a magnesium-deficient diet, plaque formation and hardening of the arteries occurs. The diet also produces a decrease in protein and energy utilization in rats.

When cattle were studied, the same results showed up. Dr. S. E. Browne (*British Medical Journal*, July 13, 1963) discovered a correlation between heart disease and soil content. He found that cattle grazing where magnesium was deficient in the soil developed calcification of the vascular walls.

Among South African Bantus and Australian aborigines, there is little heart disease. Tests show that magnesium levels in their blood are much higher than in their European counterparts.

Dr. Browne said that magnesium therapy is the answer to heart attacks. Following a heart attack, full circulation must be restored and actually increased in the smaller, peripheral vessels in order to prevent the next attack from being fatal. Magnesium does this.

Although medical doctors and cardiologists often use magnesium injections—magnesium sulphate or magnesium chloride—to successfully treat cardiac patients, Dr. Browne's observations have led him to recommend that magnesium be added to the diet. In addition, he stated that there is an "urgent need for further research into its use therapeutically."

Everyone should make sure to eat foods rich in magnesium such as the green vegetables, dried beans and legumes, peanut butter and wheat germ. These foods will help you meet your body's magnesium requirements. But it may still not be enough!

One way to make sure of getting a high level of magnesium in your diet is dolomite, a natural, safe form of magnesium that has the extra benefit of the proper ratio of calcium for balance. This balance is important because without it, the magnesium cannot be effectively used.

Be on the lookout, however, for the conditions which make the body shed its magnesium, such as gastrointestinal fluid loss, vomiting, the use of diuretics and birth control pills. The body normally throws off some magnesium through fecal excretion. This can amount to as much as two-thirds the entire amount ingested.

Contraceptive Pills Lower Magnesium Levels

Contraceptive pills lower the level of magnesium in women taking them. Drs. Naomi F. Goldsmith and John R. Goldsmith of the University of Geneva in Switzerland theorize that women taking contraceptive drugs to suppress ovulation may be in the same category as individuals living in soft water areas. Examinations of 10 ovulating women and seven women with surgical or chemical suppression of ovulation showed that magnesium levels were lower in non-ovulating women compared with ovulating women, and in users of Enovid (an oral contraceptive) compared to ovulating women. "The finding suggests that suppression of ovulation is associated with as yet poorly defined alteration of magnesium metabolism," they say. A similar irregularity in magnesium metabolism may be involved in the soft water-heart disease theory. "If this hypothesis be true, then it links these two problems in such a way that the use of the drugs could have long-term effects on cardiovascular disease mortality," Drs. Naomi and John Goldsmith conclude. Although quick to caution that the hypothesis cannot be accepted without further studies, they expressed concern about the "possible significance of a decreased serum magnesium level in millions of women who use drugs for suppression of ovulation."

Another physician, Dr. John B. Neal of Jacksonville, Florida, says that, although it is doubtful that coronary patients are deficient in magnesium from a dietary aspect, "the known physiological effects of extra magnesium from various oral magnesium compounds might be used as a therapeutic agent."

193. A Trace Of Copper For Healthy Arteries

If you remember the days when automobile tires had inner tubes, then you know that a good strong tube could be inflated to almost any desired pressure—without problems. But, if there was a structural weakness in the rubber, the tube would develop one or more bubbles popping out from the surface. The bubbles would in time give way and burst, and the tire would suddenly collapse—bang—a blowout!

Very much the same kind of thing can happen to your arteries. When a bubble occurs in an artery, it is called an aneurysm. It can lead to a blowout of the artery—a hemorrhage—and death.

The difference between an artery wall tough enough to resist aneurysm—one with the ability to stretch on demand and return to shape without tearing—and an artery wall which will bubble and tear under stress may be a simple matter of 10 ppm. of copper in your daily diet.

There is strong evidence that this trace mineral which we associate with pennies can be more precious than gold in preventing the kind of heart attack which stems from a ruptured aorta.

We have long known that copper is important in every stage of development from the prenatal state to old age, and that lack of it can be a factor in osteoporosis, anemia, vitiligo and even premature gray hair.

But research has also revealed the importance of this trace mineral to the tensile strength of the coronary blood vessels.

Heart Failure In Pigs

Dr. William H. Carnes, Professor of Pathology at the University of Utah College of Medicine, observed a cardiovascular syndrome in animals caused by insufficient dietary intake of copper, which shed new light on the importance of copper in the normal development of vascular connective tissue. Dr. Carnes reported the syndrome at the 1968 Conference on Trace Substances as one marked by internal hemorrhage due to rupture of the aorta (the large artery leading from the heart) and coronary vessels. He traced the disease to a defect in synthesis of vascular elastin apparently brought about by a deficiency in a copper-containing enzyme.

In the experiments described by Dr. Carnes, pigs were weaned at two to five days of life and put on a diet of diluted canned evaporated milk which is low in copper content. These animals soon developed characteristic cardiovascular lesions, most commonly of the aorta and coronary arteries. Death from cardiovascular rupture or from heart failure occurred usually between three and four months of age. However, lesions could be corrected and death prevented simply by supplementing the diet with copper after a deficiency had appeared.

After studying the mechanical properties of the aorta in the affected animals, Dr. Carnes concluded that rupture was due to reduced tensile strength or reduced extensibility of the vessel. In other words, the coronary vessel, instead of easily stretching to accommodate its load, would break like a balloon that is stretched beyond its ability to expand.

Dr. Carnes noted that while an extreme copper deficiency like that induced in the animals would be unlikely in humans, under some circumstances there might be a metabolic block in copper enzyme synthesis or a missing co-factor—for example a lack of pyridoxine (B_6) in a copper pyridoxal enzyme.

Dr. Boyd O'Dell of the University of Missouri, Department of Agricultural Chemistry, another conference participant, found similarities between the lesions occurring in copper-deficient animals and those seen in human subjects. As a result of O'Dell's findings, Dr. John H. Henzel, also of the University of Missouri, performed copper assays on specimens obtained from patients requiring resection of diseased abdominal aortas because of occlusive or aneurysmal disease. Nine patients were studied.

In those patients with aortic aneurysm, the copper content was significantly less. For instance, the average copper concentration in specimens from patients with atherosclerosis but no aneurysm was 26.3 ppm. For patients with both atherosclerosis and aneurysms, it was 21.2 ppm, whereas for those with aortic aneurysms without visible evidence of atherosclerosis, copper content was only 14.2 ppm. This would lead us to suspect that in those patients whose hearts were dangerously threatened yet who had no evidence of atherosclerosis, the usual precursor to heart disease, the lack of copper in the tissue, by causing a decrease in the elasticity of the blood vessel, was a prime cause of the aneurysm.

Earl Frieden, in a scholarly report, "The Biochemistry of Copper" (*Scientific American*, May, 1968), wrote that "A copper deficiency can result in the weakening of the walls of certain blood vessels, notably the aorta, rendering the vessels susceptible to aneurysms and rupture."

Are you getting enough copper? Practically all plants and animals that we use for food contain copper in varying quantities. The largest amounts are found in the young and tender leaves and in the germs of seeds of plants.

But, McHargue stated (*Kentucky Acad. of Soil Trans*. 1-2, p. 103) that "the germs of corn and other cereals contain important vitamin factors whereas the products made from the endosperm after the germ and bran have been removed in the modern milling processes are deficient in the vital factors. Then, too, the commercial fertilizers saturate the soil solution to the extent that trace minerals are not absorbed. The use of nitrogenous fertilizers is causing copper deficiencies."

According to Wintrobe, Cartwright and Gubler of the Department of Medicine, University of Utah College of Medicine, copper is found in various foodstuffs, the amount in agricultural products depending on the copper content of the soil.

Copper is so essential to life that some scientists suggest the possibility that the "curse" which led to the disappearance of the human inhabitants on Kangaroo Island off the south coast of Australia may have been copper deficiency (Bauer, 1952).

How can you make certain your diet is not copper-deficient? Foods that are rich in copper are liver, heart, and brains, seafood, yeast and kelp. Desiccated liver contains 2.5 mg. of copper per 100 grams. Green leafy vegetables and whole grains are also excellent sources if grown on mineral-rich soil without chemical fertilizers. Natural mineral supplements usually include copper.

194. Heart Attacks, Local Water And The Good And Bad Minerals

As a person sincerely interested in trying to protect and improve your health, how would you feel if someone were to tell you that your chances of being felled by a heart attack are at this very moment being powerfully influenced by rocks which lie a hundred or more feet under your basement floor? Rocks which may be hundreds of millions of years old.

Does it sound unbelievable? Incomprehensible? To some people, it may seem as difficult to believe that our health is being affected by some ancient, inert stones as it is to believe that our behavior is influenced by cosmic emanations coming from far-away planets and stars.

Nevertheless, it's true. There *is* an influence, a powerful one, in those rocks you've never seen and never will see. What's more, there is probably more agreement among top scientists and researchers as to the importance of those rocks to the well-being of your heart than there is about the importance of exercise, cholesterol and vitamins.

While controversy and many questions still swirl around the subject, what is generally agreed upon by scientists who have compiled health statistics on tens of millions of people throughout the world is this:

People who live in areas where the underlying rocks are rich in calcium and magnesium and certain trace elements seem to have significantly *less* chance of developing cardiovascular disease than people who live in areas where the underlying rocks are relatively impermeable and formed of insoluble minerals.

Rocks Give Up Mineral Content To Water

Actually, it isn't the rocks themselves that directly influence the heart and blood vessels, but the *water* which lies in these rocks or percolates through them. Water exposed to rocks rich in calcium and magnesium tends to be what is called hard water, or water rich in minerals—specifically calcium and magnesium. In carefully conducted surveys from all over the world, scientists now find that people who drink this kind of hard water stand much less chance of developing cardiovascular disease than people who drink soft water.

It is not yet known with certainty whether the protective effect is in the calcium and magnesium—often released into the water by underground deposits of a mineral known as dolomite—or if it is trace elements or other properties associated with hard water. Quite probably, the protection is in all of these factors.

An article in the *WHO* (World Health Organization) *Chronicle* of December, 1973, is an excellent review of research which WHO is sponsoring around the world to learn more about, as the article title puts it: "Water Quality, Trace Elements, and Cardiovascular Disease."

The article states that there is "a considerable body of evidence to suggest that cardiovascular mortality (i.e., deaths resulting from any disease of the heart or blood vessels, such as strokes and heart attacks) is linked in many places with the quality of drinking water; in areas where the water is hard, the death rate tends to be lower than in soft water areas. . . . This statistical association is not always significant, and in some population groups is significant for women only or for men only. . . . Generally speaking, however, the trend seems to be clear: where the water is hard, the death rate is likely to be lower.

"Water hardness results largely from the presence of calcium and magnesium salts, while softness is associated with the absence of those salts." We all know that water can be artificially softened to prevent scaling in pipes and boilers, but the article points out that it is "also possible to *harden* water artificially, and this has been done in some places, with apparently beneficial results to the cardiovascular health of the population. There are indications that a higher risk of cardiovascular disease may not depend on exposure to soft water for a lifetime or even for many years. Favorable changes have been observed in some places just a few years after the water has been hardened artificially; conversely, there have been unfavorable changes after the artificial softening of water supplied to other areas."

Heart Disease Death Rate Cut In Half With Harder Water

According to a recent article in the *Journal of the American Medical Association* (October 7, 1974) by Dr. Andrew G. Shaper of the United Kingdom, one such place where the water was changed was Monroe County, Florida. There, the water supply had been rain water with a hardness of only 0.5 parts per million (ppm). It was then changed to deep-well water with a hardness of 200 ppm. "The death rates from cardiovascular disease *dropped* from a range of 500 to 700 to a range of 200 to 300 only four years after the increase in water hardness," Dr. Shaper said in his article entitled "Soft Water, Heart Attacks, and Stroke."

Dr. Shaper, who is a specialist in cardiovascular disease, and a member of the Scientific Staff of the United Kingdom Medical Research Council in London, describes similar patterns throughout the world. In the United States, he says, information involving more than seven million people in 140 counties along the Ohio and Columbia Rivers (soft water) was compared to health statistics concerning people living along the Missouri and Colorado Rivers (hard water). In these four river basins, he writes, the death rates from diseases other than heart disease were virtually the same. But in the hard water regions, the death rates from heart disease, including the kind of heart disease related to high blood pressure, were much lower.

He also notes that recent studies in England and Wales found that middle-aged men who lived in towns with hard water had lower blood pressure, lower heart rate, and lower plasma cholesterol levels than men living in soft water towns. Not only was diastolic blood pressure lower in hard water towns, but it did not increase with age, as it did in the soft water towns.

The great American pioneer in this field is Dr. Henry A. Schroeder of Dartmouth Medical School. In 1960, he began publishing his remarkable findings about the relationship between the hardness of water and cardiovascular disease. Among other facts he brought to light is that there is a very strong and consistent relationship between hardness of water and low cardiovascular death rates when the various states of America are compared.

Dr. E. G. Knox of Great Britain recently approached the problem from a different point of view. Instead of comparing the hardness of water in different communities, he compared the total consumption of various vitamins and minerals, both from water and food, in different areas of the United Kingdom. What he found was that the strongest correlation of all was a negative one between intake of calcium and deaths from heart disease and strokes (*Lancet*, June 30, 1973). In other words, the more calcium in the diet, the lower the death rate from circulatory disease.

Magnesium was not one of the minerals he considered, but it may be significant that calcium, which is the chief mineral constituent of hard water, turned out to be the number-one protective nutrient in the whole list.

Magnesium And The Heart—A Healthy Relationship

Magnesium, the other major hardener of water, may also play a profound role. Two medical researchers from Finland compared the heart disease rate to the soil content of various minerals throughout Finland and came to the conclusion that the strongest correlation was between the presence of magnesium in the soil and a low heart disease rate. Calcium seemed to be protective, and so did potassium, but not to the extent of magnesium.

As to *why* magnesium might be so important to the heart, the two scientists, H. Karppanen and P. J. Neuvonen, suggest several possibilities. These include the possible involvement of magnesium deficiency in the development of abnormal heart rhythms and sudden heart deaths, and the fact that "some beneficial effect of magnesium sulfate on arterial diseases, including coronary heart disease, has been reported." Further, autopsies have revealed that people who die suddenly from heart disease have unusually low amounts of magnesium in their heart muscles.

This latter point was taken up by a team of researchers led by the well known epidemiologist T. W. Anderson of the University of Toronto in the same issue of *Lancet* that carried the Finnish report (December 15, 1973). Anderson and his colleagues mentioned two earlier reports which said that the heart muscle concentration of magnesium tends to be lower in people who have died from heart attacks compared to those who die from other causes. He also mentioned a study which concluded that people who live in soft water areas tend to have lower magnesium concentrations in their hearts than residents of hard-water areas. "We are able to confirm that just such a difference has been observed in a Canadian study now nearing completion," Anderson and his colleagues wrote.

Cancer And Kidney Disease Also Reduced By Hard Water

Just one more piece of evidence: calcium and magnesium, which are the major constituents of hard drinking water, have consistently negative correlations with cardiovascular-renal diseases and with cancer.

This powerful assertion comes from Herbert I. Sauer, of the Extension Environmental Quality and Environmental Health Surveillance Center at the University of Missouri, Columbia. Mr. Sauer made the statement last year at the annual International Water Quality Symposium in Washington, D.C., and his remarks were reported in *Family Practice News* (June 15, 1974).

In general, he said, the harder the water, the lower the death rates from diseases simultaneously involving the circulatory system and kidneys, coronary heart disease, and cancer in white middle-aged persons.

Whether the relatively high amounts of calcium and magnesium in hard water are directly productive of health, or whether there is some mysterious x-factor or factors in soft water that are directly toxic, has not yet been discovered. But the problem is being worked on, right now, in a number of laboratories all over the world. The feeling is that if either the precise protective factor, or harmful x-factors can be discovered, the implications will be enormously beneficial to everyone, regardless of what kind of water they're drinking.

The Acid Water Theory

There exists another major theory as to why hard water is good for us and soft water bad. This theory maintains that what is protective about hard water is not so much the presence of calcium or magnesium, but the *absence* of toxic elements usually found in soft water. These toxins may enter the water either from the soil or rocks through which the water has percolated, or from the plumbing in your home.

The key to this theory is that soft water tends to be on the acidic side. Because it is acidic, it actively attacks a number of metals and causes them to break loose from the rocks or pipes and join with the water. Chief among the suspected metals are cadmium, lead and copper. Cadmium and lead have no place at all in normal metabolism and are both recognized as highly toxic. Copper is vital to normal health, but too much of it can upset the normal balance of minerals within the system.

Scientists who favor this theory believe that while calcium and magnesium may be good for the heart, the really important role they play is keeping water sufficiently alkaline to prevent the leaching of cadmium, lead and copper out of rocks or plumbing.

This theory got a big boost from the discovery that the usual link between hard water and healthy hearts does *not* hold true for the twin cities of Kansas City, Kansas, and Kansas City, Missouri, which are on opposite sides of the Missouri River. On the Kansas side, where the water is relatively hard, the cardiovascular death rate is actually about half again as high as it is on the Missouri side, where the same water supply is artificially softened before being delivered to residents.

This finding, of course, conflicts with the great majority of other findings, but this didn't disappoint Dr. Marvin L. Bierenbaum and Dr. Alan Fleischman, of the Atherosclerosis Research Group at St. Vincent's Hospital in Montclair, New Jersey. Actually, it intrigued and delighted them, because of other findings made at the same time.

Too Much Cadmium, Not Enough Zinc

What really had their interest, according to an article in *Medical World News* (October 11, 1974) is that while the water on the Kansas side was harder, it contained three times the amount of cadmium as did the water on the Missouri side.

Even more striking, because cadmium has a tendency to accumulate in the body, people who live on the Kansas side of the river, the scientists found, have 13 times as much cadmium in their blood as the people on the Missouri side.

But that isn't the end of the story. The Kansas residents along with their high heart disease rate and high cadmium blood levels, also had only one-third the amount of zinc in their blood as the Missouri residents. It is just this relationship between cadmium and zinc which seems to offer the greatest possibility for future research.

As *Medical World News* points out, "In the past decade several investigators have induced hypertension (high blood pressure) in laboratory rats by giving them small amounts of cadmium. Others have shown that cadmium-induced hypertension can be reversed with zinc. . . "

Drs. Bierenbaum and Fleischman don't believe that cadmium is the whole answer to the hard water riddle. As Dr. Fleischman puts it, "It's just one agent." But he does say that his findings fit in remarkably well with the work of Dr. Henry Schroeder of Dartmouth Medical School, the pioneer in this field, who has emphasized that while cadmium is definitely toxic, and associated with high blood pressure and heart problems, it isn't so much the absolute amount of cadmium that's crucial, but whether or not there is enough zinc present to protect against the destructive effects of cadmium. Dr. Schroeder found that he could induce high blood pressure in test animals by giving them cadmium, and then stop the disease in its tracks simply by replacing some of the cadmium with zinc (*Journal of Chronic Diseases*, 20, 1967, cited in *Archives of Environmental Health*, February 1974, p. 108).

Why those people in Kansas had three times as much cadmium in their water and 13 times as much in their blood as their Missouri neighbors is not known for certain. However, it's believed that the major source of cadmium in water is from old galvanized pipes. These are iron pipes covered with a protective layer of zinc, but relatively high amounts of cadmium contaminate the zinc. As the pipe corrodes, the cadmium is released into the water. Ordinarily, this doesn't happen when water is hard because no corrosion takes place. Instead of metals from the plumbing leaching out and entering the water, the plumbing tends to become coated with calcium carbonate.

Cadmium-Zinc Ratio Tied To High Blood Pressure

The health-destroying effects of cadmium in water were reviewed by Carl C. Pfeiffer, Ph.D., M.D., of the Brain Bio Center of Princeton in a paper presented in 1974 at the 7th International Water Quality Symposium in Washington, D.C. Dr. Pfeiffer refers to recent findings by Dr. Schroeder showing that people who die of the complications of high blood pressure tend to have an unusually high level of cadmium in their kidneys. This has been seen in studies in at least two cities, and seems to indicate a likely causal relationship between cadmium and high blood pressure and stroke, Pfeiffer says.

The World Health Organization is funding a research project to look into this very question of zinc, cadmium, and high blood pressure because their findings, too, suggest that the kidneys of people with high blood pressure are high in cadmium and low in zinc (*WHO Chronicle*, 1973, 27, 534-538).

Copper Should Not Overpower Zinc

Zinc may also turn out to be protective against excess copper, which is easily leached from copper plumbing by soft water. The World Health Organization report notes that "Patients with either hypertension or arteriosclerotic heart disease or an old myocardial infarction generally have higher copper and lower zinc levels in the serum and toenail samples than do normal healthy people. Again, a geographical link was found with the concentration of trace elements."

That last sentence is important, because it indicates that the low zinc levels are probably not a result of heart trouble or hypertension, but more likely part of the *cause*. Dr. Pfeiffer zeroed in on the high-copper/low-zinc problem in his recent talk entitled "Does Acid Well Water Erode Plumbing, Vessels, and Sanity?" Dr. Pfeiffer declared that "With the increasing installation of copper plumbing in conjunction with the slight acidity of most drinkable water, we are getting an excess of copper which may be antagonizing the zinc we obtain from food." He added that well water from his own town of Princeton, New Jersey, contained 1.25 parts per million (ppm) of copper, which is significantly above the maximum amount of 1.0 ppm allowed by the United States Public Health Service in public water supplies.

So supplementing the diet with a little extra zinc not only protects against cadmium toxicity, but probably helps protect against copper excess as well.

Vitamin C Also Protects Against Cadmium

Vitamin C isn't found in water, but it is nevertheless proven to be a natural protective factor against cadmium. This was shown in two important studies last year, one coming from Washington, D.C., and the other from Nagoya, Japan.

In the American study, it was found that feeding cadmium to young quail produced enlargement of the heart, growth retardation, abnormality of the testicles, bone marrow and adrenal gland, and damage to the lining of the small intestine. Curiously, some of these symptoms resembled those caused by a deficiency of zinc or iron.

The effect of vitamin C on all this pathology? According to authors Richardson, Fox and Fry, associated with the Environmental Protection Agency and the Division of Nutrition of the Food and Drug Administration, "Ascorbic acid added to the cadmium-containing diet significantly alleviated or prevented almost all aspects of cadmium toxicity in quail four and/or six weeks of age. It protected against some changes that were not observed in either zinc or iron-deficient birds" (*Journal of Nutrition*, March, 1974).

The Japanese study was conducted by Maji and Yoshida of the

Laboratory of Nutritional Biochemistry at Nagoya University. They fed laboratory rats cadmium and observed the pathological effects. Then they added both vitamin C and iron to the animals' diet to determine if there was a possible protective effect.

They concluded that the supplements "overcame the growth retardation and depression of hematocrit and blood hemoglobin not only by simultaneous administration of cadmium, but also by subsequent administration after previous feeding of a cadmium-containing diet." In other words, vitamin C together with iron not only prevented most cadmium damage, but *reversed* most earlier cadmium damage as well (*Nutrition Reports International*, September, 1974).

If soft, acidic water is leaching toxic lead out of the soil, plumbing, or even the soldered joints of your plumbing, the two chief protective nutrients are calcium and vitamin C. Ample dietary calcium is also very effective in keeping lead absorption to an absolute minimum. In 1971, a study by Dr. K. Kostial and colleagues in Yugoslavia showed that extra calcium and phosphate together may be slightly more effective than calcium alone (*Environmental Research*, October, 1971). Milk and bone meal are both good sources of calcium and phosphorus, although bone meal has the higher calcium ratio that most people need. Dolomite, consisting of calcium and magnesium, is also a rich source of this mineral.

If you are in doubt about what kind of water you have, you can find out by calling the closest office of the United States Public Health Service. Perhaps a local health agency or the people who run your local water authority will be able to tell you. If you have a well, you can look for green stains if you have copper piping, or have a sample analyzed.

An analysis could include total mineral content, hardness, and calcium and copper concentration. Prices vary. The expense of running all these tests is usually unnecessary unless you suspect that your water supply is being contaminated by a nearby industry. If you have the hardness and pH tested, you can then consult a local water engineer and see if any problems with plumbing erosion are indicated.

One thing you don't want to do, is have all your water artificially softened. That's just asking for trouble, especially if you have old plumbing. If your water is excessively hard, just have the hot water you use for washing softened, and enjoy the hard water for drinking.

How To Test Your Water For Hardness

How can you tell how hard your water is? There is a simple test you can do right at home in your kitchen sink. Take a small bottle marked at the one ounce level, and fill it to that level with tap water. Then, using an eyedropper, add tincture of green soap (available at your local pharmacy), one drop at a time, shaking the bottle vigorously after each drop. The test is complete when the foam caused by the shaking stands up for two to five minutes without breaking. The number of green tincture drops it takes to achieve this indicates the number of grains of mineral salts per gallon of water. If you have 0-3 grains, your water is soft, while 3-6 grains is medium hard. Water for domestic use should contain less than nine grains, and a level around six grains is most desirable.

This simple test could save your life someday. Try it on your own tap water, and if you are already using a water softener, switch it to only hot water. If your water is soft before it enters your house, buy bottled natural spring water.

Nutritional Protection Against Toxic Minerals

As a complementary measure you can take dietary steps to minimize toxic elements which may be in your drinking water, while at the same time assuring yourself that you're getting the positive, beneficial elements which may be present in hard water.

First, make sure your calcium and magnesium intake is adequate. A study by Dr. E. G. Knox of England (*Lancet*, June 30, 1973), showed that the more calcium there is in the total diet (food and water), the less chance there is of dying from heart attack and stroke.

Magnesium is another important component of hard water and has been directly linked to the health of your heart. Since water often becomes hard by passing through underground deposits of dolomite, consisting of calcium and magnesium, using purified dolomite as a dietary supplement seems to make sense.

Eating some supplementary zinc-rich food, such as nuts and seeds, every day (which you probably need anyway regardless of what kind of water you're drinking) will put you on the right side of that critical cadmium-zinc ratio which is suspected of being a major contributing cause of high blood pressure when cadmium is overpowering the zinc. Taking the zinc will also keep the copper-zinc ratio where it should be, in light of the findings that people with clogged up arteries or high blood pressure have too much copper and not enough zinc.

Vitamin C (and probably iron) is a powerful weapon in your dietary arsenal against excess cadmium, and probably reason enough why supplementary amounts of this vitamin should be on everyone's daily menu.

Finally, the same calcium you're eating for its direct benefits will also go a long way toward reducing your absorption of any lead that may be coming into your system from your water—or any other source, for that matter. And once again, vitamin C will reduce the toxic effects of any lead that is absorbed.

195. Chlorinated Water And Heart Disease

Coronaries/Cholesterol/Chlorine (Alta Enterprises, Saginaw, Michigan, 1970) by Joseph M. Price, M.D., is a book which raises fresh doubts about the wisdom of treating our drinking water with chemicals.

For his study, Dr. Price selected 100 day-old cockerels. (The male chicken, like the male human being, is more susceptible to the development of atherosclerosis.) The methodology and results are described by the author: "Both groups were placed on a diet of cooked mash consisting of about 1:1 mixture of corn and oat meals with about five percent low-priced oleomargarine added. Pure distilled water was used exclusively. Chlorine was added to the drinking water and mash of the experimental group in the form of chlorine bleach (disinfectant), about one-third teaspoonful per quart of water. This highly chlorinated water was first given to the experimental group at 12 weeks of age.

"The results were nothing short of spectacular! Within three weeks there were grossly observable effects on both appearance and behavior. The experimental group became lethargic, huddling in corners except at feeding time. Their feathers became frayed and dirty and the cockerels walked around with their wings hunched up, their feathers fluffed up as if they were always cold (the experiment was performed in an unheated barn in winter), their pale combs drooping. This appearance is most suggestive of symptoms resulting from clogging up of the microcirculation."

The control group, on the other hand, was observed to thrive. Chickens not ingesting chlorine were larger in size and more active, with clean, shiny feathers. But as Dr. Price was to discover, the contrast was more than skin deep.

Link To Atherosclerosis Demonstrated

"No less remarkable was the gross appearance of the aortas," he notes. "The abdominal aorta (the place where atherosclerosis is known to occur in chickens) of all of the cockerels dying after four months were carefully examined. In more than 95 percent of the experimental group grossly visible thick yellow plaques of atherosclerosis protruding into the lumens were discovered! These chickens were noted to have an extremely high, apparently spontaneous death rate, and common findings on examination of the carcasses were hemorrhage into the lungs and enlarged hearts."

After seven months, he says, *every chicken* fed chlorinated water had developed atherosclerosis, while *not a single chicken* of the pure water control group had done so. When a check was made by feeding chlorinated water to the control cockerels, they, too, developed atherosclerotic lesions.

What led Dr. Price to experiment with chlorine in the first place? He was puzzled by the fantastic surge in the incidence of heart disease (heart attack, stroke, arteriosclerosis) during this century. Noting that prior to 1900 such cases were almost unheard of, he reasoned "that something has changed in the last six-seven decades of human history."

In particular, he was fascinated by evidence that heart attacks, while occurring before 1930, only reached proportions significant enough to affect mortality statistical tables at that time. He suspected that some environmental factor, crucial to the development of atherosclerosis, was being overlooked by medical science.

"Experimental use of chlorine to 'purify' water supplies began in the late 1890's," he points out. "Chlorination gained relatively wide acceptance in the second decade of this century, and in the third decade (1920's) it was found that satisfactory killing of organisms was dependent upon a *residual* of chlorine in the water above the amount necessary to react with organic impurities. When it is remembered that evidence of clinical disease from atherosclerosis takes 10-20 years to develop, it becomes evident that there is a correlation between the introduction and widespread application of chlorination of water supplies and the origin and increasing incidence of heart attacks that is exceedingly difficult to explain away."

To back up his argument, the author brings in evidence from around the globe: Japan has a low incidence of heart attack, but when Japanese move to Hawaii and drink chlorinated water, they develop atherosclerosis. Some Africans eat a very high cholesterol diet but drink no chlorinated water—and they don't get heart attacks. Irish farm workers studied by Dr. Paul Dudley

White, who drink their own well water, *never* develop coronary heart disease.

Are We Endangering Our Soldiers With Sanitation?

Finally, Dr. Price observes that during the Korean war, autopsies performed on young American soldiers killed in battle revealed over 75 percent showed evidence of coronary arteriosclerosis although their average age was only 22.1 years. Although most medical men took this as surprising evidence of the early onslaught of so-called "degenerative disease," the author offers a different explanation:

"If you ask any man who served in that war, he will tell you that the water in Korea for our soldiers was so heavily chlorinated for sanitary reasons that it was almost undrinkable. . . . Apparently, there is a direct *causal* correlation between the amount of chlorine ingested and the speed and degree of development of atherosclerosis!"

A direct causal relationship! That's a pretty strong condemnation of a chemical almost everyone else in this country considers perfectly safe. Undoubtedly, the very idea of such a health risk in chlorinated water will come as news to most people.

In the early 1950's, J. I. Rodale was alerting health-conscious people to the danger of chlorine, after coming across a question to the editor in the *Journal of the American Medical Association* (July 28, 1951). Asked about the extent of studies made to determine the harmful effects of chlorinated water used for drinking purposes, the *JAMA* writer was forced to admit: "A search of the literature did not reveal any organized investigation of the effect of heavily chlorinated water on the human body."

Long-Term Effects Are Unknown

Disturbed by this gap in medical research, Mr. Rodale said, "The more we think about it, the more horrifying it seems that all over the country drinking water is regularly chlorinated by city water departments. *And no organized investigation has ever been made of its long-term effects on the human body!* Health-conscious people can take whatever precautions they choose about the kind and quality of food they eat. But what can they do about the drinking water flowing from their faucets?

"Certainly water supply must be uncontaminated. But doesn't it seem reasonable that modern engineers could supply pure water to our cities without dosing it with chlorine? And, if we must use chlorine, shouldn't we be conducting every possible kind of test to make certain that permanent harm is not being done by drinking this water over a period of years?"

Why hasn't an acceptable substitute been adopted for disinfecting our public water supplies? The public has been subjected to chlorination of water so long that it tends to assume that the only thing wrong with water chlorination is the terrible taste and odor. But as Dr. Price's largely-unheeded findings now tend to confirm, America's future health may also be at stake.

196. Will Cutting Down On Cholesterol Help Your Heart?

More than a million Americans die of heart disease each year. In an effort to stem this tide, cardiologists for more than a decade have been urging the public to change its diet—to sharply reduce cholesterol levels by curbing intake of saturated animal fats and increasing consumption of polyunsaturated fats. Since 1968 the American Heart Association has been officially urging the public to decrease its cholesterol level. Over the decade, untold millions have responded with cholesterol-lowering dietary changes— and the heart attack rate continues to rise inexorably year by year. The failure of cholesterol-lowering diets to affect the heart attack rate makes it more and more apparent that, while there undoubtedly is some relationship, it's far from the entire story.

Responding to this awareness, one investigator, Harold A. Kahn of the National Heart and Lung Institute in Bethesda, Maryland, has taken the trouble to study and compare the American diet from 1909 to 1965. His report in the *American Journal of Clinical Nutrition* (July, 1970) points out that during the past half-century, while the death rate due to coronary thrombosis has skyrocketed from practically zero to the present rate of over one million deaths a year in the U.S., blood cholesterol levels have not increased. As a matter of fact, they have hardly changed at all. Kahn took the available data on U.S. dietary changes during this 56 year period and converted these to cholesterol changes using mathematical equations relating alterations in dietary components to alterations in serum cholesterol (the cholesterol level in the blood). For example, the average per capita per day intake of saturated fat in 1909 was 50.3 grams compared to 53.9 grams in 1965. The slight rise in cholesterol consumption, however, was accompanied by an even greater increase in consumption of linoleic acid—the main component of polyunsaturated fats—from 10.7 grams to 19.1 grams. Kahn calculated that these changes could be associated with a difference in cholesterol levels somewhere between an increase of 1.6 mg. per

100 ml. blood and a *decrease* of 3.9 mg. per 100 ml. He noted that, while heart disease has increased a few thousand times over, these data, according to the Framingham equations, may be related to an eight percent increase in risk at most.

Kahn concluded, "Serum cholesterol changes associated with changes in dietary fat have not been very great in this country for the past 50-60 years. This in turn indicates that the increased risk of coronary heart disease reported to have occurred over this period is not related to dietary fat changes to a very important degree."

However, emphasis in contemporary America has been placed on reducing blood cholesterol levels in an attempt to combat the ravages of heart disease. Scientists have shown that decreasing intake of saturated animal fats and increasing consumption of polyunsaturated fats is effective in reducing this level by as much as 13 percent. *But it is important to note that none has proved that high levels of fat or cholesterol in the blood are associated with more deposition of cholesterol in the arterial walls than are low levels.*

While many victims of arteriosclerosis and coronary thrombosis have had high levels, there are others who do not. Large portions of our population show high serum cholesterol levels on testing, yet never develop heart or circulatory disease. Doctors still can not explain why an individual person, or experimental animal, without warning, will develop a myocardial infarct (an area of the heart muscle damaged or killed by an insufficient flow of blood through the coronary arteries which normally supply it). Measurements of a patient's serum cholesterol today might be normal, yet he might go into an attack tomorrow; it may be high and he might never develop a cardiac attack.

Can We Do Without Cholesterol?

But as medical scientists still search for the definitive cause-and-effect relationship between cholesterol and heart disease, powerful public health groups have gone ahead with high powered campaigns persuading the public to adopt a diet that will reduce cholesterol levels in their blood. But you can't do without cholesterol, and a drastic change in diet in an attempt to avert heart disease could be dangerous. Natural foods highest in cholesterol are the very ones which are richest in necessary nutrients. To eliminate cholesterol-rich liver, kidneys, and eggs from the diet, for example, would be to deprive oneself of three concentrated sources of vital foods.

Cholesterol itself serves many important functions. It is the mother-substance for many hormones and is one of the substances of which the bile acids are made—those essential digestive juices which are manufactured in the liver and concentrated in the gall bladder. It is an important part of the nerve tissues. It opposes those elements which destroy red blood corpuscles.

The healthy body uses cholesterol and discards the excess automatically. And, as Kahn suggests, since the average serum cholesterol levels have not increased significantly since 1909 while death rate due to heart disease has increased way out of proportion (currently claiming 50 percent of the deaths in the U.S.), cholesterol is at best a minor factor in causing these fatalities. Kahn states that "Changes in fat consumption may well be a means of lowering present-day risk of coronary disease, but other environmental factors are more probably associated with having raised the risk from that of 50 years ago to the present level."

197. Vitamin C Battles Excess Cholesterol

Heart disease is most commonly caused by atherosclerosis, a stage of hardening of the arteries, in which fatty cholesterol deposits build up on the artery walls and narrow the passageways the blood must pass through. When this happens to the major arteries that lead to the heart, slowing down the flow during an emergency or some strenuous activity when the blood need increases, it causes heart symptoms, including angina pectoris—severe chest pains. It can lead to heart attack and death.

Cholesterol is found only in animal fat, but our bodies can make their own from sources other than fat. We need cholesterol in reasonable amounts. To eliminate cholesterol from the diet would be to deprive the body of concentrated sources of vital food elements. But if we get too much, and cholesterol accumulates in places where it has no business, it can cause serious circulatory problems.

The main trouble we have with cholesterol is in the difficulty certain bodies have in using it up. Responsible scientists have aimed their efforts at finding a way of helping the body process its cholesterol supply, so that troublesome residues will not collect in the bloodstream. One way to accomplish this is by eating foods rich in nutrients known to help the body handle cholesterol; another is by activating the natural equipment the body has for using cholesterol properly.

Dr. Emil Ginter, chief of the biochemistry department, Institute of Nutritional Research, Bratislava, Czechoslovakia, told the Fifth International Convention on Dietary Lipids (October, 1966) that vitamin C can combat the development of atherosclerosis. In his experiments he fed a cholesterol-rich diet to laboratory guinea pigs, but added a daily supplement of 50 milligrams of vitamin C. Then he sacrificed the animals and measured the cholesterol accumulation in the brain, liver, stomach and the main artery to the heart. He found that the cholesterol deposits were 30 to 40 percent lower than in control guinea pigs fed the same cholesterol-rich diet, with only five milligrams of supplementary vitamin C.

To check the vitamin C-cholesterol relationship further, a new group of guinea pigs was fed a diet completely free of ascorbic acid for two weeks. Then a normal diet was introduced, with .5 milligrams of supplementary vitamin C administered orally every day. The 30 control animals were fed the same normal diet, but received ten times as much vitamin C. After a year, cholesterol accumulation in the liver, adrenals, brain and other tissues, including the wall of the main heart artery, were 30 percent greater in the animals on .5 milligrams of vitamin C than in the better-nourished controls.

Drs. Benjamin McConnell and Boris Sokoloff reported that vitamin C supplements reduced high serum cholesterol in rabbits which had been fed high-cholesterol diets.

More important, the two researchers reported that 20 atherosclerotic human patients with high serum cholesterol experienced an *average 30 percent drop in blood cholesterol* after one month's therapy with 500 mg. of ascorbic acid three times a day (*Proceedings of the Sixth International Congress of Nutrition*, Edinburgh, 1963).

Meanwhile, in Capetown, South Africa, Dr. B. Bronte-Stewart and colleagues were studying patients suffering outright scurvy caused by vitamin C deprivation. Surprisingly, they found that abnormally *low* serum cholesterol was typical of scurvy patients. Vitamin C therapy promptly restored cholesterol to normal levels (*British Journal of Nutrition*, 1963, 17, 61). When vitamin C supplements were given to natives who had normal cholesterol levels (actually much lower than the average cholesterol level of a Westerner), nothing at all seemed to happen. This tells us that, unlike a drug, vitamin C does not simply get into the system and somehow begin destroying or washing away cholesterol. What it does is help to *normalize* cholesterol metabolism. It acts to lower it if it is too high, and to raise it if it is too low. If it is just right, it does nothing. This is a classic example of how the healthful influence of nutrients is radically different from the effect of drugs.

Clearing Out Clogged Arteries

One question that always arises in a discussion of lowering cholesterol levels is whether any reduction in blood levels of cholesterol is reflected by a reduction in the amount of cholesterol lining the arteries. A report by two Indian scientists shows that in laboratory rats, at least, ascorbic acid *does* clear out cholesterol deposits from arteries.

Drs. Bala Nambisan and P. A. Kurup worked with weanling rats and examined the large artery called the aorta for cholesterol content after one month of feeding the animals massive doses of ascorbic acid. They discovered that the reduction in cholesterol content of this vessel was significantly greater than the reduction of cholesterol in the serum (*Atherosclerosis*, 1974, 19, 191-199).

If what is true for these laboratory animals also holds true for human beings, it is good news indeed! It would mean that Dr. Ginter's patients, who reduced their blood cholesterol about ten percent with ascorbic acid supplements, achieved even more than this quite substantial accomplishment. In terms of keeping their arteries clear of cholesterol deposits, people who take vitamin C would be scoring a health improvement considerably more than the ten percent serum improvement of atherosclerotic patients treated by McConnell and Sokoloff.

In the 1950's, other experiments demonstrated vitamin C's value in keeping cholesterol levels normal. One of the most remarkable came out of Russia and showed that vitamin C can be both a preventive and a cure for atherosclerosis. According to Dr. I. A. Miasnikov (*Terapevtichevski Archiv.*, Vol. 28, page 59, 1956), within a few hours after receiving vitamin C patients showed a sharp decline in the cholesterol level of the blood. This confirmed a 1952 experiment that showed vitamin C could stop artificially induced atherosclerosis.

Cholesterol Declined In 25 Hours

Dr. Miasnikov's report covered 35 patients, 28 of whom had an excess of cholesterol; the other seven had a reading of between 150 and 180 milligrams of cholesterol (150 to 200 is considered good). In the seven patients whose cholesterol was normal, the ascorbic acid did not alter the level. However, the excessive cholesterol readings showed a considerable drop: in 15 patients the cholesterol was reduced 15 percent; eight lost 16 to 30 percent, and in five patients 31 to 50 percent of the cholesterol disappeared. A definite, sharp decline of cholesterol in the blood occurred within 24 hours after the ascorbic acid was given.

Dr. Miasnikov concluded: "Our observations indicate that ascorbic acid normalized the level of cholesterol in the blood." He also stated his belief that regular supplementary ascorbic acid will prevent the development of atherosclerosis in healthy people of advanced ages. For those who already have atherosclerosis, large doses of ascorbic acid produce therapeutic results. Patients suffering from atherosclerosis frequently develop high blood pressure. Dr. Miasnikov believes that the use of ascorbic acid reduces it and tends to maintain it at a healthy level.

To get back to the work of Dr. Ginter, he told his convention audience about a survey conducted by the Czechs, involving 1,000 school children. It revealed that 97 percent suffered from a lack of vitamin C during the winter and spring, when C-rich fruits and vegetables are less abundant. Notably, there was a corresponding rise in cholesterol levels in the winter.

198. Natural Food Elements That Reduce Cholesterol Build-up In The Arteries

Lecithin

A lot of doctors and researchers would say that one good way of keeping your heart healthy would be to find a way to keep your arteries from getting plugged up with cholesterol deposits. Often, though certainly not in every instance, major circulatory problems—including the ultimate problem of a heart attack—are caused by the failure of sufficient blood to get through the cholesterol-plugged blood vessels.

There is no shortage of suggestions on how the individual can keep his blood vessels "open," and they include everything from running several miles each day to eating a diet extremely low in fat.

There is also an impressive body of evidence which suggests that certain nutrients can have an important protective effect against cholesterol build-up in the blood vessels. Recognition of the tremendous evidence in favor of a dietary approach to protect against cholesterol build-up has come from two physicians affiliated with the Nutrition Program of the School of Medicine of the University of Alabama in Birmingham, Charles E. Butterworth, Jr., M.D., former Chairman of the Food and Nutrition Council of the American Medical Association and Carlos Krumdieck, M.D., Ph.D.

Together, these two physicians have put together a most convincing argument that lecithin has the potential to be of value in protecting against fat-clogged arteries when taken as a daily dietary supplement.

Actually, it isn't new research that Krumdieck and Butterworth report in their article in *The American Journal of Clinical Nutrition* (August, 1974). What they have done is to review a good deal of the scientific literature already published about cholesterol and lecithin and analyze it in terms of the most recent research findings in biochemistry.

Their discussion of lecithin, for example, begins with a description of the chemical structure of the group of naturally-occurring oils known as lecithins, and how this structure relates to that of cholesterol, all of which is far too technical to explain here. But what the theory boils down to is this:

There is a good deal of evidence that an enzyme known as lecithin cholesterol acyltransferase (LCAT) plays a basic role in the body's natural mechanisms for keeping cholesterol from building up on artery walls. Individuals who lack this enzyme develop hardening of the arteries at an unusually early age. And, for the body to manufacture this enzyme in the required amounts, it must have lecithin.

Further, it's been shown in rabbits (very commonly used in atherosclerosis experiments) that putting more lecithin into the system does in fact result in deposits of cholesterol being broken up and carried away. However, to do this effectively, the lecithin must be a *polyunsaturated lecithin.* In the rabbit experiment, it was this kind of polyunsaturated lecithin, derived from soybeans, that proved effective. When lecithin from egg yolks, which is a saturated lecithin, was used, it was not nearly as effective as the soybean lecithin.

In this particular experiment, the lecithin was injected into the animals, but Drs. Krumdieck and Butterworth cite other research which shows that a substantial amount of lecithin which is eaten is actually absorbed intact through the wall of the intestine.

There is also, say the authors, "some intriguing preliminary evidence" that patients who have had heart attacks or suffer from chronic coronary artery disease have unusually low levels of the lecithin-rich LCAT enzyme.

But does taking lecithin really *work?* The University of Alabama investigators mention a recent article by Jacobus Rinse, Ph.D., as an indication that it probably *does.*

Dr. Rinse, a chemist, in an article in *American Laboratory* (July, 1973), wrote that he had severe angina attacks back in 1951, which led his doctor to tell him he had only 10 years to live—providing he avoided all strenuous exercise. Subsequently, using his knowledge of chemistry, he came up with the theory that taking soybean-derived lecithin would help keep the cholesterol in his system *liquefied.* He then went on a regimen of supplementation which included one tablespoon of lecithin granules every day, along with a tablespoon of yeast, one of raw wheat germ and one of bone meal. He mixed this up with cereal and sometimes yogurt, to which he added a tablespoon of safflower or soybean oil.

In his own case, he said he was never bothered with angina after he began taking these supplements. He also reported many anecdotes of friends and acquaintances with circulatory problems who said they did much better on a nutritional program featuring lecithin.

But Dr. Rinse's experiences do not constitute the only evidence in favor of taking lecithin to protect against high cholesterol. Several earlier studies also show that lecithin is a potent weapon against excessive cholesterol. Way back in 1943, in the *Journal of the Mt. Sinai Hospital* (Vol. 9, pp. 955-956), David Adlersberg, M.D., and Harry Sobotka, Ph.D., reported on five cases of high cholesterol associated with various clinical conditions in which "a striking decrease of the serum cholesterol level was achieved by addition of commercial lecithin to the diet."

One of the five patients studied was a 55-year-old woman who was diabetic and markedly overweight. When she began taking 15 grams of soybean lecithin a day (a little more than two tablespoons of lecithin granules), her cholesterol count was 360. Six weeks later, it was down to 235, which is a little higher than ideal, but not usually considered dangerous. At that point, the doctors took her off lecithin to see what would happen and found that her cholesterol shot up again.

Another woman, 41 years old, had a cholesterol count of 620 when she began taking 12 grams of soybean lecithin a day. Two months later, it was down to 420 and a month after that, down to 300. A 35-year-old man dropped from 440 to 260 in two months while taking 12 grams of lecithin a day. Probably the most striking case was that of a 38-year-old woman who had multiple health problems, including fatty plaques on her skin as well as high cholesterol in her blood, who dropped her cholesterol from an extremely high 1370 all the way down to 445 during the period of three months in which she took 15 grams of lecithin a day.

Some 15 years after these early results were published, Lester M. Morrison, M.D., of Los Angeles reported in *Geriatrics* (January, 1958) that 12 out of 15 patients experienced an average fall of serum cholesterol of 156 mg., or 41 percent, after three months of taking soybean lecithin supplements daily. Dr. Morrison, who was one of the pioneers in using a low-fat diet to prevent atherosclerosis, also noted in this report that such a diet had failed to lower the serum cholesterol of these patients until lecithin was added to the regimen. He also notes that two of them had a history of angina pains before going on lecithin; in both, after taking lecithin for three months, "the symptoms of angina pectoris disappeared. . . ."

The initial amount of lecithin used by Dr. Morrison was relatively large—36 grams. However, he noted, follow-up work suggested that a maintenance dose of just one or two tablespoons of lecithin a day (six to 12 grams) was effective in maintaining normal cholesterol levels.

The soybean lecithin used in the clinical trials described here is prepared in a granular form and in capsulized oil form as well. It is a perfectly natural component of many foods, but is particularly rich in the oil which is expressed from soybeans. Several doctors cited here have said that their patients used the granular form, usually baked into cookies to make it more palatable. From one to two tablespoons a day seems to be an appropriate amount. About five to 10 of the high-potency capsules deliver the same amount of polyunsaturated lecithin.

New research results using lecithin to combat high blood fats were published in *Medical World News* (November 22, 1974). Doctors at the Simon Stevin Research Institute in Bruges, Belgium, reported that 100 patients who were given soybean lecithin for 14 days experienced a decided reduction in blood fat, "especially excess plasma cholesterol, which was diminished by 40 percent." The patients all had type II hyperbetalipoproteinemia. Although these results were achieved with injections of lecithin, the doctors stated that when the lecithin was given orally, they achieved "results similar to those obtained after the intravenous therapy, though not to the same degree." The exact amount of cholesterol reduction with oral lecithin was not stated in this report, but if it is anywhere *near* 40 percent, or even 30 percent, it would have to rank as an extremely potent weapon against high cholesterol.

Pectin

Researchers at Rutgers University's Department of Nutrition discovered that pectin, a carbohydrate found in the cell walls of many fruits and vegetables, may be an important factor in the prevention of heart disease. Drs. Hans Fisher and Paul Griminger, quoted in the *Farm Journal* (April, 1968), state that pectin limits the amount of cholesterol the body can absorb, and thus tends to limit the dangerous accumulation of cholesterol in the bloodstream. The high pectin count in apples, suggests the *Journal*, may be one of the reasons for its reputed ability to keep the doctor away.

The power of pectin is not a new discovery. In 1961, Dr. Ancel Keys of the University of Minnesota announced that controlled experiments on man have shown that pectin in the diet has a small but definite effect on lowering blood cholesterol levels. In these experiments carried out on four groups of middle-aged men in a state hospital, the addition to the daily diet of 15 grams (about half an ounce) of pure pectin caused the blood cholesterol to fall by an average of about five percent. When the pectin was removed from this diet the blood cholesterol promptly rose to the pre-pectin level.

Dr. Keys remarked that pectin is naturally contained in many fruits and berries, notably apples. He said that the amount of pectin used in these experiments would be provided by about two pounds of apples. "It appears probable however, that the high consumption of fruits, including apples, by some populations, help to explain the low blood cholesterol values in these populations. . . ."

Edna Brown Southmayd, Ph.D., theorized on just how pectin does its job (*Nutrition Research*, December, 1961). "As the plant matures, enzyme action within the plant releases soluble and consequently digestible pectin substances. Pectin has a strong water-binding property, which helps plants to retain their water and makes it useful in making jellies. Interestingly, it is the pectin of green fruit, which is indigestible, that has this jellying property. The pectin of more mature fruit, which we do digest, for that very reason of its solubility, is not good for jelly making. This is probably one of the important factors entering into the established fact that ripe fruits and vegetables are more fully digested than green ones."

Russian researchers say the pectin derived from sunflowers is superior, according to the USSR publication, *Labor Hygiene and Occupational Diseases*. The Russians did not state whether the pectin used in their experiments was from mature or unripe sunflower seeds. However, we have long believed that, in addition to their known superb nutritional value, there are in sunflower seeds many as yet undiscovered or unconfirmed properties.

An Italian medical journal, *Boll.* (8, 4, 1968) showed that the addition of applesauce to the diet reduces cholesterol levels considerably within 10 to 20 days, probably due to the pectins contained in the applesauce.

Three Italian doctors of Santa Anna Main Hospital, Ferrara, Italy turned the coincidence of a plentiful apple crop and a comparatively high cholesterol level in the area of their hospital to advantage. Within two to three weeks these apples alone brought about a reduction in cholesterol in 32 experimental patients.

Research began by investigating changes in the cholesterol levels of chickens when a certain amount of grated apple was added to their cholesterol-rich diet. The chickens responded so well that it was decided to take the apple approach with humans. Two to three apples after each meal were added to the diets of 26 in-patients and six out-patients at Santa Anna Main Hospital. It worked out to about 200 grams (seven ounces) of blended or grated apple pulp. Only a few of the patients actually munched whole apples.

To make certain that it was the apples alone, the full diet was continued unchanged in every other respect, including some high cholesterol foods. Tests made at the beginning and at the end of the dietetic course showed that cholesterol levels that went down with apples went up in some patients several days after the apple treatment was discontinued.

Doctors noted that the way the apples were prepared— blended, grated, or cut into chewable slices—influenced the amount of serum cholesterol differently. The finer the pulp the greater the surface of apple quickly exposed to the intestines, and the plainer were the results in blood cholesterol reduction.

The Italians were unanimous in their opinion that the pectin content of apples is the element responsible for stabilizing the cholesterol levels.

Housewives know that pectin is what it takes to make the jelly gel. In the days when pectin wasn't available commercially, cooks used to combine apples with whatever fruit they were using for jelly and jams. There was always enough pectin in the apples to get the fruit and sugar mix to gel. Of course the amount of pectin one gets in the average serving of jelly or jam is inconsequential, so don't count on it to have an effect on dangerous cholesterol levels. And don't take commercial pectin as an anti-cholesterol agent. The preparation contains, aside from "highly refined" fruit pectin, lactic and citric acid (added synthetically), plus potassium citrate and potassium metabisulfite added as preservatives.

To put these discoveries of the value of pectin to the best use, eat apples. Eat lots of apples. Eat them raw and unprocessed. Peel them, because unless they are organically grown, probably they have been heavily sprayed. If, because of some condition of health, you aren't able to chew raw apples, liquefy them in a blender just before eating them. If you have no blender, scrape the cored, peeled apple with a dull knife and eat the scrapings. You will find that raw apples are wonderfully satisfying to eat—so satisfying that you won't want to eat the pastries and other desserts that contain the overload of fat which everybody, including Dr. Ancel Keys, believes is so destructive to health. Other fresh, raw fruits and berries contain pectin, but apples are the richest source.

Garlic Oil

Two letters appeared in the December 29, 1973 issue of the English medical journal, *The Lancet*. One of the letters, signed by two cardiologists, Drs. Bordi and Bansal, came from India. These doctors had read several studies showing that when onions are taken with a meal, they counteract the usual results of high fats in the diet, which are to increase the amount of cholesterol and other fats in the bloodstream and also to increase the tendency to form clots of fibrin.

Drs. Bordi and Bansal were aware that in folk medicine, for thousands of years, garlic has had a much bigger reputation than onions, though they are closely related botanically. So the doctors tested garlic juice on five healthy subjects and found that it has a "very significant protective action." They then extracted the oil from the garlic juice and tested that on another five healthy subjects, finding that the oil alone has the full effect. Therefore, the doctors concluded that the oil is the substance that causes the physiological effect, whether taken alone, in garlic juice, or in whole garlic.

On adding 100 grams of butter (nearly a quarter of a pound) to a regular meal eaten by their subjects, the doctors found that three hours after the meal the subjects averaged a blood cholesterol of 237.4 milligrams percent. But when either the juice or the oil extracted from 50 grams of garlic was added to the identical meal, after three hours the blood cholesterol was only 212.7 milligrams percent. The butter also brought the level of plasma fibrinogen (the precursor of fibrin) to 320.9, but adding garlic reduced it to 256.4. The significance of those differences is that the garlic in both cases actually brought the levels of cholesterol and fibrinogen *below fasting levels.*

The second letter in the same issue of *The Lancet*, from three other Indian doctors, pointed out that garlic, though a little slower in its action, is as effective as tolbutamide (an oral drug for diabetics) in clearing the bloodstream of excess glucose. And blood sugar is at least as important as cholesterol, perhaps more important as a cause of atherosclerosis and heart attacks.

So here are two indications that garlic used regularly in the diet should help to prevent the development of atherosclerosis and thus should be a good safeguard against heart attacks.

The early studies made to determine what dietary differences might affect the rate of cardiac deaths, were stimulated by knowledge that Italy has a much lower cardiac mortality rate than does England or the United States. Those early studies concluded that the difference came because the Italian diet is low in cholesterol. But even while a large portion of the medical profession subscribes to the cholesterol theory today, certain flaws have rendered it unprovable. For example, the people of Ethiopia average the highest blood cholesterol levels of any nation in the world, yet that country has very little atherosclerosis.

Had the investigators overlooked a very important factor in the Italian diet—notably garlic? Italians do eat a lot of garlic and they do have a comparatively low cardiac mortality rate.

That garlic has remarkable properties has been known through all history, and forgotten only recently. In the book *Nature's Medicines* (Parker, 1968) Richard Lucas tells us that the Chinese, Greeks, Romans, Hindus, Egyptians and Babylonians all knew that garlic will cure intestinal disorder, flatulence, and intestinal worms.

During the Middle Ages garlic was considered a protection against plagues. Dr. Albert Schweitzer records that he used it with success against typhus and cholera. In fact, it is now widely agreed that garlic is a powerful antibiotic within the rather narrow spectrum of bacteria that are responsible for various intestinal disorders. According to a report in *Today's Health* (November, 1971), Russian pharmacologists are deriving an antibiotic drug from garlic.

If garlic oil had only antibiotic properties, however, we might well be able to do without it. After all, we do have many antibiotics and very effective ones too. But it is not because of bacterial disease that most people die. The leading killers and disablers throughout the United States and Western Europe are diseases of the heart and circulatory system. In Italy where they eat much more garlic than we do in the U.S.A., the heart disease mortality rate is only two-thirds as high. In Spain where they eat perhaps twice as much garlic as they do in Italy, the heart disease mortality rate is less than one-fourth what it is in the United States.

What about high blood pressure?

In 1948 in the European journal *Praxis*, Dr. F. G. Piotrowski of the faculty of medicine of the University of Geneva reported on his use of garlic on about a hundred blood pressure patients. A certain amount of high blood pressure results from disease or malfunction of the kidneys and would not be expected to respond to any dietary measure. Dr. Piotrowski eliminated those with renal hypertension from his study. That left him with about a hundred patients on whom to test the claim from folklore and from a few medical journals that garlic will lower high blood pressure. He found that in 40 percent of his cases it did exactly that.

For those for whom the therapy worked, he found that the subjective symptoms of high blood pressure began to disappear within three to five days after the administration of garlic oil was begun. Such symptoms as headaches, dizziness and difficulties in concentrating were relieved.

But will garlic oil reduce the likelihood of dying because of high blood pressure? The *Demographic Yearbook* for 1966 gave the mortality rate for hypertension, with or without heart disease, in the United States as 39.1 (deaths per 100,000 population). In Italy for the same year it was 35.4. But in Spain where even more garlic is consumed, it was only 13.9.

Garlic is not any sure preventive of diseases of the heart and arteries—after all, there are people dying of these things in Italy and Spain also, but far fewer than here. However, there is good reason to believe that a couple of perles of garlic oil taken every day will improve the chances of avoiding death by dieases of the heart and circulatory system.

199. Heart Disease In Children

Fifty years ago, the death of a child from heart disease was virtually unknown, except in infrequent cases of rheumatic fever. Heart disease was something that happened only to older people. However, we have watched with alarm as year by year an increasing number of young people are afflicted with heart disease. "Of every 1,000 newborns, eight will have heart problems. Of these eight babies, six will be all right for at least the first year of life, but the other two will give you real grief in the first days and weeks of their lives," according to Dr. Alexander S. Nadas, professor of pediatrics at Harvard University and director of the cardiology department at Children's Hospital Medical Center in Boston (*Journal of the American Medical Association*, February 25, 1974).

Bad Diet A Cause

More and more, doctors are becoming convinced that the foods we eat have a definite influence on our susceptibility to heart and artery trouble. Indeed, the modern diet for infants and growing children seems to be a prime reason behind the increased tendency these age groups have to cardiovascular disease.

High blood pressure, for example, is frequently caused by diet. A 1300-page medical text dealing specifically with juvenile cardiac afflictions, entitled *Heart Diseases in Children* (Pitman Medical Co., London) and written by Drs. Bejamin Gasul, Rene Arcilla and Maurice Levi, states that not only is hypertension (high blood pressure) a factor in the children who die in the first few years of life, but it exists unrecognized in many, many more. One way to prevent their developing heart disease is to eliminate those foods in the diet that are high in sugar, fat and salt.

Studies by Dr. Lewis Dahl, of the Medical Research Center of Brookhaven National Laboratory, have shown that today's baby foods have high sodium content, and definitely contribute to hypertension in animals.

It is significant that diets for old and young heart patients contain little or no salt. Dr. Gasul explains why salt is prohibited in cases of congestive heart failure: "This helps to reduce the elevated plasma and body sodium level which is indirectly responsible for the increased circulating blood volume. . . . Indirectly, therefore, the dietary restriction of sodium helps to lessen the load on the heart."

Dr. Gasul expressly forbids crackers, salted foods, and cow's milk. Dr. Gasul warns, "Infants who are bottle-fed with evaporated or whole cow's milk preferably should be fed some modified milk-salt substitutes. . . . The sodium content of cow's milk is nearly four times that of human milk."

Cow's milk is also poor in magnesium, which is needed to assimilate calcium. Without magnesium, calcium deposits form upon heart tissue and arteries. A chapter in the text by Ira Rosenthal, M.D., notes that although "heart attacks" are infrequent in children, "the most frequent cause of coronary occlusive disease in this age group is calcification of the arterial wall. . . ."

Sugar Intake Higher

Sugar, in combination with salt, causes hypertension faster than does salt alone. Sugar has also been observed to aggravate cholesterol deposits in the arteries. Yet our sugar intake is higher than ever.

Refining has also affected the nutritional qualities of bread. Long ago refined flour was a luxury; today a teething baby receives soft breads and salty pretzels. Notably absent from these refined wheat products is vitamin E.

An anticoagulant and antioxidant, vitamin E not only helps to reduce the demand for oxygen by the heart, but is also beginning to find its place in medicine as a recognized anticoagulant and preventative of heart disease. It is possible that if children could get enough of this element they might not develop heart disease in the first place. But bread from which vitamin E has been milled has lost its only nutritional reason for existence. What's left is a starchy loaf containing gluten, an incomplete protein that has become known as a source of allergic reactions and intestinal diseases.

Dr. Robert Levin, writing in *Connecticut Medicine* (February, 1962) stated, "Oft times I have achieved fabulous results with cardiac hypertensive patients by the simple expedient of forbidding the use of bread or flour products."

Vitamins And The Heart

Children's diets also tend to leave out the B vitamins found in eggs, meat, and vegetables. Deficiency of B vitamins usually leads to a deficiency of iron, needed for healthy blood. Dr. Gasul explains the result of this vicious cycle. "Chronic, severe anemia may give rise to congestive heart failure. This is likely to be observed in children with iron-deficiency anemia of long standing."

Another element that can help prevent conditions which lead to heart disease is vitamin C. Yet this nutrient is sadly lacking in the diets of many youngsters.

Without vitamin C in the body, bacteria have a good chance to cause damage to the unprotected heart. Bacterial endocarditis is a condition in which cardiac lesions form because of bacteria that have gained access to the heart through the bloodstream. Dr. Gasul writes that the presence of bacteria in the blood (bacteremia) may result from infections of the mouth. Yet vitamin C helps keep the oral tissues, especially the gums, healthy. This action is important, as "the frequency of bacteremia . . . is usually related to the severity of gum disease."

A diet without enough protein and vitamins invites other bacterial diseases. One is rheumatic fever, which is believed to be caused by streptococcal bacteria. This disease almost always causes serious heart injury. It is, by far, the most common cause of all heart disease in those under 20 years of age.

200. Heart Disease Strikes Women, Too

When the lightning of a heart attack strikes, its target is usually a man. Why, no one really knows, but millions of American males—many still in their 30's and 40's—are running scared from an epidemic of heart disease entirely without parallel in the history of mankind.

But few women bother their heads very much about the possibility of heart disease. In fact, articles in the lay press written by doctors and nutritionists are often addressed to women only in their role as wives, urging them to save their husbands from an early grave by chucking out all their eggs, milk, and meat; drenching all the food that remains with polyunsaturated oils; convincing their mates to run around the block a few times before sitting down to a breakfast of egg whites; helping them to quit smoking, and ceasing to endanger their hearts with unnecessary stress by denying them their favorite foods.

Such articles further support the idea that the woman, herself, really doesn't have much to fear from heart disease. But while it is true that men are particularly vulnerable to cardiac distress, women are by no means free from danger. The fact is that heart disease claims the lives of over 200,000 American women every year. Although the total deaths from heart disease are in the vicinity of one million, the toll among women is certainly nothing to be taken lightly.

Statistics in their raw form may be awesome, and usually, there is little of practical use that we can draw from them. However, when it comes to women and heart disease, this is no longer the case, thanks to a team of specialists in health statistics. Breaking down the raw data concerning hundreds of New Yorkers who belonged to a health insurance plan, and who suffered either a heart attack or angina pectoris, these researchers have been able to bring new insight into the problem of heart disease, and identify special factors which seem to create in women a much greater risk of early death.

44—A Landmark Age

One of their discoveries is that once women reach the age of 44, their chance of suffering a myocardial infarction or angina is actually increasing faster than that of men. The men are still at higher risk, but after 44, for some reason, whatever natural protection a woman has against heart disease begins to disappear at a very rapid rate.

This finding was presented to the 100th Annual Meeting of the American Public Health Association, Epidemiology Section, in Atlantic City, New Jersey, on November 14, 1972. It was just one of the highlights of a study by Eve Weinblatt and Sam Shapiro of the Department of Research and Statistics of the Health Insurance Plan of Greater New York, and Charles W. Frank, M.D., Professor of Medicine at Albert Einstein College of Medicine in New York City.

Their study found that in *some* respects, there isn't that much difference between male and female heart patients—aside from the greater and earlier incidence of the disease in men. Following a heart attack, for example, it was found that 37 percent of the women and 36 percent of the men died within one month. Likewise, the sexes were equal in the percentage of those who succumbed before reaching a hospital, and after reaching a hospital. And in both sexes, the chances of surviving an attack were lower with advanced age.

But within this generally similar picture, some very sharp distinctions showed up. Women diabetics, the researchers discovered, showed an "early mortality" following heart attack which was more than twice that of non-diabetic women suffering a heart attack. The percentages are 62 percent early mortality for diabetics and only 29 percent early mortality for non-diabetics.

In rather surprising contrast, diabetes does not seem to have much influence on whether or not a man is going to survive a heart attack. While 35 percent of male diabetics succumb within one month of a heart attack, 32 percent of non-diabetic males also succumb, which is considered a relatively insignificant difference.

Angina pectoris—crushing chest pains—works the opposite way. Half of all men who have experienced these pains before suffering a heart attack will not live more than a month following the infarct; 68 percent of those who never had the pains will survive. Women who have had prior angina are only slightly more at risk if they suffer a heart attack.

Cholesterol More Dangerous To Women Than Men

Another variable is serum cholesterol level. Women suffering from coronary heart disease have a markedly higher serum cholesterol level than men who are similarly ill. What's more, there is a very clear relationship between the degree of elevation of cholesterol level in women and their mortality after a heart attack. Women heart patients whose cholesterol level is higher than 270 are more than three times as likely to succumb rapidly to heart disease as those who suffer heart attacks but whose clolesterol level is below 270.

Again, this is in stark contrast to the picture for men. Although high cholesterol levels are believed by many to lead to heart disease, once a man actually suffers an attack, his survival seems to be totally unrelated to his cholesterol level.

Another major difference is the significance of high blood pressure. This condition is diagnosed in fully 60 percent of all women heart patients, but only in 34 percent of the men.

No one can offer easy explanations for these sexual differences. The authors of the study put it this way: "One may speculate that as a group women enter the menopause with vessels freer of atherosclerosis than men of similar ages. Parallel to the important endocrine and biochemical changes of the menopause, atherosclerosis may develop in women at a rapidly increasing rate—a rate greater than for men of the same age. This excess rate of atherogenesis in women may be reflected in a rapid rise in blood pressure levels, and a rapid rise in the incidence of clinical coronary heart disease."

Putting together these various differences, the following general principles seem to emerge:

A women is less likely than a man of the same age to have a heart attack, but after the age of 44, her arteries start deteriorating at a faster rate than a man's.

A woman with a history of diabetes is particularly vulnerable in the event she suffers a heart attack.

High blood pressure seems to predispose a woman to heart attack, much more so than a man.

A woman with a very high cholesterol level is also a poor risk to survive an attack. Often, high cholesterol levels are associated with high blood pressure, and these two factors together pose an even more serious risk.

Translating these kinds of statistical associations into practical, preventive medicine, is a tricky business at best. However, it is certainly worthwhile to investigate the possibility of what physicians call "intervention." This simply means that you aren't going to sit there and watch all these conditions run their course without at least *trying* to stop them.

To a doctor treating a patient with diagnosed heart disease, this means hormones or drugs to treat diabetes, drugs to treat high blood pressure, drugs to treat elevated cholesterol, and drugs to help the heart. Maybe he'll also try dietary intervention.

But the woman who is not under the care of a cardiologist has no particular desire to begin such a relationship. Perhaps she is under the care of a physician for diabetes or high blood pressure. She probably has no desire to escalate her case to a higher-priced specialist. What she wants is to keep herself from becoming another cardiac statistic. She *can't* prevent herself from reaching age 44, or from experiencing menopause, but maybe she *can* forestall the development of diabetes (or at least some of the complications), high serum cholesterol, clogged arteries, and high blood pressure.

This sounds like a tall order, but you can go a long way toward filling it by doing three basic things.

Get as much *enjoyable* exercise as you can. Remove highly processed foods from your diet and replace them with whole, natural foods. And maximize your nutrition with regular and sensible supplementation.

Exercise does good things for your heart—and the rest of your body. Reduction of high blood pressure and serum cholesterol are only two of the benefits of regular exercise. However, don't feel you have to jog around the block at 6 o'clock in the morning. Nine out of 10 people who begin a jogging program drop it in a week or two because they find it a nuisance, and they don't like the feeling of being out of breath for half an hour. Brisk walking, every day, is much more enjoyable, and because it is, you can keep it up week after week and year after year. Gardening is for many the most interesting and profitable way to get exercise for at least seven months of the year. The fresh, organic food you grow is probably worth as much as the exercise itself.

The Dangers Of Salt And Sugar

Salt and sugar are two chief ingredients in many, if not most processed foods, and both of these substances wreak havoc with your body's delicate metabolic machinery. It is now indisputably established that the extremely high salt intake of civilized man is a chief underlying cause of the development of high blood pressure. Why wait until your blood pressure goes sky-high and your doctor gives you a special diet to cut way down on salt? By cutting out this spice from your diet now, you could well be taking the single most important step to prevent the development of high blood pressure.

Helping Your Heart With Nutrition

There is no magical food supplement that prevents heart attacks. But virtually every vitamin and mineral known plays a definite role in maintaining the health of your circulatory system, and making certain that you have enough of each of them is simply a common sense protective measure.

Some nutritional substances have shown particular heart-helping characteristics, however, and these are discussed at length in other parts of this section on the heart. Lecithin, for example, is a very potent emulsifier of fats, keeping them broken up in tiny and separate particles, thereby preventing the fatty substances from clumping together in large masses. Magnesium has come to particular attention since, in 1970, the *Medical Tribune* reported that the hearts of patients who had died of a heart attack had 19 percent less magnesium in them than hearts of people who had died of other causes. Vitamin E, above all, has been shown to be a valuable nutritional ally in the building and maintenance of a healthy heart.

It is undeniable that for some people, heredity is going to play a very powerful role in determining how long and how well their hearts hold out. So will many other variables, including excessive weight, smoking, environmental pollution, and such elusive factors as the minerals in drinking water. Many of these variables are simply beyond our control. But diet is the one major variable which we can control and in which we can make radical modifications and improvements without having to go to any significant expense, or change our whole style of life. It may not be the best possible way, but it's just about the only way. And now the warnings are not only for men, but for all women, too.

201. Constipation Strain, A Heart Threat

Most heart patients are acutely aware of the importance of diet, and many conscientiously try to cut out alcohol and excess fat. But there is another dimension to diet which is of great importance to the heart patient, although few know much about it, and others prefer not to think about it. What happens to the food you eat—regardless of whether it is high or low in cholesterol—when it reaches your lower bowels and needs to be eliminated?

Many of us have heard of someone we knew who had a weak heart and was found dead in the bathroom. In fact, it is fairly common for people to collapse in the bathroom even when they are not known to have a bad heart.

The blunt truth is that most of these people died before their time as an indirect result of straining at stool.

The abnormal stress which straining puts on the heart is much greater than you might imagine. In fact, even people who have no signs of a heart problem can dangerously overburden their hearts when straining, according to a paper delivered by Dr. Norman Shaftel of New York to a symposium on "Pitfalls in the Rehabilitation of the Cardiovascular Patient," sponsored by the American College of Angiology in New York in 1957.

Dr. Shaftel said that tests showed that in people with no previous history of heart disorder, straining produced "important changes" in heart rate, blood pressure, and electrocardiograph patterns. Further, these changes closely resemble those which are seen in known heart patients, he said.

Specifically, about 12 percent of straining episodes are found to be of sufficient intensity and duration to produce significant abnormalities. The frequency of such incidents, he declared, *is increased five times by constipation.*

Naturally, Dr. Shaftel strongly recommended that physicians treating heart patients take every precaution to make sure these patients do not become constipated. He was unable to state precisely how common death following strained defecation is, but he did say that it "is not rare."

Embolism Can Be Provoked

An unsigned review appearing in *The Lancet* of August 15, 1959, points out that blood flow studies have shown "quite remarkable changes in the size of the veins of the limbs and of the flow of blood through them" during bathroom straining. These changes are much greater in constipation, and "may be sufficient to cause the mobilization of peripheral thrombi with subsequent embolization."

The review concludes that "early correction of constipation would seem to be a wise precaution in patients with any vascular disease liable to give rise to thrombi (blood clots)," which includes not only heart patients, but patients recovering from surgical operations where subsequent pulmonary embolisms are known to be common.

Paul M. Zoll, M.D., writing in the *Journal of the American Medical Association* (September, 1961) pointed out that because of the marked increase in pressure within the entire thoracic and abdominal cavity while straining, "a diverticulum of the bowel or an aneurysm of a major blood vessel or of the left ventricle might rupture." Straining can also bring on angina or "prolonged cardiac pain in a patient with extensive coronary disease," he warns.

Fecal Impaction Is Well Worth Preventing

Fecal impaction can result when a mass of harder than usual feces lodges in the bowels. An article by Dr. Richard W. Young in the August, 1973, issue of the *Journal of the American Geriatrics Society* warns that physicians "often overlook the obvious dangers and the frequent occurrence of fecal impaction in the aged. The chain reaction that may start from such an apparently minor disorder as fecal impaction can have many ramifications and lead to serious complications."

Dr. Young, who is associated with Villa Feliciana Geriatric Hospital in Jackson, Louisiana, explains that fecal impaction may cause, among other conditions, fever; vomiting; diarrhea (around the fecal mass) with cramps; back pains or lower abdominal pain accompanied with frequent urination; angina or abnormal heart rhythms in patients subject to these disorders; a sudden rise in blood pressure in hypertensive patients, which can lead to a stroke or heart failure; irritation or thrombosis of hemorrhoids; and rectal fissuring when the impaction is passed.

There is a happy side to all this grim business, though. In the great majority of cases, chronic constipation can be both prevented and cured by a simple and well-proven dietary expedient: adding roughage to the diet. (See Constipation Section)

202. Weather Extremes Are Hard On The Heart

Winter Cold

Winter has its special pleasures. Skiers love it, children glory in it, and all of us feel the stimulation of a bright, dry, cold winter day, when walking is a pleasure and when at night the stars come out in a special winter clarity.

But winter lasts so long! And it can be not only unpleasant but dangerous to health and to life itself.

The highest mortality from heart disease—specifically coronary thrombosis, myocardial infarction, and angina pectoris— occurs in January and February in Western Europe and northern United States, asserts *A Survey of Human Biometeorology* published in 1964 by the World Meteorological Organization, Geneva, a specialized agency of the United Nations, concerned with the relationship of man to his atmospheric environment.

The *Survey* also reports that the highest mortality from apoplexy—a rupture or stoppage of a blood vessel, such as stroke when it takes place in the brain—also occurs in the same two months, January and February.

Heart Attacks And Stroke

The coldness of winter, in and of itself, is a serious hazard to people with heart and circulatory problems.   "Persons susceptible to heart attack are liable to feel their first bout of pain (angina pectoris) when moving from a warm building into the outside air on a cold day," according to the British journal, *New Scientist* (September 12, 1968). The reason for this phenomenon is thought to be "that a nervous reflex is triggered when cold air strikes the face (especially the lips) and this produces a restriction in the vessels supplying blood to the heart."

In a healthy person, presumably, this restriction is perfectly tolerable. But in a person already having difficulty getting adequate oxygen to his heart, the narrowing of the coronary arteries can cause damage and perhaps death.

Cold weather also tends to increase the peripheral resistance of the blood vessels, the editors of *A Survey of Human Biometeorology* write. Thus the heart is taxed to pump harder to push the blood past the increased resistance offered by the arterial walls, and its need for oxygen is greater.

Heart patients should be cautious in venturing outside on bitter cold days. (So should asthma patients, incidentally; they frequently have allergic reactions to sudden breathing of cold air.) If it is necessary to make a trip, perhaps some face protection should be used. Sports stores sell protective masks. Or you can purchase a surgical mask at the drugstore. Writing in *Physical Fitness* (January-February, 1969), Curtis Mitchell speaks of doctors he knows who tie surgical masks over their mouths and noses when they go out to jog in very cold weather. A neck scarf can also be draped to protect the face below the eyes.

Internal protection, as well as external, can help the heart patient during the winter months. It was pointed out by cardiologist W. E. Shute, M.D., in his book *Medical and Preventive Uses of Vitamin E*, that this vitamin is a specific for countering the problems of restricted blood vessels. Its help is two-fold. It is a vasodilator—an agent that dilates the blood vessels—and vitamin E is an oxygen conserver—nature's most powerful guardian against loss of pure oxygen in the bloodstream.

Another vascular disturbance that mounts in the winter, according to the *Survey* compiled by the World Meteorological Organization, is fragility of the capillaries and their consequent tendency to hemorrhage.

The fact that more people have fragile capillaries in the winter than in the summer may be responsible for the high winter incidence of apoplexy, suggested the editors of the *Survey*. The types of apoplexy include the disease commonly referred to as stroke—a rupture or stoppage of a vessel in the brain. What is it about the mid-winter months that causes capillary fragility? According to the *Survey*: "It has been related to a vitamin P deficiency in winter." The bioflavonoids are commonly called vitamin P everywhere but in the U.S.

Taking adequate vitamin P is a measure to protect against rupture of the capillaries, a common occurrence in cold weather. Vitamin P occurs in foods side by side with vitamin C; like vitamin C, it is scarce in the typical winter diet.

Everyone has noticed that his hands and feet are the first to suffer from cold. They will stay warmer—and the circulation will improve—if they are exercised, or even moved around slightly;

that's because exercise creates metabolic heat. When your whole body is cold and you begin to shiver, that is nature's way of making you create metabolic heat; shivering is a form of exercise to restore the body heat to normal.

Throughout the world, in hot and cold countries, the body temperature of man and other mammals remains relatively constant at a little under 100°.

To conserve body heat, most animals grow their own outer protection, so that heat will not escape from the skin surface—the polar bear's fur, for example, and the seal's layers of fat. Humans, of course, depend on clothing. Here are some suggestions about the kind of clothing that will protect you best in bitter weather.

1. Several layers of light clothing are better than one very heavy garment. Air is an insulator, and the warm air between sweater and jacket, for example, will give you extra protection.

2. If it's snowy or rainy, it's important to wear moisture resistant clothing. Wet clothes conduct the heat away from the body, and they should be changed as soon as possible.

3. If you're going to stay out for a considerable length of time, you can best keep your hands and feet warm by again following the "layer" procedure. Two pairs of light socks are better than one heavy one. An inner glove and an outer glove can keep your hands toasty in freezing weather.

4. Make sure that your shoes are not tight—remember that circulation in the feet is a particular problem during exposure to cold, and shoes that restrict circulation are a hazard.

5. Wear a hat that can give you ear protection.

6. Protection of the legs requires really warm covering—trousers or slacks. A woman who expects to be out in the cold for any length of time shouldn't leave the house in a short dress and thin stockings.

Summer Heat

Warnings about over-exposure to the sun are usually confined to care about sun poisoning, sunstroke and possible skin cancer. These are certainly serious enough conditions, and would be enough to make most prudent persons think twice before baking themselves in pursuit of a tan. However, myocardial infarction (a clot at the heart wall) may be directly due in some cases, to over-exposure to the sun's hot rays. Writing in the *Rhode Island Medical Journal* (October, 1958) John C. Ham, M.D., and Alton M. Paull, M.D., presented evidence to support their theory.

The Heart

Two cases of myocardial infarction occurring in rapid succession, and associated with intense exposure to the sun, led the authors to investigate the possibility of naming such exposure as a definite cause of heart attack. Research soon brought out the fact that exposure of the body to heat produces changes in the physical and chemical characteristics of blood in animals and man which might tend to slow the coronary circulation and to favor blood clotting.

Experiments with rabbits, overheated for short periods of less than two hours, showed that the rhythm of their heartbeat was altered, the valves of the heart were disturbed and coronary circulation and myocardial function were abnormal. In overheated dogs, it was found that the blood chemistry was very definitely altered—the blood sugar level was changed and the salt content increased.

Ham and Paull cite a study of 44 human cases of heat stroke. In all of them, the blood chemistry had spontaneously changed, and in some cases, signs of heart failure or circulatory failure, appeared. Another report tells of three cases of heat stroke observed at various periods of time following a long march in hot weather. The subjects, all male, were 22, 23 and 30 years of age, respectively. Their symptoms included a pressure and oppressive feeling in the chest in one and a sudden loss of consciousness in another. The third patient showed strong symptoms of myocardial infarction.

Supporting Ham and Paull, H. E. Heyer, et al, (*American Health Journal*, 15; 741-747, 1953), found that the incidence of myocardial infarction in Dallas, Texas was considerably higher in the months of July and August than in cooler months. The daily temperature readings in Dallas during these months usually exceed 95°, and often 100° F. Heyer suggested that the profound physiologic adjustment one must make to maintain constant body temperature under such conditions may be a causative factor in the incidence of myocardial infarction. In none of the patients included in this study was there frank heat stroke, but a mild degree of heat exhaustion is common in Dallas. Adjustment to such a climate does cause an increase in cardiac work, often with increased output of blood volume, and transmission of a larger portion of blood through to the skin to promote heat loss. Such activity, according to Heyer, is quite likely to lead to myocardial infarction.

928

203. Obesity, The Heart-Wrecker—And How To Beat It

The overweight population of America dies from heart disease at three times the rate of the underweight population, and twice the rate of those of normal weight. A person who is 30 percent overweight at age 45 can expect to die in 12 years; a 45-year-old of normal weight has another 25 years of living to do. These statistics by the Metropolitan Life Insurance Company confirm what most physicians have known for 50 years: excess weight is a killer. And no part of the body is hurt more by overweight than the heart.

When the *German Tribune* (March 25, 1967) reported that the incidence of high blood pressure in Germany rose 250 percent since World War II, Dr. Rausch, then head of the Federal Republic's Food Council, commented that obesity was a major factor. High blood pressure, along with other coronary illnesses, accounts for 40 percent of all German deaths. The wrong diet is as much involved in the prevalence of heart disorders as the stresses of business life, said Rausch.

The Michigan School of Public Health at Ann Arbor demonstrated the blood pressure-weight relationship with a 1962 study involving 746 male workers. Their histories over 20 years were examined for blood pressure and weight changes. High blood pressure occurred more often among the men who were overweight as young adults than those who, as young adults, had been of desirable weight or slightly less. Most of the subjects were slim when young, but a majority had become obese by middle age. The small number who maintained a desirable weight throughout the 20-year period had the lowest incidence of high blood pressure. Data showed that the blood pressure rose as the weight did. The highest occurred in those with the greatest weight gain.

Reverse The Danger

One comforting fact: the damaging effect of overweight is reversible when the weight is trimmed. Typical of the many studies that support this theory is one reported in *Risk Appraisal* by Harry Dingmen, covering analyses of 9,926 random life insurance policy holders. Blood pressure increased along with age and weight increase in all of them. Based on this study the author asks, "If 1,000 heavyweight persons average higher blood pressure than 1,000 lesser-weight persons, will 1,000 persons show step-up of blood pressure when they become heavier? And conversely will there be a decrease of blood pressure with decrease in weight? Answer is yes."

A. P. Fletcher, M.D., reported in the *Quarterly Journal of Medicine* (July, 1954) on his experiment with overweight female outpatients at a London hospital. They were classified as "obese" if their weight was 20 percent over the maximum ideal weight for their age and height. They were called "hypertensive" if their blood pressure was 150 over 100. The women were put on a diet of 600 calories a day and urged to keep it. Toward the end of the dieting period the number of calories allowed was raised to 1,000. All the women who said they stuck with the diet (whether it was 600 or 1,000 calories) did lose weight, and as their weight went down their blood pressure went down also. The blood pressure of those who did not diet and did not lose weight, did not go down.

Safe And Easy Diet

The very suggestion of a 600-calorie diet defeats some overweight people. Even if they were willing to try it, they are sure they couldn't stay with it. Why not try other ways to lose weight without counting calories?

Overweight is one problem you can lick on your own. If you want to stay healthy, a sensible weight level is essential.

Eat More Often To Fight Obesity And Heart Disease

Nutritionists who used to believe that weight control was strictly a calorie counting problem in mathematics, are coming around to the conviction that the body has less tendency to accumulate fat deposits if meals are eaten more frequently and served in smaller portions—without a reduction in the daily food intake. They have also found that the meal which is most important and should therefore make the largest caloric contribution to a person's day is breakfast.

Doctors Pavel Fabry and Jay Tepperman reported in the August, 1970 *American Journal of Clinical Nutrition* that "ex-

cessive weight and, in elderly age groups, also hypercholestero-
lemia, impaired glucose tolerance, and ischemic heart disease
was more common among persons with an infrequent meal pattern than among those who customarily ate five or more meals per
day." They found, for example, that many Americans undermine
their own health when they disregard breakfast and emphasize
the evening meal as the time for their largest daily portion of
food. That this attitude toward meals may possibly be dangerous,
and might even encourage the onset of heart disease, obesity,
gallstones, and diabetes, is what nutritionists are learning from
experiments conducted so far.

It seems that if man tries to store food in the same manner that
a camel takes on water, he is headed for trouble. One experiment
after another has shown that the level of fats in the bloodstream
rises in people who eat only a couple of heavy meals a day for
their daily fuel.

Spreading out food into smaller portions throughout the day
favorably affects not only older people, but probably everybody,
according to the results of another study reported by Fabry, *et al,*
in the *American Journal of Clinical Nutrition* (May, 1966). They
found that after examining children aged 10 to 16 from three
boarding schools where the calorically-equivalent daily ration
was divided into three, five or seven portions, respectively,
throughout the day, that "in the school serving three meals per
day there was a significantly greater percentage of subjects in
whom the weight-height proportionality changed in favor of body
weight than in the two other schools . . . the increment of the skin-
fold thickness was also significantly greater compared with that
found in children of similar age who ate five or seven meals per
day." If the number of meals per day can have such an influence
on active, young children, think of what effect it must have on
older people whose activities are limited.

Sugar Is A Killer

Sugar has rightfully been called a killer. John Yudkin, professor
of Nutrition at Queen Elizabeth College, London, says in the
book *Getting The Most Out of Food* (Van der Berghs, London,
1965) that, "there are three nutritional disadvantages of a high
consumption of sugar . . . the first is that it is one of the reasons
why so many of us are taking too many calories, and run into the
problem of overweight—a problem, incidentally, that is one of

ill-health, and not merely one of poor aesthetics. Secondly it tends to displace more nutritious foods; while sugar supplies calories, or . . . energy, every single other food supplies nutrients, and calories too. . . . The third disadvantage of a high consumption of sugar is that it leads to disease. Most of us know of the connection between sugar-eating and dental decay. Less well known is the probable relationship between a high sugar consumption . . . and stomach ulcers, diabetes and above all coronary thrombosis."

So we see that not only is eating food more frequently in smaller portions better than infrequent eating, but also that a regime of only two or three meals a day containing a high amount of sugars and carbohydrates can actually be a threat to your health, and your life.

Studies so far indicate that a daily dietary regimen consisting of a substantial breakfast that provides sufficient protein followed by frequent, light meals for the rest of the day will be most helpful to your body. It will not force you to store unnecessary fats and, combined with a sensible choice of foods, will not make you a candidate for heart disease.

Further evidence of this is found in a report by Fabry *et al* in *The Lancet* (2: 190, 1968), stating that 1,359 men aged 60-64 years were examined to determine the occurrence of ischemic heart disease (caused by the decreased blood flow to the heart muscle) according to the criteria of the World Health Organization. In order to keep the evaluation as accurate as possible, 226 patients who suffered from diabetes, peptic ulcer, gastrectomy, or colostomy, all of which require special diets that influence meal frequency, were removed from the final evaluation. The study showed that 30.4 percent of those men who ate three or fewer meals a day were diagnosed to have ischemic disease while another group who ate five or more meals a day suffered a prevalence of only 19.9 percent of the disease.

How can you possibly fit as many as five or six feedings into a regular work day? The answer is that you eat lightly, and therefore quickly, each time. At home you can reach for a piece of fruit for a nutritious snack while passing through the kitchen. At work, pack a heavier lunch, and instead of just turning your back on sweet snacks during morning and afternoon break, eat an apple or munch on some nuts. You'll find your energy lasting longer, your end-of-the-morning work easier to perform, and your mealtime hunger reduced.

The prospect of eating five or more light meals and snacks of healthful foods per day is a delightful one. This program will take away the temptation to eat refined, sweet snacks between meals, and, most important, will have a positive effect on your appearance and on your health.

204. Better Hearts Through Exercise

Leave your car in the garage and walk into town or into the country, and you're doing more than conserving money and gas. You are protecting yourself from physical degeneration.

Physical activity not only burns off calories but also stimulates heart action, causing an increased blood supply to circulate through the system. Exercise helps to keep the arteries open, especially if they are already partly obstructed by excessive fat deposits. Just walking can help lower cholesterol levels and clear the arteries of plaques. For an example of what such a regimen can do for heart health, consider the Masai of central Africa.

To find a group of physically fit people practically free from heart disease has become an increasingly hard task in the civilized world. Yet one group that is remarkably blessed with this type of good health is the Masai tribe in Tanzania. A study supervised by George Mann, M.D., Sc.D., was published in *The Lancet* (December 25, 1965).

Great Walkers
Dr. Mann and his associates explain the habits of these people: "The environmental requirements of the Masai are rigorous. They spend much of their lives as boys walking with the herds. As warriors they are on the move almost daily, walking great distances in their surveillance of cattle, property, girls, and distant friends. Their exercise seems to be primarily walking which is done at a brisk, long stride" at a rate of three to five miles an hour.

The Masai are lean people. Despite a diet of meat and milk that is far from fat-free, they have low blood pressure, healthy arteries, and cholesterol levels lower than those of their vegetarian neighbors. The Masai use no salt and in fact do not even have a word in the language for this dubious substance known to raise the blood pressure. Refined carbohydrates—cakes, cookies, candies—are completely unknown. Men do not smoke until age

30. Only a very small number of tribesmen have ever had jaundice, thyroid disorders, gout, or arthritis.

Dr. Mann examined the fitness of 53 Masai males between 14 and 64 years of age. The men were asked to walk on an electrically driven treadmill until they felt exhausted. After each man stopped, his pulse rate was counted. It was found that most of the subjects could outperform "athletes of Olympic standard." Even when the men did drop out, it was because of leg pain, rather than oxygen insufficiency. This experiment was a definite indication of a group in excellent physical shape with excellent heart conditions.

Inactivity Is Dangerous

There is no reason why each of us cannot guard against death from a heart attack by changing certain habits. If you have a desk job or stay at home all the time, you are taking a risk. Dr. Mann cites the opinion of J. N. Norris: "Men in physically active jobs have less ischemic heart disease during middle age, what disease they do have is less severe, and they develop it later than men in physically inactive jobs."

While regular exercise is the best preventive medicine for heart trouble, activity after a non-fatal attack is also beneficial. In a paper presented to the Annual National Recreational Congress in Philadelphia, Pennsylvania (1962), Dr. Joseph Wolffe, of the Valley Forge Medical Center and Heart Hospital in Norristown, Pennsylvania, wrote, "Stair walking involves all systems of the body. The body is carried upward by the skeletal muscles. Groups of muscles contract while their antagonists relax. The work that is required is not limited, however, to the lower extremities; important chemical changes take place, more blood and oxygen is needed by the active muscles. The heart and vessels are gradually strengthened to meet the demand."

Walking has become very important in the treatment of heart patients. Doctors know now that it is the best way to make the muscles take over their share of the work and relieve the damaged heart. Even a little walk can improve circulation and cost the heart nothing. In fact, say Aaron Sussman and Ruth Goode, authors of *The Magic of Walking* (Simon and Schuster, New York), people whose heart rates and blood pressures are high will find that a regimen of regular walking—not necessarily far or fast—brings the heart rate and blood pressure down to normal levels.

In fact, this mildest of exercise forms has superb effects on collateral circulation and, along with the other benefits to health, it actually provides us with something that no amount of money can buy—a "second heart."

To ease the load of pushing some 72,000 quarts of blood through the system every 24 hours, nature has provided us with a "second heart" situated below the belt. This help to our heart comes from the muscles in the feet, calves, thighs, buttocks and abdomen. As these muscles work in concert and rhythmically, they contract and release, squeezing the veins, forcing the blood along. This is nature's way of moving the blood to the heart and brain against the force of gravity.

Heart Attack Patients Benefit From Walking

The key to efficiency of this system is walking—plain walking. When you walk, you force the muscles in your legs and abdomen to do their part in lending a hand to your heart. Without the push from these muscles, the blood tends to pool in the stomach area and in the feet. The heart must then pitch in with more force to move that blood which must travel the long route to deliver essential nutrition to every tissue in your body and to flush out dangerous wastes.

Most people who have suffered heart attacks are understandably reluctant to start an exercise program. They're afraid they might overdo it and have another attack. For the same reason, many doctors still hesitate to prescribe exercise. Doctors J. Schouten and J. Schreuder suggest in the *British Medical Journal* (March 9, 1968), that the doctor should take a walk with his patient after a heart attack. The patient naturally feels more secure when his doctor is present and the doctor can observe the patient to judge the safe limits of his endurance.

Drs. Schouten and Schreuder start their heart patients on exercise in bed. From there they take them walking.

Every organ in the body is benefitted by exercise of its function. This includes the heart. The question is how much exercise is beneficial before it starts to be dangerous. Most doctors would be willing to take a short walk with their patient to observe his tolerance and know how much exercise to prescribe. Start your walking program before you reach the coronary state. Chances are you will never need this kind of surveillance.

205. J. I. Rodale On Heart Disease

J. I. Rodale had a congenital heart defect, yet he was productive and active for many years beyond his predicted life span. In that time he functioned as a successful businessman, a writer, editor, publisher and world traveler. Mr. Rodale frequently wrote about his condition and credited his ability to maintain a full schedule to methods such as the ones described below.

Human Specific Gravity

A subject never discussed in connection with heart disease is the specific gravity of the human body. But it is of paramount importance with regard to the working of the human heart. In consideration of obesity, attention is given usually to a reduction in the food intake, rarely to the effect of exercise on the specific gravity of the body. Both of these are equally important in a reconstruction of the human body in order to prevent a heart attack.

But first let us see what we mean by specific gravity. According to the dictionary, specific gravity is the weight of a given volume of any kind of matter as compared with the weight of an equal amount of water. Specific gravity is a measure of the density of a substance, and for convenience it is contrasted with the density of water as a standard of comparison.

If the specific gravity of something is said to be 1.50, it means that a certain volume of it weighs 50 percent more than an equal volume of water. If the specific gravity of fresh water is one, then the specific gravity of sea water is about 1.026. Expressed another way this means that sea water is about two and a half percent heavier than fresh water. This is due to the fact that sea water contains more minerals than fresh water.

If a substance floats on water, it means that its specific gravity is less than that of water. If it sinks, then its specific gravity is higher than that of water. A fat person, for example, would have a lower specific gravity than a muscular person. This means that a cubic inch of fat tissue weighs less than a cubic inch of muscular tissue. The muscular tissue is more compact, the fat tissue less compact. Low specific gravity, that is where the tissue weighs less per cubic inch, is very disadvantageous from a health standpoint.

In considering the subject of specific gravity as it affects the human heart, John Davy said that organic disease of the heart cannot take place unless the specific gravity of the heart goes down. The higher the specific gravity of the heart, the less chance of it going bad. A high specific gravity for the heart means that it is all muscle. If the body becomes fat, some of it overflows into the heart muscle and impedes the heart's efficiency. You cannot selectively remove the fat from the heart unless you remove it from the entire body.

You may never have thought of your body as a work of engineering, but it is, and you are the engineer. You can make that body healthier by bringing its specific gravity up to the ideal figure for its best operation. Basically there are two ways to bring up a low specific gravity. One is by diet, the other is by exercise. But it should be exercise that must be taken every single day. I like walking for that purpose, and it should be for a minimum of an hour a day. Walking is the great elixir of human life! You cannot imagine how important it is.

The Pulse

In the consideration of heart disease one of the most important factors is the pulse (a high pulse being very dangerous in such a condition). Very little, however, is heard about this subject when heart disease is being discussed; therefore, I intend to go into the subject of the pulse in some detail.

According to the *Encyclopedia Britannica*, "The normal average pulse rate is 72 per minute, in women about 80; but individual variations from 40 to 100 have been observed consistent with health."

When we use the word *pulse* we are talking about what is called the heart rate, or the rate at which the heart pumps the blood. While the body is at rest, the heart will pump at an average of 90 gallons of blood an hour. During violent exercise it will pump at the rate of 450 to 600 gallons an hour, which means that the pulse goes up. But the rate at which the heart will pump differs in different people. For example, taking arbitrary figures, in one person it might take 100 beats to pump a gallon of blood while in another it might have to be done with 200 beats. The pulse beat represents the rate at which the heart pushes the blood through a network of vessels in the body. There are many factors involved in this work, but I will state as a general rule that the lower the pulse, within reason of course, the better it is for the health of your heart.

Drs. Raymond Pearl and W. Eden Moffet reported, after studying the lives of 386 men, that those who had a lower pulse by about four beats a minute lived longer—about 26 years longer—than the shorter-lived ones. Incidentally, the long-lived group weighed an average of six pounds each less than the short-lived group. If only a four beat difference had such a significant effect, what would be the effect of a greater difference? For example, by certain methods, I reduced by own pulse from 85 to about 68.

How does one go about reducing one's pulse? There are several things you can do.

First, you must reduce the quantity of food you eat per day. This should apply mainly to overweight persons so that if you are underweight, you would have to get special advice in this category.

A second means of lowering the pulse is to avoid emotional storms. Pulse acceleration is a common sequel of anger, apprehension and related moods.

A third means of lowering the pulse, if one is a smoker, is to eliminate that habit. Nicotine causes a shrinking of the arteries and will raise the pulse from five to 20 beats a minute.

Fourth, avoid the use of drugs. Physicians have observed very high pulses in persons taking antihistamines. Many persons take this type of drug for hay fever. Some sulfur-containing drugs will heighten the pulse. Digitalis, given to prevent a heart attack, has been known to accelerate the pulse.

High temperature may raise the pulse. A person who has a heart condition should not work in front of a steel furnace, or in a bakery, or in any job where the heat is high. It will raise the pulse by 10 or more beats a minute.

There are two other means of reducing the pulse which are extremely important. One is exercise, and the other is a study of one's diet to eliminate particular foods that have a propensity to raise the pulse. It is a form of allergy. The science of ascertaining these pulse-irritating foods was developed by Arthur F. Coca, M.D., and will be discussed in the following pages along with a description of how I reduced my pulse by means of exercise.

The Coca Method

Several years ago I was extremely fortunate in discovering Dr. Arthur F. Coca's work in curing allergies through the observation and control of the human pulse. Up to this time, the procedure in checking for a person's allergies was to scratch the skin with a needle, but Dr. Coca obtained results by observing the effect of each food on a person's pulse. If one particular food raised the pulse abnormally, he reasoned, there was an allergy to that food. Dr. Coca found that the average sick person's pulse was high because in his diet there were usually five or six foods which were difficult for his digestive system to handle. The theory was that in such cases the heart had to work harder to bring extra pressure to bear to complete the digestion of those foods.

To follow Dr. Coca's system you choose a time about an hour and a half after you have eaten, you take your pulse and eat a small portion of a food that you wish to test. You then take your pulse a half hour later, and again a half hour after that, recording the figures in a ruled book, with the date, time, etc., leaving room for a list of the foods eaten, and other comments. It will become a valuable record for later study.

I found that the average food raised the pulse from three to five points per minute, although there were some that did not raise it at all, but that when a food caused the pulse to run up eight or nine points, it was usually one of the allergy-causing ones. In my own case I discovered that figs, honeydew melon, hot chicken soup, onions, whole wheat and fried foods of any kind were the basic troublemakers. It was absolutely fascinating the fun there was in checking them down. For example, at first the indication showed that chicken raised my pulse unduly. But after I had accumulated sufficient records, showing in each case whether the chicken had been fried or broiled, I found that my pulse went up only when I ate fried chicken. I could eat broiled chicken without any trouble at all.

The whole thing is terrific in its implications! When one considers what a reduction of the pulse means to one's well-being and longevity, it is a wonder that so little work has been done in connection with researches on the human pulse. In my own case, merely by cutting certain items of food out of my diet, my pulse was reduced by 15 beats per minute.

If you decide to make a pulse study, my suggestion is first, for about a week, to keep a record of your pulse before and after whole meals. Take the pulse a half hour and an hour after your regular meals, without attempting to cut anything out of your diet. Later, after you have learned what foods are irritating your pulse and have eliminated them, do the same and observe the difference in the pulse increase before and after meals.

For a heart case it is of the utmost importance to make use of the Coca system for reducing the pulse, for the heart will have far less work to do if the pulse is significantly lowered.

The Reduction Of Pulse By Exercises

Before I became aware of the power of exercise to bring the pulse down, I was the most typical example of the sedentary businessman you could find. But eventually I began to realize that unless I went in for exercise, my physically inactive life would surely kill me before my time.

But here I was with a high pulse which had to come down by means of exercise, or else my life would be shortened, and on the other hand, a heart condition which might not respond too well to exercise. I had always heard that a heart case must rest as much as possible. So I decided to approach the matter warily. The first day I walked for only 10 minutes. Nothing happened! I was still alive. For the next few days I walked 10 minutes each day. Then I upped it to 15 and in about a week I was doing a full hour every morning, covering a brisk three miles and enjoying it immensely.

One day during this hourly walk it seemed that my heart began to pound a little, so I stopped and took my pulse. To my surprise, I found it to be 112. As my pulse at rest was between 76 and 80, I came to the conclusion that it was the exercise of walking that was making my heart work harder. A few hours later at rest my pulse was back to about 78. In other words, the demands that my walking made on my heart had raised it about 35 beats a minute. An interesting bit of knowledge, I thought.

Thinking that danger might be concealed somewhere in this fact, I decided from this point on to keep a record of my pulse during these walks.

A word about the method of taking my pulse. When I stop, I wait about 20 seconds, and then count the beats of my heart as I note the ticking off of 30 seconds by the watch. I then take the count of the next 30 seconds and that is the one I record. This of course, is then multiplied by two. I stop for a rest of about a half minute to a minute, halfway between each pulse stop, thus making about 20 stops in all. However, if I experience any pressure symptoms, I will stop for a moment wherever necessary.

Exercise

There was a time when I used to pooh-pooh the value of exercise, and I used to tell the story of Chauncey Depew, the famous financier of the last century, who lived to be way over 90, and who always deprecated the importance of taking exercise. "The only exercise I get," he used to say, "is to act as pallbearer for friends who used to take exercise."

Perhaps he didn't take exercise as such but I'll wager he was a big walker, for those were the days before the auto was known. He was a stockholder in many corporations and was known to attend many board meetings, going from one to another, sometimes merely to show his face and to collect the director's fee. But there is a reason why some persons live to 90 without exercise, and why others die at 50. It is a matter of the vitality endowment at birth, the condition of the glands, chest expansion, width of arteries, etc. If a man has chosen the right ancestors and received a good share of their physical perfection through the accident of birth, then he can break many health rules and still live to a ripe old age.

One need not spend hours in daily calisthenics. Walking furnishes a very interesting form of exercise, although at least 10 minutes of daily setting-up exercises can be very valuable. I strongly recommend a walk of at least an hour a day. Some people seem to forget that they have feet. They forget that there is such a thing as walking. The other day in visiting a hospital I walked down two flights of stairs, and a nurse remarked, in amazement, "Are you *walking* down?"

A doctor in a medical journal says, "The popular picture of the coronary heart disease victim is that of a burly business or professional man, fat and soft from overeating and lack of exercise." Another expresses it this way, "Motion is the essence of life. Like all things pertaining to life, we know little concerning it. It is an inherent characteristic of all animate things to move through space with ease and power, not only for protection but for the pleasure of doing so." I have learned to love my daily hour's walk, and wouldn't miss it for anything except rain or snow.

Dr. Paul D. White, world renowned heart specialist, told a House Appropriations Subcommittee, "Coronary thrombosis is an epidemic . . . . Wise exercise is one remedy."

As far as I'm concerned, I'm conscious of the fact that I have to move about as much as possible, in order to keep the fat out of my heart muscle. I have my telephone at another desk. Every time it rings I have to walk 15 feet to it and 15 feet back. My office is on the third floor and every day I walk up and down to and from it at least four or five times—sometimes more, because I purposely do not have a buzzer system. When I want to talk to one of my people, I go to them. I do not make them come to me.

Exercise—What It Does

The most important thing that exercise does is to oxygenate the body which is most desirable to a heart case, for it is lack of oxygen which is an important element in inducing a heart attack. Oxygenation of the body may be compared to the draft of a boiler which burns up the refuse and slag in the body.

Dr. William B. Kountz, Professor of Clinical Medicine at Washington University, at a public meeting said that the medical profession has long been aware that a decline in the body's oxygen consumption causes such ailments as hardening of the arteries, heart disease, body-wasting and other typical manifestations of old age. This is important, he said, in the maintaining of the burning or oxidative process of the body. When the oxygen supply to the tissues goes down, the number and size of the cells also decreases. This causes tissue atrophy, or aging. Thus, by taking exercise, and insuring the oxygenation of the body, one might age more gracefully.

Angina pectoris, a disease marked by a sudden or periodic chest pain, sometimes with a feeling of suffocation and impending death, is due most often to lack of oxygen in the muscular substance of the heart; that is, the heart muscle.

Another effect of exercise is to maintain the general muscular tone throughout the body. This includes the heart muscle, the importance of whose tone can well be realized. An important muscle is the diaphragm which, if its muscular tone improves, will enable a person to breathe more efficiently. This means healthier lungs. The diaphragm works like the piston of a pump, and if it has good tone, it can more efficiently cause the suction of blood into the heart via the great veins. Exercise breaks up congestion in the lungs; breathing becomes easier.

The effect of exercise is to quicken the circulation. In a man at rest about a gallon of blood is circulated every minute. Approximately the entire blood supply visits the tissues once every minute. With vigorous exercise these visits may be eight or nine times as frequent. The blood, instead of traveling at a rate of 55 feet a minute in the large arteries, may move 450 feet a minute. This makes possible a more rapid and complete removal of waste from all parts of the body, and increases the amount of oxygen in parts of the body depending on it. Exercise taken simply and regularly tends to keep the arteries soft, warding off arteriosclerosis or other old age conditions.

Exercise improves bowel function and digestion. It also helps to induce sleep. It controls obesity and, most important, takes the fat out of the walls of the coronary and other important arteries. This is one of the most important rewards of exercise. It reduces the cholesterol level of the blood.

Besides lowering the cholesterol level of the blood, exercise increases the specific gravity of the body, making the tissues more compact. This is highly desirable in connection with the body's general economy, but especially in regard to the functioning of the heart.

Is Exercise Harmful To A Heart Case?

I think common sense would dictate that a person who has heart trouble should eliminate strenuous forms of exercise, such as hockey and basketball. In our discussion we will include such exercises as walking, golf, horseback riding, and setting-up exercises. I would say that 99 percent of heart cases can safely exercise.

It used to be thought that the average heart attack came in the throes of severe activity, but recent studies indicate that this is not so.

When Dr. Arthur M. Master analyzed 2,200 heart attacks, he found 23 percent occurred during sleep, 29 percent while at work, 24 percent during mild activity, 13 percent during walking at an ordinary pace, nine percent during moderate activity and only two percent during unusual exertion.

The question naturally arises whether there are certain kinds of heart conditions where caution should be the rule on the question of exercise. There are a few. Where there has been some kind of incident in connection with the heart, conservatism would call for prudence in connection with exercise. In such cases the physician will usually advise the proper course.

Walking For The Heart

The historian George Macaulay Trevelyan once said, "I have two doctors, my left leg and my right"—a very witty statement, but powerfully true. In the case of a heart condition, these two "doctors" can save the life of the patient. Movement, that's what a heart case needs. Keep the heart pumping and teach it to like it.

People have said to me, "I'm so busy, when will I have the time to walk?" Squeeze the time out somehow. Everything else will get done, you will see. Here is an interesting plan for the beginning walker. Start off by walking 15 minutes before going to work. Then do 15 minutes during the lunch period, and 15 minutes before or after the evening meal. Slowly these periods can be lengthened until one finds that he is going two hours a day without any trouble at all.

If there is something about your kind of heart condition that you think contra-indicates walking, you will know it after your first 15 minutes. But it would be best to clear it with your doctor first—and then follow some kind of plan.

At the beginning it would be best to search out a flat terrain, otherwise heart cases will experience angina symptoms. Expect also that you will have more difficulty at the beginning of a walk than in the second half. If pressure pains occur, rest a moment or two. At the beginning of muscular exertion, time is required for the adjustment of the circulation to the increased oxygen demand. But this initial period of oxygen deficiency soon passes. The taking of vitamin E, which increases the oxygenation of the body, is very helpful to walkers.

There's a great advantage to heart cases in walking regularly, rather than merely at weekends. Give the heart a daily treatment. It is just like taking vitamins—you must do it every day. The cumulative effect on the heart's action will soon be noticeable. After a while you will develop a kinesthetic sense, that is, a sense of surefootedness, a sense of perception of muscular movement. It will create grace in the motions of the body.

Section 37
Hemorrhoids

206. The Best Things To Do About Hemorrhoids

According to conservative estimates, half the adults in this country over the age of 40 suffer from hemorrhoids, which are simply varicose veins of the anal region. But, even though hemorrhoids afflict one out of every two, they can be prevented and cured—with improved diet, exercise, and careful attention to cleanliness.

In 1974, Dr. P. Muller and his associates of the Hospices Civils in Strasbourg, France, reported to *Family Practice News* (March 15) that when they successfully administered flavone compounds (another name for bioflavonoids) to women with gynecological problems, those women who had hemorrhoids experienced relief from this problem, too.

To appreciate the vital importance of these flavones found in berries, in buckwheat, and in the pulp and inner rind of citrus fruits, it helps to understand a little about the anatomy of the hemorrhoid.

Architectural structure has something to do with these lesions. Gravity imposes a constant load on the delicate veins which supply the anus, the puckered valve at the end of the 25-foot-long digestive tract. While most veins have check valves to prevent backflow of blood and keep it moving toward the heart, there are no check valves in the column of blood which extends through the veins down the abdomen to the hemorrhoidal area. Therefore, the entire weight of this column of blood bears on these tiny blood vessels.

When pressure causes an excessive flow of blood to the rectal area, the normal channels are unable to handle it all and the smaller veins get the excess.

When pressure is strong in the abdomen, thus constricting the veins, some of the blood that would ordinarily return through the abdominal veins goes instead to the alternative system. These alternative veins begin to stretch and stretch like a balloon. Sometimes they lose their elasticity and remain engorged—they

948

may protrude and cause external hemorrhoids. They may tear and bleed. Blood loss may not seem like much—but if it persists it can cause anemia.

While straining at stool is the prime cause preventing the blood from getting through the larger veins, straining applies to conditions other than a difficult bowel movement. Lifting a heavy object, and even coughing tightens abdominal muscles, thus squeezing on these veins.

Dr. John E. Eichenlaub gave this advice many years ago in *Today's Health.* "While lifting, breathe freely to eliminate any abdominal pressure on the hemorrhoidal veins." Inhale and exhale constantly. The idea, while lifting or during bowel movements, is not to hold your breath—a common practice among those who strain at stool.

Drink lots of liquids—water and fruit juices. Avoid sugar and refined foods made of white flour. Among people who live on unrefined foods, such as the Zulus in Africa, hemorrhoids are virtually unknown. Eat high-residue foods like fresh fruits, vegetables and bran. Use the unprocessed or coarse bran. The greater water-holding capacity of coarse bran makes it preferable for the treatment of all colonic disorders, it was revealed in a study on the action of different bran preparations conducted at the University of Edinburgh, Western General Hospital, and reported in the *British Medical Journal* (October 26, 1974).

A doctor in Switzerland reported he cured thousands of patients suffering various types of hemorrhoids with orally administered trioxyethylrutin, a bioflavonoid sometimes referred to as P_4 (*Current Therapeutic Research*, August, 1963).

The reputation of rutin and the other naturally occurring bioflavonoids for strengthening capillary walls led Dr. Bernard A. L. Wissmer of the University of Geneva to use this food component in his efforts to relieve hemorrhoids. The aim in the production of P_4 was to step up the efficiency of rutin so that even the most serious conditions might be saved from surgery.

Dr. Wissmer's experiment included 250 patients with various types of hemorrhoids. Each patient's progress was watched through anoscopic and rectoscopic examination for about six months. Each patient received P_4 orally in capsules containing 100 mg. of the medication. The usual dose was four to six capsules every day for a week, then the dose was reduced to two or three daily for a period of three or four weeks or more.

Complete disappearance of symptoms and bleeding occurred

in 97 out of 148 patients treated with P_4 for chronic internal hemorrhoids. Of the remaining cases, 32 experienced significant improvement; however, slight bleeding persisted occasionally. In 16 cases there was partial improvement—reduction of pain, less frequent bleeding. Only three of the 148 cases showed no improvement whatsoever and eventually had to have surgery. For the majority of patients, an end of pain and bleeding occurred in only two to five days. An objective examination after only one or two weeks showed remarkable changes in the rectal area as it returned to normal.

In 32 cases of chronic external hemorrhoids (piles), which are more difficult to treat, there were 28 complete remissions without evidence of recurrence, and only four failures.

Another group of scientists used rutin rather than P_4 to correct capillary fault.

Griffith, Krewson and Naghski, who documented their findings in their book *Rutin and Related Flavonoids* (Mack Publishing, Easton, Pa., 1955) started their patients on 20 mg. three times daily, and tested them every six weeks. Every time a test was found to be abnormal, rutin dosage was increased. Since rutin is not toxic, the final dose may be high, in their series as high as 600 mg. per day.

Adding to the re-awakening interest the medical profession is showing in the therapeutic possibilities of onions for treatment of high blood pressure and other problems of the circulatory system, there appeared in the *Canadian Medical Association Journal* (April 5, 1969) a letter from Dr. M. Valeriote of Guelph, Ontario. Dr. Valeriote pointed out that he had been chronically troubled over a long period of time with bleeding hemorrhoids. In 1945 he had an operation which corrected the situation temporarily. Two years later, though, the bleeding recurred "and since then there has been evidence of bleeding with almost every bowel movement."

Dr. Valeriote made an unexpected observation, however. "About 18 months ago, after a particularly severe bleeding, there was no bleeding for two days. This was unusual. It occurred to me that possibly this had some relation to the fact that I had just eaten a very large helping of fried onions. When the bleeding recurred I again ate a large helping of onions and again the bleeding stopped. I found that I was able to control the bleeding by eating onion soup or fried onions. In December I began a three-week holiday and made a point of eating onion soup every day (a practice which I have continued) and there has been no bleeding for over two months."

Dr. Wilfrid E. Shute, who was chief of cardiology at the Shute Foundation for Medical Research in Toronto, Canada, tells of his successful treatment of many cases of varicose veins in this book written with Harald Taub, *Vitamin E for Ailing and Healthy Hearts* (Pyramid House, 1969). Since hemorrhoids are, in fact, varicose veins of the anal canal, it would certainly make sense to increase your intake of this versatile vitamin which can be very helpful to you in yet another area. Vitamin E has demonstrated time and time again its remarkable ability to prevent and dissolve blood clots. It may well help to eliminate the clots which make piles so painful.

For relief of pain from hemorrhoids and for lubrication, try A and D ointment, vitamin E ointment, or a vitamin E suppository which contains no drugs.

Improved diet, more exercise and cleanliness comprise a self-help program which will help prevent and in some cases, even cure a case of hemorrhoids.

If, however, you have rectal bleeding, with or without pain and with or without any sign of hemorrhoids, have it checked out by a doctor. One of 50 people complaining of hemorrhoids actually has a tumor. If you are the one in 50, catching it early may save your life.

Section 38
Hernia

207. What Are Hernias? Might You Have One?

Most persons who have never actually experienced a hernia, or rupture, as it is commonly called, are not very clear on just what it is. Technically, hernia is the escape or protrusion of an organ, or part of an organ, from its natural cavity. By the terms of its own definition, a hernia can occur almost anywhere in the body—the brain, the lungs, the iris of the eye, etc. Each of these is an organ contained in a specific area of the body, and if some part of one of them should spill over the bounds set by nature for its containment, or should push through the skin walls that hold it in place, a hernia of that organ has occurred.

More commonly a hernia refers to the escape of some part of the intestine from the abdominal cavity, through an opening in the abdominal wall. It then pushes out from the inner body, often to a point just below the surface of the skin. When it reaches this point, a hernia is usually visible. At first it is about the size and shape of a marble, and grows larger as more and more intestine escapes. The victim often notices a "dragging" feeling in the abdomen, coupled with severe constipation and tenderness.

Sometimes the hernia is not visible and can only be discovered by a physician examining the common sites of hernias. This is especially true of the hernia sites in the thigh, groin and navel regions, the three most common sites of hernias in the lower abdomen. However, detection of the hiatal hernia, the primary hernia of the upper abdominal region, is extremely difficult, even when the doctor is specifically examining for one. But hernias of the lower abdomen are much easier to detect. Although not always visible externally, the doctor can detect them by placing his hand over the suspected area and asking the patient to cough. The sudden increase of abdominal pressure created by the cough creates a "pulse" that can be felt if the hernia is present.

There are three areas in which the occurrence of intestinal hernias of the lower abdomen are most likely: the groin or the base of the abdomen, the point at which the legs and torso meet (inguinal hernia); the upper part of the thigh (femoral hernia); the region of the navel (umbilical hernia). In each of these cases, some loop of the intestine will have broken through the abdominal wall and followed the easiest path to one of these points.

The inguinal hernia occurs most frequently in men. The inguinal canal is a passage, from the abdominal wall to the groin, through which the unborn male's testes descend to the scrotum, and certain ligaments in the female descend to the genital area. Normally this canal closes once its purpose has been accomplished. However, if the closure is not complete, it can be seen that the passage would offer an excellent avenue for the descent of an escaping intestinal loop. In the male, this loop can descend into the scrotum, and remain painful and undetected until the patient undergoes a physical examination.

There is also a type of hernia more peculiar to females. Most female hernias are of the femoral type. The femoral canal leads from the pelvis into the thigh, and serves as a vascular channel for the main vein, which returns blood from the leg to the heart. Normally this vein and a few small lymph glands are the sole occupants of the canal. However, when a hernia develops here, a sac composed of a weak portion of the inner abdominal tissue, and a small segment of the intestine, pushes into the canal, causing a visible and painful bulge on the upper inside part of the thigh.

The umbilical hernia is the result of a giving way of the abdominal wall tissues near the site of the navel, a weak area in many infants. The protrusion is usually quite visible, and sometimes easiest to treat.

208. The Varying Causes Of Lower Abdominal Hernia

The causes of lower abdominal hernia vary, but most of the immediate causes relate in some way to sudden or unusual pressure on the abdominal wall. The most widely recognized cause is heavy lifting, and putting the weight of the object on the stomach muscles instead of the stronger arms, shoulders and legs. Another frequent cause of lower abdominal hernia is constipation, and the resultant straining at stool. This puts a tremendous strain on the abdominal wall, and is a dangerous practice which should be carefully avoided. Excessive coughing can result in hernia, and vomiting is another physiological activity which puts great pressure on the tissue that keeps the intestines in place.

The accumulation of fat in the intestinal area causes a downward pull against the abdominal wall which can result in hernia. Persons who are heavy about the middle should make every effort to reduce, lest hernia be added to the other problems of overweight. Pregnancy can effect a similar strain on the abdominal wall; however, if proper nutritional procedures are followed, the body can compensate for this natural condition with ease.

Jumps from high places to solid surfaces should also be avoided. The intestines' weight is augmented by a high jump and sudden stop. Again the abdominal wall must, so to speak, "catch" the intestines when one lands. If the tissue is weak, this type of activity can easily lead to a hernia.

The intestines are rather like a long hose coiled carefully within the abdomen. If a hernia should occur, and a part of the intestinal hose should escape, it is like a hanging loop. If caught soon enough, it can be pushed back through the hole and into its normal position quite easily by simple surgery. If the hernia is neglected, it can grow and become twisted, just as garden hose can become twisted, so that no blood can pass through it. The result can be infection and gangrene. Therefore, it is extremely dangerous to ignore a hernia, for, unless it is repaired, it can become serious enough to cause death.

209. Using A Truss For Lower Abdominal Hernias

Where does the truss fit into the hernia picture? The truss is a pad of some kind (wood, hard rubber, plastic, etc.), usually fastened to a belt which fits around the waist. The pad is placed at the site of the hernia to push the intestine back toward its normal position. If used properly it can relieve much of the discomfort and pain of a hernia, but it is not a cure. Usually it is used as a temporary measure in case surgery might not be readily possible, for one reason or another.

In a small child, the truss is sometimes used to better effect. Children are often born with hernias around the navel. If the hernia is properly supported, the tissue from which it escaped, may, due to the youth of the child, grow properly over it. Doctors often allow up to three years for this to occur before resorting to surgery.

Avoidance of hernia begins in the womb. The proper diet of the mother-to-be can assure her child of sufficiently strong and properly developed abdominal walls. Protein is the main need here. Such tissue strength is normal enough, as is the proper closing of the inguinal canal. If the materials are available, the developing baby will make use of them, it is certain.

Continued high protein intake will keep the abdominal wall in good repair, and the proper amounts of vitamin C will help in keeping the cells, which make up this tissue, tightly knit.

Exercise And Avoid Colds

Exercise, with special emphasis on the abdominal muscles, is another preventive measure that should be taken by all health-conscious persons. Such exercises as sit-ups, in which one rises from a supine position to a sitting position without use of the hands, are especially useful in this.

Since coughing can contribute to intestinal strain, colds are to be especially avoided in the light of what we know about hernias. Vitamin A and C are two excellent preventives. To keep clear of constipation, a diet high in protein, natural bulk and unprocessed foods, especially raw fruit and fresh vegetables, will help. Also, try for foods rich in the B vitamins, for they aid in maintaining friendly organisms in the intestinal tract, which helps in digestion of foods.

In lifting, follow the rules offered in the United States Public Health Service pamphlet, *Workers Health Series #3*:

1. In lifting heavy weight, face the object, keep the feet close to it and space them about 18 inches apart.
2. Lift from the floor with knees bent, using leg rather than back muscles.
3. Don't reach too high for heavy packages.
4. Carry loads on the shoulders where possible, rather than on the hips.
5. Get someone to help you if you need it.
6. Use mechanical devices where you can—hoists, elevators, trucks, etc.

210. Rules For Heavy Weight Lifting (An Illustration)

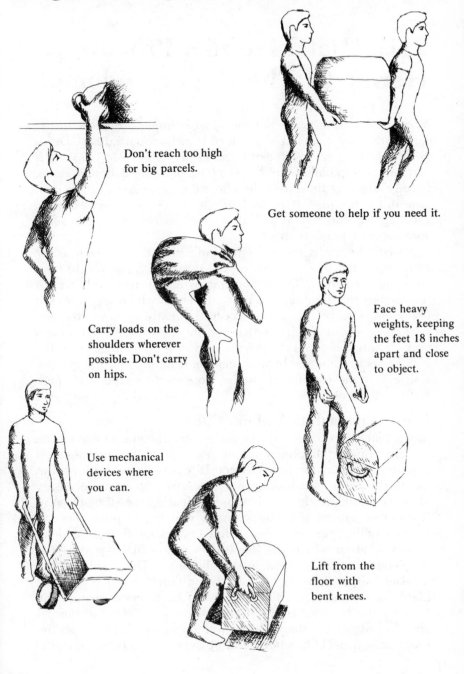

Don't reach too high for big parcels.

Get someone to help if you need it.

Carry loads on the shoulders wherever possible. Don't carry on hips.

Face heavy weights, keeping the feet 18 inches apart and close to object.

Use mechanical devices where you can.

Lift from the floor with bent knees.

211. Hiatal Hernia: Primary Hernia Of The Upper Abdomen

The hiatal hernia is one of the most common "defects in the gastrointestinal tract in the Western world," reported Drs. Denis Burkitt and Peter A. James in *The Lancet* (July 21, 1973). It is virtually symptomless and occurs in both men and women, mainly affecting those people who are middle-aged and in poor condition. Because it is so difficult to detect, doctors often misdiagnose this hernia as indigestion, heartburn and, in some instances, even heart attack.

A hiatal hernia is the movement of either the stomach or the esophagus (the tube connecting the throat to the stomach) from its normal position. These two organs are surrounded at their junction by the diaphragm, a muscular sheet which separates the abdomen from the chest and controls breathing. One common reason for hiatal hernia is that the muscles of the diaphragm surrounding the connecting point between the stomach and the esophagus become flabby and relax their tight structure, permitting either the esophagus or the stomach to squeeze through until it is out of place.

Bad Eating Habits A Major Cause

Since hiatal hernia is caused mainly by the loosening of the muscles in the diaphragm, your eating habits and physical condition have a significant effect. If a person stuffs himself at meals, drinks too much or becomes overweight, an unnecessary strain is placed on the diaphragm by bloating the stomach. And it's almost natural that the stomach will try to push through because of the pressure of expansion. Or, in another type of hiatal hernia—that in which the diaphragm is too high—part of the esophagus can be trapped in the abdomen. The result? If the stomach slips through, it can be divided in half by the diaphragm—the stomach acids tend to be trapped on top, the food on the bottom. In addition to slowing down the normal speed of digestion, the collection of acid may slip through the esophagus, especially when bending over, causing the regurgitation of acid into the throat. If the diaphragm is too high and part of the esophagus is trapped with the stomach, other problems might occur. The stomach walls are coated with thick mucus, to protect them from the effects of powerful stomach acids, but the esophagus walls are not. And when the stomach acid touches the walls of the esophagus, it stimulates the nerve endings there—an extremely painful condition—and possibly can cause esophageal ulcers.

The symptoms are not always easy to recognize, and when they do occur, they are often mistaken for something else. Dr. T. W. Challis of Queen's University, Kingston, Ontario, estimated that about half of the people whose hiatal hernias were discovered accidentally had no signs of the problem. And it's best if it is diagnosed early—waiting can lead to complications, including infections of the esophagus and hemorrhage. Irritation of the esophagus by the stomach acids can cause spasm or involuntary contraction of the muscles there, producing pain quite similar to that of a heart attack.

Nor do your symptoms deceive you alone. There is a very good chance that a doctor, as well, could be deceived by the symptoms of hiatal hernia into providing a totally mistaken diagnosis and treatment. If a patient goes to the doctor with symptoms of heartburn, the doctor could prescribe an antacid and say to call again in the morning. Although that antacid will probably reduce the patient's pain temporarily, he could pay heavily for it. A report published in the *New England Journal of Medicine* (February 22, 1968) showed that continuous use of antacids can deplete the body's phosphorus, possibly causing loss of teeth, cavities or, worse, osteomalacia, an adult form of rickets. So if the patient suspects a hiatal hernia, it's always wise for him to mention it to the doctor so that he looks specifically for it.

212. Sensible Regimen For Hiatal Hernia

If you don't have your hiatal hernia repaired by surgery, there are other things you can do. To reduce the condition, you should take better care of yourself, watch your eating habits, and follow a few simple steps:

Lose weight! This cannot be stressed enough. If you have built up layers of flab, your diaphragm is almost certain to rebel against you. And it should—you're preventing it from getting its proper exercise and helping it to get flabby, too. If you lose weight, chances are your hernia will reduce.

Avoid acid-producing foods. In most people, acid doesn't present a problem. In fact, some take extra acid into their systems to help their digestion. But when you have a hiatal hernia, acid certainly is one of your worst enemies. You need just enough acid to digest your food, but no more. Coffee, alcohol and spicy foods all stimulate your stomach to produce extra peptic acid, which can eat through the walls of your esophagus, cause you discomfort and increase many of the symptoms of hiatal hernia. Antacids which some doctors might suggest, shouldn't be necessary if you watch your diet.

Eat less at each meal. The more you eat at one sitting, the more pressure there is to force the stomach acids you *do* produce into your esophagus. If you're still hungry, you can eat more meals per day—but eat lightly enough so that your stomach is only about half full. You won't get that bloated feeling, and your hiatal hernia will do its best to ignore you.

Put more food fiber and roughage in your diet. Drs. Denis P. Burkitt and Peter A. James reported in an article in *The Lancet* (July 21, 1973) that the hiatal hernia is caused by the typical Western low residue diet, which is now listed as one of the main causes of diverticulosis, an inflammation of the bowels caused by the infection of several tiny herniated pockets formed on the inside of the bowel. Drs. Burkitt and James, who were among the first to note the correlation between a low residue diet and diverticulosis, believe that the hiatal hernia is caused by raised intra-abdominal pressure due to long periods of straining at the stool, a typical result of the constipation caused by low residue diets.

Leave a good deal of time between the time you eat and the time you lie down. It's as logical as the force of gravity—lying down helps the backward flow of your stomach contents, helping the stomach acids to enter your esophagus. Leave about two to four hours for your stomach to digest what you've eaten. That way, the stomach has a chance to cut off some of its acid production.

When you lie down, try to keep the upper part of your body higher than the lower part. It all comes back to gravity. If your head is higher than your feet, the force of gravity will naturally help keep the acids in your stomach, where they belong. How do you do it? Put two or three bricks under the legs at the upper part of your bed or stack some pillows under your back.

Don't wear anything tight around your waist, including tight belts, tight pants, or slimming underwear. If you take off some weight, they won't be tight! And that's one of the best things you can do for a hiatal hernia. The squeezing of tight clothes and belts is the same as the pressure of overweight.

These suggestions might force you to change some of your well-established habits, but it's a lot better than facing a hospital stay! There are, however, some cases in which surgery is unavoidable—such as when the irritated esophagus begins to form scar tissue.

But certainly it would be ideal to avoid the problems of a hiatal hernia completely. And the best way to do that is to eat a balanced diet, keep your weight down and exercise regularly. Keeping your body in shape could prevent your diaphragm from weakening as the years go by, and keeping your weight down will reduce the pressure on your stomach and keep it from pressing on your diaphragm. If your body is strong and your stomach and diaphragm aren't under the strain of over-eating and overweight, hiatal hernia should be something that happens to other people—not to you.

Section 39
Hospital-Caused (Nosocomial) Infections

213. You May Get More Out Of Your Hospital Stay Than You Bargained For!

213. You May Get More Out Of Your Hospital Stay Than You Bargained For!

Why do you go to the hospital? To be treated in a safe, clean environment, you say? Then perhaps you have not heard that "the problem with hospital infections is not only a 'full blown national epidemic' but also a worldwide one in institutions that care for the sick." That was the opinion of David Feingold, M.D., of the Beth Israel Hospital, Boston, in summary of the International Conference on Nosocomial Infections (*New England Journal of Medicine,* December 17, 1970).

A study performed at the Ottawa General Hospital and reported in the *Canadian Medical Association Journal* (April 6, 1974) revealed that 58.5 percent of infections suffered by patients at that hospital were of nosocomial origin. Further, one of every 13 patients admitted to the hospital became infected while undergoing treatment there. The researchers found their statistics to be comparable to infection rates in many American hospitals.

And you need not be a patient to suffer hospital-related problems. Dr. Henry D. Isenberg, attending microbiologist at the Long Island Jewish Medical Center, New Hyde Park, New York, warned in an interview (*Geriatrics,* May, 1971) that "today's medical institutions might serve as significant vectors in nosocomial diseases that pose a potential threat to the community." Indiscriminate use of antibiotics, he says, can endanger not only those patients taking them directly, but those nearby and visitors as well. So even if you're lucky enough not to be hospitalized yourself, you could be affected by breathing the antibiotic-polluted air while visiting a friend. And while your friend's infection is being treated, the treatment may be helping to develop a new, resistant strain with which the patient can afflict the community upon leaving the hospital. This has already happened—there are now staph organisms which are resistant even to the semisynthetic penicillins.

Dr. Isenberg said that in the average hospital, about one-third of the patients receive antibiotic injections three or four times each day. The clearing of the needle, a process which sprays a small amount of the contents into the air before each injection, can lead to 30 or 40 liters of "high-potency antimicrobial agents" being added to the air each year. The result of this liberal use of antibiotics: An upset of your body's balance of bacterial agents, a building of microbes and development of new, more difficult strains—all this in the supposedly antiseptic citadel of good health, your local hospital.

But back to your friend. Let us assume the doctor administered a common antibiotic for an infection, and it cleared up with the typical speed "miracle drugs" offer. But without warning, several days later at home, your friend suddenly begins to complain of genital and rectal itching and bleeding. What's the cause? That antibiotic! How does it happen? According to R. R. Willcox, M.D., of St. Mary's Hospital in London, when susceptible bacteria are suppressed by antibiotics, other immune yeast-like organisms such as *Monilia* (*Candida*) *albicans* may appear and cause unpleasant side-effects. Vaginal and rectal infections are common effects.

Despite this knowledge, doctors appear to be favoring broader exposure to antibiotics—not only as the panacea for every infection (which they certainly are not), but also as a preventive measure (which can be downright dangerous). Microbes that in the past presented no problem now thrive in an atmosphere wiped clean of their enemies by antibiotics. According to an editorial in the *Archives of Environmental Health* (June, 1966) by Hobart A. Reimann, M.D., of Philadelphia's Hahnemann Medical College, "Relatively few infections can be cured, and rarely can any be prevented, with antibiotics." Yet doctors all over use them in an attempt to prevent oncoming infections. He also warned that "probably 90 percent of antibiotics are applied unnecessarily" and that the thought that antibiotics "can do no harm" is a myth: About 300 deaths annually are caused by penicillin, and less serious harm from antibiotics occurs in 15 percent to 30 percent of the recipients.

Then why do so many doctors advocate antibiotic use? Because it's easier. Wrote Dr. Reimann: "Physicians often mistake spontaneous recovery for antibiotic cure and by doing so encourage the neglect of proper diagnoses, supportive care, and preventive measures." Statistics bear him out: The mortality from bacterial infections in hospitals is about the same as it was in 1930, *before* the advent of the antibiotic "wonder-drugs!"

In other words, hospitals are not really better at treating bacterial infections—a patient will probably be cured of the infection he entered with, but it's quite possible that he'll leave with something worse!

But antibiotics aren't the only culprit in hospital-caused infections. Many recall the reports in March, 1971, of 350 cases of blood infection and nine deaths resulting from intravenous fluids by a major drug manufacturer. The contamination of the bottles was shocking—but even more shocking was the finding, when 81 hospitals were randomly polled, that 43 percent were still using the solution and of these, 8.6 percent were not aware of an infection problem associated with the use of the solutions, and approximately 25 to 50 percent of the 35 hospitals were not following one or more of the specified precautions outlined in an earlier warning by the Center for Disease Control in Atlanta, Georgia.

In addition to the bloodstream, major targets of hospital-caused infections include the urinary tract, the lower respiratory tract and surgical wounds.

Hospital procedures provide many opportunities for the transmission of infections. Simple logic might tell you that in an institution where a different disease lurks in every bed, there's a chance that hospital personnel could transmit an infection from one patient to another. Of course, we assume that hospital personnel scrub before going from patient to patient, but even if their hands are clean, they can carry germs on their clothes. A report on hospital infections by W. A. Altemier, M.D., of the University of Cincinnati College of Medicine and the Cincinnati General Hospital says, "Most of the staphylococci dispersed by personnel seemed to come from their clothing."

The patient undergoing an operation runs not only the standard surgical risk, but also is threatened by the possibility of a carrier in the surgical team—even if he's not near the table. An article in the *Journal of the American Medical Association* (December 7, 1963) stated that an infected hospital staff member "conventionally masked, gowned and shod, in any part of the operating room is a hazard to the patient." Or there may be an infection lingering in the air from previous surgery. What are the patient's chances of contracting an infection from this operation? Common estimates range up to about one in five.

The most innocent looking hospital fixtures might be the downfall of many patients, as a story in the *New England Journal of Medicine* (August 31, 1967) pointed out. In one New England hospital, six of 13 patients in an intensive care unit came down with fever, shaking and chills, mental confusion and temporary low blood pressure—and one died. The cause: about 60,000 organisms of *K. pneumoniae* and *citrobacter* per milliliter in the hand cream dispenser used by about 62 percent of the nurses in that unit.

Other sources of risk for the patient: ice from hospital ice machines, woolen blankets, insects, food, air; floors and other surfaces; water, faucet aerators and sinks; oxygen humidifiers and ventilation systems. Indwelling catheters, which are artificial tubes inserted in the body to provide constant drainage, are especially susceptible starting points for bacterial infection, and these bacteria often carry with them high mortality rates. Inhalation equipment, multi-bed rooms or wards, and long hospital stays themselves also contribute to infection risk.

Some parents have lost their newborn children through infections transmitted to them by the nurse in the obstetrical ward. In one incident, 11 newborn infants were infected with *P. mirabilis* causing bacteremia, meningitis and osteomyelitis—leading to the deaths of four out of 11. It was discovered the infection came from the delivering nurse! Overcrowding of nurseries, common in many hospitals today, also increases the chance of infection for newborns.

What Hospitals Can Do

By now you may be asking, "What can be done to prevent hospital infections?" The Ottawa researchers believe that the problem is not lack of knowledge, but a failure to apply knowledge that is responsible for the spread of infections in hospitals. They suggested four steps that could be taken toward eliminating nosocomial infections: (1) modernizing archaic hospitals and hospital facilities, (2) establishing efficient surveillance programs in all hospitals, (3) instituting better catheterization techniques to prevent infections of the urinary tract, and (4) establishing control programs in hospitals which would require a specific explanation for every infection that occurs in every hospital.

The American Hospital Association published a book, *Infection Control in the Hospital* (1970), designed as a "handy desk reference" for hospital personnel to help them prevent these diseases.

The AHA's picture of an ideal hospital appears to be one in which: "Not merely cleanliness but sterility is sought whenever the threat of infection is present. Air-conditioning and heating units with humidity control are commonplace, and air filtration has recently been introduced to eliminate microorganisms. Dust is proscribed. All linen coming in contact with patients is washed thoroughly and is often sterilized. Drugs and fluids given to patients are controlled and inspected by pharmacists, manufacturers, and government agencies. Food and water are clean and generally free of potential pathogens. Patients with known infections are carefully isolated from others to prevent spread of disease. Even those patients peculiarly susceptible to infection are protected against acquisition of pathogens from their environment and from other persons."

The process for prevention is complex, with each administrator and each department assuming some responsibility for keeping patients free of hospital infections, and this complexity may serve as rationale for some hospitals who could say it is unfeasible for them to try it. The system, however, seems reasonable in most respects. The AHA also suggests an integrated hospital infection committee to coordinate all activities meant to keep you from being infected while (and because) you're in the hospital.

Other methods of infection control, suggested by Dr. Ruth B. Knudsin, a research associate at Harvard Medical School's department of surgery, include use of autoclaving or dry heat sterilization; ultraviolet radiation; clean, laundered gowns, caps and gloves worn by all personnel who might come in contact with infection. She adds that bacteria on air, floor and equipment must be monitored "at least on a weekly basis."

Chicago's Presbyterian-St. Luke's Hospital instituted an infection control program in 1968. A study of the program conducted from 1969 to 1973 and reported in the *Medical Tribune* (April 16, 1975) showed that the program, in addition to saving lives, saved patients almost $650,000 a year.

Dr. Larry D. Edwards, epidemiologist at the hospital during the study, stated, "The average patient stay in the hospital was 11-12 days during the study, varying from year to year. The average stay for patients with hospital onset infections, on the other hand, was 33 days, or an additional 21 days. . ." Reducing the rate of infections meant that fewer patients had to stay the extra number of days, and thus, costs were lowered.

Unfortunately, few hospitals will see the initiation of programs like the one in Chicago, or the implementation of the AHA's and Dr. Knudsin's recommendations in the near future. In the meantime, if you go to the hospital, take adequate amounts of vitamins A, C and D. Although they don't themselves kill germs, studies have shown them to be effective in building your body's resistance. And ask for alternatives to antibiotic treatment. Be careful of with what and whom you come in contact, and keep your visitors to an absolute minimum—they can bring infections into the hospital from outside.

Section 40
Insomnia

214. The Frustration Of Sleeping Problems

No one yet knows why we sleep or how much we really need to sleep. Scientific thoughts on the origins of sleep vary remarkably. Some scientists think sleep provided early man with a protective nocturnal "low profile," while others argue that sleep has always been a useless habit, a freak of evolution because sleeping beings are so vulnerable.

Sleep research, still virtually a new field, depends heavily on electronic brain scanning devices that require the subject to sleep with wires taped to face and head. Prior to the 1930's, researchers had no such devices: the sleeper's functions could be measured only by waking him. Although the modern sleep laboratory features a comfortable bed and a homey "sleepful atmosphere," most people do not wish to sleep in an unfamiliar place with wires pasted all over their heads, in spite of researchers' assurances that the wires cannot possibly deliver electrical shock or twist in the night to cause discomfort. As a result, most sleep research to date has been performed only on people seeking relief from a large variety of sleep disorders, and on college students anxious to earn a few dollars as guinea pigs at the university sleep laboratories. So research into human sleep patterns is somewhat narrow, with theories of what constitutes "normal" sleep based on studies of intelligent young adults and on subjects of all ages with existing sleep disorders.

Our knowledge of sleep is based on centuries of prejudice, and a body of incomplete data collected during the past four decades from which a few substantial theories have evolved, along with a number of conflicting methods of treatment for the myriad of sleep disorders ranging from insomnia to hypersomnia.

Thanks to electronic break-throughs that now allow sleep research without interrupting sleep, we have been able, during the past two decades, to gain major insights into sleep. Current research into its causes and effects is at an all time high.

215. How Do We Sleep?

Sleep is not just one long period of unconsciousness even for the best sleepers. Electroencephalograph (EEG) tracings of the brain waves of subjects in sleep labs show that sleep is divided into four stages collectively called "orthodox" sleep, and periods of dreaming. We pass through all the stages several times a night, and don't feel fully rested if the pattern is disturbed.

Just before the onset of the actual sleep cycle, we experience a period of relaxation during which the EEG shows the frequency of brain waves to be in the alpha rhythm, indicative of a relaxed, pleasurable state. As our muscles become even more relaxed, the body temperature begins to fall, and pulse and respiration become slow and even. We enter stage 1, the lightest phase of the sleep cycle. Our brain waves gradually widen and slow down as we sink deeper into sleep and descend through the second, third and fourth stages. When we reach stage 4, sleep is at its deepest. After about 90 minutes we enter another type of sleep known as REM (rapid eye movements). During this phase, the brain waves resemble those of a waking state, and the eyeballs dart back and forth. This is the stage of sleep in which we dream. REM lasts for about 10 to 15 minutes, then we begin the complete cycle over again, beginning with stage 1, and descending through the other stages. The entire cycle is usually repeated three or four times in the course of the night.

We always experience both orthodox and REM sleep, unless under the influence of certain drugs or a goodly quantity of alcohol. Orthodox sleep normally takes up three-fourths of the total sleep time, and REM the other quarter, in a healthy adult who is a good sleeper.

Laboratory studies have demonstrated that while orthodox sleep is necessary for physical health, REM sleep is just as essential for mental and emotional well-being. During the deep stages of slumber, the body's cells metabolize energy for the day ahead. We need more stage 3 and 4 sleep after heavy exercise, after physical injury, or after experiencing severe pain. We need REM sleep to maintain the ability to concentrate our attention, and to preserve emotional stability. Our need for REM increases after a day full of stressful concentration, important decision-making or intense learning.

The good sleeper will descend through the sleep cycle at regular intervals throughout the night, and gets the right proportion of REM and orthodox sleep. His body functions slow markedly during sleep, and he doesn't toss around much in bed.

On the other hand, the poor sleeper is irregular in his sleeping patterns. He wakes often during the night, and spends less time dreaming than his well-rested counterpart. He is more physically active during the night, taking longer to fall asleep and tossing and turning after he has.

216. What Is Insomnia?

An insomniac is anyone who believes he needs more, and sounder, sleep. Problems he has with falling asleep, staying asleep or sleeping soundly enough are classed as insomnia.

Experts recognize three types of insomnia: acute, chronic and intermittent. Acute insomnia is widespread, but of brief duration. It is usually due to a personal crisis, and when the crisis is overcome, the insomnia disappears.

With chronic insomnia, the sufferer never seems to get enough sleep. It may be due to a long-term illness, or it may have no apparent cause. Chronic insomnia can last for years or a lifetime.

In intermittent insomnia, the person sleeps quite well every night for weeks or months, then suddenly experiences many nights of wakefulness. Intermittent insomnia, like chronic insomnia, often has no evident cause, and so it is difficult to treat.

Usually, the more the insomniac searches out the phantom sleep, the more elusive it becomes. The lack of sleep takes its toll in appearance and attitude. Women, especially, suffer cosmetically from lack of sleep. A line or two on a man's face may go largely unnoticed, but a line on a woman's face is immediately obvious, and usually a cause of distress.

Cosmetic damage is only the superficial evidence of more serious physical and psychological problems caused by prolonged insomnia. Medical and psychological evidence shows that extended sleep loss causes changes in behavior. Insomniacs tend to be irritable and find it difficult to concentrate on simple tasks. Four or more days of complete sleep deprivation have caused visual and auditory hallucinations, and personality collapse in laboratory subjects. Luckily, few insomniacs will ever experience symptoms that severe. An insomniac may believe he hasn't slept a wink, but he is almost always a victim of self-deception. Furthermore, it takes only one night of sound sleep to recover from several nights of poor sleep.

As part of the research conducted in sleep laboratories, the subject's ability to perform various tasks after a sleepless night is monitored. Surprisingly, most people are able to function well in challenging situations that arouse their interest, such as the student who must take an exam. It is in performing routine, boring, repetitive chores, such as adding long columns of figures, that the insomniac's efficiency suffers.

Is It Really Insomnia?

Reports of human beings who claim to live without sleep have never been confirmed to the satisfaction of medical researchers. While there are several documented cases of people who sleep only two or three hours per 24, scientists believe that those who say they never sleep simply doze off without realizing it.

The poor sleeper tends to overestimate the time it takes him to fall asleep. Because he spends most of his sleep time in the lighter phases of sleep, the insomniac feels he has not slept at all, when actually he has spent several hours in stages 1 and 2. Since the light stages of sleep are close to the waking state, they don't provide a feeling of real rest and refreshment unless followed by deep sleep and REM. Hence, the "insomniac" may sleep for hours and wake up feeling like he has been awake all night.

Another type of false insomnia is generated by the myth that everyone needs eight hours of sleep. The person who consistently sleeps five hours a night may come to believe that he is an insomniac, when in reality he is simply a very efficient sleeper who passes quickly into the deep stages of slumber. He may not even stop to consider that his "insomnia" has not interfered with his health or his ability to do his job.

Sleep patterns depend on both personal and cultural forces. The fixed amount of sleep demanded by many individuals seems to be determined by society's timetable for working hours, school, leisure time, and so forth.

Where did we ever get the idea that everyone requires eight hours of sleep? And why must it be at night? If we are individual enough to be hungry at different times and to prefer different foods in different amounts, if some of us can yearn for exercise while others avoid it, why can we not accept personal attitudes toward sleep?

Just because you sleep less than seven hours a night does not necessarily mean you're harming yourself. Famed architect R. Buckminster Fuller took a half hour nap every three hours around the clock, for a total of only four hours sleep out of every 24. Yet, he thrived on this schedule for a full year, giving it up only because it was so out of tune with the pace of the world around him. On the other hand, you may be getting a full eight hours of sleep every night when you really need 10 for peak health and productivity. People who require 10 or 12 hours of sleep are no less vigorous than anyone else—it just takes them longer to recharge their batteries.

Many times it is our *worry* about not getting enough sleep, rather than simple lack of sleep that causes insomnia problems. In the midst of a sleepless night, the insomniac concludes that he'll be good for nothing the next day, only to discover that, although somewhat groggy, he is able to manage quite adequately. If we can still function well despite all our sleeping difficulties, our fear of not getting enough sleep should be eased considerably.

Variations in our sleeping patterns should be no cause for alarm. Researchers have found that we all need more sleep (and often get less) in times of anxiety and stress, when we change jobs, quarrel with our families, or become depressed. Some women need more sleep on premenstrual nights, and many people must sleep more when they are trying to lose weight. However, we need less sleep when things are going well. No one needs exactly the same amount of sleep every single night.

217. What Causes Insomnia?

Insomnia has many causes. Its origin can be psychological, medical, dietary, environmental or purely physical.

Psychopathological insomnia is perhaps the most widespread, and is the most difficult to treat. In such cases, the insomniac has no medical problem, his own thoughts simply keep him awake. When we are worried about finances, job-related problems, our relations with others—any distressing daily conflict which occupies our minds, we are likely to become victims of psychologically-caused insomnia. When the sleeplessness persists, however, we must seek ways to quiet the mind and relax enough to sleep. Prolonged insomnia endangers health and may well lead to behavioral problems. Three-fourths of the psychiatric patients being treated for mental and emotional disturbances have trouble sleeping, and had the same trouble for some time prior to treatment.

Medical causes of insomnia are many and varied. In one type of disorder known as sleep apnea, breathing stops during sleep for several seconds up to more than two minutes. When the person stops breathing, he awakens and may have trouble getting back to sleep. Some people with sleep apnea wake up as often as 250 times a night.

A disease accompanied by physical pain and discomfort will often cause insomnia. Many cardiac patients, for example, find it quite difficult to get a good night's sleep.

A third cause of insomnia lies in our daily diet. Many foods and beverages can act as stimulants, and prevent sound sleep.

Very little has been written about the kind of nutrition that will promote a good night's sleep. And yet, if you eat the usual TV snack like pretzels, potato chips and salted nuts, you might as well curl up with a good book or start knitting a large afghan. Morpheus has just gone out the window.

There are some foods which help you relax and sleep, and others that stimulate activity. Some foods shoot high octane into your bloodstream; others have a tranquilizing effect that helps you slow down, turn off your motor, relax and sleep.

Everyone knows that coffee is an enemy of sleep. Caffeine in any form stimulates the adrenals to produce more hormones which send a message to the liver to break down glycogen into glucose which flows into the bloodstream and makes you want to get up and go. This is why a cup of coffee "gives you a lift"—far away from the Land of Nod. Bear in mind that cocoa, tea and soft drinks also contain caffeine and should be especially avoided if sleep is your objective.

While every insomniac knows about the wide-awake tossing he suffers in the still of the night because of unwise indulgence in caffeine, not many night tossers realize that a close runner-up to caffeine in the ranks of the sleep destroyers is salt—common everyday sodium chloride, the stuff you put in your soup, on your potatoes, tomatoes, eggs and radishes; the stuff that comes with your pretzels and potato chips.

And yet, when you stop to think about it, it is not surprising that a diet rich in salt should keep you awake nights. Salt is a stimulant. It is pointed out by Henry Bieler, M.D., in his book *Food Is Your Best Medicine* (Random House, 1965) that salt stimulates the adrenal glands, just as caffeine does. In fact, salt is a two-time offender to the insomniac. It leads to high blood pressure which in itself is an enemy of restful sleep.

In the book, *Sea of Life* (David McKay Co., New York, 1969), Dr. William D. Snively reports a study of a large group of Americans questioned about the amount of salt they normally use. Out of 100 who reported that they never salted their food at the table, only one had high blood pressure; among 100 who added salt to taste, eight had high blood pressure; among 100 who added salt even before tasting, 10 had high blood pressure.

Why does excessive salt cause your pressure to go up so that you simply can't sleep? There is an old aphorism "Water goes where the salt is." Because sodium clings to water, when an excessive amount enters the extra-cellular fluid, it carries extra liquid with it. This naturally increases the volume of the plasma. In order to distribute the expanded blood, Dr. Snively explains, the heart must create additional pressure and therefore pumps harder. It is this pumping that has you counting sheep till you need a computer.

A French army doctor, Professor Ciorault, at a conference on mental hygiene, in relating insomnia to salt intake pointed out that sodium and potassium are natural antagonists in the body's chemistry because a cell is in a state of repose when it is rejecting sodium and accepting potassium. It is in an active state when it is accepting sodium. He said he successfully cured his patients of sleeplessness simply by eliminating salt from their diets. (*Salt and Your Health,* Hearthside Press, Inc., New York, 1965.)

Insomniacs would be well-advised to avoid such sodium-rich foods as smoked, canned, spiced and pickled meats, bacon, ham, sausage, bologna, shellfish, all processed fish, frankfurters, liverwurst, salami, canned vegetables, sauerkraut, regular commercial bread and rolls, salted crackers, canned soups, salted nuts, pretzels, chips, all salted cheeses, commercial ice cream and salted butter. Also, olives, ketchup, mayonnaise, pickles and relishes. Because softened water has a high sodium content, use only hard water for drinking and cooking.

Insomnia can also be caused by purely physical or environmental factors. For example, if you habitually sleep with your arm tucked under your pillow, cutting off the circulation in your arm, the sensation of numbness may be enough to wake you. Heat, cold, humidity, noise, a too-hard or too-soft bed, insect bites, and becoming entangled in the bedclothes—all these environmental influences commonly disturb sleep.

218. Drugs Are Not The Answer

Americans who believe they can substitute drugs for a well balanced nervous system spend hundreds of millions of dollars a year on compounds they hope will give them a good night's sleep. They may get just what they bargained for—a few nights of well-earned rest. But for many, the first packet of sleeping pills is a ticket on a vicious merry-go-round that can lead first to dependence, then to addiction and finally to death. In their book *Sleep* (Coward & McCann), Gay Gaer Luce and Julius Segal state that for every five deaths caused by acute alcoholism there are now four deaths from barbiturate poisoning.

Taking drugs to overcome insomnia is adding insult to injury. A sleeping pill paralyzes that part of the brain that controls dreaming and does not produce a restful sleep, but rather a state of rigid unconsciousness resulting in a tired, unrested body and mind.

Barbiturates and the other hypnotic drugs depress REM sleep. When the afflicted person stops taking the drug, he suffers "REM rebounds," and dreams incessantly, as if his brain was trying to make up for lost dreaming time. The dreams are not pleasant, but usually take the form of intense, terrifying nightmares. After a night of rebound sleep, the person may well decide that he really does need the drug, and resumes taking it.

Sleeping pills can intensify depression. Depressed people often suffer from insomnia, but when they are given hypnotics to induce sleep, their depression frequently becomes far more severe.

Prescription sleep drugs are highly addictive. In many people, the addiction begins simply and innocently enough, with a doctor who prescribes barbiturates to a patient because the patient says he can't sleep. The trouble is that dependence on them sneaks up fast. To the body the drug is a poison to be neutralized, and soon the drowsiness and loss of consciousness (actually toxic effects of the drugs) are eclipsed by body defenses. The patient must take a double dose to get the same effect. Most sleeping drugs begin to lose their effectiveness in two weeks. Luce and Segal warn that, "Millions of people drift down this path so gently they do not realize what may be happening to them."

Some people rely on over-the-counter sedatives sold without prescriptions. The sleep ingredient in such products is usually an antihistamine or scopolamine, a derivative of belladonna. According to the book, "These are mild and harmless enough if ingested according to directions. But the mildness is a problem, for the drowsiness caused by antihistamine would hardly benefit anybody with severe sleep difficulties. In large doses they induce side effects—dizziness, blurred vision, nervousness, blood changes."

Whatever type of sedative a person takes to improve his sleep (phenobarbital compounds are the most commonly prescribed), it is likely to leave him sluggish and fuzzy in the morning. To wake up fully, sleeping pill patients frequently turn to amphetamines, central nervous system stimulants, of which Benzedrine and Dexedrine are the most familiar.

A sleeping pill addict starts with a couple of capsules to get to sleep, and a Dexedrine or two in the morning to wake up brightly. By evening it may take a larger dose of barbiturates for sleep, and then more Dexedrine to wake up. He needs more and more pills just to keep going.

Patients who develop dependencies on these drugs may not notice the gradual changes in their personalities. Paranoia, aggressiveness and loss of judgement are generally exhibited by those dependent on sleeping pills. Elderly people, especially, are strongly affected by hypnotics; they often become confused and intoxicated the next day.

Alcohol seriously complicates the problem. A temporary psychosis frequently occurs when alcohol is combined with barbiturates and other sleep drugs. The alcohol multiplies the effects of both itself and the hypnotic, and can cause death.

This pernicious mixture of drugs is responsible for many suicides, both intentional and accidental. Sleep reports that, "Barbiturates can have psychological effects that may indirectly cause a fatal overdose. They can emulsify a person's sense of time and perception of his surroundings. A lamentable death may occur long before this stage when an insomniac awakens, unable to recall how many pills he took and how long he slept. In a state of confusion he may swallow more, without counting."

Despite all the certain and potential hazards which accompany the use of sleeping pills, thousands of people continue to ask for them. A patient would be astounded if he went to his doctor complaining of stomach pains and the doctor wrote out a prescription for a pain killer without investigating the cause of the pain. Yet, insomniacs expect to be given drugs simply because they can't sleep, without exploring the cause of their wakefulness.

Hypnotic drugs treat the symptoms of insomnia, but do not solve the problem. If the insomniac really wants to help himself, he should first try to ascertain the cause of his trouble, and then seek a non-pharmaceutical means of treatment. There are many other effective ways to help yourself to better sleep. And unlike drugs, these methods are harmless, and do not disrupt the natural, necessary sleep cycle.

219. Learn To Sleep YOUR Way

Insomnia generally occurs either in the first part of the night, or after early morning. For some there is a waking period in the middle of the night. Dr. Roger Williams, professor of biochemistry at the University of Texas, is convinced that if people would accept recurring periods of sleeplessness as normal to *them*, and catch up with the sleep they lose at some other part of the day, they would find a new sleep rhythm and be done once and for all with drugs and other sleep aids.

If you find that you are habitually awake during your first hours in bed, chances are that you should be up and doing things until you feel tired enough to sleep. Are you the type who can't sleep past five o'clock in the morning? Don't try. Get up. This may be the most productive part of the day for you.

Dr. Williams, in his book *You Are Extraordinary* (Random House), confesses that he is a middle-of-the-night insomniac. "I do not regard my condition as a disease; if it is, it is an attractive one for me. My mind is clearest during this hour or so and I reserve this time to do my best thinking. I go to bed with problems unsolved, but when I get up in the morning, after having had this quiet hour in the night, the best solution I can devise inevitably comes to me. . . ." Sometimes an hour's nap after lunch or before dinner will fill in the missed sleep-time nicely. Some people just don't need any more.

In a survey of college students, asked to register anonymously how much daily sleep they would like, the answers ranged from three, four or five hours up to 11 or 12. Some people go through life with no more than two or three hours of sleep a night. They get along fine, even though medical science can't explain how they do it.

Explanations are not always necessary. The insomniac who tosses and turns all night worried that he won't be able to function the next day, loses more sleep over the worry than over the insomnia. Actually, most so-called chronic insomniacs function quite efficiently through the working day. They complain for years over the lack of sleep, the tossing and turning they do half the night, yet they never fall asleep at work, and may never even think of sleeping again until it is bedtime for the rest of the household.

The animal world presents a variety of sleep habits. Chickens, for example, do all their sleeping at one time, but cats are notoriously "polyphasic" sleepers, getting their sleep in a series of "cat-naps." We all know people who wouldn't think of taking a nap during the day, and others who can't get through the day without one.

Everyone knows "night people" who hate to go to bed early and don't "come to" until noon. Others are the early-to-bed, early-to-rise type. The lucky ones work at jobs that accommodate their individual peculiarities—"day people" make good milkmen, and a "night person" is perfect for the late shift in a diner. The rest of us can fill in the ordinary nine to five working day.

An interesting experiment with individual sleep patterns was set up by Professor Nathaniel Kleitmen of Chicago, a prominent sleep researcher. He and an assistant secluded themselves deep in Mammoth Cave in Kentucky, far away from daylight influences. They set up quarters and attempted to alter their sleep patterns. They kept track of their body temperatures: body temperatures go down in sleep. The professor and his student were trying to acclimate themselves to a 28-hour day, adding up to a six-day week of 168 hours.

The student easily made the switch. Within a week his body temperature was going down *six* times during the 168 hours and he slept accordingly. The professor couldn't adjust. His body temperature always went down *seven* times during the 168 hours. He was out of phase. He couldn't sleep when he was supposed to on the new schedule. His temperature wouldn't go down at the right times. Nor could the professor stay awake when he should; that was the very time his temperature went lower.

Newborn babies present a common example of varied sleep patterns. "He has his days and nights mixed up," says the mother. Some babies fall right into the parents' sleep pattern almost at once, and others take years to get the hang of it.

Do you know your own sleep pattern? Give yourself the chance to find a sleep rhythm that suits you personally. If your sleep pattern is unusual, try not to let it worry you. Unconventional sleep patterns are not rare. If you can't sleep at first, wait until you're tired before you go to bed. Don't try to sleep, because you're almost sure to fail. "Trying" implies the opposite of relaxation, and unless you're relaxed, sleep won't come.

Psychologist Richard R. Bootzin developed an effective method of curing insomnia by training the individual to use the bed only for sleep. In Bootzin's treatment, the patient may not stay sleepless in bed longer than 10 minutes. After 10 minutes of lying awake, he must rise and leave the bedroom, returning only when he feels sleepy again. Further, no matter how little sleep he gets, he must rise at a regular hour each day.

On the first night of treatment, the patient may not sleep at all, and will feel exhausted throughout the next day. The following night, because he is more tired, he will probably fall asleep in the early morning hours. On each successive night, the patient will fall asleep at an earlier hour. After a few days, when he realizes the treatment is working, he will stop worrying about his insomnia, and can fall asleep with even greater ease. In a few weeks, most chronic insomniacs can be trained to fall asleep as soon as they get into bed.

The Right Foods Can Help You Sleep

Just as some food substances rev up your motor and prevent restful sleep, other substances have a peaceful, tranquilizing effect and hasten your trip to the pleasant Land of Nod.

Chief among these tranquilizing substances is calcium. A constant supply of calcium is required in the circulating blood for the building of bone and the control of electronic impulses transmitted through the nerves. If the concentration of calcium ions in the blood plasma falls below normal, the nerves lack the basic material that quiets them down. Muscle cells, as a result, often go into continuous contraction—the condition known as tetany. Before the calcium deficit reaches the bankrupt stage that brings on tetany, you could experience what is commonly referred to as a case of nerves. You feel jumpy. No wonder. Your nerve and muscle cells are screaming for calcium.

When you lie down to sleep, unless there is enough calcium in your bloodstream to meet the demands of your muscles and nerves, there won't be enough reaching your brain to shut off the constant signals that are keeping you awake. On the other hand, when your calcium supply is optimal, the blood delivers enough of it to satisfy all your body's needs, the nervous system ceases to send out its frantic calls for calcium and you are on the train to slumberland.

The older you get, it seems, the more calcium you need because your ability to absorb this mineral diminishes as the years pile up. This increased need for calcium in the latter years may be one reason why older people suffer from insomnia much more than younger people.

Women during the menopause frequently have difficulty sleeping. This is because sex hormones apparently play a role in the bone building process. When these hormones diminish as they do in the case of women at the time of menopause, you need to make doubly sure that calcium is plentiful to continue the bone building work and thus prevent the fragile bones, easy fractures, nervousness and sleepless nights that so many women suffer during and after the change of life.

Make sure that your diet is enriched with calcium-rich foods—especially green leafy vegetables. Don't overlook seeds—especially sesame seeds which are extremely rich in calcium.

Bone meal is an excellent calcium supplement to help you to sleep soundly with the added advantage of a range of other minerals that help keep bones strong and sound.

One of these is magnesium, which works in partnership with calcium and is absolutely essential to healthy nerves.

There are other food elements which are vital to a good night's sleep. Are you getting them?

Are you, for example, getting enough pantothenic acid? Without it, you can be sleepy but have trouble falling asleep. This member of the B family, usually sold as calcium pantothenate, is most abundant in liver, kidney, heart, yeast, wheat germ and bran, whole grains and green vegetables.

Another of the B vitamins that is important to a good night's sleep is B_6. For people who suffer from nervousness and insomnia, this vitamin often acts like a tranquilizer. Niacin, too, is necessary to a good night's sleep. Mushrooms are a good source of niacin, and so are heart, liver, wheat germ and brewer's yeast.

Brewer's yeast supplies all the B vitamins that promote bedtime tranquility. Enjoy a cup of broth made with two heaping tablespoons of brewer's yeast before you retire and you'll probably be half way to slumberland before you hit the pillow.

Everyone has heard that drinking a glass of warm milk before retiring will help you doze off faster. This seems like a perfect example of an old wives' tale, but there is scientific evidence to show that drinking warm milk actually does help you fall asleep.

Insomnia

Dr. Julius Segal, head of program analysis and evaluation activities at the National Institute of Mental Health and the author of several books on sleep, suggests that milk is actually a mild, natural sedative (*Family Practice News*, Feb. 11, 1973).

Milk, he points out, is a protein-rich food which contains large amounts of amino acids, including tryptophan. Tryptophan is a substance used to manufacture serotonin, the chemical substance in the brain which scientists believe is related to sleep. Tryptophan is found in foods like cheese and meat, in addition to milk. It is taken from the food into the blood, and is carried to the brain to be converted into serotonin. The groggy feeling sometimes noticeable after a heavy meal is caused by the tryptophan in the food.

This amino acid was given to volunteers in recent sleep research experiments. Dr. Segal says that the volunteers fell asleep with unusual speed, awoke less during the night, and spent more time than usual in the deep phases of sleep.

Dr. Segal recognizes that it is likely that a warm glass of milk may also have an emotionally soothing effect, but he thinks its sedative quality is probably a result of the large amount of tryptophan in milk. Even animals can be sedated with large doses of tryptophan, he says, and it seems unlikely that any psychological effect would be involved.

Some practices for gaining sleep, when it doesn't come easily, stem from old fashioned nostrums. Perhaps the success of some of these favored remedies lies in the mind-over-matter approach. Others carry relaxing, drugless, sedating qualities. In any event they are harmless and often successful in their application.

Hops are used as a sleep inducer by many who cling to folk-ways. Seldom grown these days, except commercially, the hops vine with its trailing flowers was once quite important to the American colonial garden. Early Americans brewed a tea of the flowers and even made pillows of the dried hops, saying it brought comfort to the soul and sleep to the searching mind.

One of the most unusual folk remedies for insomnia involves the lowly onion, a vegetable whose oil is a unique soporific. In soup or salad, stewed or raw, two to three onions a night will put you right to sleep. If the prospect of rising sleepless to peel onions at midnight puts you off, try onion jelly, which you can prepare in advance and store in the refrigerator until needed. As recommended in Mai Thomas's *Grannies' Remedies* (Grammercy, 1965) the following recipe is one of the smoothest ways of getting those big pills down. Two to three good-sized onions are grated into enough stock to barely cover them and the potion is stewed until tender. The juice of half a lemon is added, which makes the potion digestible to any stomach. By adding as much hot water as desired, and boiling for 10 minutes, with a small dab of butter just before you take it off the fire, you'll have an onion soup all but guaranteed to nudge you into stage one.

Herbalists have long heralded camomile tea as a sleep inducer and a protection against nightmares. Dr. R. Swinburne Clymer in his book *Nature's Healing Agents* (Dorrance and Co.), which first appeared in 1905 but was reissued in 1963, says that camomile acts to soothe the nerves, relax the body and eliminate stomach problems. In small amounts, camomile tea can be safely given to children without fear of side effects.

Just recently, a medical team from New York City was astonished when they accidentally discovered just how effective camomile tea is as a sedative.

Lawrence Gould, M.D., and colleagues, writing in the *Journal of Clinical Pharmacology* (January 10, 1974), were running a series of tests to measure the effects, if any, of camomile tea on cardiac patients who had undergone ventricular catheterizations as part of their treatment.

The tests showed that drinking camomile tea had no significant cardiac effects. But there *was* a positive reaction of a different kind: "A striking hypnotic (sleep-inducing) action of the tea was noted in ten of twelve patients," the medical team reports. "It is most unusual for patients undergoing cardiac catheterizations to fall asleep. The anxiety produced by this procedure as well as the pain associated with cardiac catheterizations all but preclude sleep. Thus," the report continues, "the fact that ten out of twelve patients fell into a deep slumber shortly after drinking camomile tea is all the more striking. Further investigations of the role of camomile tea as a hypnotic are therefore warranted."

It seems that if someone can fall asleep right after undergoing such painful, anxiety-producing medical procedures, the garden-variety traumas of everyday life ought to be easy work for a nice warm cup of camomile tea.

If you would like to try this soothing drink, look for the camomile flowers packed loose in an air-tight container, rather than in tea bags. Add half a dozen or so flowers to a cup of boiling water, cover, and allow to steep for five minutes. Drink while the liquid is warm, about thirty minutes before bedtime.

Other herbs which contribute to sleep include henbane, catnip, lady's slipper, yarrow and mullein. One concoction that is supposed to bring sleep is a tea made from lettuce leaves. Use any of the heavier green-leafed types of lettuce, not the iceberg variety. The leaves are chopped very fine and steeped in boiling water for five minutes or more. Strain and drink.

Exercise Can Be Important

Dr. Segal, who found milk to be an effective and mild sedative, is a great believer in exercise. "Sleep can be improved dramatically by daily exercise," he declares. Again, he found that "folklore knowledge" could be corroborated by scientific experimentation.

But this doesn't mean you should exercise before going to bed. On the contrary, Dr. Segal says, exercise at this time "may act as a stress, blocking rather than easing sleep." He recommends mild exercise in the morning, such as a long walk, as a good means "to produce refreshing sleep at night."

Learn How To Sleep

If none of these methods work for you, you must *learn* to go to sleep. You can do this just as you learn to play ball or to dance. You learn "not to do," says Dr. Samuel W. Gutwirth in *How To Sleep Well* (Vantage).

The method requires regular practice sessions aside from bedtime, of about 45 minutes a day. In a quiet room, the subject lies on his back, outstretched. He tenses each group of body muscles for several minutes (the arms, legs, trunk, facial muscles, eye muscles), then relaxes them, consciously allowing them to grow more and more limp. Dr. Gutwirth says this emphasizes the contrast between tension and relaxation. Once the sensation of complete relaxation is firmly embedded in your mind, you need only point your consciousness in that direction and sleep will follow.

The late J. I. Rodale had the soul of a true researcher, and investigating the mystery of sleep was especially attractive to him. Here is a typical sample of his reports on the subject—personal, amusing and informative. Are you exposed to enough sound to get a sound night's sleep?

220. Tick Tock Your Way To Sleep

J. I. Rodale

I have made a very interesting observation about sleep. . . . I can sleep better with the sound of a clock's mechanism in my ear. Some people use alarm clocks to awaken them. I use one to sleep.

I had occasion to visit in another city, and I had the best night's sleep there that I could remember in years. When I awoke I marveled at it. Then I noticed an old-fashioned loud-ticking clock that had ticked all night long on a bureau that was practically just above my head. When I got home I referred to the 10 books on sleep in my library, but not one of them had anything in it about the effect of sound on sleep.

I recalled Mark Twain's famous comment about his sleep experience. When he lived in New York City, next to an elevated railroad, he had no trouble achieving perfect slumber, but when he moved to the quietness of Hartford, Connecticut, he became an insomniac. To counter the quiet, Twain said he hired a boy to stand all night outside his bedroom door pounding on a big tin pan, which soothed him into a hypnotic sleep. He claimed he never had any sleep trouble after that. But bear in mind that Mark Twain also said, "Don't go to bed, because so many people die there!"

I decided to experiment and bought myself a loud-sounding tick-tock clock and put it next to my bed that night. It bothered me. I moved it to about three feet from my ears, and the result was a wonderful night's sleep. . . . a sleep of the just, as they say.

I began to speculate as to why a steady sound could soothe one to sleep. Could it be hypnosis? This is something for medical experts to experiment with . . . especially those who write books on sleep. It might lead to the general study of sound as a therapeutic agent for many states of illnesses.

I began to think of sounds . . . various kinds . . . and their effects on man: very noisy sounds, especially in industry, the harsh deafening noises of high-powered machines that could lead to deafness and damage to the nervous system. But on the other side of the coin were the soothing sounds such as rain, which comforts one in the security of one's bed. Is there anyone who does not love that sound, and who cannot sleep sweetly through it? We probably inherited our love of that sound from primitive man who slept through the sounds of rain and wind in the trees and the surge of the ocean seas, but awoke when he heard the lion's roar. One sleeps well amidst the music of crickets at night in the country, and the noise of the bull-frogs, but let one tiny mosquito begin to buzz in your ear and sleep becomes impossible.

Come Father's Day and one of my children, knowing of my new interest, presented me with a Metronome. But it was nothing like my loud clock. Where the latter went tick-tock, the Metronome seemed to go click-clack . . . a big difference! In fact, in my sleepy mind, the clock sounded more like a soothing tickety-tockety; but when I woke up it became tick-tock again, but at least not click-clack!

Now, like Diogenes with his lamp, I set out, armed with the knowledge of my observation, to question people, seeking more information.

One friend said, "Your experience reminds me of the fact that when they take a puppy away from its mother, they put a ticking clock near it. The regular tick-tock reminds the puppy of the beat of its mother's heart. But it could be also that the ticking sound lulls it to sleep."

One day on my usual walk, I came across a man fishing on the banks of a stream, right next to a bunch of rocks where the water going over it produced quite a gurgling sound. I stopped and asked him, "If it were night and there were a bed here, do you think you could sleep with all that noise of the water going over those rocks?"

"You bet I could" he replied. "In fact, let me tell you, at home I have a large window fan in my bedroom and when it goes all night I can sleep better than when it is quiet. Also, when I go to the seashore, where we have a bungalow right next to the beach, I find that the roar of the ocean puts me to sleep quickly and keeps me sleeping."

I then decided to interview the occupants of the seven or eight bungalows located at the side of the brook where I had talked with the fisherman. They all said that they slept extremely well, and that the rippling sound of the waters did not disturb them. Did not disturb them? I told them it probably helped them and they did not disagree. One of them said that visitors from the city always remarked how well they slept, attributing it to being in the fresh air of the country, not realizing that it might be because of the eloquent voice of the brook.

A friend related an experience in a silk mill where he used to work. To one who has never heard it, let me say that the noise there is terribly loud. In this mill each worker was supposed to watch five or six looms. If there is a break in the thread, the loom automatically stops, and the worker repairs the break. One of the men there regularly used to fall into deep sleep amidst all that noise. But let one of his looms suddenly stop, and he was awake like a shot. Evidently his subconscious mind was listening for him.

I am reminded of one of my own experiences with my clock . . . I forgot to wind it one night, and it stopped in the middle of the night. From about 3 A.M. on I tossed fitfully.

A chiropodist friend (podiatrist he calls himself) told me that his wife always goes to bed first, puts on the radio and sleeps soundly to its music. When he comes into the room and either shuts it off or reduces its volume, she awakens with a start.

This is a subject worthy of investigation because insomnia is a major public enemy in this country. I feel that all kinds of sounds should be experimented with as sleep inducers. Phonograph records of ocean waves, and brooks rippling, and rain pitter-pattering on window panes, and such, might be used. The way I look at it now, the fallacy of counting sheep to get to sleep is that they are silent sheep. A device that gives the sound of the sheep's baa-ing as they jump over the hurdles could be a very effective sleep inducer. And the electric clock—the mistake of that instrument is that it is taking the tick-tock out of our lives.

The sick room is a place where sound might be used therapeutically. How unscientific it is to throw a patient into a hospital room with only a radio or television with their untherapeutic sounds to alleviate the pain. What kinds of sounds are pain relievers, or balm to the bed-ridden?

I want to stress here, in case you are not a good sleeper, and the clock method does not help you, that you probably sleep more than you think you do. And this reminds me of a story. In the morning at breakfast, grandpa listened to the family talking about heavy rain and lightning and thunder during the night. He became very angry. "Why didn't you waken me?" he demanded. "You know I can't sleep during a storm!"

In conclusion may I suggest that if one kind of noise does not put you to sleep, another kind might. The problem is to find your kind of sound!

221. Seven Ways To Sounder Sleep

1. Don't take sleeping pills. Besides being addictive and dangerous, many of them prevent dreaming and that can destroy your mental health. Without dreams, the day's tensions have no outlet.

2. Don't eat salty foods, especially before bedtime. Salt stimulates the adrenals, and restricting intake is all that some insomniacs need to get a good night's sleep.

3. Increase your intake of calcium, which helps calm nerves. Bone meal is an excellent source; so are sesame seeds. Mixed together in homemade yogurt, they're even better.

4. Be sure you're getting enough B vitamins. Two heaping tablespoons of brewer's yeast in some broth before retiring will take care of this nicely.

5. If you smoke, stop or at least cut down. It's been proven that heavy smokers generally have a harder time falling asleep, hardly ever dream, and may not get any "deep sleep" at all. Immediately after giving the habit up, they sleep easier, longer, and begin resting their minds with dreaming, at first dreaming excessively, but in a few days, quite normally (*Medical Tribune*, Nov. 24, 1969).

6. If you wake up in the middle of the night and can't fall asleep again, don't fight it. Your "internal clock" may be convinced this is a great schedule, so get up and do some work or reading. You'll probably soon be asleep again.

7. Take afternoon naps, or at least lie absolutely still with all noise shut out. Rather than interfering with your nightly sleep, you will find that you fall asleep more easily if you are well rested. Try to nap at the same time every day; retire for the night at a regular time too.

222. Narcolepsy And Hypersomnia

Hypersomnia is characterized by excessive sleep, whereas the sleep of narcolepsy is irresistible and of short duration, in unpredictable "sleep attacks." These attacks are most frequent after meals, and when the victim is involved in monotonous tasks throughout the course of the day. One to five hours pass between such seizures, and the patient usually awakens feeling rested.

Narcoleptic attacks usually occur with the patient immediately entering REM sleep, as opposed to the sixty to ninety minutes of orthodox sleep which are typical of normal sleep.

Narcoleptics often appear lazy to themselves and to associates, and experts point out that proper diagnosis of this disorder is important so that such people are not unfairly labeled unreliable. Auxiliary symptoms occur in ninety-five percent of all cases, and include cataplexy (usually in response to sudden stimulation— most often laughter), hypnagogic hallucinations, and sleep paralysis. Once diagnosis is obtained, patients should not drive or operate dangerous machinery unless medication arrests the problem.

Like insomnia, hypersomnia is often secondary to depression. It is different from narcolepsy because the sleep is not irresistible and lasts much longer—sometimes as long as several days. Complete waking from sleep is difficult. There are no auxiliary symptoms as there are in narcolepsy. Chronic hypersomnia can be a symptom of central-nervous system abnormality from traumatic or pathological causes. The sleep cycles of hypersomniacs are normal, with sleep beginning with the light stages, and all stages holding their regular cyclic and proportional relationships. Unfortunately, little research has been done in the area of hypersomnia.

Sleepwalking

Sleepwalking is most common among males, more common in children than adults, and occurs among an estimated one to six percent of the population. There is more likelihood of sleepwalking if the patient is under stress.

Sleepwalking occurs during the deep stages of orthodox sleep; incidents may be provoked by lifting the young sleepwalker to his feet during stage 4 sleep. Such incidents cannot be provoked among normal children. To date, research among adult somnambulists is very sketchy.

Sleepwalking episodes last from thirty seconds to half an hour or longer. Many researchers believe it is impossible to sleepwalk while dreaming, since the body's muscles are paralyzed during REM sleep. Hence, the sleepwalker is most probably not "acting out a dream" even though some episodes among children are accompanied by screaming, crying or wetting. In laboratory tests, sleepwalkers have displayed complete amnesia in regard to sleepwalking incidents.

The biggest problem with sleepwalking children is their parents, who need to be assured that in almost all cases, the disorder will be outgrown if left to run its natural course. Further, among children and adolescents, somnambulism does not indicate psychological disturbance. With adults, however, it has been linked to neurotic character disorders.

The first consideration in sleepwalking is the safety of the sleepwalker, and the only point on which all doctors agree is that sleepwalkers should not sleep in potentially dangerous locations. They should not, for instance, sleep in towers; sharp objects ought to be placed out of reach and somnambulistic children probably should have a room on the first floor. In some cases, perhaps, windows and doors ought to be discreetly locked at bedtime. No further treatment is indicated for children, but adults with persistent or severe sleepwalking incidents ought to seek medical help.

Night Terrors And Nightmares

Night terrors occur during stage 4 sleep, and are distinguished from nightmares, which are a REM phenomenon. Night terrors, which occur most often in children, are very like somnambulism, and often occur simultaneously with sleepwalking episodes. Fortunately, like somnambulism, these early sleep disorders are usually outgrown, and are thus considered evidence of delayed maturation of the central nervous system. During night terror episodes, heart rate increases to 150-170 beats per minute, and vocal activity is common in the form of screams or gasps.

Night terrors last only a few minutes. The victim breathes quickly, feels anxious and has a sense of impending doom. Many night terrors are forgotten, and memories will be of only a single frightening image.

Recommended treatment for night terrors and nightmares (which cannot be distinguished except by careful professional diagnosis) is to make light of such incidents among children, who will probably outgrow the problem. Where night terrors or nightmares persist in children, and where their occurrence is frequent among adults, psychologic evaluation and treatment are indicated.

Section 41
Kidney Disease

223. Living With Nephritis—The Kidney Destroyer

No other system in the human body is more intricate or hardworking than the blood-purifying apparatus of the kidneys. Nestled on each side of the spinal column in the mid-back region, these two deceptively compact organs continuously filter wastes and impurities out of the blood and excrete them in the urine.

Because we are totally dependent on this filtering mechanism for continued life, any impairment of the kidneys becomes a very serious matter indeed. The National Kidney Foundation estimates that there are about 60,000 deaths due to kidney disorders in the United States every year. That makes renal or kidney disease one of the major causes of death, on a par with cancer and cardiovascular disease.

Nephritis is the general term used to describe the many forms of renal disease that cause inflammation and can ultimately destroy the tiny membranes and microscopic filtering units, or nephrons, inside the kidney. Unfortunately, the damage done by nephritis is usually irreversible. In the final stage, the kidneys begin to fail and uremia occurs. Toxic waste products accumulate to dangerous concentrations in the blood.

There is no known cure for nephritis. Before about 1960, victims of terminal kidney disease would sink into a coma and die. Doctors could do nothing. Now, as we'll see, there is new hope for kidney patients in the form of life-prolonging dialysis and even organ transplants.

Analgesics Can Damage The Kidneys

At this point, the causes of kidney disease are not fully understood. Some problems start with a simple lower urinary tract infection that spreads. Or the disease may strike seemingly without warning. However, there is considerable evidence that self-inflicted drug damage—overuse of aspirin compounds, especially those containing phenacetin or acetominophen—may be responsible for as many as 20 percent of all kidney disorders in the United States.

That's the opinion of Dr. John J. Murray of the University of Pennsylvania in Philadelphia. Dr. Murray found in a study that 20 out of 101 cases of chronic kidney failure were the direct result of use of large doses of analgesic compounds. He says it's not aspirin alone that causes the problem, but compounds containing aspirin and the other mentioned painkillers.

Women are especially vulnerable to this kind of kidney problem. Nearly all the patients in Dr. Murray's study were middle-aged women who took the painkilling compounds for recurring headaches or backaches. They were using 10 to 12 tablets a day, and have been following that routine for four or five years. All had taken compounds containing the equivalent of seven pounds of phenacetin during their lifetimes.

Examination of 300 damaged kidneys over a two-year period at the South African Institute for Medical Research disclosed that eight percent were damaged by aspirin, Dr. Cyril Abrahams told a conference on rheumatism, arthritis and allied disorders (*Medical Tribune*, November 21, 1968). He said that the amounts of analgesics taken by some of these patients over periods ranging from three to 22 years were "tremendous." Some had taken the equivalent of 60,000 tablets, though damage can result from as few as 3,000 tablets.

Dr. Abrahams described a vicious cycle in which some patients took aspirin for headaches and excessive use of the aspirin caused new headaches. Naturally the patient took more aspirin to get rid of the headache, which disappeared for a while only to return, along with kidney disease.

Kidney Poisons Are All Around Us

Other substances that are capable of causing serious kidney disorders are also increasing yearly in our environment. In an effort to alert physicians to the danger, George E. Schreiner, M.D., listed the following sources of toxic nephropathy in the *Journal of the American Medical Association* (March 8, 1965):

Ingestion of bichloride of mercury, other heavy metals and carbon tetrachloride cause almost immediate tissue or functional changes in the kidney. Dr. Schreiner warned that antihypertensive drugs that reduce circulation can cause tubular changes such as salt-wasting. The kidneys are also affected by sulfonamides, bee venom, poison ivy and other "nephroallergens." Frequent use of certain laxatives which can cause a potassium deficiency are likely to result in renal disorders.

The main complaint of Dr. Schreiner is the fact that many years elapse between the introduction and widespread use of a dangerous compound and the accumulation of enough evidence to show that it is a serious threat to the kidneys. Because the kidney metabolism and its structures are extremely complex, the kidneys are ever in danger of damage from a variety of compounds.

Animal studies have demonstrated that a deficiency of choline, one of the B vitamins, can also destroy the kidneys. In her book, *Let's Get Well*, nutritionist Adelle Davis says that the kidneys are affected first when choline is lacking: "Even when adequate protein is given, young, rapidly growing rats on a choline-deficient diet develop nephritis (inflammation of the kidney) within four to seven days, and most of them soon die, their fat-filled kidneys swollen, discolored and containing large areas of dead tissue."

Choline-deprived, damaged kidneys also cause a rise in blood pressure, which can be reduced by adding choline to the diet, as shown by Y. Nishizawa, et al. (*J. Vitaminol.*, 3, 106, 1957). When 158 patients suffering from hypertension were given choline, those who suffered from headaches, dizziness, palpitations and constipation got partial or complete relief within ten days. Blood pressure in all the patients dropped by the third week, at which time it was down to *normal* in one third of the patients.

Sweating Assists Kidneys

Patients in the earlier stages of kidney disease can sometimes be benefited by use of the sauna. When the kidneys are unable to flush sufficient wastes from the blood, these materials can build up and cause very serious reactions. In some cases, however, the wastes can also be released through sweating.

At Peter Bent Brigham Hospital in Boston, patients with kidney failure were put on sauna therapy for half an hour every day. Tests indicated that urea nitrogen, a waste product usually eliminated from the body through urine, but which remains in the blood when the kidneys do not operate properly, was secreted from the sweat of the patients in concentrations 10 times that of controls.

The sauna also remarkably reduced the itching sensation

which often accompanies chronic uremia. In six patients, the itching eventually disappeared entirely.

The study was reported in the April 25, 1966 issue of the *Journal of the American Medical Association.*

Once renal disease progresses to the terminal stage, however, more drastic measures are needed. About 20,000 persons in the United States suffering from total kidney failure are being kept alive by a process known as hemodialysis. Three times a week, their blood is filtered and purified by an artificial kidney machine. This therapy can be performed at home or at one of numerous dialysis centers. Without regular dialysis, these patients would die of uremia in three to five days. Approximately 5,000 more Americans owe their lives to transplanted kidneys, often "spares" donated by close relatives. Such heroic measures—undertaken at great expense—are keeping kidney patients alive, hopefully until medical researchers find the key to this disastrous disease.

224. Magnesium And B$_6$ Discourage Kidney Stone Formation

There's good news for many people suffering from kidney stones—those who, for little understood reasons, tend to form stones (or calculi) from mineral salts in the urine. Primarily produced in the kidneys, urinary stones often must be removed surgically or, if they're small enough, they pass out of the body through the urinary tract, frequently causing excruciating discomfort in the process.

But, says the good news, calcium oxalate stones, the most common kind, can be prevented. It appears that they occur, in the vast majority of cases, because of a double nutritional deficiency. Adequate daily supplements of the two deficient nutrients—magnesium and vitamin B$_6$—may be all that's needed for a person to rid himself of this often agonizing ailment.

The most encouraging part about this good news is that it isn't really "news" at all. It's time-tested. The finding was first reported in 1967. And the latest report is simply this: a broader study than the first, involving many more patients and doctors, confirms the benefit of magnesium and B$_6$ in the prevention of urinary stone formation.

Complete Relief In Many Cases

Harvard investigators Drs. Edwin L. Prien, Sr., and Stanley F. Gershoff, first announced their successful use of the double supplement in the *American Journal of Clinical Nutrition*, (May, 1967). Of 36 patients who previously had formed at least two urinary stones a year, the investigators reported, 30 either had no further stone recurrence or markedly decreased recurrence during the five years or more they were protected by a daily supplement of magnesium oxide and pyridoxine (B$_6$).

In another article published in the *Journal of Urology* (October, 1974), the same authors report on an expanded study, involving the cooperation of 64 urologists and (initially) 265 carefully selected patients, all with a long history of chronic stone formation. In the course of the five-year investigation, 98 patients were lost to the study for a variety of reasons.

Of those who stayed with the program and continued to take the protective nutrients, only 17 were considered failures and continued to form stones as in the past. Eighteen others continued to have pain symptoms (though milder than before) and probably—say the investigators—passed small fragments of stone or "gravel" in their urine. The remaining 132 were symptom-free and stone-free.

This is quite a record! All of 89 percent benefited, and 79 percent found complete protection—simply by regular ingestion of two harmless nutrients!

"A number of patients, having become free of stones," Prien and Gershoff write, "stopped treatment and began having stones again within a few weeks, only to become free of stones again when they resumed treatment."

What's In A Stone?

Before we can get a clear picture of just how these nutrients work to protect against urinary stones, we need to understand something about how stones are formed and what they're made of. The content of stones varies geographically and even with the stage of "civilization" a country has reached. But in North America, the Harvard researchers say, the major substance making up urinary stones is calcium oxalate. "About a third of the urinary calculi are composed of this substance and another third contain major amounts, usually associated with calcium phosphate," they note. Oxalic acid and calcium—both normal constituents of urine—combine to form this relatively insoluble crystal.

You've probably heard of oxalic acid in connection with certain foods. Chocolate, cocoa, tea, rhubarb, spinach, chard, parsley, and beet tops are all noted for their high oxalate concentration. If you eat a lot of these foods without increasing your calcium intake, you run a very real risk of calcium deficiency. That's because the mineral binds so readily with oxalic acid, and when it's tied up in this combination, it's mostly lost to the body. It can't be absorbed and passes out uselessly via the intestinal tract.

But oxalic acid from the diet forms only a minute portion of the oxalic acid present in urine. Drs. Louis Hagler and Robert H. Herman, Army research scientists writing a three-part series on oxalate metabolism in the *American Journal of Clinical Nutrition* (July, August, September, 1973), explain that only about two percent of dietary oxalate is absorbed and eventually excreted in the urine. Most of the urine's oxalate is of endogenous origin— that is, it's synthesized by the body itself. Ascorbic acid and a substance called glyoxylate, are the main—though not the only—precursors that provide raw material for oxalate production.

The two kidneys, where urine is formed, remove oxalic acid from the bloodstream. When blood arrives at the kidneys, complex mechanisms go to work to sort out all the various constituents of the fluid. Materials that the body needs are then restored to circulation. Wastes and other unwanted factors, including surplus nutrients and surplus water, are collected and allowed to dribble down a tube (ureter) to the bladder, whence they are excreted (via the urethra) during urination.

Urine Is Supersaturated

Since both oxalic acid and surplus calcium are directed into the urinary pool by the hard-working kidneys (they process between 400 and 500 gallons of blood a day!), you can see that the stage is set for these two urinary components to combine into calcium oxalate. And, in fact, they do just that—not only in chronic stone formers but in normal individuals as well. All of us.

"The urine is normally supersaturated with respect to calcium oxalate," Drs. Hagler and Herman state. When a solution is "supersaturated," as we learned in high school chemistry, even the slightest jiggle can trigger the sudden precipitation of the solid. In light of this uneasy situation, the puzzling question is not why *some* people form urinary stones—but why such stones aren't formed by everyone. Why do most people *not* get urinary stones, the authors question, and "in what ways do stone formers differ from the normal?"

It seems very clear that nature must normally provide some protective device so that, despite the supersaturation of urine with calcium oxalate, most of us never have kidney stone trouble. And if this natural protection is largely provided by dietary magnesium and vitamin B_6, we might guess that stone formers "differ from the normal" in terms of their greater requirement for these two nutrients.

Not that they need extravagant amounts. Not at all. In working with stone-forming patients, the Harvard team successfully used

300 mg. of magnesium oxide. (The Recommended Daily Allowance of magnesium for adult males is 350 mg.; for females, 300 mg.) As for vitamin B_6, patients received 10 mg., which is five times greater than the RDA. But much recent research on this B vitamin suggests that 10 mg. is probably much closer to the human physiological need for the nutrient than the meager two mg. declared adequate by the National Research Council and the Food and Drug Administration.

It's a comment on the deficiency of the American diet that these patients needed only relatively modest quantities of two key nutrients to control their stone-forming activity. If the food industry's refined, processed, and chemicalized products truly provided "all the nutrients you need"—as the FDA claims—there's a good chance many of these patients would never have formed stones to begin with.

Nutrients In Action

Finally, let's get to the question of how these two nutrients work in protecting against stones.

Magnesium, Drs. Prien and Gershoff have shown, makes the urine more solvent in respect to oxalates. With greater solvency, the fluid can hold the crystals in solution with less risk of precipitation or aggregation—that is, the clumping together of particles.

Vitamin B_6, on the other hand, has no effect on the solubility of oxalate in the urine, but appears to help control the body's production of oxalic acid and therefore to limit the amount reaching the kidneys. While human studies are somewhat conflicting on this question, the researchers say, "It has been conclusively shown in animals that vitamin B_6 deficiency is accompanied by a marked increase in endogenous oxalate excretion."

Dr. Gershoff makes this comment on the human need for vitamin B_6 (quoted in Dr. John Ellis's book, *Vitamin B_6: The Doctor's Report*, Harper & Row, 1973): "It would appear that for many, if not all, individuals, the dietary level of vitamin B_6 needed to ensure minimal oxalate excretion is greater than the amount needed to protect against most other known manifestations of vitamin B_6 deficiency." In other words, not only stone formers but others as well probably need five times the official RDA of B_6 in order to properly control the body's synthesis of oxalic acid.

Our two nutrients, as you can see, make a great team. First we have B_6 cutting down the amount of oxalic acid in the urine. Second, the oxalic acid that does reach the urine is made more soluble by the action of magnesium.

If this were the whole story—if deficiency in magnesium and B_6 were the sole cause of kidney stones—then undoubtedly all patients in the Prien-Gershoff study would have been cured of their ailment. But kidney stones are a complex disorder with the relationships of a number of nutrients involved—calcium, phosphorus and sulfur, for example, in addition to magnesium and vitamin B_6. Other factors, too, enter the picture—heredity, geography, metabolic disorders, and others. So the simple double-nutrient preventive approach won't help everyone. But the large proportion of kidney stone patients who could be expected to benefit by the recommended nutritional therapy is good news indeed.

As you've undoubtedly noticed, the Harvard doctors use magnesium oxide as the magnesium supplement, rather than dolomite. Since dolomite contains calcium as well as magnesium and reduced calcium intake is usually advised for stone formers, it would be best for kidney stone patients to follow the researchers' advice. "Magnesium oxide is now available in 140 mg. capsules," Drs. Prien and Gershoff say, "and two per day should be adequate."

Apart from this one caution about calcium restriction, the recommended nutrients for chronic stone formers is sound advice for everyone. We all need these full physiological levels of magnesium and vitamin B_6 to maintain optimum health.

225. Cystitis

Cystitis is an infection of the bladder which is characterized by inflammation, a burning sensation during and after urination, and a need to void frequently. The bladder may have a full feeling even when it has just been emptied. When the infection is severe enough to affect the kidneys (which is rare) fever is usually present.

The urethra is the route by which the infection travels to the bladder. Since the female urethra is only about one and a half inches long and the male urethra is approximately eight and a half inches long it is much easier for germs to reach the female bladder. So cystitis is more common among females.

If bouts of cystitis recur and it becomes a chronic malady, a cystoscopy (an internal examination of the urethra and bladder) may be done on the patient to determine whether there is an abnormal bladder condition which creates an atmosphere conducive to infection.

Antimicrobial drugs are generally prescribed for treatment of cystitis. But, as with all drugs, they take their toll on the body's resources, particularly the B vitamins and intestinal flora.

In his book, *The Healing Factor*, (Grosset and Dunlap, 1972) Irving Stone recommends vitamin C for the treatment of genitourinary diseases. "Large doses of ascorbic acid are administered, preferably orally and in solution, at frequent intervals. The doses will be of the order of two grams about every two hours."

Irving Stone, who has for over 40 years been researching the benefits of ascorbic acid, claims that when taken in mega doses it builds up in the urine to the point where it detoxifies the poisons.

Section 42
The Liver

226. How Your Liver Rules Your Life

After the skin, the liver is the next largest organ of the human body, and, next to the brain, perhaps the most versatile. It acts as the body's master laboratory, filtering out undesirable substances, neutralizing waste materials, manufacturing organic compounds, storing nutrients and releasing them to the bloodstream when the body needs them. It has about 500 recognized functions.

In its role as a gland, the liver manufactures and secretes bile for digestion and stores it in the gallbladder. When food reaches the acid-laden stomach, the liver and pancreas receive a signal. By the time food reaches the first part of the small intestine, the duodenum, the liver has signaled the gallbladder to release the necessary bile. The bile joins the equally alkaline pancreatic juice and intestinal fluids. Together, they tear into acid-saturated foods and break them down into their components, preparing them for utilization by the body.

As the food is broken down, the sugars rush ahead from the intestine into the liver via the bloodstream. Aside from the leftover fats that are sent throughout the body by the lymphatic vessels, everything else proceeds to the liver for the inspection and processing of food particles, fatty acids and glycerol. At this juncture, after the digestive process has reduced the ingested food to a rubble, the liver makes sense out of it by assimilating it into compounds which the human body can use.

In order to perform its myriad number of chemical functions, including many that science has never been able to duplicate, the liver makes its own enzymes which act as catalysts. The enzymes that the liver produces are organic catalysts that provide an encouraging atmosphere enabling organic substances to rapidly change their structural makeup.

Because of the incredible speed with which the liver can produce these catalytic enzymes, it is ready to work on the amino acids and sugars as soon as they arrive after racing through the capillaries from the intestine, entering the liver through the great portal vein. The liver rearranges these amino acids into new and usable proteins.

When the skin is broken, the liver is called upon to control the bleeding by clotting. To do this, it manufactures the coagulant prothrombin. It also helps in preventing the dangerous thickening of the blood in the arteries by manufacturing two anticoagulants, heparin and antithrombin.

When the muscles call for energy, which is often the case after exercising, the liver taps its supply of glycogen, converting glucose and releasing it into the bloodstream. When the muscles, in turn, throw off poisonous lactic acid, the liver draws it back and reconverts it to glycogen.

Even when your body's red blood cells have served their purpose and died, they are salvaged in part by the liver—at the rate of approximately ten million per second! The liver does this by sending them first to the spleen, which breaks them down into their components, and then using the raw materials for building new blood cells and other body components.

However, the liver cannot use everything that is sent its way. What the body doesn't need, such as waste nitrogen, is turned into urea and sent to the kidneys for elimination. The liver is also instrumental in regulating the balance of salt and water in the body by building amino acids into albumin; it balances the sex hormones to keep the sexual urge from increasing or decreasing; and it destroys excess thyroxin that would throw the growth processes out of control.

As blood passes through the liver on its way toward the heart and the rest of the body, it picks up nutrients and vitamins that the liver stores—vitamins A, D, the B complex and such minerals as zinc, iron and copper. And, of course, the liver has the job of removing toxic substances from the blood before sending it on, which means eliminating poisons from such substances as alcohol, nicotene, caffeine, drugs, industrial poisons, sprays and solvents.

If it sounds like a great deal of blood passing through the human liver, it is! The liver in the average human weighs approximately five to eight pounds and is capable of containing at any one moment a quarter of the body's blood—only the lungs receive more blood than the liver.

The liver receives fresh arterial blood from the heart via the capillaries and then sends it back to the heart through the veins. It also receives venous blood, which must be cleaned before it can safely go any farther. The liver also serves as an internal sentry for the heart. It catches any unanticipated amount of excess blood before it can flood the heart and perhaps interfere with the pumping action of that organ. The liver can do this because it can stretch large enough to hold any excess blood. It then releases this excess accumulation of blood in a steady stream that will not overtax the heart.

The Healthy Liver Regenerates Itself

Aside from filtering out poisons and wastes for the body's protection, the liver itself possesses innate safety factors. The liver has the remarkable power of regeneration. In some way still not fully understood by physicians, scientists and medical researchers, if a portion of the liver is removed by surgery or destroyed by infection, the remainder of the liver works as if nothing were missing and, within a short period of time, grows back what was lost. Its ability to function while the liver tissue has actually been destroyed provides another enormous margin of safety. According to Dr. Carl J. Wiggers in *Physiology in Health and Disease*, it has been proven that the liver can actually function and maintain life even if 80 percent of the tissue is missing or unable to function for some reason.

The Warning Signs Of Liver Disease

The human body cannot do without the liver's operations even for an instant. If any part of the liver malfunctions, the chances are that it will remain undetected until the condition becomes quite serious; however, there is one good indicator of liver ailment that will alert the victim quickly—jaundice.

Jaundice, now recognized as a symptom, not a disease, occurs when the liver malfunctions and bile pigments build up within the bloodstream giving the skin a yellow color; in fact, all body tissues turn a sallow yellow, including the whites of the eyes. The condition may be caused by diseases destroying the red blood cells, an obstruction in the gallbladder, an infectious inflammation, or a fat buildup in the liver itself, retaining the pigments that are normally discharged.

The most common types of liver disease are cirrhosis and viral hepatitis. Cirrhosis of the liver occurs when the liver cells gradually stop functioning and are replaced by hard fibrous tissues while the organ itself shrinks. In cases of viral hepatitis, which may be infectious, or serum hepatitis, the liver becomes inflamed.

227. Hepatitis—It Can Happen To Anyone

There are 70,000 new cases of hepatitis reported annually in the United States, according to Dr. Fenton Schaffner (*The Toronto Star*, February 15, 1973). Dr. Schaffner, professor of medicine and pathology at the Mount Sinai School of Medicine, stressed that these figures represent only a small part of the actual number of cases. "There are possibly ten times that number," he warned.

There are two types of hepatitis: infectious and serum. Infectious hepatitis, contracted by eating tainted shellfish, drinking contaminated water, eating contaminated foods, or inhaling airborne germs from infected individuals, is considered much less dangerous than the sometimes fatal serum hepatitis. The latter is spread by transfusions of contaminated blood and by injections with unsterilized hypodermic needles. When hepatitis does occur, the first classic symptom is a gradually increasing weakness and dizziness which may seem to be the first stages of the flu or a bad cold. Soon utter and complete fatigue takes over, along with nausea, pains in the stomach, tenderness and swelling in the area of the liver and an unconquerable loss of appetite. The urine is noticeably darker in color because the virus acts to destroy the tissue of the liver and interferes with the liver's ability to process waste materials of the body.

Such attacks impede the liver's ability to manufacture important blood components and the storage and processing of certain vitamins. The liver must eliminate poisons which come to the body through polluted air, foods and drugs. If it is not functioning, all of these elements pile up in the body and can poison the entire system, causing constant deterioration of the liver, because under such circumstances, its amazing ability to regenerate is impeded. Chronic hepatitis, which lasts for more than three months (some cases have been known to last up to two years), is considered more dangerous than acute cases of hepatitis since longer bouts of the disease can very easily turn into cirrhosis, a disease with a high fatality rate.

Treatment For Hepatitis

Fortunately, in most cases of acute hepatitis the liver is able to restore itself if a strict regimen of no alcohol, sound nutrition and plenty of rest is followed. The biggest obstacle to regaining health through this regimen is that the hepatitis victim is always short on appetite and finds it difficult, if not impossible, to eat the food he needs to supply the liver with the necessary nutrients for self-repair. Along with vitamins C and E, a fat intake not to exceed eight grams a day and large amounts of distilled water to flush the kidneys of any toxic substances, recommended nutritional consultant Richard J. Turchetti. Turchetti, who co-authored *New Age of Nutrition* (Henry Regnery Co., Chicago, 1974) with Joseph J. Morella, advises that ". . . a good treatment for hepatitis is a high protein diet: one gram of protein per day for every pound of body weight. Brewer's yeast, wheat germ, egg yolks, are good sources of high quality protein and excellent sources of the B-complex, which helps combat the stress damage."

Infectious Hepatitis And Shellfish

Shellfish are succulent, delicious and even nutritious, but they may harbor infectious hepatitis and other diseases whose viruses are found in the raw sewage that is part of the off-shore waters that is the natural environment of shellfish. This aspect of their environment is a danger; the fact that bivalve shellfish are filter feeders only compounds the danger. According to Dr. John R. Mitchell of the Michigan Department of Health, in an article in the *Archives of Environmental Health* (Vol. 12, May 1966), both clams and oysters have the ability to take up viruses and bacteria from contaminated water and concentrate these microorganisms in their own tissue at levels 60 times greater than the surrounding water.

Officials Claim No Adequate Test For Hepatitis

Under present regulations, the Food and Drug Administration is responsible for making sure that all shellfish reaching American tables are untainted. However, the FDA has given the states the duty of enforcing these regulations. Many states, in turn, have left the policing of harvesting beds in the hands of local municipalities. Often, there just aren't enough inspectors to do an adequate job. Consequently, sporadic cases of shellfish poisoning continue to occur.

"The problem is that there is no laboratory method test today that will detect the presence of hepatitis organisms in shellfish," an FDA spokesman said. "The number one priority of the FDA is to come up with a test to find out if shellfish are contaminated before they are eaten. Right now, the only thing we can do is wait for an outbreak of hepatitis to occur and then trace it back to the bed from which the shellfish came. And sometimes," he added, "we aren't all that successful."

In states where shellfishing is a significant part of the economy, surveillance tends to be strict. State regulatory agencies continuously monitor all areas along their coastlines for pollution. The beds or flats are patrolled by state wardens. When a flat yields polluted clams, the area is posted and clam-digging is prohibited. Anyone found clamming in prohibited areas faces a fine.

Heat Shellfish Thoroughly To Be Sure

Aside from stricter regulatory controls and just plain abstinence from eating shellfish, just what can individuals who like clams and oysters do to avoid the menace of hepatitis? Proper and lengthy steaming is the answer, according to Dr. David Snydman, epidemic intelligence officer with the Viral Disease Division at the Center for Disease Control in Atlanta, Georgia. Hepatitis can be avoided, says Dr. Snydman, if shellfish are steamed from four to six minutes or more.

This advice is confirmed by Drs. John A. Bryan, deputy director of the Viral Disease Division of the C.D.C., and J. Clark Huff, writing in the *Journal of the American Medical Association*, October 29, 1973.

They cited studies showing that during steaming, it takes at least four minutes for the temperature inside the clam meat to rise to the temperature of the steam. But clam shells usually *open* within the first minute of steaming. "Therefore," they warned, "when clams are steamed only until the shells open, the internal temperature is not high enough to inactivate the infectious agent of hepatitis."

Thoroughly steamed, clams may not be as tender as they would be with a light steaming, but that is the price of safety. Further evidence that thorough heating is the key to safe shellfish enjoyment was provided by Irwin M. Arais, M.D., writing in the *Journal of the American Medical Association* (October 5, 1963). In answer to a question about polluted shellfish beds around Pascagoula, Mississippi, and Mobile and Troy, Alabama, he said that "frying of clams and oysters from each of these areas apparently inactivated the hepatitis virus; however, milder treatment such as preparation of stews and chowders did not inactivate the hepatitis virus."

Because of the serious pollution affecting our coastal waters, and the ability of shellfish to absorb and concentrate pollutants, a regular diet of clams, oysters or any other shellfish is a risky diet. If you have friends or relatives who do eat shellfish, it would be wise to pass the word along. Eat them if you must, but be sure they're cooked properly.

228. Cirrhosis Of The Liver

Cirrhosis of the liver is of very gradual onset and occurs when liver cells, unable to renew themselves, become replaced by hard, fibrous connective tissue. For reasons still unknown to scientists, the remarkable regeneration capabilities of the liver are unable to overcome the cirrhosis of the liver cells—the term cirrhosis is actually a medical term for the formation of scar tissue anywhere in the body. The scar tissue, which actually forms as the liver shrinks, impairs circulation within the liver and leads to serious liver malfunction. In advanced cases of cirrhosis of the liver, the liver has a hobnailed appearance, with scar tissue actually segmenting it.

This disease of the liver is now among the ten leading causes of death in the United States. According to a census by the National Center for Health Statistics in 1972, cirrhosis of the liver was the cause of 32,000 deaths, ranking fourth in order after heart disease, cancer and diabetes mellitus. It appears that cirrhosis of the liver is not confined to the middle-aged and older, according to Dr. Charles S. Lieber, chief liver specialist at the Bronx Veterans Hospital and professor of medicine at the Mount Sinai School of Medicine. He stated that cirrhosis of the liver was the third or fourth leading cause of death among people between the ages of 25 and 65 in the city of New York (*Evening Chronicle*, Allentown, Pennsylvania, September 9, 1974).

According to *The Merck Manual of Diagnosis and Therapy* (Twelfth Edition, Merck and Co., 1972) alcoholism, malnutrition, severe hepatitis, the prolonged obstruction of the flow of bile, congestive heart failure and syphilis are listed as the diseases which may lead to cirrhosis of the liver; however, scientists are still not sure of the actual disease-causing mechanism.

According to an article in the *New England Journal of Medicine* written by Drs. Charles S. Davidson and George J. Gabuzda, cirrhosis of the liver is a widespread disease in parts of the world where there is little animal protein in the diet; that is, the people eat largely carbohydrate diets. It does not seem to matter how fine a source of carbohydrate they may have or how natural all of their foods are. If animal protein is lacking, cirrhosis of the liver is most likely to occur.

Symptoms Of The Disease

Cirrhosis of the liver provides many outward physical signs. Here is a list compiled by Dr. A. E. Read and published in the *British Medical Journal* (February 17, 1968). *A note of warning*—if these abnormalities are noticed, you should see your physician immediately. Beginning with the head and progressing to the feet, they are: *Head*—thin hair; exophthalmos (bulging eyes); jaundice; facial telangiectasia (reddish areas caused by dilated blood capillaries); and spider nevi or Nevus (pinhead dots from which blood vessels radiate). *Trunk*—spider nevi of the collar bone region; gynecomastia (enlargement of the male breast); swollen liver; collateral veins (secondary blood vessels formed when the main blood vessels are broken); ascites (abnormal accumulation of fluid in the abdomen); small testes; and absent or reduced pubic hair. *Limbs*—muscle wasting; clubbing fingers; opaque nails; edema; and pupura (bluish skin caused by hemorrhage). Long before these symptoms mature, subtle and vague signs like upset stomach and perpetual fatigue persist.

Choline Deficiency And Cirrhosis Of The Liver

It is believed that cirrhosis or scar tissue of the liver replaces fat deposits in the liver. It is known that *steatosis*, or fatty degeneration of tissue, occurs in the organ when the body is deficient in choline, a member of the B complex vitamins. This medical fact was reported in the *Federation Proceedings* (January-February, 1971), a report of the American Institute of Nutrition.

"It is known from histological and biochemical evidence that withdrawal of choline from the diet in one single meal causes accumulation of lipid in the liver," reported Sailen Mookerjea, of the medical research department of Charles H. Best Institute, University of Toronto. He said that experiments conducted by him and his colleagues, as well as those of Rosenfeld and Lang (*J. Lipid Res.*, 7: 10, 1966), show that "the increase of liver lipids within one or two days of choline deprivation, uncomplicated by unnecessary manipulations, has always been an irreproachable fact."

Dr. Richard Follis, Jr., explained why in his book, *Deficiency Diseases* (Charles C. Thomas, 1958). He said that fats must leave the liver in the form of phospholipids. When choline is deficient in the diet, this phospholipid turnover is reduced. Choline, he added, also enables the liver to burn up fatty acids.

"By these two mechanisms," wrote Dr. Follis, "the liver cells are normally able to clear themselves of fatty acids which are brought to them by the bloodstream, whether from ingested lipids or from the breakdown of fats elsewhere, particularly in the deposits of subcutaneous tissues and other areas." But if choline is not available, fat droplets settle within the liver cells, where they may form cyst-like structures. This fatty infiltration renders the liver helpless to detoxify substances that enter the bloodstream, or to metabolize proteins and carbohydrates, or to regulate the electrolyte balance in the body's tissues. In time, the whole body may eventually become diseased by poisons that the liver has been unable to eliminate.

Such a situation is less likely to occur if your diet contains a maximum of choline and a minimum of fats. A study demonstrating the effect of a combination of choline deficiency and excessive fat upon the liver was conducted by N. W. King, an assistant pathologist at the U.S. Army Medical Research and Nutrition Laboratory in Denver, Colorado, and reported in *The American Journal of Clinical Nutrition* (January, 1965).

Dr. King observed that rats fed the choline-deficient diet developed "severe" damage—30 to 40 percent of the cells composing the liver lobules became infiltrated with fat. Half the rats in this group also received fat injections which caused 75 to 80 percent of these cells to fill up with fat droplets. When choline was added to the diet, the changes were not so severe. The livers of rats fed the choline-rich diet throughout the duration of the experiment appeared normal in every way. In humans, also, choline supplements have been found to diminish steatosis of the liver. *The American Medical Association Journal* (February 24, 1951) reported that two groups of infants suffering from this ailment were put on a high-protein, low-fat diet. The group receiving choline supplements, in addition, "had less fatty infiltration after a given length of time." Choline is a basic constituent of lecithin, the emulsified phospholipid (combination of fatty acids and phosphorus) that in the average diet is found only in egg yolk, although abundant supplies of lecithin are also contained in soybeans. Most important to the study at hand, however, is that human breast milk also contains lecithin, while cow's milk is lacking in it.

Treatment

If cirrhosis of the liver is recognized early enough and proper treatment begun, the disease may be arrested but not reversed. The scar tissue will remain a permanent part of the organ. In arresting the disease in the early stages, the sufferer may be able to lead a normal life if he follows a simple regimen under the supervision of a physician. The patient should eliminate all toxins from the diet, especially alcohol, and include a diet rich in protein, including meat, fish, eggs, fruit, green vegetables, and vitamin and mineral supplementation.

Alcohol And Cirrhosis

Although not all alcoholics are victims of this form of cirrhosis, there is a high incidence of the disease among moderate and heavy drinkers. The relationship between alcohol and cirrhosis is a logical one, since the liquid diet of the alcoholic is pure carbohydrate, which can only be detoxified by the liver at a fixed rate. The alcohol that cannot be processed by the liver progressively destroys liver cells, creating large fat deposits which eventually become hard and turn a tawny yellow. The mechanics of the relationship between cirrhosis and a fatty liver are still unknown, but large fat deposits usually precede cirrhosis.

Alcohol is also known to be an antagonist of the B complex vitamins which are so essential to the good health of the liver. According to Dr. Carroll M. Leevy, a professor at the New Jersey College of Medicine, alcohol can markedly reduce absorption of thiamine hydrochloride (vitamin B_1) and other nutrients. This indicates that malabsorption may lead to a deficiency state which could initiate liver injury despite a normal diet. Deficiency in vitamin B_1 can cause confusion and memory loss, gastric distress, stomach pains, constipation, heart irregularities and tender muscles.

Once the damage has been done, the effects from long-term excessive drinking cannot be reversed, but further damage can be arrested if the habit is kicked—not just tapered down, but cut off. "Cirrhosis of the alcoholic is not spontaneously progressive," Dr. Leevy explained. "Abstinence from alcoholic beverages and provision of a nutritious vitamin-supplemented diet lead to stabilization of the process in its early phases and cause a significant reduction in morbidity and mortality."

Section 43
Miscarriage

229. Preventing Miscarriage

229. Preventing Miscarriage

What should be done in the case of spontaneous abortion or miscarriage (the spontaneous interruption of pregnancy up to the twenty-eighth week)? Can it be prevented? Should it be prevented? What work has been done in this area?

Spontaneous abortions are generally estimated to occur in about ten percent of pregnancies. Some doctors believe this is an unrealistic figure. They cite the large number of abortions not reported, and those which occur before a physician has been consulted.

In 1972, Irwin Stone commented in his book, *The Healing Factor* (Grosset and Dunlap) on the importance of the work of Dr. F. R. Klenner in proving the effectiveness of vitamin C in preventing miscarriage. Dr. Klenner prescribed large doses of ascorbic acid in the cases of over 300 pregnant women. The patients ingested from four to 15 grams of ascorbic acid daily, on an escalating basis, for the duration of their pregnancies.

During the first third of gestation, they took four grams daily, six grams daily for the second trimester, and 10 to 15 grams daily (depending on the individual mother's requirement) for the remaining months of pregnancy. There was not one miscarriage in this entire group of women.

Considering that (as has been stated earlier) 10 percent of all pregnancies are terminated by miscarriage, this is a remarkable study.

Dr. Carl T. Javert of Cornell University claims that vitamin C and bioflavonoids prevent miscarriages. In a study of 1,334 patients, he found that 45 percent of three groups tested were deficient in vitamin C. Giving large doses of vitamin C and the bioflavonoids to 100 pregnant women with histories of habitual abortion, he achieved a successful pregnancy in 91 percent. These patients took a diet rich in vitamin C (350 milligrams) plus a supplement containing vitamin C and the bioflavonoids— making a total of 500 milligrams of vitamin C per day. The vitamin C or bioflavonoids alone did not do the job. But the combination of the two worked the miracle.

Dr. Robert Greenblatt of the Medical College of Georgia also advocates using vitamin C and the bioflavonoids for habitual abortion. He says a group of women who never had been able to carry their children to term and bring them into the world alive were examined to determine the state of their capillaries—the tiny blood vessels that spread through every inch of our bodies. It was found that they suffered from capillary fragility. The walls of these tiny vessels burst easily, causing bruised areas. Vitamin C and the bioflavonoids were given to them with excellent results. Eleven of the thirteen patients who had experienced two previous miscarriages delivered live infants.

Why are the capillaries so important? This network of tiny blood vessels provides the working barrier separating the blood from the cellular elements and tissues. Across the walls of the capillaries must pass all life-giving ingredients found in the blood whether they are in the form of gases or solids.

The most important part of the capillaries is the layer in their walls which contains the intercellular cement. Any change in the composition of this cement is bound to have a tremendous effect on how substances pass through the capillary wall into and out of the blood. The composition of the cement is influenced largely by vitamin C and the flavonoids.

According to researchers who have experimented with these two food substances, there is no diseased state in which the capillaries are not harmed, and there is no diseased state that will not be improved by improving the state of the capillaries. In the case of habitual abortion, the capillaries are failing. So vitamin C and the bioflavonoids should be used.

What foods contain bioflavonoids? The substance used by many researchers comes from citrus fruits—it is contained in the white underskin and segment part of the fruit—not in the juice. The edible part of the orange contains a tenfold concentration of bioflavonoids, compared to the quantity in strained juice. In the freshly peeled orange there are 1,000 milligrams of bioflavonoids and about 60 milligrams of vitamin C. In the strained orange juice there are only about 100 milligrams of bioflavonoids. This is an excellent reason for not juicing citrus fruit. When you eat it, don't remove the white layers under the skin and around each segment of fruit. Lemons, grapes, plums, black currants, grapefruit, apricots, cherries and blackberries also contain flavonoids. The flavonoids may also be called rutin, hesperidin or vitamin P.

Smoking increases the odds of miscarriage. *Good Housekeeping* in its August, 1963 issue quoted Dr. Jay Zabriskie who had reported on what he had learned from 2,000 consecutive births in an Army hospital. Half the women smoked. "On the average these women bore babies half a pound lighter than those of nonsmokers and gave birth prematurely two-and-a-half times as frequently. Smokers had had miscarriages in 12.6 percent of previous pregnancies, compared to 8.8 percent for those who did not smoke." Cigarette smoke contains toxic chemicals and it depletes the body's supply of vitamin C.

But the question remains: Should an attempt be made to save a fetus if a woman shows signs of miscarrying? It is the view of many physicians that spontaneous abortion is nature's way of rejecting a fetus which has been poorly formed, or had an unhealthy start. They say, if spontaneous abortion or miscarriage begins, it is best to let it run its course, rather than trying to save a fetus which might be born abnormal if carried to full term.

The well-known Dr. Evan Shute is not of this opinion, and quotes figures to show that this is far from the rule. He refers to E. S. Burge who, in the *American Journal of Obstetrics and Gynecology* (44: 973, 1942), remarks that of the threatened abortions in 12,000 cases, no more than 1.5 percent ended in the birth of major defectives. On that percentage, Dr. Shute suggests that, of 100 mothers threatening to abort, 98.5 should produce babies free of any major defect. Such odds offer every reason for attempting to avert threatened abortion, says Dr. Shute. It is not at all a rule that congenital defects are bound to appear in infants whose spontaneous abortion was reversed.

Dr. Shute then goes on to tell of his 25 years experience, in which he has administered vitamin E routinely to every private obstetrical patient registered with him, from the beginning to the end of the pregnancy. The doses have ranged from two drams of wheat germ oil to 50-450 milligrams of vitamin E per day.

Of 4,141 private, consecutive, unselected cases, all given alpha tocopherol, there have been 134 recognized abortions and miscarriages, an incidence of 3.2 percent. Dr. Shute suggests that this percentage be raised to 5.2 percent to account for abortions reported over the phone before there has actually been time for an office visit, and for incidents casually mentioned at a later office visit. The 5.2 percent figure is still only about half of that reported in literature generally. This lends support to the idea that alpha tocopherol is helpful in preventing abortion in a large number of cases treated both preventively and therapeutically.

Of Dr. Shute's 4,141 patients, there were 139 threatened

abortions and 98 threatened miscarriages (the term differs only to designate the first three or second three months of pregnancy), and the abortion or miscarriage was reversed in 76 percent and 96 percent respectively. Therefore, 182 normal children were born, in comparison to 13 abnormal children, six of whom died at birth.

Dr. Shute further holds that the administration of alpha tocopherol just before or just after conception is helpful in the prevention of congenital defect, and this theory has been borne out in literature concerning animals made vitamin E-deficient by special diets. The placenta is the foundation of good circulation for the fetus. Presumably, if there is a good foundation, a good infant will develop and the mother will remain normal. On the other hand, a defective placenta may alter the whole pregnancy and its product for the worse.

The placenta provides the embryo with nutrients of all types, but especially oxygen. Alpha tocopherol has been shown time and again to be an oxygen-conserving agent. This alone would make it a valuable agent in pregnancy.

The placenta can also be regarded as a great sponge, a net of capillaries. Keeping these capillaries intact is vital to the life of the fetus. Alpha tocopherol has unique properties for preserving normal capillary strength and in maintaining their proper width.

But before the placenta takes over, the ovaries are most important. Progesterone is the specific hormone of pregnancy. It is released during the menstrual cycle, at the time when the egg is traveling toward the uterus, and continues in production while the pregnancy lasts. One of its functions is keeping the muscles of the uterus from contracting. The initiation of labor, some authorities believe, is caused by a dwindling progesterone supply.

Estrogens are also essential for maternal maintenance of the developing fetus. A drop in estrogen levels during pregnancy is a clear signal to doctors that something has gone amiss and the baby is threatened.

The placenta plays a very important role in maintaining hormonal balance in pregnancy. This organ serves as an endocrine gland, synthesizing hormones throughout pregnancy. Released into the mother's bloodstream, the placental hormones direct the special body chemistry necessary for carrying the child safely and for preparation of the breast for milk production.

The placenta begins to synthesize its first hormone immediately after attaching itself to the wall of the uterus—an event that occurs some seven days after fertilization. This initial placental hormone stimulates the manufacture of female hormones by the mother's ovary.

There's a moment—about the time of the woman's second missed period—when the placenta stops synthesizing this first hormone in significant quantity and takes on the job of manufacturing estrogens and progesterone. At this time, there's a shift from ovary to placental control of pregnancy. According to Dr. K. J. Catt in his book, *An ABC of Endocrinology* (Little, Brown and Company) this is when the risk of miscarriage is greatest, because declining output of female hormones by the ovary may not be countered instantly by the initiation of production by the placenta.

Dr. Isobel Jennings, British pathologist who has made a study of the nutritional needs of the hormone system, has noted (in *Vitamins in Endocrine Metabolism,* Charles C. Thomas) that vitamins A and B_3 (niacin) are necessary for the synthesis of the sex hormones, and that vitamin C also probably plays a role. Since these hormones are a constant requirement throughout pregnancy, it is obviously important that the vitamins needed for their synthesis should be constantly and adequately included in the diet. But of all times to make sure you're getting your fish liver oil for vitamin A, enriching your diet with such B complex supplements as yeast, wheat germ, or desiccated liver, and getting your vitamin C in fruit, vegetables, and rose hips, it would seem especially vital to do so at the risky time of the second missed period.

Aside from vitamin E, vitamin C and bioflavonoids, the B vitamins, notably vitamin B_1 and niacin, have shown themselves to be of value in maintaining a normal, comfortable pregnancy. A diet which is rich in foods containing these nutrients, as well as supplementary dosage, is the best guarantee a woman can have for a successful pregnancy.

Section 44
Mononucleosis

230. Fighting Mononucleosis

230. Fighting Mononucleosis

Mononucleosis is an acute infectious disease, which comes upon a person suddenly, with accompanying fever, aching joints, a skin rash, dizziness, an inability to swallow, a general feeling of weakness and inflammatory swelling of the lymph nodes, especially those of the neck. It is a miserable and debilitating disease for which there is no proven treatment as yet. The best a person can do is get plenty of bed rest and fluids and wait till the self-remedying disease runs its course. Of course, a well-fortified system is safer than one run down by poor diet and lack of proper rest.

Doctors at Johns Hopkins University, Baltimore, Maryland, were the first to describe the disease accurately in 1920, noting that students had such symptoms as gland swellings, and blood tests showing an abnormally high count of white blood cells. "The normal white cells were overshadowed by large cells with a single nucleus—'mononuclear' cells; thus the name," according to Dr. Halberstam reporting in *Today's Health* (December, 1974).

In the 1950's the disease became known as the "kissing disease" after Dr. Robert Hoagland, then chief physician at the United States Military Academy at West Point, noted that cadets who had contracted "mono" had admitted kissing girls while on leave who had also come down with the disease. According to reports in the *Southern Medical Journal* (December, 1955), Dr. Hoagland's first case was a cadet who became ill in February, 1951, and who had spent some hours on the train before Christmas in company with a female medical student whom he had never seen before. They engaged in intimate kissing, permitting the mixing of saliva. In later correspondence, it appeared that she developed the disease three days before her contact with the cadet. They both were also exposed to a bottle which was passed around among a group of train acquaintances. This cadet contact thus had an incubation period of 47 days.

"In his 73 cases, Hoagland found that all except two had engaged in such intimate oral contacts 32 to 49 days before illness. Three had had only one such contact 42 to 45 days previously. Of the two without a history of kissing, one frequently drank from bottles passed to him by friends. He explains the February and August incidence in his cases by the fact that the semiannual vacations fall some weeks before this time, which, because of the restricted life at the Academy, offers practically the only possibility of the necessary exposure. . . ."

Oral contact with communal drinking utensils and kissing are not the only ways in which the disease is spread from one person to another; there is evidence of sporadic outbreaks of the disease attributed to the use of blood transfusions. Although occasional cases are seen in young children and in adults over 35, 95 percent of the proven mononucleosis cases are found in patients between the ages of 17 and 30, according to Dr. Halberstam.

Noting that "most patients who have 'mono' are back in perfect health within two or three weeks of the peak of their disease," Dr. Halberstam also puts to rest another mistaken notion about the disease: that it is oftentimes fatal. "Despite legends to the contrary," he said, "mononucleosis *is* a benign disease. Among the millions of cases, a few rare fatalities have occurred—almost always due to rupture of the enlarged spleen which often marks the illness. Like other viral illnesses, mononucleosis can affect various organs within the body. Jaundice, rashes, decreased blood platelets with a consequent bleeding tendency, neurologic abnormalities—all have occurred in tandem with 'mono,' but such complications are very rare and disappear when the 'mono' does."

Although the cause of mononucleosis has remained a mystery for more than 40 years since doctors in Baltimore first described its symptoms, researchers now believe that the probable cause of the disease is a virus known as the Epstein-Barr (EB) virus. According to Dr. Alfred S. Evans, of the Yale School of Medicine, New Haven, Conn. (*Modern Medicine,* January 7, 1974), freshmen entering the school who had EB antigens in their blood were immune to mono. And independent studies have proven that when persons lacking the EB antigen in their blood are injected with the virus, they readily come down with the disease.

Since a bout of mononucleosis provides the striken person with a permanent immunity against the disease in the future because of the resulting automatic inclusion of EB antigens in their bloodstreams, it remains a mystery to scientists as to just how certain people who have never had the disease come to possess the EB antigen. All that is known, according to Dr.

Evans, is that those groups least susceptible to "mono" because they possess the EB antigen usually come from the lower socioeconomic levels. College students who come from a "more hygenic and higher socioeconomic level" (especially those from Ivy League schools) have the "greatest risk" of encountering mononucleosis, noted Dr. Evans. Research into vaccines which will provide safe inoculations containing the EB antigens is hampered in the laboratories; it appears that mononucleosis does not occur naturally in test animals.

The best medicine for mononucleosis is *no* medicine. According to Dr. Halberstam, medications containing antibiotics are harmful, since they seem to "provoke more skin rashes" than would occur under ordinary circumstances. The best remedy appears to be plenty of bed rest and fluids. It would also be wise for prevention's sake to remember two of the ways by which the disease is transmitted: using communal drinking utensils and kissing. As for drinking from a cup which is being passed around, it is best just to avoid it completely. But kissing is another question entirely. The late J. I. Rodale had some very good advice on the subject of mononucleosis and kissing among young people: "So—what do I suggest? That all young folks who expect to indulge in kissing go into training for it—that is, take plenty of vitamin C, and a few other vitamins for good measure, and cut down on the artificial sweets—the colas, ice creams, candies, etc., and other refined foods—make their bodies strong and healthy through good nutrition and exercise, build up a resistance to germs, and then they won't have to fear kissing..."

Section 45
Motion
Sickness

231. Help For Troubled Travelers

231. Help For Troubled Travelers

Your inner ear contains the balance mechanism that keeps you from falling over when you stand up or walk. In some people, if this mechanism receives too much stimulation from motion not in their control, such as the movement of a bus, car, boat or plane, its signals spill into various centers of the brain that make one feel depressed, nauseous and sweat but still feel cold. Women are especially susceptible to motion sickness, and so are those of both sexes who suffer high blood pressure, sinusitis or migraine headaches.

If you know from experience that motion makes you queasy, there are several precautions you can take to ease your journey. Sit in the front seat and watch the road when traveling in a car. When you travel by air, ask for a seat in the center of the plane, over the wing, because motion is less pronounced there than in the nose or tail sections. On shipboard, amidships is best, and if at all possible, avoid the bow.

Vision plays a role in motion sickness. Ask anyone who has stood at the bow of a ship and watched the horizon bounce as ocean swells carried the ship up and dropped it down. So if the view outside the window of a plane or ship visually confirms the vehicle's dips and rolls, *don't look out!* When riding in a car or bus, try to focus your gaze on the horizon or some far away object, and keep your head steady while the vehicle is turning.

Lying back in your seat with your head in a reclining position will minimize the effect of movement on your inner ear, and lessen the chance that it will trigger motion sickness.

Many experts suggest keeping mentally occupied with word games, conversation or anything else to distract the mind from motion. However, reading should be avoided.

Eat lightly and simply—steer away from heavy foods with rich sauces if you're going to travel. Don't drink any fizzy or alcoholic beverages, and don't smoke. Proper evacuation of the bowels before leaving also helps decrease the likelihood of motion sickness.

How about anti-nausea drugs? None of them are without unwanted side effects, so unless experience has taught you that you invariably *do* get motion sickness, skip the medication and assume that, like the majority of travelers, you're going to be okay. If you don't want to take that chance, carry the medication for use *if* needed. These drugs take effect quickly, so if discomfort should come, relief is readily achieved.

And here's something worth investigating: pyridoxine, vitamin B_6, has been successfully used to prevent nausea in pregnancy and also to forestall post-surgical vomiting, according to Dr. Paul Gyorgy in Sebrell and Harris's *The Vitamins* (vol. II, Academic Press, New York, 1968). It seems reasonable to expect that B_6 might also protect against motion sickness. So why not take extra supplements of this safe and helpful nutrient before and during your trip?

Section 46
Multiple Sclerosis

232. Diet Deficiency Long Suspected As Cause Of Multiple Sclerosis

Multiple sclerosis is a disease of the central nervous system, in which myelin, the protective covering of the brain and the spinal cord, becomes damaged (demyelination). As a result, the nerve impulses are blocked or distorted and the body cannot properly respond to them.

The disease starts inconspicuously, with occasional moments of weakness and numbness in the limbs, disturbances in the sense of balance and dizziness. As multiple sclerosis progresses, the victim's walk becomes unsteady, his mind is affected and emotional changes occur. Vision is sometimes impaired. Gradually, the disease spreads to the brain, bone marrow and other vital areas of the body, with increased paralysis throughout the body. The disease moves into its most critical stages when the lungs and the heart muscles become affected.

Nobody knows the cause or the cure of multiple sclerosis, nor why it usually strikes people between the ages of 20 and 40.

Equally mysterious is the benign course the disease takes in some people, with unexplained periods of complete or partial remission of the debilitating aspects of the illness. These periods last as long as 20 years in some patients, while in others the period may only be for a few years or a few weeks. These remissions occur suddenly, and while they last there is no sign that the patient was ever attacked by multiple sclerosis. However, not all MS patients encounter remission, and for them the disease can mean a relentless decline, progressing from loss of coordination, through paralysis to eventual death.

The possibility that multiple sclerosis may be due to a diet deficiency has been a theory pursued by several medical researchers. A five-year study conducted at Northwestern University, Evanston, Illinois, suggested that a diet rich in seed oils and fresh fish, especially if eaten by pregnant women and by children, would reduce the incidence of multiple sclerosis. Drs. Joseph Bernsohn and Leo Stephanides reported their findings in *Nature* (January 22, 1967) based on the initial discovery that polyunsaturated fatty acids are necessary to the development and integrity of the brain and spinal cord, the two vital areas affected by multiple sclerosis. Linolenic acid, a polyunsaturate, is particularly important to the brain, but the body cannot manufacture it. We must get linolenic acid from food. Fresh fish and seed oils—safflower seed, corn, sunflower seed, cotton seed and soybean oils—are particularly rich in linolenic acid.

If this link between unsaturated fats and MS does indeed exist, the researchers believe that a lack of linolenic acid in the diet of newborn children can lead to structural defects in the nervous system. Pregnant women deficient in linolenic acid might pass these same defects on to the fetus. The defects would be difficult to detect until the child is 15 or 16, the age at which the human brain is fully developed. At this point the brain and spinal cord are susceptible to "demyelination," destruction of the fatty sheaths around the nerve fibers which is a characteristic of multiple sclerosis.

Victims of MS do show below normal amounts of linolenic acid in their brains. Conversely, in certain geographic areas where there are large amounts of linolenic acid in the diet, MS is rare. In Japan, for example, people consume great amounts of raw fish and multiple sclerosis is almost nonexistent. The same is true in Africa and Southeast Asia where the diet is composed largely of berries, unprocessed greens and nuts.

In 1973 a team of British doctors (*British Medical Journal*, March 31) reported studies showing that two tablespoons of sunflower seed oil taken twice a day led to a considerable reduction in the severity of multiple sclerosis and increased the period of remission in humans.

This beneficial effect of sunflower seed oil was determined by Dr. Harold Millar and his associates at the Royal Victoria Hospital in Belfast, Northern Ireland, after a carefully developed double-blind study conducted over a two-year period under a grant from the Multiple Sclerosis Society.

Seventy-five patients with multiple sclerosis were admitted to the trial which was carried on in two cities—Belfast and London. The patients were divided at random into "treated" and "control" groups. Only patients who could walk, with or without aid, were included. All were at a clinically-inactive phase of the disease at the start. Any patient who had already taken sunflower seed oil was excluded.

Two doses of an oil mixture were taken each day, morning and evening, for a period of two years. For the treated group, each dose consisted of 30 ml. (two tablespoons) of a sunflower seed oil emulsion providing 8.6 grams of linoleic acid. The control group received two daily doses of an emulsion similar in appearance and flavor but containing olive oil instead of sunflower seed oil. Each dose of this emulsion provided 3.8 grams of oleic acid (a non-essential fatty acid which can be synthesized by the body from saturated fatty acid) and just 0.2 grams of linoleic acid. Thus, the treated group got 43 times as much linoleic acid as the control group.

Patients were seen at intervals of two to three months and the severity of the disease at each visit was determined by reference to a specially-devised scoring chart. Their progress was assessed according to sensory function, bladder and bowel functions, visual and mental function and the patients' ability to cope with ordinary day-to-day tasks.

Dr. Millar's group determined the effect of the linoleic acid by counting the number of relapses suffered over a two-year period by the patients in both groups. There were 62 relapses among the 39 patients who did not receive the sunflower seed oil. There were only 41 relapses among the 36-member group who did get the sunflower seed oil.

Not only were relapses less frequent in the treated group, they were much less severe. In fact, relapses—such as temporary loss of vision or weakness in the legs—were judged twice as severe in the untreated group and much longer in duration.

It was also determined by measuring fatty acid levels in the subjects' blood that there was no defect in the absorption of linoleic acid, in the doses used, as a consequence of multiple sclerosis. In the patients receiving sunflower seed oil supplements, the mean serum linoleate level rose from 28.6 percent (linoleic acid expressed as a percentage of the total fatty acids) to a value of 35.2 percent after three to five months, and to 36.3 percent after nine to 12 months. The serum oleic acid levels in this group fell from 28.5 percent to 25.2 after three to five months and to 24.3 percent after nine to 12 months. Thus there was an increase in the proportion of saturates in the blood of treated patients.

In the patients receiving the olive oil supplements, on the

other hand, the values of both linoleic and oleic acid in the serum remained almost unchanged. The probability that the increased intake of oleic acid might be responsible for the more frequent and more severe relapses in the control group was ruled out. It is more likely, the investigators concluded, that the linoleic acid supplements afforded a measure of protection during the two years of the trial.

233. Can Vitamin D And Calcium Prevent Multiple Sclerosis?

When humans migrated from the tropics to northern climates many thousands of years ago, not everyone fully adapted to diminished sunshine. And this maladaptation, inherited today by a small proportion of the population, may hold the secret of why some young men and women—seemingly healthy and in the prime of life—are mysteriously stricken with the crippling neurological disease, multiple sclerosis.

This is the theory of the cause of multiple sclerosis (MS) advanced by Dr. Paul Goldberg, a research scientist in Cambridge, Mass. According to Goldberg, a plentiful year-round supply of the sun's ultraviolet rays, which trigger the production of vitamin D in human skin, is the reason why multiple sclerosis is "almost non-existent" in tropical regions. In temperate and northern climates, he argues, the disease strikes those who inherit an unfulfilled need for the high levels of vitamin D that the sun bestows on tropical humans (levels of some two to four thousand International Units a day, in contrast to the official Recommended Dietary Allowance of 400 I.U.).

While these susceptible individuals receive enough vitamin D from diet and the northern sun to prevent a recognized deficiency disease, Dr. Goldberg proposes that subtler damage may be taking place. He suggests that, especially during the growth spurt of adolescence, their *relative* deficiency in vitamin D interferes with normal development of the central nervous system; consequently, poorly constructed neural tissue breaks down in later years, causing the debilitating symptoms of MS. Calcium, whose absorption and utilization is triggered by vitamin D, is possibly another major factor in the MS story, according to Dr. Goldberg.

If his theory proves valid, multiple sclerosis would be as easy to prevent (though, unfortunately, not to cure) as scurvy or beri-beri or any other deficiency disease, by providing adequate supplements of the deficient nutrients. Dr. Goldberg offers the hope that, by stepping up vitamin D intake to "natural" tropical levels during adolescent growth, we might absolutely eliminate the threat of multiple sclerosis to susceptible young people.

Pinning Down The Cause Of MS

The Cambridge scientist presented his views in a two-part series published in the *International Journal of Environmental Studies* (1974, Vol. 6, Part 1 pp. 19-27, Part 2 pp. 121-129).

Dr. Goldberg concluded from his research, which encompassed a broad review of world literature about existing epidemiological and biochemical evidence pertaining to multiple sclerosis, that the probable cause of MS was a relative vitamin D deficiency and associated calcium deficiency. Some of the associations which led to his final conclusion follow:

The geographic distribution of MS has striking patterns, which must be accounted for in any theory of the disease's cause. As noted earlier, MS is primarily a disease of cold countries with relatively sparse yearly hours of sun. "Prevalence is greatest in the northern latitudes of Europe and North America," Dr. Goldberg writes, "where rates can exceed 100 per 100,000 population. In regions south of 40° N (a latitude running through Kansas City and Philadelphia in North America, through Spain and Greece in Europe) the risk of acquiring the disease diminished toward zero as the equator is approached."

In latitudes where MS occurs, there is anything but uniform geographic distribution. Rather, there are pockets of high concentration of MS cases, and other areas where prevalence is low. What Dr. Goldberg calls the "fine structure" of MS distribution, as established in painstaking epidemiological studies in Norway, Sweden, Finland, Denmark, Great Britain, and Switzerland, shows puzzling differences between even neighboring communities. In the Oarkney and Shetland Islands off the coast of Scotland, for example, MS prevalence is four times higher than in the nearby Faeroe Islands.

The risk of getting MS depends not on the prevalence of the disease where a young person *now* lives—but on where he grew up. Citing the research of J. F. Kurtzke who in 1972 reported on "Migration and Latency in Multiple Sclerosis," Dr. Goldberg states: "A population raised, for example, in a zone of high risk retains that risk despite emigration to a region of low prevalence."

Multiple Sclerosis

MS strikes primarily at young adults between the ages of 20 and 40. It is extremely rare in childhood.

There's an inheritance factor in MS. While no clear genetic pattern is evident, Dr. Goldberg says, "the risk for a first degree relative of a patient with MS is at least 15 times that for a member of the general population."

Studies in Switzerland show there's a strong correlation between MS rates and altitude. On the high mountain ranges, MS is rare, whereas all regions where the disease is prevalent are located at lower altitudes—1000 meters (3280 ft.) above sea level or less.

Studies in the U.S. indicate that people brought up in large urban areas have a higher risk of contracting MS than those who are reared in the country. In northern Europe, there's no such pattern, and in fact some studies show just the opposite.

The Safety Belt

While there is much to puzzle over in this collection of sometimes contradictory findings, one fact remains constant: the equator offers what amounts to absolute protection against the disease. The protective environmental factor at the equator apparently is sufficient to overcome all other possible contributing causes—including the genetic factor and various currently proposed causes. (These include a "latent virus" as the causative factor and there's also a theory of "autoimmune reaction," in which it is hypothesized that the patient's own immune mechanisms attack the myelin tissue.)

Focusing on the area where nature itself protects against MS, and isolating abundant sunshine as the obvious environmental factor that distinguishes the tropics from other parts of the globe, Dr. Goldberg concluded that the further away from the equator and its year-round sunshine, the greater the incidence of MS. Moreover, a number of scattered investigations—in the U.S., Australia, and Israel—showed that in a given group of individuals, the prevalence of MS correlates significantly with sunniness of the "home towns" of the group. Where many came from sunny regions, MS prevalence was low—and vice versa.

Dr. Goldberg concluded that a vitamin D deficiency indirectly affected the myelin sheaths which insulate the central nervous system, since it's the vitamin which is essential for the body's utilization of the mineral calcium. And calcium, according to Dr. Goldberg, has an integral and dual role in the make up of the body's central nervous system: as a component of enzymes participating in myelin synthesis and as an actual part of the myelin sheath itself. There's a small amount of calcium in all human myelin, and because of the special biochemical properties of this mineral it could provide these fatty structures with needed mechanical rigidity and stability, says Dr. Goldberg.

If, as Dr. Goldberg proposes, vitamin D and calcium promote "the normal metabolism of myelin lipids," it follows that deficiency of the nutrients will lead to abnormalities. It's during growth and development of the central nervous system that the damage is done, Dr. Goldberg argues, rather than at the time the symptoms appear. Though imperfectly constructed, newly synthesized myelin continues to protect the CNS nerve axons while the brain (including myelin, which also forms part of the brain's "white matter") is still growing. It's after brain growth has pretty well stopped that symptoms usually appear, a result of the breakdown of poorly constructed tissue. Children almost never get MS, yet childhood environment relates to the risk of the disease in later life. And MS strikes predominantly at young adults. All these age-related findings are consistent with Dr. Goldberg's theory.

Dietary Vitamin D

But if vitamin D from sunshine is the protective factor during the growth of the CNS, why are there communities with notably low MS rates in the far north where sunshine is scarce? Dr. Goldberg answered this question by conducting a detailed examination of diet, and other factors, in northern areas where the "mini distribution" of MS has been plotted. In communities where fish (and therefore dietary vitamin D) is an important part of the diet, MS prevalence is low; in the example cited earlier—the islands off Scotland—the Faeroe Islands have a large and active fishing industry and very little MS. In the nearby islands of Shetland and Orkney, fish is reported to be consumed in far less quantity, and on these two islands MS rates are among the highest in the world.

In Norway, fishing communities not only consume more fish than elsewhere but more margarine (in place of butter) as well, and in Norway margarine contains a significant proportion of fish oil—the richest source of dietary vitamin D. In such coastal areas the MS incidence is low, whereas it is high in Norwegian agricultural communities.

Dr. Goldberg also analyzed the estimated grain consumption in low- and high-MS areas. Particularly barley and oats, he noted, have a high content of phytate, which is "antagonistic to vitamin D"—that is, it binds calcium in the digestive tract and makes it unavailable for the body's use. The high phytate regions in northern Europe also correlate fairly consistently with the high MS regions.

As an ultimate example of a region afflicted with every environmental factor that deprives humans of vitamin D and calcium, Dr. Goldberg points to northern Scotland: "The high consumption of oats in northern Scotland, combined with a diet low in vitamin D (low in fish and fish oils) and very little sunshine may explain why MS rates there are the highest thus far recorded for any country."

Though of paramount importance, diet is not the only factor that influences vitamin D intake at northern latitudes. In Switzerland, high altitude (where the sun's ultraviolet rays are more plentiful) is protective and reduces MS risk. Industrial smog in U.S. urban areas reduces ultraviolet penetration and increases MS risk. However, in northern Europe (which lies at considerably higher latitudes than the U.S.) diet rather than sunshine has to be the decisive factor, so there we find no such correlation between high MS risk and urbanization.

Heredity And MS

Dr. Goldberg's theory appears to tie up loose ends and conflicting facts that have baffled and intrigued MS researchers for many years. The final fact that needs explaining is why, in light of this theory, so few people contract the disease. Even in the highest risk zones, MS prevalence is only about 100 per 100,000.

Dr. Goldberg accounts for this rarity in terms of heredity. On available evidence, other scientists have postulated a hereditary factor or gene; Dr. Goldberg argues that the gene predisposing individuals toward MS is one that dictates a high demand for vitamin D. Everyone inherits a distinctive pattern of nutritional demands—as distinctive as each individual's finger prints. And for every nutrient there is a small fraction of the population whose need is far greater than average. Those with such a high demand for vitamin D, it is proposed, can contract MS if neither sun nor diet supplies the ample quantity they need. But for the great majority, with more average needs, MS presents no risk.

Heredity probably explains the low incidence of MS in Japan and other Far East countries, Dr. Goldberg concluded.

Not A Cure, But A Hope For The Future

Unhappily, the theory offers no hope as an MS cure. Present sufferers cannot benefit from it. It's just possible, though, Dr. Goldberg said, that a young patient who is just beginning to get symptoms might be able to slow or stop the progress of the disease. "Brain growth, and probably myelination, often continues well into the third decade, . . . and conceivably, supplements might restore some of the damaged myelin tissue, if the new patient started the program soon enough," he reported.

As for protecting the adolescents in your family, remember this is still only a theory—though a highly plausible one. On the other hand, it may very well be possible for some doctors to administer Goldberg's suggested preventive regimen of vitamin D, calcium, and perhaps magnesium, another mineral of vital importance to normal nerve function, to children over the age of ten who seem to be at especially high risk—because of where they live and because of a history of MS in their families. If they are worried about the aspect of taking excessive vitamin D, they could make periodic tests, and also shun the synthetic vitamin D in favor of natural vitamin D from fish liver oil, which is safer and has the same chemical structure as the vitamin D humans synthesize themselves.

At the very least, Dr. Goldberg's epidemiological theory of MS can benefit all potential victims of this disease by stimulating more discussion and research of the problem among medical scientists.

234. Megavitamin Therapy For Multiple Sclerosis

Dr. Frederick R. Klenner of Reidsville, North Carolina, uses massive doses (megadoses) of B complex vitamins to treat multiple sclerosis and other nervous disorders affecting body muscle such as myasthenia gravis, a nervous disorder which can immobilize muscles in the neck and face, and for which there is no generally accepted cure. Dr. Klenner not only uses megadoses of B vitamins but he also employs other nutrients, including minerals, trace elements, oils and amino acids. Many of these are also given in enormous amounts.

Reporting in the *Journal of Applied Nutrition* (Vol 25, No. 384, 1973), Dr. Klenner stated that nutritional therapy must figure prominently in dealing with diseases of the nerves and muscles. He has found in case after case that by *saturating* the body with these nutrients, such as he does in treating cases of myasthenia gravis, the "roadblocks" that disturb the metabolism can be overcome by sheer quantity, so that a sufficiency of energy can be produced.

The megadoses of nutrients which Dr. Klenner administers to his patients—for early cases of multiple sclerosis, as well as myasthenia gravis—can and should be administered only by a physician. Nevertheless, Dr. Klenner's clinical experience in using nutrients to overcome the symptoms of these terrible diseases underscores the role these same nutrients play in preventing nervous disorders in every living being.

Dr. Klenner reports that some patients he treated 20 years and more ago remain in excellent health. He tells of a man with a diagnosis of multiple sclerosis who was confined in a wheelchair at a veteran's hospital for two years. During a 30-day vacation in which the patient returned home, Dr. Klenner treated him with large doses of nutrients every day. When he returned to the hospital, the physician in charge immediately recognized the dramatic improvement and advised his patient to return home and continue the treatment. "After three years he was given a clean bill of health by three neurologists and was given a responsible position," Dr. Klenner declares. Today, more than 20 years after he began treatment, the man continues to do well, with a modified form of therapy.

Although Dr. Klenner's work with early MS and myasthenia gravis patients is highly encouraging, he has never done "controlled" studies—in which some patients are treated, others not treated, and the results compared—simply because he sees himself as a healer, not an experimenter. On the other hand, Dr. Klenner, before taking his medical degree, did several years of postgraduate study in chemistry and physiology, which give him unique qualifications to use and accurately observe nutritional therapy in a variety of ailments. In fact, he has already won wide recognition for his clinical observations with megadoses of vitamin C to help in the treatment of acute conditions. In his new study, Dr. Klenner zeros in on neuromuscular disorders and the need they create for extraordinary amounts of nutrients, especially, the B complex family. Even more specifically, he emphasizes the crucial role of thiamine hydrochloride, or vitamin B_1, in the combustion of nutrients to provide usable energy.

Section 47
Muscular
Dystrophy

235. A Family Of Disorders Characterized By The Severe Degeneration Of Muscle Tissue

235. A Family Of Disorders Characterized By The Severe Degeneration Of Muscle Tissue

Muscular dystrophy literally means "faulty nutrition of the muscles." It encompasses a number of similar and chronic diseases (dystrophies) whose common symptom is the progressive wasting and weakening of healthy muscle tissue, and its replacement by useless fat and hard fibrous tissue. The disease is considered largely hereditary, although abrupt and spontaneous occurrences of muscular dystrophy, resulting from unexplained genetic mutations, are not uncommon. The disease affects more than 200,000 people in the United States, and the vast majority of the cases are children. However, a form called "muscular dystrophy of late onset" occurs in adults between the ages of 40 and 50. This form is not considered hereditary.

Muscular dystrophy and multiple sclerosis are often associated in people's minds incorrectly. True, they both affect muscle function, but in quite dissimilar ways. Multiple sclerosis attacks the entire central nervous system, indirectly affecting muscle tissue since it attacks neural cells and thus impedes muscle movements, causing muscles to atrophy from disuse. Muscular dystrophy, on the other hand, attacks the healthy muscle tissue directly, causing a progressive deterioration of the cells which make up muscle tissue. Some researchers believe that muscular dystrophy may be caused by a malfunctioning of the central nervous system, but the majority of researchers believe that the disease begins within the walls of the muscle cell itself.

According to the Muscular Dystrophy Associations of America, there are five major types of muscular dystrophy: Duchenne (pseudohypertrophic), Landouzy-Dejerine (facio-scapulo-humeral), Limb-Girdle, Steinert's Disease (myotonic dystrophy), and Muscular Dystrophy of Late Onset; and three less common dystrophies: opthalmoplegic, distal and congenital. Each dystrophy is distinct and has its own peculiar pathology: one might affect sufferers at a specific different age; another involves the weakening and degeneration of a specific region of the body's musculature, and still another has a singular pattern of progression. In all but dystrophy of late onset, the dystrophies can be traced according to hereditary patterns of the parents.

Distal dystrophy, which affects the small muscles in the hands and feet, progresses slowly and is relatively benign or painless; but the Limb-Girdle dystrophy, which affects both the pelvic and shoulder muscles, is also benign in nature but its progress can be either slow or rapid. Nevertheless, whether the muscular impairment is light or crippling, there is no remission. Certain forms of muscular dystrophy may stop progressing, but none will ever go into remission.

Genetic Counselling: A Wise Precaution

Although it is not one-hundred percent effective, one of the best preventive measures now in use against hereditary forms of the disease is genetic counselling among parents who suspect they may be carriers of the genes responsible for muscular dystrophy. This is especially true of Duchenne dystrophy, the most severe and most ravaging of all muscular dystrophies. Named after Guillaume-Benjamin-Amant Duchenne, its discoverer and an early French pioneer in the field of neurology, it occurs only in young boys, usually before the age of three.

The Duchenne gene is recessive and transmitted by unaffected females. According to Dr. Walton, "women who already have an affected boy and have another affected male relative in the female line of inheritance are definite carriers of the gene. They can be advised that each pregnancy has a one in four chance of producing a further affected child and a one in four chance of producing another female carrier . . . Women with a brother or uncle affected with the disease are possible carriers."

Intensified efforts are underway, Dr. Walton wrote, to improve the carrier detection rates in genetic counselling. Researchers, he reported, are using estimations of the body's potassium levels, rubidium turnover rate, the analysis of specific muscle antibodies, investigations of electrocardiograph abnormalities and a number of other sophisticated methods in efforts to improve the detection rate of suspected carriers. "The object of this research," stated Dr. Walton, "is to reduce to zero the number of carriers which go undetected, and thus to reassure female relatives of patients that they have no more chance of having an affected child than any other member of the population."

Muscular Dystrophy Treated With Vegetable Oils

The Muscular Dystrophy Associations of America (MDAA) was founded in 1950. Since its inception, the MDAA has been instrumental in improving care for muscular dystrophy victims as well as providing the first large fund expenditures for research. During the past quarter century the MDAA has funded several animal test studies, providing information which may one day lead to a cure for human muscular dystrophies.

In 1967, during an international science conference held in Montreal, Canada, it was announced that Drs. Ethel Cosmos and Jane Butler, members of the Cell Biology Division of MDAA's Institute of Muscle Disease, had derived substances from vegetable oils which had reversed the process of muscular dystrophy in experiments with afflicted chickens. This was the first time a reversal had occurred in any animal species suffering from a hereditary form of muscular dystrophy.

Follow-up studies of the research confirmed the initial findings. While conditions in test animals were not identical to those found in human sufferers, the animal experiments "yielded important information about the morbid process" of muscular dystrophy. "It has been demonstrated repeatedly that the administration of these oils will reverse the dystrophic process, giving the striking picture of regeneration of muscle in an area where the original muscles appeared to have completely degenerated and had been replaced by fat. More recently, specific substances in the oil have been identified. These compounds produce regeneration that is even more striking than that produced by the oil itself."

Muscular Dystrophy—A Multiple Deficiency?

Researchers agree that any cure for muscular dystrophy will have to provide a substance which will regenerate wasted tissue and enable it to maintain its cohesion. In typical dystrophic tissue in humans, the muscle cell membrane becomes increasingly permeable and muscle enzyme substances originally contained within the cell seep out into the blood serum. In fact, the measurement of muscle enzymes in blood serum samples is commonly used to diagnose muscular dystrophy. Scientists believe that body nutrition may hold one of the answers to this complex problem.

In a study recorded in the *Journal of Nutrition* (July, 1954), Drs. E. L. Hove and D. H. Copeland, of the Alabama Polytechnic

Institute, reported that muscular dystrophy in test rabbits was caused by a diet low in vitamin E. One might presume that the same thing could be true for human beings, except for two things: first, most human beings get *some* vitamin E, no matter how poor a diet they eat; second, most human beings do not get enough of the other vitamins necessary for good nutrition. Laboratory animals which live on carefully planned diets get plenty of all these. So perhaps the answer lies in combinations of vitamins.

In their study, Drs. Hove and Copeland noted that progressive muscular dystrophy in rabbits came as a result primarily of a chronic choline deficiency. Choline is a B vitamin. These authors noted that one of the functions of vitamin E in the body is to bring about the synthesis of a substance called acetylcholine from choline and acetate. This shows that vitamin E is bound closely with this particular B vitamin, choline, in at least one important body function. Another B vitamin, pantothenic acid, is also involved to a certain extent.

Therefore, the authors said, a deficiency in choline should produce muscular dystrophy as well as a deficiency in vitamin E. To see if it did, they designed a diet in which there was little or no choline, and placed a group of laboratory rabbits on this diet. Other groups of rabbits, eating the same diet, were given choline so they would not have this deficiency. *All of the rabbits whose diet was deficient in choline developed muscular dystrophy between the seventieth and hundredth day on the diet.* The symptoms of muscular dystrophy were identical in all respects to those of the dystrophy of rabbits deficient in vitamin E. When choline was added to the diet, all signs of muscle weakness disappeared in four days. When the rabbits were examined at post-mortem, it was found that the degeneration of muscle which had taken place was similar to that found in vitamin E-deficient rabbits.

Then the investigators tried something else. They knew that a deficiency in choline produces damage to the liver. Damage to the liver interferes with the body's assimilation of vitamin E. Perhaps, reasoned the researchers, the muscular dystrophy produced by lack of choline was really the same thing they had seen before. Maybe the lack of choline simply resulted in a lack of vitamin E—and what they actually observed was the same thing they saw in rabbits who received no vitamin E in their diet. They had to devise some way to test the choline-deficient diet only.

So they began giving their rabbits vitamin E in large quantities—about ten times the amount they knew was needed. Interestingly enough, they knew, from former experiments, that animals who developed liver disorders as a result of choline deficiency had a greatly increased need for vitamin E! So, at the same time their liver disorder is preventing them from making use of whatever vitamin E is in their diet, this same disorder is causing them to need more vitamin E than they normally would!

By giving large doses of vitamin E, the authors of this article managed to see to it that the animals were not deficient in vitamin E. They could tell this by testing the vitamin E content of their blood. In this way, they knew for certain that the disease was not produced by a vitamin E deficiency, but by a deficiency in choline. In some respects, they said, the kind of disorder produced by choline deficiency is more like that seen in human beings. The significance of their findings, they noted, is that dystrophy may result from dietary deficiencies other than a vitamin E deficiency. However, in human muscular dystrophy, there is not usually evidence of severe liver damage.

We have here another chain in the link showing the complexity of nutritional relationships and the harmfulness of tampering with food. Vitamin E (a fat-soluble vitamin) is closely related in its function to one of the minor B vitamins. Perhaps a deficiency in both of them might be partly responsible for human dystrophy.

We Are Deficient In Vitamins B And E

Would it be possible for a modern human being to be deficient in both vitamin E and choline, one of the B vitamins? It is not only possible, but almost completely certain that anyone who eats refined foods regularly is bound to be short in both these vitamins. They are most plentiful in the germs of cereals—those living parts of our grains which we remove and discard when we make white flour, white rice, when we produce cold breakfast cereals, refined corn meal and all the many products made from these devitalized foods. Cereal products are enriched by replacing synthetically a few of the vitamins and minerals that have been removed when the germ is removed. Iron and a few of the B vitamins are added. *Vitamin E is not replaced. Choline and all the other minor members of the B complex of vitamins are not replaced.* Since cereals are our richest, most practical, everyday source of both these food elements, do you see what damage may have been done by food refining—especially to those people who may have abnormally large requirements for one or both of these vitamins?

In addition, remember that both vitamins are destroyed by a number of chemicals to which most of us are exposed frequently. Chlorine destroys vitamin E. Most of us are eating many foods that have been bleached with chlorine compounds. Rancid fats destroy vitamin E. Foods fried in fats used over and over again are bound to contain rancid fats. How many Americans eat fried foods almost every day?

Section 48
Parkinson's Disease

236. New Hope For Parkinson's Victims

236. New Hope For Parkinson's Victims

Parkinson's disease, also called "shaking palsy" or *paralysis agitans*, is a disorder of the central nervous system which usually attacks people between the ages of 50 and 69. An estimated one out of every 1000 people develops the illness. Sometimes Parkinson's disease appears in persons who have had encephalitis, but in most of the cases, no cause can be found.

Although the cause is indeterminate, symptoms of the disease appear when there is an imbalance of two substances in the brain, dopamine and acetylcholine. These two substances transmit messages between nerve cells, which in turn control the function of muscles throughout the body. In healthy people, dopamine and acetylcholine balance one another, and nerve impulses are successfully passed along. But in the person with Parkinsonism, the amount of dopamine in the brain is somehow decreased, the balance is lost, and nerve signals become confused. No one knows what causes this lack of dopamine, but when it occurs, the symptoms of Parkinson's disease appear.

The early signs of the illness usually develop gradually, making early diagnosis difficult. Generally, the upper body is affected first. The hands and arms show a slight tremor, and the patient finds it hard to perform simple manual tasks, such as buttoning a shirt or tying a shoe. As the disease advances, the trembling becomes more pronounced, and is the most severe when the limb is at rest. Tremors are most noticeable in the hands and feet, and in a back-and-forth motion of the head. Muscles become rigid, resulting in slow and jerky movements. Routine acts such as getting up from a chair become difficult. The patient walks with slow, shuffling steps, his body bent forward as though he is about to fall.

Parkinsonism patients often develop a blank, wide-eyed facial expression, and may stare straight ahead without blinking for long periods. Salivation increases, and the skin usually becomes quite oily. The rigidity of the muscles often causes cramp-like pains in the arms, legs and spine.

When the full range of symptoms has appeared, the disease is readily diagnosed.

Treating Parkinsonism

Many treatments have been used for Parkinsonism since James Parkinson wrote the first essay on shaking palsy in 1817. Some years ago, it was common practice for surgeons to insert a small needle into the brain to freeze or incise nerve cells in the part of the brain which governs the symptoms of the disease.

More recently, drug therapies have been developed in an attempt to restore the balance between dopamine and acetylcholine in the brain by inhibiting the action of the acetylcholine. Many drugs have been tried, but most proved to be largely unsuccessful due to dangerous side effects or simple lack of effectiveness. Such diverse drugs as antihistamine amantidine, and even amphetamines have been used at various times in the treatment of Parkinson's disease.

The first breakthrough came in the late 1960's with the development of levodopa, more commonly known as L-dopa. The principle behind levodopa is that of boosting the amount of dopamine in the brain to a normal level. Dopamine, itself, cannot be administered because it cannot cross from the bloodstream into the brain, but the body can convert levodopa to dopamine after it reaches the brain.

L-dopa has been more successful in alleviating the symptoms of Parkinsonism than have other drugs, but the course of treatment is arduous. Because much of the drug is converted to dopamine by various body tissues before it ever reaches the brain, L-dopa must be taken in large amounts. The usual dosage necessary for relief is from four to eight grams every day.

Patients must be slowly accustomed to the drug because it causes serious side effects; dosages start low and are gradually increased until the patient can tolerate the amount necessary to ameliorate his symptoms.

Even when patients are accustomed to L-dopa, its numerous side effects persist. Nausea and vomiting are common, along with low blood pressure and irregular heartbeat. Many people also experience anxiety or depression, and abnormal motor coordination.

A few years ago, a team of British researchers published results of a study in which they found that the beneficial effects of levodopa diminish with prolonged use, especially after two years (*Lancet*, Oct. 27, 1973).

Nutrition becomes a problem for people taking L-dopa. Large amounts of protein in the diet tend to block the effects of the drug. Substantial doses of vitamin B_6 also interfere with levodopa's effectiveness, and patients must sometimes restrict their intake of vitamin B-rich foods—an undesirable practice.

In a letter to the *Lancet* (March 1, 1975), two researchers from Rockland State Hospital in New York suggested that adding extra vitamin C to the diets of L-dopa patients could decrease the drug's side effects. The researchers reported success with vitamin C supplementation in an elderly Parkinsonism patient who suffered severe side effects from levodopa. However, apparently no other serious research into the role of nutrition in treating Parkinson's disease has been conducted in recent years.

A New Drug

To increase the efficiency of L-dopa and eliminate some of its side effects, a new drug called carbidopa has been developed to accompany levodopa therapy. Carbidopa prevents L-dopa from being broken down by body tissues, allowing more of the drug to reach the brain intact. This means that smaller amounts of L-dopa can be taken with greater effectiveness. When the two drugs are taken in combination, the unpleasant nausea and vomiting caused by levodopa are alleviated, and symptoms of Parkinsonism are diminished more quickly. However, other side effects such as abnormal muscle function, anxiety and depression are still encountered.

There is still no entirely successful therapy for Parkinson's disease. Drugs cannot completely eliminate the symptoms of the illness, and treatment remains, at best, a compromise between symptoms and side effects.

Section 49
Prostate
Disorders

237. Prostate Enlargement Symptoms Are Pain And Inconvenience

If you have ever had to drive for miles and miles while the need to urinate kept building up and no filling station (perhaps it should be called an emptying station in this case) in sight, then you know exactly where your bladder is. It is at that point in the lower abdominal cavity where you felt all that pressure.

Right at the central point where the pressure was most intense, is the exit of the bladder. It empties into a long, narrow tube called the urethra which carries urine out through the penis in a man.

It is through this same urethra that seminal fluid is ejaculated during sexual intercourse. Obviously, the sex glands must be intimately connected with the urethra and must empty their secretions into it. That is why a malfunction of the prostate, which is a sex gland surrounding the urethra just below the mouth of the bladder, is most frequently experienced as problems connected with urination.

Fertility Depends On Prostatic Fluid
The prostate manufactures the liquid which acts as a vehicle for the sperm cells of the male. Without this important fluid there is no way of transferring the sperm into the female vagina for the purpose of fertilizing the female egg, and hence no way of carrying out the normal process of reproduction. Without the prostate gland to manufacture this essential fluid, the male becomes sterile.

Slightly above and behind the prostate, on either side of the urethra, there are two tiny sacs called the seminal vesicles. These are a storehouse for the sperm cells that are produced in the testicles. The fact that the sperms have to make their way up from the testicles to get into the seminal vesicles provides the guarantee that the sperms stored there will be alive and active.

The seminal vesicles do not empty directly into the urethra, but rather into the prostate. What happens is that at the moment of orgasm, the muscle tissue surrounding these glands contracts. Sperm cells are forced into the prostate and mixed with prostatic fluid which is forced into the urethra and by a series of contractions ejaculated through the penis.

The basic composition of semen is similar to that of the egg, being largely albumin which is the most complete and highest grade protein known, and lecithin, a compound of the essential fatty acids. In addition there is an enzyme called acid phosphatase that maintains a low acidity of the prostatic fluid. Other investigators have found substantial amounts of vitamin C and A, both of which are prime fighters against infection and toxicity. The minerals zinc and magnesium are also present in unusual concentration.

Enlargement Triggers Urinary Difficulties

A normal prostate is about the size of a walnut. We can picture it as consisting of bunches of tiny bulbs resembling bunches of grapes, fitting snugly around the urethra so that it can empty prostatic fluid into that tube at the moment of the male orgasm. Because of its anatomical position, when the prostate enlarges it puts restricting pressure on the urethra, and a man first notices that he may be developing a prostatic problem when he finds that it takes him longer to empty his bladder. The more the prostate enlarges, obviously, the greater is the pressure and the more difficult it becomes to get the bladder completely empty. As described in *Gray's Anatomy*: "In consequence of the enlargement of the prostate a pouch is formed at the base of the bladder behind the projection, in which water collects and cannot entirely be expelled. It becomes decomposed and ammoniacal, and leads to cystitis." Cystitis is the formation of crystals in the bladder, which subsequently lead to pain and infection. This in turn can affect the kidneys and lead to a buildup of urinary wastes in the bloodstream. So we can see that even what is known as benign prostatic hypertrophy, meaning simple enlargement without any infection or malignancy, is a serious affair and not to be taken lightly.

In addition, the enlargement of the prostate gland is an indication of reduced activity, and there is every reason to believe that in addition to its necessity to male fertility, the prostate also secretes hormones that are fed into the bloodstream and are concerned with general health and well-being. A reduction in the production of these hormones would then have a generalized effect on health.

In the early stages, the symptoms of enlarged or inflamed prostate (prostatitis) are rather vague—a feeling of congestion and discomfort in the pubic area. There follows a constant feeling of fullness of the bladder, with frequent, urgent trips to the bathroom. Once there, however, there is often difficulty in starting a stream, and sometimes no urination at all. The recurring need to void during the night is also common. Eventually, a residue of urine that has not been expelled is collected in the bladder and dribbling occurs. This is the unconscious release of urine, in small amounts, forced out by a full bladder. When the urethra is interfered with to the extent that very little or no urine can escape from the bladder, the serious problem of possible uremic poisoning arises. This can occur when such large amounts of fluid accumulate that the bladder can hold no more. With the normal avenue of release through the urethra shut off, the urine floods back into the kidneys, presenting a grave danger of poison to the system.

What is the general procedure for dealing with prostate problems? There are several courses of treatment. For immediate relief of a full bladder, a catheter is employed. Usually it consists simply of a sterile rubber tube which is inserted into the opening of the urethra and gently pushed along its length to the mouth of the bladder. The bladder empties through the tube quickly and with ease. Of course, this method is excellent for emergency treatment, but not for constant repetition. For one thing, it is painful, and the chance for infection as well as damage to delicate tissues is very real. For another, the bladder fills quickly, and catheterization would have to be repeated frequently if relief were to be maintained.

Another means of relieving the symptoms of swollen prostate is to massage the gland. This can be accomplished by a physician, and is often effective in reducing the swelling. But the treatment must be repeated periodically. So-called sitz baths in which one soaks only the lower portion of the trunk, have a soothing effect and often reduce the swelling, but are obviously inconvenient.

When Is Surgery Necessary?

The average doctor's final opinion on what to do about prostate trouble is "have it removed." The operation is reasonably safe and relief is sure. Of course, sterility is an inescapable aftermath of the operation, though this does not mean that there is any lessening in the patient's desire for sexual activity. The person who has had prostate surgery is usually perfectly normal in this respect, but for the fact that he can't father a child. It is understandable, however, that men are anxious to find some other way to solve the prostate problem.

A word should be said here about cancer of the prostate. For some unknown reason this gland is extremely susceptible to malignancy. When prostatic difficulties do occur, it is wise, therefore, to make certain through a medical examination by your doctor that no cancer is present. Sometimes surgery is the only recourse in such cases.

Although much is known about the function of the prostate, and it can be said with assurance that this gland is vital to fertility in the male, our knowledge is by no means complete as yet. Many medical researchers believe that at least one hormone concerned with the general health and functioning of the body is manufactured in this gland. So that even though it is possible to lose one's prostate without loss of potency, there is every reason to believe that when this gland is removed, far more than fertility vanishes with it. Loss of the prostate is a serious matter, even though there is little reason to fear that the operation will be fatal. Its removal can sometimes be necessary, but should be thought of only as a last resort. Only if the organ should actually be cancerous is there any reason to hasten into surgery.

Be Alert For Symptoms Of Trouble

This does not mean, however, that difficulties with the prostate should be taken lightly or ignored in the hope that they will go away. Some kind of remedial action is always indicated. There is always the danger that the ailing prostate will enlarge and constrict the urethra and impede or completely stop the passage of urine. Such a condition can be extremely painful and even fatal if not treated.

Any of the following symptoms are an indication that it is time to visit your doctor for a check on the condition of your prostate:
1. Low back pain.
2. Blood in the urine or in the seminal fluid.
3. An increase in sexual excitability or frequent erections that come without any special stimulation.
4. Pain during the ejaculation of the seminal fluid.

1069

5. Impotence or premature ejaculation.
6. A chronic sense of fullness in the bowel and difficulty in defecation.
7. Any decrease in control over urination, such as difficulty in starting or stopping the stream or inability to slow the stream.

When you consider that though it is not probable, it is at least possible that difficulties with the prostate might indicate an acute infection, an attack of tuberculosis, a veneral disease that you might not have known you had, or even cancer, it should be obvious that if you even suspect that there is anything wrong with your prostate, the first thing to do is get to a good doctor for an accurate diagnosis of just what the trouble is.

238. Pollen As A Treatment In Prostatitis

Prostate trouble is a common occurrence in men as they grow older—in fact it is almost taken for granted. An estimated 60 percent of North American men over age 60 have some enlargement of the prostate, and by age 80 the proportion rises to 95 percent. In short, prostatic hypertrophy (enlargement) appears to be one of those unpleasant physiologic changes that inevitably occur in people as they grow older.

Yet this has not always been the case, according to a paper published in 1960 in *Grana Palynologica* by Erik Ask-Upmark, M.D., of the University of Upsala in Sweden. Titled "On A New Treatment of Prostatitis," Dr. Ask-Upmark's paper starts with the intriguing statement that: "Prostatitis represents a relatively new pathologic entity. When I was studying medicine, one heard of its existence, but chiefly as a patho-anatomic curiosity. It was not, on the other hand, seen in the clinics, at any rate not in medical ones."

It would seem clear that within the past century there has come about some fundamental change in our way of living that has made alarmingly commonplace what was once a rare disease. Most of us know that the most fundamental change in way of life during this period has been the shift in eating patterns from the consumption of fresh whole foods to the use of canned or highly processed foods which, in the course of commercial handling, are robbed of much of their nutritional virtue. There are indeed a range of nutrients processed out of our food that are vital to prostatic health. Prominent among them is magnesium, whose deficiency in the American diet is estimated at 200 milligrams a day. Vitamin F, the essential fatty acids, is commonly converted into hydrogenated fats that are damaging to the human system. Zinc is removed from flour by processing and has become generally deficient in our diets as well.

Thus it is really unnecessary to look any further than our change in eating habits, which has robbed the prostate gland of some of the nutrients it requires most for health, to understand why prostatitis has become generally deficient in our diets as well.

Thus it is really unnecessary to look any further than our change in eating habits, which has robbed the prostate gland of some of the nutrients it requires most for health, to understand why prostatis has become something close to a universal affliction of aging men.

Pollen Contains Nutrients Important To The Prostate

This understanding also provides insight into why it is that pollen should have been found to have a particularly beneficial effect in alleviating prostatic infection and hypertrophy. Although there has never been anything like a complete analysis of the remarkably complex components of a grain of pollen, it is certainly rich in essential fatty acids and in minerals, some of which occur only in unbelievably small traces, but among which zinc and magnesium are relatively plentiful.

The possibilities of pollen in this regard first emerged in 1957. In that year, Dr. Ask-Upmark had a patient with a particularly intractable prostatic infection that he had been trying to treat for five years. ". . . at intervals of six to eight weeks, sometimes more often, an acute exacerbation occurred, with fever and marked local symptoms. Chloromycetin proved to be the only antibiotic capable of overcoming the acute attacks. It was not, however, able to prevent recurrences, despite the fact that on one occasion as much as 150 grams was administered in the course of two months."

Dr. Ask-Upmark goes on to describe how this patient decided that he needed something to improve his general strength, and on his own initiative began to take six tablets a day of pollen extract. The improvement was like a miracle. "Since then—thus for three years at the time of writing—he has had only a single recurrence. This was in the beginning when, in connection with a journey, he neglected to take the pollen preparation for two weeks. Otherwise, he has taken the preparation daily." And taking the pollen, this patient had no trouble with his prostate.

Prostatitis Can Be Chronic Or Acute

As Dr. Ask-Upmark describes prostatitis, it occurs "both in an acute form and as a chronic disease, in which acute exacerbations are highly characteristic. The local symptoms can most simply be described as those of cystitis, i.e., a continual urge to void, and discomfort on urination. Prostatitis has, however, certain typical features. Firstly, the discomfort on urination consists far more of pain than of burning. Secondly, this pain is often referred to the tip of the penis, approximately as in the presence of an advanced vesical calculus (stone). Thirdly, the patient may have a sensation of fullness in the rectum, which can reasonably be ascribed to bulging of the swollen prostate gland into it. This makes the patient try to relieve his discomfort by (unsuccessful) defecation. These local symptoms are accompanied, in the acute phase, by systemic disturbances in the form of fever. . . ."

The above remarks by Dr. Ask-Upmark led another Swedish physician, Gosta Leander, to undertake a fuller investigation. Dr. Leander studied 179 cases, all of verified prostatic infection. The study was set up as a double-blind test, using both pollen extract and placebos with neither the patients nor the doctors aware until the conclusion of the test of who was getting which kind of tablet.

Describing how he evaluated the study, Dr. Leander says "When an infection is in progress, the prostate and the vesicles have doughy consistency, they are tender when palpated and they contain a more or less pus-filled secretion. When therapy is successful, evacuation is improved and, consequently, the secretionary stasis is eliminated. This can be easily confirmed by palpation. Concurrently, the secretion reverts to normal and this, too, is easily confirmed by direct microscopy." In other words, the criteria used were strictly objective. It was not just a question of the patient's feeling better, but actually being better as shown by physical and microscopic examination. And what did Dr. Leander find? He found that by adding pollen to the diets of his prostate patients, the results he achieved were 60 to 80 percent better than with conventional therapy alone.

Valuable As Sole Therapy

With more and more European urologists becoming interested in this new therapy, a corresponding group of twelve urologists in Germany and Sweden carried on further studies, using pollen extract alone. One hundred seventy-two patients were divided into two groups according to whether or not they had ever suffered from urinary or focal infection. In group one, those cases that were not known to ever have had urinary or focal infection, 56 of 114 (48 percent) showed definite substantial improvement. In group two, 35 percent of the cases improved.

The above study took place over the short term—a period of

three months—and it was pointed out that the results were not necessarily conclusive because the trial period was so short.

One of the doctors involved, Professor G. W. Heise of the Magdeburg Academy of Medicine, carried on the trial with his nine patients for a full year. As he describes it, all nine of the patients had similar symptoms. They all experienced difficulty in urination (pain, urgency, frequency). They all had definite difficulties during coitus, and examination found leukocytes (white blood cells) in the ejaculates of all. "All the patients were found to suffer from lowered libido and painful orgasms, and six of them exhibited manifestations of impotence."

After a period of treatment as long as a year, Dr. Heise found that "comprehensive reexaminations revealed that *all the patients had responded with a definite improvement.*"

He goes on to explain that in all cases, examination of the ejaculates showed them to be free of leukocytes and bacteria after a protracted course of one tablet of pollen extract taken three times a day. There were no longer any pathogenic bacteria of any kind to be found in the urine or ejaculate. All the patients exhibited a considerable improvement both mentally and physically, "cohabitation difficulties no longer occur and pains radiating to the perineum and sacral region have disappeared. Micturition (urination) disturbances could no longer be observed. . . ."

No Side Effects Were Observed

Furthermore, it is noteworthy that neither Dr. Heise nor any of his predecessors saw any side effects of any kind occurring with the pollen extract treatment.

Thus far we have dealt with the ability of pollen to overcome actual infections of the prostate gland. It should therefore be emphasized that pollen is not in itself any kind of antibiotic. This is a matter that is simply determined by laboratory testing, putting an active solution of pollen into direct contact with various types of common bacteria. The tests have been made and the pollen has been found to have no effect on bacteria.

This makes it all the more remarkable that when there is a known bacterial infection of the prostate, treatment with antibiotics will clear it up only temporarily and the infection can be expected to return. Yet the addition of pollen to the diet, which does not kill the bacteria, somehow so strengthens the prostate's own ability to fight against infection that it has been found frequently to result in permanent improvement.

1074

What element in the pollen has this effect? Is it the magnesium? The zinc? Perhaps the polyunsaturated fatty acids or—another strong possibility—a tiny yet potent amount of sex hormones that analysis has more recently found in pollen.

In 1971 a Yugoslav scientific journal, *Experientia,* published the results of an analysis performed at the University of Zagreb by three members of the faculties of pharmacy and biochemistry.

Meticulously reporting their methods, the Yugoslav scientists reviewed existing data relating to the finding of estrogens in pollen, and went on to report that they had also found traces of testosterone, epitestosterone, and androstenedione in the pollen of the Scotch pine. The quantities are incredibly small: 0.8 micrograms to 5.9 micrograms in 10 grams of pollen. A microgram is a millionth of a gram. Yet, if one of the causes of prostatic difficulties is a man's dwindling production of sex hormones, the addition of such microscopic quantities of the hormones might have a strengthening and invigorating effect.

Noninfectious Cases Helped Also

If any case, it is well established that pollen is a definite aid in the treatment of prostatitis and brings far greater success to the overall treatment. The next obvious question to be asked is whether the same natural substance would also help in disorders of the prostate where no infection exists.

This question was examined by L. J. Denis, a urologist at the military hospital in Antwerp, Belgium. His report was published in *Acta Urologica Belgica* (January, 1966).

Dr. Denis started his study with 31 patients diagnosed as suffering from chronic prostatitis. Their conditions were carefully evaluated by chemical analysis and microscopic studies of their urine and prostatic secretions. Out of the 31, only ten were selected as showing no signs of bacterial infection whatsoever, yet still suffering from the symptoms of chronic prostatitis. These ten were treated with four tablets a day of pollen extract.

Describing the prostate patients in whom "no evidence of infection was detected," Dr. Denis says: "The mean age was 36. Slight urinary problems were present in each instance which was mainly the reason for their reference. These included frequency (4), urgency (4), hesitation (2), discomfort when urinating (7). None of them complained of urethral discharge. Three of them complained of loss of sexual desire and four had regular pain in one of the testicles, groin or perineum."

Prostate Disorders

Subjective relief—that is, the patients themselves believed they had improved and no longer complained of the same symptoms—was obtained in all cases.

It would, of course, be extremely difficult and probably impossible to conduct a study of whether the regular consumption of pollen will prevent prostatitis from ever occurring. Such a study could only be made on a statistical basis, comparing the incidence of prostate difficulties among pollen takers as contrasted with those who do not take it. It would involve enormous numbers of people followed up over a period of perhaps twenty years. It is beyond the scope of any capability that we know of. Nevertheless, when a material has proven of substantial benefit to prostatic health, both in permitting the gland to fight off infection and improving the noninfected condition that is generally known as benign prostatic hypertrophy, it seems reasonable to suppose that the same material, included as a regular part of the diet, might well forestall and prevent prostate problems.

239. Zinc Is Important To A Man's Energy And Sexual Vigor

Every man knows that his vigor, his mental energy, his aggressiveness and his general well-being are all intimately connected with sexual health. Nor is there any doubt that at times when men experience symptoms of dwindling sexual health, they also find themselves short of energy and drive all too aware of getting older.

Although every man possesses a variety of sexual organs, it is the prostate gland that seems to be the overall controller of sexual health. One good demonstration of that is the absence of any important effect on health, that any medical inquirer has ever been able to determine, of the sterilizing procedure called a vasectomy. This operation prevents sperm cells from traveling from the testicles to the seminal vesicles. The disruption of this fundamental reproductive function and the reduction of the testicles to virtual uselessness does not seem to have any effect on potency, virility or overall health. But when the production of prostatic fluid dwindles, so do a man's desires and his capabilities. And for reasons not yet determined, so does his vitality and his drive. If the prostate enlarges, that creates an impediment to complete emptying of the urinary bladder, which has an overall deleterious effect on health. And while there is no proven connection, many men believe that they have found lowered resistance to disease to run parallel to decreased activity of the prostate.

Zinc Is Concentrated In The Prostate

It has been known for more than 50 years that the prostate accumulates high levels of zinc—more zinc than any other organ of the body. It has therefore been supposed that there is a connection between the health of the prostate and its containing adequate amounts of zinc. But there has been no actual demonstration until a study done, as a cooperative effort by personnel of the Chicago Medical School, Cook County Hospital, Hoktoen Institution for Medical Research, Cook County Graduate School

Prostate Disorders

of Medicine and Mt. Sinai Medical Center in Chicago. In a report titled "Zinc: A Key Urological Element," Dr. Irving M. Bush and his seven associates make a number of important points, one of which is of particular interest. In order to determine what are the normal concentrations of zinc in the prostate gland and in the semen, which receives its zinc from the prostate, they checked the levels in a total of 210 healthy men of various ages. And one of their findings was that "initial results indicate that seven percent of males have low semen and prostatic zinc levels. In addition, 30 percent of males may have borderline values."

Normally there is eight times as much zinc concentrated in the prostate as there is in the other tissues of the human body. That much has been known since 1921 when it was reported to the French Academy of Science by Bertrand and Vladesco. It was not until 30 years later in 1951, however, when two scientists with Canada's Chalk River Atomic Project made a study of zinc levels in various organs of the rat, that it began to seem likely that there was an intimate connection between the health of the prostate and the concentration of zinc it contains. A year later the same scientists reported that they had observed in humans that where there is benign hypertrophy of the prostate, the zinc concentration is a little lower than normal. In addition, they found that in conditions of chronic prostatitis in which there is not only an enlargement but also infection, the zinc concentration is even lower, and where the prostate has become cancerous, the zinc concentration is lowest of all. The study constituted a clear indication that making sure your diet contains abundant zinc might be a very good way of avoiding trouble with the prostate in later years.

Further knowledge that zinc plays an important role in male sexual health emerged in an important study made in Egypt and published in the *American Journal of Clinical Nutrition* (December, 1966). Titled "Zinc Levels and Blood Enzyme Activities in Egyptian Male Subjects With Retarded Growth and Sexual Development," the report by a group of U.S. Navy Medical Research officers dealt with an unusual frequency of dwarfs in villages of the Nile Valley. These dwarfs were not only retarded in growth but also in sexual development, having the genitals of children and no facial or pubic hair.

Comparing these retarded people with normal male Egyptians and Americans living in Cairo, it was found that the retarded males had abnormally low zinc levels, due primarily to zinc loss because they were infected by a parasitic disease, schistosomiasis. Since their diets were not particularly high in zinc to begin with, the losses induced severe zinc deficiencies, because of which their sex organs did not mature at all. And because the sex organs did not mature, their bodies generally did not mature.

A Promising New Therapy

This study left little room for doubt about the intimate interconnection between zinc nutrition and the health of the sex organs. Since then there have been numerous studies confirming that conclusion.

But the study in Chicago has opened a new and highly significant area of investigation. Granting that zinc is involved in proper sperm function, sexual health and several basic genital hormone systems, and that the man who is deficient in zinc is prone to develop health problems in connection with his prostate, can zinc be used as a treatment or cure for those problems after they have developed? The Chicago investigators attempted to find out.

They took 194 patients suffering with various illnesses of the prostate, 32 of them having cancer in that organ. The patients were divided into groups and treated with various therapies, one of them being zinc (50 to 220 mg. a day) while others were treated with two forms of synthetic estrogen, a common medical procedure, or with an antibiotic, tetracycline. Ninety-six healthy men of various ages were used as a control.

In chronic abacterial prostatitis, which is to say chronic inflammation of the prostate that is not caused by bacteria, it was found that treatment with zinc for two to 16 weeks relieved the symptoms in 70 percent of the 40 patients treated. Whether it actually effected a permanent cure of the infection or merely relieved the pain and the urinary difficulty temporarily was not determined. The estrogen and antibiotic treatments did not help at all.

Fifteen patients with simple enlargement of the prostate who were treated with zinc all reported improvement in the symptoms. After two months of treatment, actual shrinkage of the prostate gland occurred in three of the 15 patients. This would indicate that in prostatic hypertrophy zinc will improve the overall condition, but will return the prostate to normal size in only 20 percent of the cases treated.

Put More Zinc In Your Diet

In their conclusion the investigators promised to pursue further the question of how effective zinc is as a treatment for other genito-urinary diseases and how it should be used. Their work so far does hold out the strong possibility that even if you have begun to age sexually and to develop the ills and degenerative diseases that accompany such a condition, you still have a reasonable chance of reversing that tendency if you make sure that you get plenty of zinc in your diet. For the purpose, of course, you will never get enough in food alone. Nevertheless it will certainly be a help to eat as many as possible of the zinc-rich foods in your daily diet. Such foods include brewer's yeast, nuts, molasses, eggs, rice bran, onions, rabbit, chicken, peas, beans, lentils, wheat germ, wheat bran, beef liver and gelatin. Oysters are very rich in zinc—more than any other food—but those who eat them risk the danger of their coming from contaminated water.

A daily supplement of zinc gluconate is by far the most reliable source, giving you the zinc in an absorbable form and as much of it as you require.

And of course, if you are fortunate enough still to be in excellent sexual health without any problems, that is probably the best indication of all to include a daily supplement of zinc in your diet. All the studies make it next to certain that if you keep your prostate well endowed with zinc it will have less tendency to enlarge and weaken in function as you grow older.

Section 50
Rabies

240. Prompt Treatment Needed For Rabies

240. Prompt Treatment Needed For Rabies

Rabies, according to medical terminology, is a "virus-produced disease which causes swift destruction of the nerve cells in the hindbrain." Although it is usually carried to man by dogs, other animals also spread the infection. After a person is bitten and infected, the disease usually develops in four to eight weeks, but it may lie dormant for as long as a year. If the offending animal can be located, it is quarantined and observed for signs of the rabies. The problem comes when the animal remains at large and it is not known whether rabies is present.

Pasteur is given credit for developing the first vaccination for rabies. He inoculated a boy, Joseph Meister, who had been bitten by a rabid dog. Joseph recovered and Pasteur's serum was acclaimed.

It was soon found, however, that the Pasteur treatment could have serious and often fatal side effects.

The insidious thing about rabies is that the treatment must start before the disease is evident. Once a person manifests symptoms of the virus it is too late to initiate treatment. There is only one case on record of someone surviving rabies when the treatment was started after the onset of the symptoms. And there is some speculation as to whether that patient actually had rabies.

Pasteur's treatment has always been very controversial. A report in the *Journal of the American Medical Association* for January 14, 1956 relates the happenings of a meeting of the Academy of Medicine in France, where a Dr. Hasegawa and his co-workers spoke sharply against the use of the Pasteur vaccination. They pointed out that it may be followed as long as 20 years later by a disorder called Korsakoff's psychosis, which is a state of delirium. They also said that, in a study of 460 patients treated with the Pasteur injection after being bitten by a rabid animal, 20 died.

There have been improvements in the rabies vaccine since Pasteur. Right after World War II, doctors started administering an anti-rabies vaccine made from the blood of horses that were immune to rabies. This serum works by releasing antibodies that fight the rabies virus. This is only the initial phase of the treatment. It must be followed by a series of vaccinations with an inert rabies virus, which produces a permanent, or at least long-range immunity to the rabies virus.

Unfortunately, this vaccine produced severe negative reactions in about a third of the people who received it. The older a recipient, the greater his chances of a negative reaction to this serum. The reactions caused by the serum include chills, nausea, anaphlactic shock and, in the extreme, death.

In 1974, Dr. Victor J. Cabasso, a leading virologist, developed Hyperab, an anti-rabies globulin of human origin. This serum does not produce the side effects which made the other serums dangerous. It's given in two stages. The first globulin injection stimulates the immediate growth of antibodies to fight the attacking rabies virus. This is followed by a series of vaccinations for long-term immunity. This guards against the rabies virus which may lie dormant in an affected person for as long as a year after the initial bite.

This human globulin was used with a rabies vaccine of duck-embryo origin in a series of carefully controlled studies. These studies revealed that an initial dose of both these vaccines resulted in an ample level of passive rabies antibodies within 24 hours of the injection. This was true throughout all the studies which were conducted by the researcher, Hattwick.

The only problem seems to be in obtaining sufficient serum, since it comes from humans, hyperimmunized with rabies vaccine. And only a small percentage of those immunized produce sufficient antibodies to be donors for Cabasso's serum.

Section 51
Sexual
Disorders

241. Impotence, Frigidity, Infertility

241. Impotence, Frigidity, Infertility

Impotence

The term impotence refers to the male's inability to achieve an erection of the penis and, in most cases, the resulting inability to convey semen. There are two main categories of impotence: (1) *primary impotence*, in which the male afflicted has never been able to achieve an erection because of a birth defect or the result of a lifelong abnormal hormone chemistry; and (2) *secondary impotence*, a much more common affliction whereby the male, who was at one time able to achieve and maintain an erection, loses the ability due to physiological or emotional disturbances. *Secondary impotence* is often temporary in nature and can be alleviated with professional help. The term used in a clinical manner does not refer to the production of spermatozoa; a male could very easily be quite fertile and at the same time impotent, and vice versa.

The Incidence Of Impotence Increasing At An Alarming Rate

According to Dr. A. C. Kinsey, a noted researcher of American sexual mores and author of *Sexual Behavior of the Human Male* (W. B. Saunders Co., 1948), the occurrence of impotence in men under 35 at the time of his study was only 1.3 percent, but a poll taken in 1970 by *Psychology Today* reported that an incredible one-third of its readers responding to the poll "had difficulty achieving ordinary erection." Impotence affects a significant number of males in all age groups. "Impotence is the most common sexual disorder in men over 45 years of age," according to an article in *Geriatrics* (vol. 30, #4, 1975).

The problem of "impotence has become the least publicized epidemic of the past decade," according to Dr. Harvey E. Kaye, author of *Male Survival* (Grosset and Dunlap, 1974). But what is the cause of this remarkable increase in impotence? The underlying problems are both physiological and emotional. Psychiatrists and sex researchers say that some of the causes include guilt stemming from parental prohibitions; the emergence of the liberated woman who demands sexual performances that are sometimes beyond the powers of her partner; and the ever-growing fear of just plain failure in sexual endeavors. The latter usually involves a male who, for any number of reasons, may have a transient encounter with impotence while attempting intercourse. However, one such experience may permeate his psyche and result in a pattern of impotence which becomes more ingrained as time goes on, unless professional help is sought.

Causes Of Impotence Are Many And Complex

Whatever the major cause of impotence is, it is apparent that it is a complex problem involving many interrelated factors. "Impotency results from a multitude of stresses exerted on the penis, arising from any one of a multitude of causes. Physical illness, diseases such as diabetes, thyroid insufficiency, multiple sclerosis, to mention a few, are rare although possible etiological factors. Drug intake is a somewhat more common cause," according to Dr. Kaye.

Drugs Can Cause Male Impotence

According to Helen Singer Kaplan, M.D., Ph.D., and author of *The New Sex Therapy* (Brunner-Mazel Publications, 1974), there are a number of drugs which can decrease the sex urge, resulting in impotence. Among those drugs are alcohol and barbiturates; amphetamines, which when chronically used can "diminish libido and sexual functioning"; antabuse, which is prescribed for alcoholics; and presate, which is used for weight reduction. Sedatives made from belladonna derivatives, sold over-the-counter without prescriptions in pharmacies, are also the cause of some temporary impotence.

Drug-induced states of impotence are mainly temporary and disappear once the noxious drug is discontinued—all except the chronic use of alcohol. According to an article in *Family Practice News* (Vol. 4, Sept. 15, 1974), which reported on an address given by Dr. Randle E. Pollard before the National Medical Association, alcohol can cause definite impairment of the male's masculinity, causing impotency. "The liver damaged by alcohol abuse has a reduced ability to conjugate estrogens, causing a man to become more estrogenic, and thus less male," the article reported.

Middle Age And Impotency

Many men delude themselves by believing the myth that impotence, no matter how transient, is a normal occurrence of the aging process. This belief is totally unfounded if the proper precautions are taken, according to sex researchers Dr. William H. Masters and Virginia E. Johnson. "Masters and Johnson found men sexually active into the 80th and 90th years—but invariably they had kept in condition by making love a regular part of their life." (*Family Health*, May, 1974)

It is true that the bloodstream levels of testosterone, the male hormone, decrease with aging, but research has shown that this does not affect erectile impotency. "Apparently the penis requires only a minimal amount of testosterone for successful operation, and the somewhat lower levels in older men may indicate little more than sexual apathy. . . ." reported Dr. Kaye.

Abstinence from sex and the resulting impotency pattern may be helped along by the ignorance of the family physician who is unaware of data discovered by recent sex therapy and research, indicating that although the arousal time for an erection may become slower, loss of potency is not "a natural consequence of aging." According to an article by Saul Kent in *Geriatrics* (April, 1975) entitled "Impotence: The Facts Versus the Fallacies," many men, thinking that impotence is natural, give up pursuing sex long before they ordinarily would have to, and the blame often falls on their family doctors. "Physicians may contribute to this decline in sexual activity by telling their aging patients exactly what everyone else is telling them: 'You're too old for sex. Why persist in trying to fight nature? You'll just have to accept your impotence as inevitable.' When a man hears this from a physician, he understandably may be convinced that his sex life is over."

Frigidity

Frigidity in women is analogous to impotence in males. The syndrome is characterized be a coldness or total aversion to sex. The cause can sometimes be physical, but in the majority of cases, it is emotional in nature and professional guidance is often needed.

Aside from the myriad emotional problems which can precipitate a distaste for sex in frigid women, there are some physical problems which may lead to incipient frigidity that can easily be avoided. A primary cause of female sexual inadequacy is dyspareunia, or pain during the sex act. This pain may have a real physical origin or it can originate in the mind. Mild pain is actually the worst, for severe pain will call attention to itself until professional help is sought. But mild pain, vaguely felt, is often ignored. Yet, if it continues for any length of time, a woman will respond negatively to the prospect of intercourse.

Such physical pain can be caused by scar tissue from rape, abortion or bruised remnant of the hymen. But the chief cause of scarring is the routine reliance on episiotomy (surgical incision of the vulvar orifice) to facilitate delivery during childbirth. Because the anesthetized mother is unable to cooperate with contractions, the obstetrician widens the passage by cutting and uses forceps to pull the child out. And while any tissue damage is usually skillfully repaired, blunders do occur. The result may be pain or flabbiness of the vaginal wall, two conditions which destroy sexual pleasure. Of course, these pitfalls can be avoided in natural childbirth.

Another frequent cause of pain is loss of vaginal tissue elasticity, especially common among post-menopausal women. Smegma around the clitoral area can be a cause of minor but long-lasting dyspareunia. Smegma is a cheese-like substance, an accrual of dead epithelial cells. Superficial exterior cleanliness is always a good practice.

Lack of vaginal lubrication is another basic cause of pain during intercourse. Although it is necessary and usually present, lubrication can be blocked by various factors. Fear of pain, pregnancy, and disease can impede lubrication, and stop it altogether. So can a physical defect, which can only be determined by a gynecologist.

Infertility: A Problem Of Both Sexes

Infertility, or sterility, is a problem which is growing in significance every year. This poignant problem is casting a long shadow over the lives of over ten million American couples who long for a baby. For generations childlessness has been attributed to the female, but this is just another lingering Victorian myth. It was reported at the World Congress of Fertility and Sterility held in Stockholm (February, 1967) that as much as 50 percent of the time, the male may be the infertile partner in a childless marriage. Infertility, like impotence, is becoming a pressing problem for the American male.

Zinc Also Aids Fertility

But there are clues to the mystery. It has been demonstrated that the mineral, zinc, may have an important influence on infertility. Zinc is found in very high and active concentrations throughout the male reproductive system in prostate seminal fluid, especially the sperm, which contains the highest concentrations of zinc of any type of cell in the human body. In Iran and Egypt where many people subsist on zinc-deficient diets, medical researchers found that boys who were undersized and immature grew rapidly and matured sexually once they were put on an improved diet with increased iron and zinc. Dr. A. A. Prasad and his colleagues found that the 40 boys admitted to the research ward of the U.S. Naval Medical Research Unit in Cairo, U.A.R., suffered both growth retardation and hypogonadism (retarded genital development). Further testing showed that while the iron and improved diet aided growth, *it was the zinc supplementation which promoted the greatest degree of sex maturation.*

You might well wonder what this dramatic finding on the other side of the world among undernourished boys has to do with the increased rate of impotence and infertility in our own country. A great deal. Although we are not suffering with frank malnutrition that is easily diagnosed, many of us are suffering marginal deficiencies that may lie at the root of many of the mysteries currently baffling the medical profession—the increased rate of infertility and the growing problem of lack of sexual spark among young men in their prime.

"Physical examination of the infertile male often reveals obvious hypogonadism which is generally associated with poor sexual performance but neither the husband nor the wife may be aware of it," observed Dr. Charles W. Charney in the *Journal of the American Medical Association* (November 30, 1963). Through Dr. Prasad's study of the Egyptian boys, we know that zinc plays an important role in the growth and maturity of the gonads—the sex organs. It is also known that a deficiency of zinc can lead to unhealthy changes in the size and structure of the prostate.

Zinc then is a necessary element for fertility and male vigor. Like every other mineral element, zinc is concentrated in the bran and germ portion of the cereal grains. So it is obvious that any man who is concerned with maintaining or improving his fertility should make certain to have a regular and generous intake of unprocessed grain foods.

Section 52
Shingles

242. Shingles (Herpes Zoster) The "Exquisite-Pain Disease"

242. Shingles (Herpes Zoster) The "Exquisite-Pain Disease"

Shingles is an infection of a major sensory nerve by the herpes zoster virus. The disease (also called *herpes zoster*) begins with a severe pain in the chest or lower abdomen, accompanied a few days later with a localized concentration of chicken-pox-like blebs or blisters over the painful area. The rash appears on either side of the waist or chest—hence the name zoster, from the Greek word for girdle. The virus sometimes attacks nerves in the face, and serious visual impairment can develop if the eyes are affected.

The pain of the inflamed nerve (actually a form of neuralgia) can be excruciating—"exquisite pain" as some doctors describe it. Often it is accompanied by excessive sensibility of the skin, where even the touch of clothing is unbearable. For some patients the pain is not so severe, but rather a dull nagging or burning sensation.

Young people are apt to recover from a shingles attack in a week or two, or a month at the most. But some 30 percent of patients over 40 continue with lingering pain, and among patients over 70, almost 50 percent continue with pain for a year or more. Although they are rare, there have been reported cases of postherpetic neuralgia lasting for as long as 15 years. Particularly for older persons, then, shingles is anything but a trivial disease. Unfortunately, there is no agreed upon preventive or remedy.

Despite the medical profession's failure to date to come up with the "perfect pill" to counteract herpes zoster, there may very well be other non-traditional methods that will work. There is case history evidence that vitamin C given in massive doses can limit the infection of shingles. Vitamin B_{12} also has been used with good results by a number of practitioners. The standard physician's guide, the *Merck Manual*, cites reports that there is improvement in shingles following large doses of this B vitamin.

But, beyond these two specific vitamins that have been used therapeutically for shingles, there are other vitamins (and minerals as well) that have proven significant in maintaining a healthy nervous system. It is reasonable to suggest that these nutrients should be helpful in repelling a viral attack on nerve cells. And it is reasonable to suppose that they would be beneficial in healing the damaged nerves that cause pain after the active phase of the disease is over. Of all the viral diseases, shingles seems the most likely to yield to nutritional therapy, which is based on building the body's own natural defenses against infection and disease.

The Double Action Virus
Children can come down with chicken pox after they've been exposed to an adult in the active stage of shingles; also, an adult can come down with shingles after contact with children suffering from chicken pox. This phenomenon has been the source of long-standing controversy over whether the viruses of the two diseases were identical or only very similar. But modern laboratory examination of the viruses recovered from the skin lesions of patients of both diseases, along with comprehensive blood serum tests, strongly suggest that the two infecting agents are the same. The common virus is called the varicel-zoster virus.

Researchers believe that the virus usually first infects a person during childhood and causes chicken pox. Although the person then becomes partially immune against a recurrence of chicken pox, the varicel-zoster virus remains dormant and a potential cause of shingles. Presumably, then, the virus is present in everyone who has ever had chicken pox. However, in most of us, apparently the virus stays dormant since only approximately 83 in 100,000 people contract shingles.

So it is obvious that some breakdown in normal body defenses permits the virus to "wake up" and inflict its second-round damage. Bearing out this thesis is a list of adverse conditions, which tend to break down natural resistance, and can initiate an attack of shingles: injury, debilitating disease, certain drugs (particularly the immunosuppressive medications) and a variety of poisons—for example, carbon monoxide poisoning.

In other words, it's not the presence of the virus, which has been there all along, but the condition of the host that causes this disease. It would appear then that vitamin therapy, which aids the body's own defenses, offers the best defense.

Vitamin Therapy Found Effective
Dr. Frederick Klenner, a North Carolina physician, successfully used massive doses of vitamin C in treating patients who were

suffering from acute cases of shingles, (*The Key to Good Health: Vitamin C*).

Vitamin B_{12}, known for its importance to nerve health, has also been found therapeutic in the treatment of shingles. Drs. A. K. Gupta and H. S. Mital reported in an article in the *Indian Practitioner* (July, 1967) that they had observed a "dramatic response to vitamin B_{12} therapy as judged by relief of pain and the speed of disappearance of vesicles" in the case of 21 herpes zoster patients. Improvement usually began, they said, on the second or third day following daily injections of 500 mcg of the vitamin. Most importantly, follow-up study showed no development of postherpetic neuralgia in any of the cases. In this respect, as in the initial response to therapy, the authors noted their experience confirmed reports of earlier experimenters.

Though this therapy has not been proven in controlled tests, it would seem to carry great promise. If you should feel the pain of shingles and find the tell-tale rash breaking out, it would be wise to ask your doctor to look into the possibility of megavitamin therapy as soon as possible since the sooner the therapy starts, the better the chance of complete recovery.

What About The Lingering Pain?

Pain killing drugs are usually unsuccessful in treating the lingering pain of postherpetic neuralgia. In severe cases, where the pain is unbearable, surgery is sometimes used to cut the root of the nerve. It is then also important to improve your nutrition so that your damaged nerve is given the utmost support in the healing process.

We have already noted the importance of B_{12} but in fact every element of the B complex is important to central nervous system activity.

Organ meat, particularly liver, is a major source of the B vitamins. You may want to take your liver in desiccated form. Brewer's yeast and wheat germ are also rich in this nutrient. All green vegetables (particularly broccoli) have stores of vitamin C, as do most fruits. Rose hips, as a supplement, are one of nature's richest sources.

Two minerals that should get your special attention are calcium and magnesium. As Dr. Willard Krehl pointed out in *Nutrition Today* (September, 1967), "magnesium deficiency unquestionably causes changes in nerve conduction, transmission at the myoneural junction and muscular contraction." And calcium, reported Drs. Ferris Pitts, Jr., and James McClure, Jr. in the *New England Journal of Medicine* (December 21, 1967), combines with lactate around the sensitive endings of the nerves, preventing the acid from irritating the nervous system. Calcium is also necessary for the transmission of nerve impulses.

White milk and other dairy products are the best food source for calcium. Bone meal contains both calcium and phosphorus and other minerals, including magnesium. You'll get magnesium in raw or lightly cooked vegetables, whole grain cereals, and raw nuts. Dolomite is a convenient magnesium supplement.

For people who have never had shingles, such a diet might be the best possible preventive. For remember, that virus is always present in your body if you've ever had chicken-pox, and only your own good health and the health of your nerve cells keeps this enemy at bay.

Section 53
Sinusitis

243. Why Your Sinuses May Ache

Just about everyone has awakened one morning with a headache and a stuffed nose. If the symptoms persist and if we have been in the habit of paying attention to TV drug commercials, we might well call the doctor for an appointment and inform him that our sinuses are "acting up" again.

Perhaps our self-diagnosis would be correct, but the odds are it wouldn't. Says one doctor, Byron J. Bailey, writing in the December, 1973 issue of *American Family Physician*, "Of every 100 patients who come to see me complaining of 'sinus trouble,' less than 10 have sinusitis."

Jerry C. Freeman, M. D., and colleagues put it even more pointedly in the October, 1972 issue of *The Nebraska Medical Journal*:

"A tremendous number of people today claim to have 'sinus' and cling faithfully to their symptoms of nasal obstruction and intermittent headache, becoming somewhat like Linus deprived of his blanket when one suggests that their problems are, with rare exception, due to conditions almost wholly confined to the nose and their psyche.

"Thus, a complete compendium of sprays, drops, salves, injections, insufflations, and irrigations have arisen to produce an almost voodoo cult of practitioners in the art of relieving 'sinus.' The term 'sinus,' so commonly used, I carefully place in quotes to differentiate it from primary disease of the sinuses, *sinusitis*, a distinct, but frequently mis-diagnosed condition." The distinction is, of course, of immense importance. What the average person might interpret as a sinus problem could be nothing more than an uncommonly bad common cold. And fortunate indeed is the person who gets off with a mere cold, for a genuine dose of sinusitis can, in extreme cases, require surgery and even lead to cancer.

Still, the layman cannot be blamed for his mistaken diagnosis.

Even a highly trained physician can't be sure he is looking at a sinusitis case merely on the basis of apparent symptoms.

How Doctors Diagnose Real Sinusitis

Any of the following symptoms could indicate sinusitis:

—Decreased hearing acuity, hoarseness and sore throat, but no other pain; a constant draining of mucus in the throat.

—Difficulty in breathing through the nose; dull to extremely severe headaches, usually beginning about midmorning and gone by late afternoon; sensitivity around the cheekbone.

—Ultimately, sinusitis can produce a high fever, restlessness and delirium. Nasal discharge may contain pus and be flecked with blood. According to J. D. K. Dawes, M. D., writing in the April 2, 1966, issue of the *British Medical Journal*, "Recurring acute exacerbations may physically and mentally exhaust the patient to the point of chronic illness, and, failing relief, irritability and anxiety may incur the label of neurosis."

"In fact," says Dr. Eugene E. Mihalyka (*The Plain Dealer*, August 19, 1965), "I have had members of the family of a severe sinusitis victim tell me that the patient's whole personality changed violently when he had an attack of sinusitis."

According to Dr. Byron Bailey, three symptoms are common to all sinusitis cases: a clogged nose, a continuing flow of mucus down the throat (known as postnasal drip) and headache. While in some cases the headache is little more than a dull annoyance, in others it is severe and the most obvious symptom.

That fact was illustrated by Joseph Lubart, M. D., in the February, 1974 issue of the *New York State Journal of Medicine*. One of his patients, a man approaching 50, suffered headaches for six years before the problem was diagnosed as sinusitis and treated successfully. The pain usually began with an ache in the upper teeth of the right side of his jaw. From there it spread to the temple and right eye, which grew red and painful. Finally the pain shot to the ear and down the neck. The right side of the nose became blocked. The severe suffering usually lasted for 15 minutes.

Several of Dr. Lubart's patients had been diagnosed previously as migraine victims. One attended a headache clinic. Several were given thorough examinations. Yet, until they reached Dr. Lubart's office, none of the patients had been diagnosed as having sinusitis. In all cases, that was the cause of the headaches, he said. Therapy, including surgery to remove bony abnormalities, eliminated the suffering.

What Causes Sinus Infection?

Sinus irritation and infection can be caused in many ways. There are eight sinuses—or cavities—plus a complex system of air cells in the normal human head, every one of them a potential site for infections. All of these various holes are grouped about your nose—in the forehead, between the eyebrows, under the eyes, beside the nostrils, etc. Secretions drain from them into the nasal passage.

The sinus openings into the nasal passages are seldom larger than the thickness of the lead in a pencil. It takes no great imagination to envision the traffic jam that can build up in a sinus exit once a cold or other infection causes an abnormally high flow of mucus.

Ordinarily, nature has a marvelous solution—we blow our noses. The forcible expulsion of air through the nasal passage creates a vacuum which sucks the mucus out of the sinus and into the nasal cavity.

The sinusitis sufferer isn't so fortunate. For one reason or another, either the exit holes from the sinuses or the nasal passage itself is jammed. The fluid secretions collect in the head, and the pressure of the fluid causes the pain and other symptoms associated with sinusitis.

Sometimes—rarely—clogging of the nasal passage is a result of a physical deformity in which a bone in the nose obstructs drainage from the sinuses. In cases of this sort, surgery is the only permanent solution.

Far more commonly, however, sinusitis is the result of an infection. In fact, according to Dr. Bailey, "Sinusitis almost always occurs secondary to acute viral or bacterial infections of the nose. Because of the direct continuity of the respiratory epithelium, it is likely that all nasal infections involve the sinuses to some degree.

"Infection spreads from the nose by direct continuity into the sinuses through their small ostia (openings) and may be hastened by nose blowing, sneezing or swimming and diving while one has an upper respiratory infection."

Rapid change in barometric pressure, which occurs frequently in airplane flights, can cause damage to the membranes lining the sinuses, and the injured tissue is a marvelous breeding ground for bacteria. Abscessed teeth can also infect the sinuses.

However the bacterial or viral infection comes about, the body immediately takes steps to destroy it.

Mucus, A Natural Germ-Killing Defense

The body's first-line defense weapon is mucus. This is a thick, sticky substance secreted by the mucous membranes of the sinuses, and contains a powerful antibacterial agent called lysozyme.

It is an almost perfect system, considering the fact that with every breath of air we breathe, billions of potential disease-causing bacteria and viruses enter our nasal passage. Most of these invaders are immediately trapped on the sticky mucus like a fly on flypaper and then destroyed by the lysozyme. The ones that begin to multiply by attaching themselves to a sinus wall are wiped away by an increased excretion of mucus from the sinus membranes.

The mucus must then be helped along its route through and out of the nasal passage by countless tiny little fingers called cilia. And sometimes they break down. This is the reason that the process is not quite perfect.

The way cilia function is one of the most fascinating subjects in biological science. Cilia are amazingly small—no more than .0000078 inches in diameter and .000585 inches in length. Yet, when they are healthy, they work with great efficiency.

Controlled by a process still not understood, the tiny hairs brush the mucus forward "metachronically." That is, instead of all the cilia moving forward and backward simultaneously, they cooperate, passing the mucus forward to the next set of cilia, which repeat the process. The cilia hairs work together like waves to keep the mucus flowing continuously.

The Goal—Get Those Cilia Working!

Now, the cilia play a crucial role in the development as well as the prevention or cure of sinusitis. In the words of Dr. Mihalyka, "Treatment (of sinusitis) must aim to reduce the congestion of the mucous membranes so that the sinuses can empty and get rid of this mucus discharge properly." Under normal circumstances, that is possible only if the cilia are functioning properly.

So the question, "What causes sinusitis?" is frequently the same as, "Why aren't the cilia working properly?"

Says Kaye H. Kilburn in the June 18, 1965, issue of *Science*, "... smoke from filtered and unfiltered cigarettes stops ciliary activity and mucus transport." Even if the cigarette smoke destroys only a portion of the cilia, it has been found that the metachronic wave will stop at the damaged cilia and not continue beyond them. This may well be an explanation for the common smoker's cough upon awakening each morning—since the cilia are not functioning, the phlegm and mucus gather in the throat and sinuses overnight and only violent coughing can dislodge them.

According to Dr. Bailey, alcohol is another enemy of cilia. So is most air pollution.

Far more serious, because they are totally unsuspected by the average layman, are the very drugs used to clear a stuffed nose—the nose drops and nasal sprays. Referring to these, Dr. Mihalyka warns that "many popular remedies do actual harm while giving you only temporary relief." And Dr. Bailey adds that the use of a topical decongestant is controversial because of the harm it does to the cilia.

"While they (the drops and sprays) may be of some benefit for relief of acute obstruction," says Dr. Jerry Freeman, "their long-term use results in sensitization of the nasal mucosa with rebound engorgement of the vessels and a resulting rhinitis medicamentosa that is worse than the primary disease. Combinations containing antibiotics, antihistamines or corticosteroids are of no additional benefit, and dangerous sensitization to antibiotics may occur following their repeated use in this manner."

While a genuine crisis may require drugs, or even surgery, generally the wisest policy is not to purchase immediate relief at the price of long-term suffering. Fortunately, as we'll see in the next chapter, there are wiser alternatives.

244. Vitamin A And Zinc For Healthy Sinuses

What should you do for sinusitis? The first step, particularly if your sinus problem involves great pain, is to have a physical check-up which should include a thorough examination of the sinuses. The major reason for this is to rule out the possibility of a malignancy, a polyp or bone growth. In these comparatively rare cases, nothing short of surgery is likely to help.

Beyond that, the goal must be to give the mucous membranes and hair-like cilia lining the sinuses a fighting chance against viruses, bacteria and the poisons in our air. One way we can do that is to eliminate unnecessary poisons like cigarette smoke and alcohol.

Another step—the major one—is to provide in abundance the nutritional elements needed by the mucous membranes and cilia. That will allow them to work at their optimal level.

The cilia particularly need potassium and calcium. Without these nutrients, the cilia cannot function. But if there is one nutrient that might be considered the backbone of the mucociliary system it is vitamin A.

"Deficiency of vitamin A," writes Dr. Gerald H. Clamon in *Nature* (July 5, 1974), "causes a well-defined lesion, namely keratinized squamous metaplasia. . . .In this lesion, the normal columnar ciliated and mucous cells of the epithelium, which depend on vitamin A for their formation, are totally replaced by squamous cells which produce keratin."

Mucous Cells Die Without Vitamin A
In lay terms, Dr. Clamon and his associates are saying that without adequate amounts of vitamin A, cilia and mucous cells die off and are replaced by hard, scaly (squamous) cells which produce keratin, the major protein in ordinary skin cells.

Doctors don't know why the specialized cilia and mucous cells fail to grow without vitamin A—but fail they do. Fortunately, says Dr. Clamon, "Addition of vitamin A to the organ cultures after development of such lesions causes reversal of the process of keratinization and replacement of the squamous cells by columnar ciliated and mucous cells."

Thus, even those cilia destroyed by cigarette smoke, alcohol, nose drops and nasal sprays can be replaced with healthy young cilia, provided that the potassium, calcium and vitamin A they require are present in the diet—and the toxins removed.

But adequate amounts of one more nutrient—zinc—are also essential. According to J. Cecil Smith, Jr., writing in the September 7, 1973, issue of *Science*, vitamin A cannot do its job if zinc isn't also present.

Says Dr. Smith: "Zinc is necessary to maintain normal concentrations of vitamin A in plasma. By using animals deficient in both zinc and vitamin A, it was demonstrated that zinc is necessary for normal mobilization of vitamin A from the liver."

Dr. Smith's experiments were not limited to animals. Studying 61 Baltimore, Maryland, children, Smith and his colleagues found that only when levels of zinc increased in the blood did the liver release its stores of vitamin A so that it, too, could enter the bloodstream and be carried to the organ where it was needed.

Proper Humidity Is Important

The whole subject of sinusitis remains shrouded in controversy. Some doctors feel that it is often diagnosed when it really doesn't exist; others point to cases of people who suffered for years because their sinus inflammation was never diagnosed. The controversy extends right down to the question of whether increased humidity is beneficial or harmful. Some doctors recommend using a humidifier for sinusitis patients, while at least one researcher found that high humidity slows the mucus flow. In all likelihood, a comfortable relative humidity of between 30 and 50 percent will help many sinus sufferers. Certainly, the extremely dry air which exists during wintertime in unhumidified homes (typically around five to 10 percent relative humidity) can only dry out the membranes, harden mucus and immobilize the cilia.

On the other hand, excessive or uncomfortable humidity will also cause problems. This will generally occur during the summer months. Inside the home, humidity can be reduced to more comfortable levels with a dehumidifier or air conditioner, but outdoors, you're out of luck.

Some doctors recommend antibiotics for sinusitis; others say they are useless or downright harmful. The same is true of nasal decongestants. And in some cases of sinusitis, a bone abnormality is found which must be corrected surgically.

What all this boils down to is that sinusitis requires diagnosis and evaluation on a very individualized basis. There is no single prescription that can be handed out to all sufferers.

But in the midst of this disagreement, two incontrovertible points stand out—and they are important ones:

—The single most important step in bringing relief is to clear the sinuses and nasal passages of mucus and the germs the mucus has trapped.

—Only healthy mucous membranes and cilia can perform this function on a day-to-day basis. And to do the job they must be kept healthy through proper nutrition—eliminating toxins such as alcohol and cigarette smoke, and assuring adequacy of vitamin A, zinc, calcium and potassium.

Section 54
The Skin

245. Fighting Acne?—Try These Simple Weapons

Acne begins when the tiny channel or follicle leading from a sebaceous (oil) gland in the skin to the skin surface becomes plugged up. Ordinary dirt can plug it up, but far more frequently skin cells themselves are responsible.

The top layer of skin, epidermia, also called the *stratum corneum*, is hard and horny. Ordinarily these outer skin cells are continually being brushed away by clothing, bathing, etc. But in certain individuals, especially during adolescence, for some reason, they tend to adhere to each other. Then, instead of being sloughed off, they lodge within the small follicles leading from the sebaceous glands.

Each hard little plug is known as a comedone. These comedones can turn into blackheads when the plugged sebum turns black because of oxydation, not dirt. The plugged condition is called keratosis. When an individual has an excessive number of plug-like comedones he is said to be suffering from hyperkeratosis of the sebaceous ducts or follicles.

The sebaceous glands ordinarily secrete a lubricant called sebum, a thick fluid-like substance containing fatty materials and soft cellular debris from the lower epidermal layers. Even when the follicle is plugged shut, the secretion continues. This causes swelling and irritation. A papule, or small pimple, results. If the pimple contains pus, it is called a pustule. Sometimes even a cyst forms. In a typical acne case, that process is repeated hundreds of times on the face and neck.

Since acne occurs most commonly during adolescence, striking 95 percent of all adolescents, it is generally accepted that the gland changes taking place at this time must have something to do with its causation. Sex hormones are developing; a child's body is becoming the body of an adult. As childhood falls behind and a youngster's body continues to grow and develop, hormone production is greatly increased. This increase during puberty induces changes throughout the body, one of them being increased output of oil by the sebaceous glands.

There is good reason for believing that the psychological stress of adolescence may be a factor in the development of acne; however, there is abundant evidence that a diet lacking in certain vitamins and minerals can also lead to acne. Unfortunately, little serious effort is made among physicians and health agencies to *prevent* acne by educating parents and children to anticipate these needs.

In recent years, X-ray has been used as a treatment—even though most experts are strongly opposed to radiation exposure except in life-or-death situations. Some doctors administer broad-spectrum antibiotics—tetracycline has been in use continually for several years—although there is no real evidence of their effectiveness. Oral contraceptives are even prescribed for some female teenagers to help them fight acne.

It has been the trend among dermatologists to treat acne externally. They prescribe lotions, or a combination of lotions with sunbaths. Sulfur, quartz lamps, lotio alba, tincture of green soap, hot or cold compresses—any of these might be a daily ritual for an acne sufferer, who usually goes right on developing more and more pimples.

Most doctors agree that the tried and true old-time remedies work as well as any. A report issued by the Kansas State Department of Health quoted one physician's opinion that, "Twenty-five percent of acne can be managed successfully by washing the face four or five times a day . . ." But this cleansing should *not* be done with soap. (A soft white cloth soaked in warm water is best.) The sebaceous glands are irritated by soap, and the irritation causes the glands to secrete still more sebum than normal. This excessive secretion is what creates the unsightly blotches and blackheads characteristic of acne.

The irritative qualities of soap, and the harsh effect it has on the skin have been demonstrated frequently in medical literature. Why presume that these objectionable qualities are suspended when soap is used on the face?

Acne Yields To Vitamin A Acid Treatment

The best of the old-time acne therapies still seems the best today—vitamin A. Perhaps the most exciting therapy of all for acne is vitamin A in its acid form. This is not taken orally, but applied directly to the skin (topically), and it can only be obtained by a doctor's prescription.

The early weeks of treatment with vitamin A acid therapy may prove a disappointment because the acne condition is aggravated: scores of new comedones stud the skin surface and can be wiped away with the fingers; slight pimples develop into full-blown and open comedones; and new pustules and papules suddenly appear. This condition continues for approximately six weeks. The explanation, according to researcher James E. Fulton, M. D., is that, "Under the influence of vitamin A acid, comedones, inert for weeks or months, suddenly 'blew-up.' As a rule, these inflammatory lesions were rather small, implying that the acid was exciting inflammatory explosions at an earlier stage than would occur naturally." Vitamin A's value against acne, according to Dr. Fulton, lies in its action to control the overproduction of sebum and the resulting "hyperkeratosis of the sebaceous follicles."

Dr. Fulton and his superior, Albert M. Kligman, M. D., carried on their studies with 229 adolescent patients at the Acne Clinic, attached to the University of Pennsylvania. The patients were divided into four groups: 37 patients were given a traditional remedy, sulfur resorcinol; 49 received benzoyl peroxide, apparently the favorite acne treatment among most doctors; 40 more were control subjects; and vitamin A acid was used on the remaining 103 patients.

Every week the patients came to the clinic, and the number of comedones, papules, pustules and cysts were carefully counted. Between three and four months later, the degree of improvement was evaluated. The results were impressive. Among the controls, there was a total improvement of 8.3 percent—presumably, this is a natural rate of improvement without therapy. Of those on the sulfur-resorcinol, total improvement averaged 15.9 percent. Those receiving bensoyl peroxide, the current medical favorite, showed 31.9 percent improvement. However, on vitamin A acid, improvement virtually doubled—to 61.9 percent. Almost 40 percent of these secured an excellent result.

More Than Vitamin A Acid Is Needed

But vitamin A acid is no panacea for acne. Most patients are improved, but not all, and not everyone can tolerate some of its irritant effects. Furthermore, if the application of vitamin A is stopped, the acne will probably return, usually within three to six weeks. However, Dr. Jon D. Straumfjord, originator of the treatment, said that oral vitamin A supplements may keep acne away, once the condition is cleared up and the acid applications are discontinued.

Daily oral doses of vitamin A and diets high in that nutrient combined with soapless face-washing several times daily may spare youngsters now entering adolescence the misery of an acne condition.

Vitamin D Treatment Recognized

At about the time vitamin A therapy for acne was first discussed, vitamin D was receiving attention as an acne treatment. Unfortunately it is almost completely ignored today. Dr. Merlin Maynard of San Jose, California, reported in a 1940 issue of the *Archives of Dermatology and Syphilis* on the successful treatment of acne using vitamins D and calcium. In addition to receiving vitamin D, Dr. Maynard's patients followed a special diet, accenting lean meats, fresh fruits and green vegetables, with a minimum of carbohydrates; no sweets, chocolate, pastries, greasy or highly seasoned foods or soda fountain drinks.

Dr. Maynard concluded, "The greatest benefit of using vitamin D in acne, in my opinion, has been the avoidance of roentgen therapy (X-ray) which too often becomes the master rather than the servant of the physician. And certainly my satisfaction with vitamin D treatment has been great. The other vitamins have an irrefutable place, but their use is by no means as general as vitamin D." Despite this optimistic report, little meaningful research on vitamin D and acne has appeared since.

The Role Of Other Vitamins

The role of other vitamins in controlling acne conditions has been indicated in the studies of several physicians.

Vitamin C's role in *controlling* acne was demonstrated by Dr. George E. Morris of Boston. He found that 43 of 53 acne patients showed improvement after four months of receiving two eight-ounce glasses of citrus juice and three grams of ascorbic acid each day. Dr. Samuel M. Bluefarb of Northwestern University found that a combination of one gram of vitamin C, orange juice—plus 100,000 units of vitamin A administered daily—benefits adolescent acne. After observing 96 patients over a period of eight years, Dr. Louis Tulipan, of New York, reached the conclusion that vitamin B deficiency is the main cause of *acne rosacea*, a form of the disease prevalent among adults 25 to 45 years old. The skin thickens and becomes bright, purplish-red over the nose and on the cheeks and chin. He credited his success in treating this ailment to using brewer's yeast, which contains all the B complex of vitamins, rather than just one or another of the B vitamins alone.

Dr. Paul Kline treated 25 patients with multivitamin injections over a period of eight months. Twenty-four of the patients responded with satisfactory improvement. There was very little tendency for the acne to return after the injections were stopped. The younger the patients, the better their response.

These encouraging results with vitamin therapy are reported in medical journals, but rarely come to the attention of the public. Instead, the public is exposed to material which claims acne is hereditary, can be controlled by strict non-nutritious diets, and can be treated through the use of several irritating chemical lotions and salves.

Dr. L. Edward Gaul suggested in *The Journal of the Indiana State Medical Association* (January, 1966) that excessive use of salt may be related to acne. Adolescents on low salt diets have shown improvement within two weeks, and in two months, the acne bumps have disappeared entirely, according to Dr. Gaul. His article indicates that adolescents get excessive salt with such popular snacks as french fries, popcorn and potato chips. It is worth noting that all of these snacks are also heavy on residual hydrogenated fats.

Few adolescents are willing to forego snacking entirely. But snacking habits can be improved to satisfy ever-active appetites and provide nutrition at the same time, by including fresh or dried fruits, nuts and raw vegetables.

Acne Caused By Cosmetics

It is unlikely that a medicated cosmetic would clear up a case of acne or balance the oily nature of an individual's skin, when the cause is actually internal and not merely a surface condition. Keeping the skin clean is important in the treatment of acne, but applying a coverup for appearance is certainly *not* therapeutic.

Research into acne caused by cosmetics was the subject of an article entitled *Acne Cosmetica* which appeared in the *Archieves of Dermatology* (December, 1972). The authors, Drs. A. M. Kligman and Otto Mills, researchers at the well known acne clinic of the Department of Dermatology at the University of Pennsylvania in Philadelphia, noticed an "acne form rash" from certain "beautification" lotions which patients at the clinic were using at home. They first became aware of what they termed *acne cosmetica* when the number of post-adolescent women showing up for treatment at the acne clinic began to steadily increase in number. These figures also included a number of female hospital personnel.

Acne cosmetica, which strikes between the ages of 20 and 50, does not have the characteristic large lesions and huge blotches which cover the face, arms and back. It arrives unobtrusively. The small embarrassing bumps gradually increase in size and number. Week after week the patient uses more and more makeup to cover more and more bumps. Stretch the skin and they show up as solid whitish grains. (Blackheads are not part of the *acne cosmetica* syndrome.) The daily struggle to cover up is futile, for as Dr. Kligman noted, "The most extensive eruptions occurred in women who were trying to mask the lesions under heavy coatings of cosmetics."

The lesions tend to cluster on the chin, occasionally marring the cheek, but for some unknown reason, lesions usually do not appear on the forehead. Although it is rare, oiliness may be a symptom. Women with dark complexions and large pores are more likely to contract *acne cosmetica*. One prominent feature is the noticeably dark follicles, which are thought to be "clogged." But the researchers' report cautioned that, "washing and squeezing accomplishes nothing." Yet it is these conspicuous follicles which give the face a coarse appearance, which is often the most distressing aspect of *acne cosmetica*.

Many of the outpatients at the hospital who were treated for *acne cosmetica* had experienced acne in their teens. Usually this typical teenage acne has disappeared by the time the new trouble erupts. Imagine the dismay of these women when at the age of 25, 35, or even 45, they have a recurrence of acne. This, it is reported, may be caused by the heavy use of cosmetics to cover up previous scarring, since those with a history of severe acne had the most severe cases of *acne cosmetica*. But, the report stressed, "it must be made unequivocally clear that many women who had no previous history of acne also developed *acne cosmetica*."

Half Of All Cosmetics Cause Pimples

The pimples of *acne cosmetica* may crowd in at times, vanish at others. The eruptions may disappear for months and even years and then slowly redevelop. The researchers postulated that this fluctuation may be the result of using many different cosmetics. The patients the doctors observed were using so many different kinds of cosmetics that the doctors were unable to say that any particular kind or brand or even price range was especially culpable. However, when they purchased 25 different brands of cosmetics at random, and tested them on the ears of rabbits, they discovered that 56 percent of those tested produced some lesions on the rabbits' ears.

Although acne afflicts both sexes during adolescence, there appears to be a low grade, persistent comedonal acne in adult women that simply does not exist in men, according to Dr. E. Epstein reporting in the *Dermatological Digest* (July, 1968). In his research he found that 18 percent of the women between the ages of 26 and 35 whom he saw in his private practice had acne, while only two percent of the men he saw in this age group had it. Between the ages of 36 and 45, he said, acne occurred in 14 percent of his women patients and in only four percent of the men. The only difference, it appeared, was that the women use artificial cosmetics and most men do not.

246. What To Do About Cold Sores, Fever Blisters And Canker Sores

There are several internal and environmental alterations ranging from menstrual disturbances to antibiotic therapy that can account for the annoying skin disturbances known as cold sores, fever blisters and canker sores. These ugly lesions, which are acutely painful and exquisitely tender to the touch, usually afflict the soft membranes of the mouth, lips, nose or even the genital regions.

Some people appear to be especially prone to developing these painful ulcers, and if you are one of them, you may have tried everything from camphor compounds to vaccinations and psychotherapy. In any case, you don't need to be told any more about the itching, burning, and the usual one to two weeks of misery until the condition subsides—if it does at all.

There *is* something you can do to swiftly clear up and, even better, prevent fever blisters and canker sores. And that is to acquire a yogurt maker, some yogurt-starting culture known as *Lactobacillus acidophilus*, make yourself some yogurt, and eat it every day. A simpler way is to order a bottle of tablets made from yogurt and the active *L. acidophilus* bacteria. For people who don't like the taste of yogurt, the tablets are a desirable alternative.

According to studies published in the medical literature, the chances that yogurt culture will quickly clear up your fever blisters are about nine to one in your favor. After ingesting the tablets, and within a very short time, typically two or three days, the sores are either gone or going fast.

Some of the first case studies were presented by Dr. Donald J. Weekes, when he was associated with the Department of Otolaryngology at Harvard Medical School and the Department of Surgery at Peter Bent Brigham Hospital in Boston. Writing in the *New York State Journal of Medicine* (Vol. 58, No. 16, Aug. 15,

1958), Dr. Weekes described how treatment with a living culture of *Lactobacillus acidophilus* and the related *L. bulgaricus* affected half a dozen patients.

Dramatic Cures

Among these early cases was a 39-year-old physician's wife who had been complaining of almost continuous *aphthous stomatitis* (canker sores) for two years, which had developed following treatment with an antibiotic for an acute upper respiratory infection. Her sores had not responded to any medication that her doctor husband could obtain. After suffering for two years, she began taking two *Lactobacillus* tablets dissolved in the mouth with milk four times a day and her symptoms were promptly relieved. Another case involved a 35-year-old bus driver who had been suffering with canker sores for three days and was sufficiently annoyed by them to seek medical help. *Lactobacillus* tablets completely relieved his symptoms in two days. Another case was that of a 42-year-old graduate nurse whose canker sores were so excruciatingly painful that she had been unable to take any nourishment or fluids for several days before admission to the hospital. "Forty-eight hours after treatment with *Lactobacillus* therapy all ulcers had healed, she was taking fluids well, and urine volume returned," Dr. Weekes reported.

The Real Nature Of Fever Blisters And Canker Sores

Fever blisters or cold sores, also known as *herpes labialis*, are eruptions caused by the virus *herpes simplex*. Canker sores probably are not of herpetic origin, but are extremely difficult to distinguish from truly herpetic lesions, and very often accompany them. Both conditions are sometimes lumped together in the term *gingivostomatitis*. Both lesions are painful and typically persist from seven to fourteen days.

The odd thing about these flare-ups is that they are not caused by infection, at least a new infection. It has been shown repeatedly that most of us pick up the *herpes* virus at a relatively young age and carry it with us for many years, if not for life. When normal defense mechanisms break down, the virus suddenly becomes active and the result is a crop of tender blisters on the gums, mouth, or genitalia. After these blisters break, they may ulcerate and cause terrific pain. Conditions which may trigger these flare-ups include cold wind, sun, menstrual difficulty, and antibiotic therapy, as well as upper respiratory infections, sudden onset of fever, infected teeth, a sore throat, gastrointestinal upsets, emotional states, exhaustion, ingestion of certain foods or drugs, poor nutrition, and moderate social drinking. The nature of the connection between this wide array of challenges and the flare-up of the *herpes* virus is not clear, but it definitely exists.

Now that we have some idea of what seems to be involved in *herpes* sores, we want to know what there is about *Lactobacillus acidophilus* that causes them to disappear. This, researchers are not yet prepared to explain, but they have made some reasonable postulations as to how they inhibit *herpes* infections. It is possible that the power of *L. acidophilus* to "take over" the lower intestine and inhibit the growth of undesirable bacteria is also somehow responsible for inhibiting the virus sores of *herpes*.

Crowds Out Other Bacteria

Lactobacillus acidophilus is a bacterium which is normally found in very large numbers in the large bowel of a healthy person. There, it performs many vital functions. One of them is to manufacture B vitamins which are crucial for the production of antibodies which protect us from infection. *L. acidophilus* is also highly antagonistic to other forms of bacteria which may occur in the gut and are harmful or distressing instead of helpful. Specifically, when *L. acidophilus* breaks down the lactose in any dairy product, or the pectin or fiber in bulky foods, it produces lactic acid. Lactic acid, it has been shown in test tube experiments, is a potent killer of undesirable bacteria.

An article by Dr. H. L. Wollenweber published in *Office Pathology* (November, 1965) noted that, "Reduced numbers of *Lactobacilli* apparently have an effect on the ability of the host to mobilize leukocytes into an area of injury . . . Enhancement of leukocytic exudation, brought about by intestinal flora, may be one explanation for the influence of microbial flora on host resistance to an infection." Still another factor which may be at work is the fact that *L. acidophilus* produces large amounts of lactic acid as it feeds on lactose from dairy products. The increased acidity in the lower gut may well be responsible for many of the beneficial effects of *Lactobacillus* therapy.

However, there is one very specific mechanism which Dr. Weekes found to be at work in patients treated with *L. acidophilus*—that is a very dramatic rise in their level of salivary acid phosphatase. It has been shown, said Dr. Weekes, that phosphatase can inactivate *herpes simplex* (H. Amos, *Journal of*

Experimental Medicine, 98:365, 1953). Why salivary acid phosphatase should become lowered in an individual, and how the level is restored by *L. acidophilus* therapy are mechanisms not yet known.

95 Percent Success

More important, perhaps, is that enough *is* known about *Lactobacillus* to make its therapeutic use highly advisable for fever blisters and canker sores (not to mention gastrointestinal upsets). About five years after his earliest experiments, Dr. Weekes published the results of much more extensive tests using *L. acidophilus* and *bulgaricus* in tablet form to treat *gingivostomatitis* (*E.E.N.T. Digest*, Vol. 25, No. 12). Among the 64 patients treated for *herpes simplex labialis* (fever blisters or cold sores), 37 were completely free of the symptoms within one to four days. Another 24 showed dramatic improvement and suppression of the lesions. Altogether, 61 patients, or 95 percent of all those treated, experienced favorable results. Dr. Weekes was particularly impressed with the fact that *when the tablets were taken during the early burning and itching stage, therapy actually blocked the development of the sores.*

The response of the group treated for canker sores was also impressive but not quite as dramatic as that of the *herpes simplex labialis* group. "Of the 97 patients in this group, 40 were cured and 37 showed a definite improvement within four days. Local soreness usually disappeared within 24 to 48 hours." This represented a favorable response of about 80 percent. Dr. Weekes theorized that the reason for the somewhat lower success rate in treating canker sores is that some of them may not be of herpetic origin, but due to diet or allergic factors. He also noted that the lesions which usually fail to respond are those which have persisted continuously for years.

Six patients with *herpes* lesions on their genitals responded favorably, as did six of seven patients treated for *herpes* lesions on the cornea of the eye. Another study of the effectiveness of viable or living yogurt culture in treating *gingivostomatitis* was published by P. L. Abbott in *Journal of Oral Surgery* (19, 1961). When given during the early burning or itching stage to patients with recurrent canker sores, the treatment blocked eruption of blisters in all 22 patients.

In their article "Treatment of Oral Ulceration With *Lactobacillus* Tablets" (*Oral Surgery, Oral Medicine and Oral Pathology*,

Nov. 1965), Baltimore oral surgeons Leonard Rapoport and Walter Levine reported that 38 of 40 patients whom they treated achieved relief of pain within 48 hours, while 36 reported the total disappearance of all lesions within five days of treatment. Their patients took from two to four tablets three times a day, depending upon the severity of the lesions and physical size of the patients.

In light of all this evidence, there is no reason for anyone to go on suffering from the discomfort of fever blisters or canker sores. Nor is there any reason to experiment with patent medications and powerful drugs. According to Dr. Weekes, therapeutic measures recommended during the past half century have included chemical burning with silver nitrate, sodium perborate, gentian violet, camphor, hydrogen peroxide, alcohol and zephiran. Systemic medications recommended have included estrogenic and progestrogenic hormones, steroids, antihistamines, amino acids, antibiotics, sulfonamides, arsenic solutions, vaccinations, X-rays, and more. But not one of these treatments has a record of success even approaching that of *L. acidophilus.*

Commercial yogurts are not recommended for this purpose. For one thing, prolonged chilling of yogurt culture tends to sharply reduce the number of living *Lactobacilli.* Secondly, commercially available yogurts almost never contain *L. acidophilus.* Some contain a certain amount of *L. bulgaricus*, but other strains of bacteria are also usually present, and the effectiveness of these strains in fighting *herpes* has never been demonstrated.

It is best to use *L. acidophilus* exclusively, because this culture—to a certain extent at least—tends to implant itself in the intestines and continue to grow and promote its beneficial effects over a period of time. *L. bulgaricus* simply does its work and then disappears.

Whole Yogurt Or Tablets

The best course of action, it seems, is to purchase some *L. acidophilus* yogurt starting culture, and make your own yogurt for consumption during the next day or two, while the number of beneficial bacteria are still high.

If the ulcer is actually in the mouth, it would be a good idea to take a little yogurt or even buttermilk as frequently as possible, allowing the food to cover the ulcer for a minute or two. Because these cultured milk products are already rich in lactic acid, they should accelerate healing, according to Dr. H. Kragen (*Zahnarztliche Welt*, 9:1954).

If you already have a cold sore, or if you get them on a regular basis, tablets of concentrated living yogurt culture may be the best and most convenient answer. You can take the tablets with you and eat them wherever you may find yourself at meal time. In fact, if you are regularly afflicted by *herpes* sores, you may have to take the cultures, either as fresh curds or in tablet form, every day in order to prevent new lesions, because the *Lactobacilli* inactivate rather than destroy the *herpes* virus.

There is the possibility that people with an intolerance to the lactose in milk products may experience difficulty with this treatment, because the *Lactobacilli* need lactose in order to go on living and producing the valuable lactic acid. However, in all the studies cited here, the investigators reported only a very small number of instances in which patients complained of gastrointestinal upset. In these instances the tablets would appear a more desirable remedy.

If you do take the tablets to abort an erupting *herpes* lesion, or cure one which has already appeared, a dosage of about 10 to 15 tablets daily has proven effective. That may sound like a lot of tablets, but remember, this is not a drug, but a *natural* food substance which is eaten daily by millions of people all over the world.

247. Eczema Yields To Vitamin Therapy

The term "eczema" was indiscriminately used in the past to describe any number of superficial skin diseases characterized by patches of scaling, areas of fluid discharges ("weeping sores"), blisters and sore red blotches which could appear anywhere on the skin surface. If the condition couldn't be diagnosed as psoriasis, *acne vulgaris*, or a contagious skin disease, then it was generally, and often quite erroneously diagnosed as eczema.

However, physicians are now more careful in what they diagnose as eczema. They realize that there are various forms and stages of eczema, ranging from a constant irritation to sudden recurrences, but the same pattern of symptoms appears to emerge in all forms. The disease is identified by dry patches of skin, crusted and scaly with cracks or breaks that at times may "weep." The rash produces severe itching and burning in the affected area. This itching and burning sensation sets the disorder quite apart from psoriasis, which is much less painful.

Eczema is not known to be caused by any virus or infection, but is more the result of an allergic reaction among certain individuals to some external irritant which initially manifests itself in the epidermis, or the upper layer of the skin. Because it appears to be hereditary and victims have a previous history of allergies such as hay fever and asthma, it is generally felt among many medical researchers that certain people have a definite predisposition to eczema.

One of the most common types of eczema results from certain external irritants. These irritants can be poison ivy, certain dyes, detergents, chemicals used in the conditioning of perma-press fabrics and other chemical irritants. Unlike *contact dermatitis*, which has similar symptoms and is sometimes caused by the same external stimuli, eczema causes a permanent inflammation of the affected skin area, or, at the very least, chronic recurrences. Contact dermatitis is a painful, but short-lived, skin reaction and irritation; eczema is a distressing affliction.

Diversification And Classification Of Eczema Types

According to Drs. Hillard H. Pearlstein and Robert Auerbach writing in *Postgraduate Medicine* (March, 1972), "there is no completely satisfactory classification of all clinical variations" of the skin diseases classified under the general heading of eczema; they are several in number and affect people of all ages and in almost every region of the body. However, they note that the most painful type of eczema is called "atopic," and it "is the most common type of infantile eczema."

Prurigo (itching), oozing sores, prickly heat, secondary bacterial infections caused by the scratching of itching sores, and occasional cataracts are just some of the symptoms of this painful disease usually afflicting children before the age of two. Although the researchers offer no cure for this painful form of infantile eczema, they do recommend several precautionary steps which may ameliorate its intensity and degree: the avoidance of hot and humid climates which tend to increase sweat retention; cool baths and showers should replace bathings with hot water, which tend to irritate the itching and weeping of the sores; and the avoidance of any chemical irritants, whether in the form of "superfatted soaps" or ordinary household irritants such as aerosol spray products. Drs. Pearlstein and Auerbach also advise that if the eczema occurs in tandem with an attack of asthma, hayfever or any other dust allergies, then a change of climate would certainly be to the sufferer's advantage.

Seborrheic dermatitis is another common form of eczema. Often accompanied by acne, this type of eczema forms sore, scaly, yellowish or reddish blotches laden with sebum, a thick fluid-like secretion composed of fat and epithelial debris secreted by the sebaceous glands. The lesions form on the scalp and facial regions. This form of eczema is almost indistinguishable from psoriasis.

The *Journal of The American Dietetic Association* (September 1959) reported that certain kinds of eczema may have improved with pyridoxine (vitamin B_6) treatment, even after other treatments had failed. Dr. W. A. Krehl of Yale University, author of the article, reported that good results had been achieved when 24 to 50 milligrams of pyridoxine were given intravenously or subcutaneously and that "many of these cases of seborrheic dermatitis responded well to the local application of pyridoxine."

Saturated Fats And Eczema

Authors Bicknell and Prescott, in their book *Vitamins in Medicine,* report many cases where ingesting unsaturated fatty acids greatly improved eczema. What are unsaturated fats? They are the ones that stay liquid at room temperature. The oil you use in salad dressings is unsaturated. So are the liquid cooking oils (soybean oil, wheatgerm oil, sunflower seed oil, corn oil, etc.).

Since the earliest investigations, in 1933, researchers have known that unsaturated fats can be used to treat eczema. The Lee Foundation Report (February, 1942) reported that 87 chronic eczema patients, who were seen over a four and a half year period, responded to treatment with corn oils, though standard treatments used for years had failed. *The American Journal of Diseases of Children* (January, 1947) issued a similar report on 171 children suffering from eczema and treated with unsaturated fatty acids. About half of these (none of whom had shown any response to other treatments) improved markedly.

Another approach to treating eczema, used in Russia, is vitamin A extracted from pumpkins. In *Abstracta Dermatologica* (September-October, 1965) Russian scientists reported that patients were given 20 to 40 drops of carotene (the provitamin that occurs naturally in yellow vegetables and is converted into vitamin A by the body) from stored pumpkins. This was taken twice daily by mouth, and an ointment made of the carotene was rubbed on the affected part of the skin. According to the abstract, "Apparent cures or considerable improvements were observed in 16 of 19 patients with eczema (including infant eczema), in 24 of 33 patients with microbial eczema . . . and in six of seven patients with serious manifestations of hyperkeratosis (scaliness) of the skin."

Finnish Physician Reports Success With Vitamin B₂

Dr. R. Patiala, of the University of Helsinki, Finland, conducted studies with vitamin B₂ and reported these findings in 1966: "For about three years I have undertaken, partly in the cutaneous disease section of the clinic of the University of Helsinki, partly on the outside, the use of vitamin B₂ preparations in the treatment of infantile eczema and diathetic Besnier's *prurigo* (chronic itching skin inflammations).

"The patients studied represented five cases of severe infantile eczema, and 21 cases of Besnier's *prurigo,* of which three were associated with attacks of asthma. The ages of the patients ranged between six and twelve months for the infantile eczema, between three and 32 years for *prurigo*.

"Of the subjects overtaken with *prurigo*, 17 were of the female sex and four of the masculine sex. One notes in the previous hereditary history of the majority of the patients some eczema, some asthma and occasionally both. . .

"The eczematous patients presented head and especially facial eruption, associated in some with an eruption of the bend of the arms, of the elbows and of the back. The condition of the patients overtaken with Besnier's *prurigo* varied considerably in intensity according to the case, but all offered typical lesions at the bend of the arm and at the back of the knee and often at the lateral part of the neck. The hermatologic (blood) examination showed an eosinophil (white corpuscle count) varying from four to ten percent."

In all cases of infantile eczema, Dr. Patiala administered vitamin B$_2$ intramuscularly (½ to one ampule every two days according to age); the series was composed of five ampules. By contrast, Besnier's *prurigos* were treated by intravenous route and as much as possible daily, at the rate of two ampules of riboflavin, or one ampule of lactoflavine. If necessary, a second identical series was administered a month after the end of the preceding one and in some cases even a third after a delay of two to three months.

The tolerance was always perfect; no patient found discomfort even after the dose (exceptionally administered) of four ampules at one time. During the first five injections no local care was used. Then some creams or soothing pomades were applied. It is, furthermore, probable that a smaller dose of vitamin B$_2$, for example a half ampule two times per week, would have been sufficient.

The therapeutic action of riboflavin and of lactoflavine being identical, there is no place to separate the results that they give. Their rapid efficiency in the case of infantile eczema was evident; as early as the fourth day after the first injection the skin was dry, still a little scaly, but the improvement was still better characterized by the disappearance of itching; the infants, previously restless and agitated, ceased to scratch, remained quiet and slept again. When the treatment was undertaken at the acute phase, the cure occurred without relapse after a single series, and with two children, without any additional local care. In chronic eczemas of the type of Besnier's *prurigo,* the improvement was manifested by the improvement in appearance of the outbursts of acute itching.

The action of vitamin B₂ on the nervous condition merits particular mention. Disappearance of restlessness and the return of sleep were particularly noted in the children of seven to nine years of age. This and a good appetite were considered the essential ingredients for improving the general condition. The cure obtained by the riboflavin or the lactoflavine has, however, been lasting only iⁿ two cases; in the other cases relapses have occurred, but they were generally weaker than the initial attacks. In the three intricate cases of asthma with eczema, the asthma yielded first and improvement of the cutaneous symptoms followed.

Although lasting results have not always been obtained in infantile eczema and diathetic prurigo treated with riboflavin or lactoflavine, it is permissible to say that this medication represents a major contribution in the treatment of these rebellious diseases and that it helps the patients to recover from the extreme discomfort of attacks of acute itching.

Soy products appear to have some value in treating eczema. The January 10, 1957, issue of *Medical Science* carried Dr. Sidney Kane's observations on 102 infants, aged one week to nine months, whose symptoms of asthma, eczema, nasal discharge, and irritability were traced to a sensitivity to cow's milk. After soy milk was substituted, 75 of the 76 infants with eczema improved greatly.

Soybeans should always be cooked since raw soybeans contain a factor that inhibits trypsin, an important enzyme needed for protein utilization. Raw soybeans also interfere with growth by tying up such minerals as calcium and phosphorus in the body.

248. Fungus Infections: Some Are More Than Just Skin Deep

Whenever people mention fungus infections, they usually refer to fungus disorders, or mycoses, such as athlete's foot, ringworm or moniliasis, certain fungus infestations of the genital areas, infections of the mouth (causing thrush) or painful inflammations under the fingernails. These are all cutaneous (appearing on the skin) mycoses. There are, however, mycoses which appear beneath the skin, referred to as subcutaneous, which are much more dangerous and increasing in frequency, and are often misdiagnosed by physicians. These include such difficult to diagnose fungus infections as histoplasmosis, coccidioidomycosis, blastomycosis and cryptococcosis.

What has brought about the proliferation in this low form of plant life? Medical authorities are finding that the overuse of antibiotics, which weaken the body's natural defenses, is contributing to the sharply increasing incidence of a new order of diseases ranging from superficial skin infections to life-threatening lung and systemic disorders.

Fungus diseases, when they are caught early, have a good prognosis. Because they can exhibit symptoms similar to cancer, tuberculosis, brain tumors and even insanity, fungus infections present a diagnostic challenge and constitute a far greater health problem than most authorities realize, according to Dr. Libero Ajello, chief of the mycology section of the National Communicable Disease Center, Atlanta, Ga. Dr. Ajello made these comments at the Pan American Health Organization's International Symposium on the Mycoses, February 24, 1970.

It is impossible to make an accurate estimate of the prevalence of these cunning masqueraders because these mycoses mimic other diseases causing frequent misdiagnoses.

Some people afflicted with fungus infections are languishing in mental institutions and tuberculosis sanatoriums. The National Tuberculosis Association estimates that some eight thousand patients with mistaken diagnoses are still being admitted to tuberculosis sanatoriums every single year.

Some patients, because of mistaken diagnoses, are subjected to needless surgery. The case of one such example was reported in *Everywoman's Family Circle* (June, 1962). The patient, identified as Mrs. Martin, had a bad cough, looked run down, and had a fever at suppertime each evening. Chest X-rays showed a shadowy region in the upper portion of the right lung and some enlarged lymph storage cells. Even though the tuberculin test was negative, doctors considered that there was sufficient evidence to perform surgery immediately. It was then that Mrs. Martin's doctors discovered they had made an inaccurate diagnosis. The pathologist could not find a single tuberculosis germ on the tissue taken from her lung. It was diseased—but not with tuberculosis. The serum test which should have been done before surgery was ordered after the needless surgery. The verdict was clear: Mrs. Martin had histoplasmosis, considered the most common systemic fungus disease. Her doctors had been caught off guard because Mrs. Martin lived in Boston and the doctors were under the impression that histoplasmosis was found only in the Ohio and Mississippi valleys. The doctors had thought it had to be tuberculosis because of the X-rays, but this disease, like others that begin in the lungs, often fools the X-ray.

And yet, X-ray alone, without serum or skin sensitivity tests for fungus, is the major factor in establishing medical diagnosis for tuberculosis. Some patients are suspected of having lung cancer when they really have histoplasmosis.

Thousands of persons who think they have the flu or bronchial infections actually have histoplasmosis. Dr. Michael L. Furcolow, formerly chief of the United States Public Health Service, Kansas City Field Station, and now professor of community medicine at the University of Kentucky, is firmly convinced that the presence of histoplasmosis should be considered "in any patient with a persistent influenza-like illness—especially if it occurs in the summer or if there are several similar cases around. Systemic histo in very young persons," Dr. Furcolow said, "is often confused with leukemia because the organisms may grow in bone marrow."

Fungus diseases take on many disguises, too, according to Dr. Furcolow. "The fungus disease may be taken for typhoid if the patients have diarrhea and the physical examination shows enlargement of the liver and spleen," he said.

Histoplasmosis of the nervous system may also produce focal granulomas mimicking brain tumor, according to Drs. H. H.

White and T. J. Fritzlen writing in the *Journal of Neurosurgery* (19: 260-263, 1962).

Benign Bacteria Needed For Control

People who are on antibiotics and other drugs may recover from the original ailment only to fall victim to a devastating fungus infection. Drugs and radiation upset the body's natural population of microbes and thus may give fungi a foothold ordinarily denied them. These resulting fungus infections may sometimes take the life of the patient even though the medical treatment is effective against the original disease condition. For instance, invasive pulmonary aspergillosis, a fungus lesion of the lungs which resembles tuberculosis, almost always follows antibiotic or steroid therapy and is definitely increasing in incidence, reported Drs. H. Sidransky and M. Pearl in *Diseases of the Chest* (39: 630-642, 1961).

It is now known that antibiotics can impair the body's natural defense system because they destroy not only the cause of a particular distress, but also very valuable intestinal bacteria. It is your own normal population of bacteria that wars on fungal invaders and thus builds immunity. When these bacteria have been wiped out by drugs such as antibiotics, your defenses are down and you are vulnerable to attack by fungi. It could be any one of the large family of fungus diseases—depending on which one is slinking around in your neighborhood. It could be *tinca pedis* (athlete's foot) or *candida albicans* which can cause moniliasis, or it could be one of the serious systemic mycoses which are attacking more and more people, and which often mimic other diseases.

What most people do not realize and what may be an important factor contributing to the increasing incidence of fungus diseases, is that all of us are eating antibiotics without a doctor's prescription and without even being aware of it.

Penicillin and other antibiotics are sold by the pound to farmers and by the ton to feed manufacturers, it was reported in *Environment*, (January-February, 1970). Almost all of the antibiotics used in human medicine are being used as supplements to animal feeds or to treat diseases of animals.

It is a distinct possibility that the antibiotics we unknowingly eat in animal products are depleting our own native populations of bacteria and thus opening the way to infestation by the tiny fungus spores, some native and some foreign. The fungus *can-*

dida albicans, for instance, normally exists harmlessly in body openings that have damp mucous linings. When this fungus gets out of hand it causes moniliasis, which in women affects the vaginal tract and in men frequently infects the intestinal tract. No known drug is more than temporarily effective against it, while replenishment of the intestinal bacteria gets it permanently under control.

If you use commercial meats or if you have had an illness which required taking antibiotics, as soon as you go off antibiotics, try taking yogurt or acidophilus milk to help replace the friendly bacteria that help to guard you from fungus invasions. Raw fruits and vegetables, yeast, wheat germ and a good supply of vitamin A and the B vitamins also help to replenish your valuable intestinal flora.

249. Ichthyosis—The "Fish-Skin" Disease

Ichthyosis is an especially unpleasant skin disorder. It is characterized by widespread dry patches on the skin that turn dark and scaly. The skin, where it is affected, resembles fish skin in appearance, which is how the disease got its name: *ichthus* is Greek for fish.

It is not a fatal disease and its effects appear to be chiefly psychological, occasioned by the distress of the exceptionally ugly appearance of the affected skin areas. American medicine has paid little attention to ichthyosis, although thousands suffer from it. The long held belief that ichthyosis is a hereditary and incurable disease has been generally accepted among physicians.

In Egypt, however, where ichthyosis is widespread and where the extreme dryness of the climate makes it far more uncomfortable and more frequently painful to those whose skin is attacked, there was a good deal of pressure placed upon Egyptian doctors to produce a cure for ichthyosis. After much experimentation, that is just what they accomplished. In the *Egyptian Pharmaceutical Bulletin* (44, 4, April, 1962) Dr. M. R. Zawahry of Ain Shams University reported that "niacin is probably the most valuable therapeutic agent in ichthyosis. . . . Cases have been cleared entirely after a period of treatment with this vitamin. Such cases always recur when the treatment is discontinued . . ."

B₃ Deficiency

When a doctor is able to cure any disease by administering a nutrient and the disease recurs when there is a discontinuance of the nutrient, it makes for a very strong supposition that the disease is actually a deficiency of the particular nutrient. The question then arises, is it the type of deficiency that comes about because the patient has not eaten enough of the nutrient in his diet, or is it the type that occurs because of a physiological defect that makes it impossible for him to utilize the nutrient normally?

To test this question, Dr. Zawahry took a number of ichthyotic patients of various ages from three to 24 and checked urinary excretion of N-methyl nicotinamide, the final degradation product of vitamin B_3 in the body. Dr. Zawahry reasoned that if it could be shown that the nutrient, when eaten or administered, was eventually excreted as its final degradation product, then it must have gone through all the chemical transformations within the body that are necessary for the proper metabolism of that vitamin.

No Heredity Involved

Dr. Zawahry found that while the original vitamin B_3 levels of the ichthyotic patients were low, administration of large doses resulted in perfectly normal serum levels that matched expected limits of normalcy.

Dr. Zawahry demonstrated that if ichthyosis is indeed a deficiency of niacin, it is not due to any hereditary fault in the metabolism. It is simply a failure of the patient to get enough niacin in his diet. Niacin, one of the B complex vitamins, is found in supplements of desiccated liver, brewer's yeast and wheat germ. Ichthyosis is not a disease we see often, and perhaps we never thought of preventing it by watching our B complex intake.

250. Types Of Burns And Their Treatment

Serious burns are usually classed as second, third and fourth degree burns. The higher the degree, the greater the depth and severity of the burn. Most of us have experienced a first degree burn, the type in which the skin becomes reddened and irritated, but does not blister or break. An ordinary sunburn is considered a first degree burn. In second degree burns there is partial destruction of the skin, but it is not lifeless. Blistering is the most common indication of a second degree burn. In third or fourth degree burns, the skin has been destroyed through its full thickness, sometimes through underlying tissues down to the bone. It is dry and firm, leathery to the touch. A charred-appearing skin is the mark of a fourth degree burn.

Techniques used in the treatment of burns have improved in recent years and have increased the chances of survival considerably. Fifteen years ago, recovery from burns which covered one-third, or more, of the body was uncommon. Today, even if one should sustain serious burns that cover as much as half of the body area, the possibility of recovery is strong.

There are three main phases in the clinical history of serious burns. The first is a period of shock, in which there are pronounced shifts in body fluids and electrolytes in the burned area, a loss of plasma and protein, and possible damage to various organs, as well as the involved tissue. This period, which is in force from the moment the burn is incurred, is followed by a critical second period during which secondary anemia usually develops and infection of the injured area is likely. This stage lasts for about 10 days to two weeks, and is followed by the final period of healing and repair.

One often sees the term "shock" used in connection with severe burns. Shock is a condition in which the blood pressure is reduced to a point of severe danger. This reduction may be the result of a loss of blood through a break in the skin, a constriction of the blood vessels, or a loss of body fluids that rush to nourish some injured part of the body.

This last is the case with shock due to burns. Body fluids are dispatched to the burned tissue to supply nourishment to the cells. These fluids seep through the skin and are lost. If they are not quickly replaced through transfusions, the body's process can be so impaired by lack of blood supply that death soon follows. Shock is, therefore, the most important single consideration in the first moments after a victim incurs a severe burn.

Many physicians rely heavily upon extra doses of proper food elements in treating burns: a high protein intake is generally considered essential to the cure of burns, and as much as 400 grams of protein per day may be prescribed, and with it, one gram of ascorbic acid (vitamin C) daily, and large doses of the B vitamins.

The burn patient's nutritional state is of extreme importance so that healing can come from within. The use of drugs often closes wounds superficially, then they show infection at a later time and must be treated by grafts and diet.

One of the nutrients hailed specifically for its effectiveness in treating burns is vitamin E (alpha tocopherol). Wilfred E. Shute, M.D., in his book "Vitamin E For Ailing and Healthy Hearts" (Pyramid), writes: "I have learned that vitamin E is of maximum use in treating burns, from the small domestic burn, due to contact with a heated iron or a stove burner or scalding steam and water, to the most severe third degree burns. Here the results are more important, because the scars that result from vitamin E treatment are unique and uniformly render unnecessary the usual costly, protracted skin grafting with resultant pain and agony to the patient."

One consequence of severe injuries from burns is to force potassium out of damaged cells and sodium from the blood stream into them. The excess potassium then meanders through the body, slowing down heart action. At the same time, to replace the sodium lost to the cells, the blood stream taps its own reservoirs of salt water. This results in falling blood pressure, kidney slow-up and even fainting spells. Drinking literally gallons of saline solution (adults with severe burn have spontaneously swilled down more than 10 quarts in a twenty-four hour period) enables the blood stream to replenish its stock of sodium, blood pressure goes up again and the kidneys speed up in pumping the potassium out of the body. It is all simply a matter of keeping the vital sodium-potassium-water balance of the body normal.

Fortunately, for most of us, our experience with burns is limited to the painful but minor consequences of contact with hot pots, matches and radiators. First aid remedies for these vary from house to house and doctor to doctor. Most people put some kind of grease over the burn, some do nothing and "let the air get at it," in spite of instinct which tells us to plunge the burn into cold water to take the heat away. The *American Medical Association* recommends ice water as the best first aid measure for burns covering up to 20 percent of the body.

Soak the burned area immediately in a basin containing tap water, ice cubes and a disinfectant. For burns of the head, neck, chest, etc., where immersion is impractical, apply towels chilled in a bucket of ice water. The cold treatment is continued until it can be stopped without return of pain—usually within 30 minutes to 5 hours. Although the primary injurious effect of the burn has taken place, the usual inflammatory process secondary to the burn can be reduced in degree and at times reversed by ice-water therapy. The time factor between injury and treatment determines the result. This treatment should be initiated at once. This would be far more effective first aid treatment than applying butter or grease which will only have to be painfully removed by the attending physician.

Preventing burns is easier and less painful than treating them: It is sad to report that 70 percent of all burns occur in or near the home and involve children under five years of age. The number one cause of these fires is clothing which becomes inflamed when it brushes burning trash, a fireplace or is ignited in that most fascinating and disastrous of all childhood games, playing with matches. Because they are usually fuller and frillier, girls' clothes more often figure in accidents of this type. It is up to the parents to see that their children learn to respect fire and to stay away from it. It is hard to think of any time in a child's life when there is a need for him to deal with fire: oil lamps and gas lights are no more; fireplaces, which are rare, should never be lighted by children and should be kept screened when burning. Most furnaces are now automatically fired and a child need not even be aware of their existence.

As for the ever-present fascination that matches seem to exert, the problem must be met before trouble starts. The child must be made to realize that matches are out of the domain of his playthings, that they are not to be touched by him. After you feel that this lesson has been carefully impressed upon the child, resolve to keep temptation out of his way. Remove all matches from places accessible to him, and make sure that they are not left by someone else in a place he might be able to reach.

It is difficult to exaggerate the dangers of hot liquids when children are around. A few basic precautions can prevent tragedy. First of all, keep children out of the kitchen when hot liquids are being handled; children can easily bump or trip you and the hot stuff might spill down on them. If your stove is such that the handles to cookpots can protrude over the edge, always make certain that the handles are turned in, toward the back of the stove. A child's fingers, tipping a pan in curiosity, can lead to a serious accident. Don't let children try their hand at cooking unless you can spare the time to supervise and give them your full attention. Stoves and children are a hazardous combination.

251. A Prickly Heat Treatment That Works

Prickly heat, technically known as *malaria rubra papulosa,* is a common summertime ailment affecting both infants and adults, although in temperate climates such as ours, infants suffer from it more frequently than adults. When it does afflict adults, it is usually restricted to the inside of the thighs at the groin.

The rash itself is composed of tiny, slightly inflamed pimples which develop on the skin surface, accompanied by a tingling and itching sensation. In a few days the pimples become blisters containing a milky substance. Once the pimples break and disappear, which is usually quite soon after they first appear, they leave tiny scabs which flake off.

The rash usually develops very quickly as a result of excessive sweating, and can occur wherever such sweating takes place. For instance, if one side of a baby's face is pressed against the pillow or a nurse's body for any length of time, prickly heat can be expected. If a diaper is tight and warm and produces profuse sweating, the rash will probably develop.

The irritating itch of the rash, especially in children, becomes unbearable. The youngsters scratch the irritation, it becomes infected, and a much more serious problem then ensues. Parents usually resign themselves to the idea that prickly heat, when it develops, must be allowed to run its natural course. In the interim, they may use cooling and allaying agents to lessen the itching, such as the excessive use of talcum powder. According to recent findings on talc, it would appear that the cure is worse than the disease since talc is linked closely with asbestos, a mineral fiber known to have carcinogenic capabilities.

A wise and cautious substitute that parents will find just as effective as talcum powder, and just as effective in the pain relief it can provide, is natural cornstarch.

Vitamin C As A Treatment
Aside from cornstarch, there may be an even more natural and positive means of curing, and even preventing, the irritation of

prickly heat—vitamin C. Dr. T. C. Hindson, a British dermatologist in Singapore, gave evidence of vitamin C's value in an article entitled, "Ascorbic Acid for Prickly Heat," published in the British medical journal *Lancet* (June 22, 1968).

Dr. Hindson had a large number of patients in Singapore— including some adults—who suffered from intractable prickly heat. One of these patients was an Australian Air Force officer whose acute case of intertriginous dermatitis, or prickly heat, suddenly cleared up after he took one gram of vitamin C daily to help get rid of a cold.

To determine if this was a true cause-and-effect relationship or a mere coincidence, Dr. Hindson designed a classic double-blind trial using 30 children ranging in age from four months to eight years, all of whom had suffered from prickly heat for at least eight weeks. He geared the dosage to what the Air Force officer had taken, which amounted to 15 mg. of vitamin C for every 2.2 pounds of body weight. In other words, a child weighing 19 pounds received a daily dose of 125 mg. of vitamin C. "Where a child was too young to take tablets," Dr. Hindson noted, "parents were instructed to administer them crushed with food."

After only two weeks, 14 of the 15 children who had been taking vitamin C were improved or completely free from the bothersome rash. In the group of 15 other children who had been given dummy pills, only four improved. All 30 were then given ascorbic acid. Examinations conducted one month and then two months after this time revealed that not one patient had signs of prickly heat. During the periods between examinations, only a very few of the children had minor recurrences of the rash.

Dr. Hindson isn't sure why the vitamin works. Past research, however, suggests that prickly heat occurs when the sweat glands in a particular area of the body stop working. These glands usually stop functioning because of fatigue. They have been overtaxed and overworked for too long and just become inactive. That is why prickly heat and similar irritations of the groin are common in hot climates where the sweat glands are continually taxed.

While admitting that the exact mechanism by which vitamin C prevents prickly heat has not been established, Dr. Hindson said that vitamin C acts as a hydrogen ion carrier for certain enzyme systems which relate to the sweat glands. When the sweat glands are overtaxed, perhaps a shortage of the vitamin develops and the enzyme does not function properly.

The Skin

Another possibility Dr. Hindson suggested is that "the vitamin in large doses might take over the action of, or replenish some essential but fatigued enzyme system—such as the succinic-dehydrogenase system—which Dodson (1958) showed was the first to disappear on excess sweating. . ."

Dr. Hindson reported that vitamin C levels have never been determined in sweat collected from individuals on high ascorbic acid intake. But what this researcher has proven rather conclusively is that, "Ascorbic acid, when given in high doses, is effective in the treatment and prevention of prickly heat."

252. Pruritus Ani

Pruritus ani, itching or burning of the rectum, is a condition commonly experienced but generally neglected in magazines for the public. The rectum is a very likely location for this type of contact dermatitis. Not only are the sources of contact more numerous than one would imagine (soap, clothing, toilet tissue, enema nozzles, suppositories, orally administered antibiotics which have passed through the digestive system and laxatives), but the area is moist and covered, so that germs and fungi have an excellent breeding ground. The residues of the foods we eat, which pass out of the body in fecal matter, might also cause a reaction with the tender skin of the rectum. This is especially true of such foods as mustard, horseradish and hot peppers.

Moisture, which is usually aggravating to skin rashes, is constantly present in the rectal area due to a system of sweat glands which are part of the sexual glandular system. These glands are highly responsive to emotion or sexual tension, so that a person in a highly emotional state or one who is excited sexually exudes large amounts of perspiration in this region. The perspiration which is released here is high in protein and carbohydrates, two elements which favor the growth of bacteria. This increased moisture also leads to the release of dyes from clothing worn in this region, and these dyes can initiate or aggravate a condition of pruritus ani. Once the condition exists, the itching is more severe than in most areas of the body, due perhaps to the abundant nerve supply and the delicacy of the skin. Few victims can resist scratching, and the added irritation only causes a worsening of the condition.

Diet And Pruritus Ani

It is known that pruritus ani is sometimes coupled with a lack of certain dietary constituents. Vitamin A and the B complex, as well as iron, are often mentioned in this connection. Diabetes is frequently accompanied by a fungus infection of the rectum, due to the high sugar content of the skin, which favors the growth of fungi. Good diet would be the very first thing to check— sufficient B vitamin foods (liver, brewer's yeast, wheat germ, sunflower seeds) and those rich in vitamin A (carrots, squash, dark green vegetables) and iron (grapes and raisins, celery, liver). Some researchers have found that excessive use of citrus juices could cause an irritation of this area.

Effective treatment of this condition is based on these general principles: keep the area clean by careful removal of all fecal matter and sensible hygiene habits; do not scratch through clothing, as harmful dyes are readily introduced in this way (white underclothes should be worn to lessen this possibility); the area should be kept as dry as possible, and no ointments or greasy salves should be used.

253. Safe, Effective Psoriasis Therapy

More than six million Americans suffer from the chronic anguish of psoriasis. Irregularly shaped and slightly raised dull red blotches appear on the sufferer's skin. These characteristic patches of psoriasis are covered by grayish or silvery scales, which if scratched, will peel and flake off like dandruff. This skin disorder can afflict people at any age, and although it is not contagious, it does appear to run in families.

The lesions of psoriasis, which in the early stages can be misdiagnosed as ringworm, may appear anywhere on the body but the face, which for some unknown reason seems immune to the unsightly blemishes of psoriasis. However, psoriasis does afflict certain parts of the body more than others, such as the scalp (psoriasis of the scalp is often mistaken for dandruff), elbows, knees and the trunk of the body.

The medical profession ascribes no definite cause to this embarrassing and unsightly disease, and no sure cure either. "Psoriasis is an antidote for the dermatologist's ego," remarked Dr. P. Bechet, an eminent dermatologist and medical historian. This vexatious scaling disease forces its sufferers to try everything in the dermatologist's chemical arsenal—tar, mercury Chrysarobin and phenol. These may bring some measure of transient relief, but in recurrent outbreaks the repulsive blotches are there again in full bloom, bigger than ever, redder and itchier. In some instances dermatologists resort to X-ray therapy, which carries the obvious risk of dangerous side effects.

Unfortunately, one of the medications in current use that brings the most relief, also exacts the highest price in side effects. It is Methotrexate, a highly toxic anti-cancer drug which is known to cause severe liver damage. Conceived for the treatment of leukemia, this drug, an anti-metabolite, has been used against psoriasis with FDA blessing long enough to cause the death of dozens of psoriasis patients. While the drug is recommended only for severe, recalcitrant cases of psoriasis, it was reported at the Fountain Subcommittee Hearings held in July,

1971, that between 50,000 and 100,000 psoriatic patients were receiving this drug which can cause ulcers in the mouth, esophageal bleeding, bone marrow damage, and severe liver damage including cirrhosis.

Other drugs frequently prescribed are steroids, such as ACTH (a synthetic hormone) and cortisone, and their derivatives. These sometimes lead to problems far worse than the original ailment. But most psoriasis victims are so desperate that they willingly take the calculated risk inherent in the steroids. Unfortunately, any positive result is generally temporary. Steroids often lead to severe recurrences and adverse reactions. Cortisone causes urinary losses of calcium and phosphorus, resulting in demineralization of the bones which can become so porous that an exertion no stronger than a sneeze might break a rib. An added problem with steroid therapy is severe depression; it invites ulcers and adrenal exhaustion with a subsequent drain on recuperative powers. It also weakens the body's defenses so that dormant, forgotten infections can take hold once more.

A Successful Treatment

There is one successful "drug," however, that has the approval of the FDA but, ironically, is rarely prescribed by physicians. It is the topical application of vitamin A acid, the salvation of the acne patient. The advantages of vitamin A acid for psoriasis were first observed in double-blind controlled studies by Drs. Phillip Frost and Gerald D. Weinstein, both of the Department of Dermatology, University of Miami School of Medicine. The doctors discovered that vitamin A, in its acid form, brought remarkable relief from the itching and unsightliness of psoriasis in 24 out of 26 patients, and these effects were noticeable after only a week's treatment (*Journal of the American Medical Association*, March 10, 1969).

Prior to their clinical studies, Drs. Frost and Weinstein first compared the effects of several commonly available forms of topically administered vitamin A (vitamin A acid, vitamin A aldehyde, vitamin A alcohol, and vitamin A acetate) on three patients who had extensive psoriasis and three patients with ichthyosis (dry scaly skin). After one week, the area which had vitamin A acid applied to it showed markedly decreased scaling among the patients with the dry, rough, scaling skin of ichthyosis and much less redness among those patients with psoriasis. No changes were discernible where the other forms of vitamin A had been applied.

The superior healing properties demonstrated by vitamin A acid in this simple patch test encouraged Drs. Frost and Weinstein to make a more extensive evaluation of vitamin A acid. They chose patients with those skin conditions most resistant to all kinds of treatment—10 with epidermolytic hyperkeratosis, in which the skin becomes hard and loose; 24 with some form of ichthyosis and 26 with extensive psoriasis. Vitamin A acid scored major points in almost every patient, especially those with disorders which do not usually respond to the dermatologist's efforts. The improvement was dramatic in patients with psoriasis. It is interesting to note that the improvement resulting from vitamin A acid usually lasted 10 to 14 days after discontinuing therapy.

Of course, the very vitamin from which vitamin A acid is derived has been shown as effective in the treatment of psoriasis. Halibut liver oil is an excellent source of both vitamin A and its working partner, vitamin D, which might also have an ameliorative effect on psoriasis. D is the sunshine vitamin, and it has been observed that psoriasis improves in the summer because of day to day exposure to the sun. It almost never appears on the face and hands, which have more exposure to the sun than the rest of the body.

Physicians have given 200,000 vitamin A units daily for six months, according to J. M. Lewis and colleagues, writing in the *Journal of Pediatrics*, (31, 496, 1947) without observing any signs of toxicity. However, it is considered advisable to limit intake of less than 50,000 units of vitamin A daily, unless you are being supervised by a physician.

Years ago it was determined that what sometimes seems to be a deficiency of vitamin A, may be a deficiency of vitamin E. Unless vitamin E is amply supplied, the vitamin A obtained from both foods and supplements, the vitamin A already in the blood, and that which is stored in the liver and other body tissues, is quickly destroyed by oxygen (*Biochemical Journal* 34, 1321, 1940).

Good Nutrition Is Vital

While stressing the use of ointments, salves and medicated poultices which afford only temporary relief at best, physicians all too often overlook the patient's diet in treating psoriasis. Medical research has more than amply shown that psoriasis is, at least to some extent, an affliction involving defective metabolism and a faulty diet. Of those researchers who have treated the disease successfully, many have concerned themselves chiefly with the element of diet involved in fat metabolism.

More than twenty years ago, Doctors Paul Gross and Beatrice M. Kesten, both with the Department of Dermatology at the Columbia-Presbyterian Medical Center, reported success in treating psoriasis with soybean lecithin. Lecithin supplements are almost always derived from the soybean plant, but lecithin also occurs naturally in unrefined grains such as wheat germ, nuts, seed foods, whole grains and vegetable oils.

In their studies the doctors eliminated eggs, fatty meats, poultry, fish, cheese and excessive amounts of butter and cream from their patients' diets in order to run the experiment on a strict low fat regimen. The lecithin was distributed to the 235 subjects, along with vitamins A and D and the B vitamins thiamin, pyridoxine, riboflavin and pantothenic acid. Because of the restricted diet, the doctors considered it important to administer vitamin supplements, but felt certain the lecithin was responsible for the therapeutic results in this case. Out of the total figure, the researchers considered that 155 were adequately treated. The rest either did not cooperate or abandoned the diet before any conclusions could be drawn. The majority of patients experienced satisfactory control of their psoriasis, and 66 subjects showed some improvement, but required therapeutic ointments in addition to the lecithin in order to bolster their progress.

The researchers concluded that "this form of therapy is capable of correcting some of the metabolic defects but not the actual cause of the disease." They recommended a low fat diet, plus a lipotropic, or fat-emulsifying substance such as lecithin to control psoriasis.

In 1965 Dr. Daphne Roe, a dermatologist and nutritionist at Cornell University, told the annual meeting of the New York State Medical Society that psoriasis may be more serious than is usually assumed. Dr. Roe warned that the continual loss of skin tissue can cause enormous losses of vitamin and mineral nutrients. Even people who eat a normally good diet, she said, might develop nutritional deficiencies in the wake of psoriasis.

The use of B vitamins in treating psoriasis can't be overlooked. *The Journal of Investigative Dermatology* reported that riboflavin (vitamin B_2) taken both orally and by injection, seemed to help in some psoriasis cases. Dr. Merlin Maynard, who conducted the research, reported that this treatment healed lesions in 25 percent of the patients, and improved most of the rest. In some cases the beneficial results lasted for two years after the treatment was discontinued.

Dr. John F. Madden, a physician in St. Paul, Minnesota, has achieved positive results in treating psoriasis with vitamin B_1 (thiamin), an ointment and a low fat diet. Reporting in the *Journal of the American Medical Association*, he said that, after experimenting with various treatments, vitamin B_1 was the most beneficial, bringing definite improvement to one-third of the patients who tried it. In addition to thiamin and riboflavin, some physicians have reported good results with vitamin B_{12}, when continued for as long as 30 days.

Psoriasis sufferers should really be conscious of every mouthful of food they eat. They should avoid meat and dairy fats. The only acceptable fats are unsaturated fats, such as those in eggs, salad oils and other vegetable sources such as sunflower seeds, avocados and raw nuts. Not only are they valuable for psoriasis, but they also help melt fat deposits and keep cholesterol emulsified, circulating and supplying energy instead of menacing health.

Patients should avoid hydrogenated shortenings, the thick white ones many people use for frying and baking. Margarine is also hydrogenated. Psoriasis sufferers will do well to shun the hidden fats which they are bound to encounter if they buy any packaged foods at all or if they eat in restaurants. Crackers are crisp because of the hydrogenated shortening they contain.

Food supplements can supply vitamins A and D (plentiful in fish liver oils), and the B vitamins (wheat germ, brewer's yeast or desiccated liver are the best sources); lecithin and/or the unsaturated fatty acids are available in flakes or in capsules. These lecithin supplements, derived chiefly from soybeans, should be a staple in the diet of every psoriasis sufferer.

254. Purpura: The Bruising Disease

Purpura, commonly known as the bruising disease, is a hemorrhagic disorder characterized by spontaneous bruising or bleeding, petechiae (tiny bumps) in the skin and mucous membranes, and sometimes a marked decrease in circulating platelets. The disease, once considered rare, appears to be increasing in frequency, especially among women.

According to researchers, it appears that this increase is due to the heavier use of estrogens, both for birth control and as adjuncts in the treatment of menopausal side effects. Estrogen, it has already been determined, is a vitamin E antagonist. It can cause a deficiency of this important nutrient which, among other well documented benefits to your body, can actually help to preserve the integrity of the capillary walls.

Purpura, according to a study published in the *Journal of Vitaminology* (18, 125-130, 1972) could very well be a colorful manifestation of a vitamin E deficiency. The ability of vitamin E to erase those purple spots and correct thrombocytopenic purpura in animals was demonstrated more than 20 years ago by Dr. Floyd Skelton when he was a research assistant to Dr. Evan Shute at the Shute Institute. Dr. Skelton used estrogen to induce thrombocytopenic purpura in dogs. He subsequently cured them with vitamin E and, by using large doses of vitamin E, was able to prevent purpura even when estrogen was administered (*Vitamin E For Ailing and Healthy Hearts*, Pyramid, 1969).

People with purpura, however, are still being subjected to steroid therapy with its devastating side effects. While the spots frequently provoke a shower of insinuating jests, anyone who's ever had it knows that purpura isn't funny. But purpura need not be tragic or tiresome, now that it can be cured with medications without dangerous side effects.

Japanese Study
Vitamin E as a treatment for purpura was first tested on patients in Japan. Dr. Takaaki Fujii of the Utsunomya Hospital used

vitamin E on seven patients with purpura between the ages of 16 and 54. All of them appeared to be well nourished and showed no signs of scurvy (capillary fragility, sometimes a precipitating factor in purpura, and the result of a vitamin C deficiency). When Dr. Fujii administered vitamin E to all of these patients in dosages of 400 to 600 milligrams orally every day, he noted quick recoveries and disappearance of all spots in two to four weeks.

Estrogen is not the only drug which is a vitamin E antagonist. A 16-year-old boy treated by Dr. Fujii had a sore throat, cough, headache and high fever due to an upper respiratory tract infection for five days, and then developed extensive multiple petechiae on his arms and his legs. Physical examination revealed nothing else of significance other than a slight swelling of both tonsils. Vitamin E therapy was started two days after the petechiae developed. Four hundred milligrams were given every day for one week. At the end of the week, most of the petechiae had disappeared. At the end of two weeks on the same dosage, there were no petechiae.

Another patient, an 18-year-old boy, had no fever or any sign of infection prior to the onset of the little purplish-red spots. His family doctor had been treating him with a series of drugs including a cortisone derivative. Despite the treatment, the petechiae did not disappear completely and the young man came to Dr. Fujii's hospital where he was started on vitamin E therapy immediately. After 400 milligrams of vitamin E were given daily for one week, most petechiae disappeared and two weeks after the therapy began, none remained.

Another patient, a young woman of 22, had had a sore throat and fever for three days, then developed edema (swelling) around the eyelids, red colored skin eruptions accompanied by swelling on her face and extensive urticaria (elevated itching patches of skin) and petechiae over her whole body. From the physical findings and the blood examination, the edema, eruptions, urticaria and petechiae were considered to be due to increased permeability of the walls of the blood vessels. Vitamin E, 400 milligrams daily, was started on the day she came to the hospital, and after five days, the edema around both eyelids and the red colored eruptions of the face disappeared completely. Most of the petechiae also disappeared and in Dr. Fujii's words, "she looked to be an entirely different person." After 10 days, the urticaria and the petechiae also disappeared completely.

While the mechanism of the anti-purpuric action of vitamin E for vascular purpura is not entirely clear, Dr. Fujii feels that, since vitamin E was also effective in improving local edema, urticaria or skin eruptions in addition to its effect on petechiae, this would suggest that vitamin E has an "inhibiting action on the increased permeability of the capillary walls due to various factors such as infection, drugs, and others." He noted that Dr. M. Kamimura has observed in his experiments on human skin that when he used various chemicals such as histamine, acetyl-choline, and a-chymotrypsin he was able to stimulate capillary permeability and was then able to reduce this permeability by using alpha tocopherol acetate, 300 milligrams, for five to seven days (*Vitamins*, 28, 129, 1961).

255. Something Can Be Done For Vitiligo

Vitiligo is a painless disease that usually afflicts people between the ages of two and 30 and is characterized by the sudden appearance of light blotches on the skin. The light patches enlarge slowly, marked by a dark border. The white patches occur because the skin, for some still unknown reason, is unable to manufacture melanin, or pigment, creating an embarrassing piebald pattern on the skin surface. It afflicts people with all skin tones, although it is more pronounced in people with dark pigmentations.

There is little discussion of the disease in medical textbooks, except for detailed descriptions of it. The impression is that the medical profession sees little to be done for the victims of vitiligo except to recommend cosmetics (usually for those with light skin tones) and caution against sunbathing, since a tan only heightens the contrast between those areas with vitiligo and those that can form normal pigment.

Several years ago, Dr. Benjamin Sieve, a professor at Tufts Medical School, compiled a comprehensive history of the treatments in use dating back to the 1930's and 1940's, and the then-current thinking on the subject. Among the treatments described by Dr. Sieve was one used by Dr. H. W. Francis. He thought the disease was due to the absence of free hydrochloric acid in the stomach, since he had vitiligo and found the acid absent in himself. He took 15 cubic centimeter doses of hydrochloric acid at each meal for two years and noted that the light areas completely disappeared. He used the same therapy on three other patients and reported similar results. Dr. Sieve suggested that the effect of the hydrochloric acid might have been to aid in the processing and absorption of necessary nutrients.

Nutrition as a factor in preserving skin pigment was reported in the *Archives of Dermatology and Syphilology* (March, 1937), where researchers detailed experiments using vitamin C to restore skin color. The following year a German medical journal carried an article also recommending vitamin C as a treatment for vitiligo.

Para-amino-benzoic acid (PABA), a B vitamin, has been mentioned repeatedly in connection with the treatment of vitiligo. Dr. M. J. Costello, in the *Archives of Dermatology and Syphilology* (February, 1943) reported success in treating vitiligo of the eyelids in a two-year-old child with 100 mg. of PABA daily. Dr. Sieve was impressed with the potential of PABA, and set up an experiment to observe its effect on 48 cases of vitiligo.

The group consisted of 25 females and 23 males, ranging in age from 10 to 70 years. The vitiligo condition had persisted from two to 28 years. Most of the patients showed evidence of a chronically poor diet and a history of gland imbalance. Fatigue, irritability and emotional instability were common among them, as were constipation, weight gain, arthritis and various types of headaches. Physical examinations presented classic findings consistent with an underactive thyroid condition in many of the subjects. Along with these came a preponderance of brittle nails, coarse and thickened skin and varying degrees of hypertension (high blood pressure).

After only partial success with administering a patent combination of B complex vitamins, Dr. Sieve instituted injections of the vitamin, coupled with monoethanolamine (to help the vitamin remain in the blood longer) twice daily—morning and evening—and a 100 mg. tablet of PABA to be taken at noon and at bedtime. He soon observed new pigmentation in the depigmented areas. Within four to eight weeks the milk white areas of vitiligo turned pinkish. In six to 16 weeks after therapy was started, small islands of brown pigment were usually noted within the areas of vitiligo. Soon streaks were thrown from these islands and the streaks reached out to join other islands. Eventually the islands disappeared and the repigmentation became complete. The results of the therapy in all 48 patients were termed "striking" after six or seven months.

Dr. Sieve stressed, time and again, the important part diet plays in vitiligo. In his opinion hormonal imbalance can also cause the disease, and contributory factors can be wounds, infections, pressure points and light rays. The problem of vitiligo is more complex than the simple lack of the B vitamin PABA. According to Dr. Sieve's research, dietary deficiencies must be corrected, hormonal imbalances righted and local infections cleared up before a single specific vitamin can be expected to have any effect. He also emphasized that the injections to supplement the tablets are essential, because the vitamin alone, taken orally, does not remain in the blood stream for a sufficient length of time to act effectively.

256. Warts—Resistance Is The Answer

The common wart, although uncomfortable, unsightly, and often excruciatingly painful (when they are on the bottom of the foot), may be nature's way of signaling trouble ahead. Philadelphia radiologist Dr. Robert P. Barden demonstrated that an eruption of warty growths, or dermatomyositis, might herald a hidden malignancy. However, this is not to say that everyone with warts is harboring a pre-cancerous condition. It does mean, though, that the appearance of warts has an important biological significance which it would be wise to investigate.

Why is it that of all the so-called wart cures, no one method is effective in all cases? The answer to this therapeutic riddle, according to Dr. Daniel Hyman of New York City's Roosevelt Hospital, lies in the viral origin of warts. They disappear when the body's immunologic mechanism is stimulated. The patient himself produces the antibodies. These agents interfere with viral propagation or actually destroy the viruses outright.

Vitamin A Improves Resistance

Now, what are these host-produced biologic agents and why do some people seem to have an ample supply while others do not? Whatever these still poorly defined immunologic agents are, their power is enhanced when the body is amply supplied with vitamin A, long recognized as the special guardian of eyes, teeth, bones, skin and soft tissues—the anti-infection vitamin.

Dr. B. H. Kuhn, writing in the *Southern Medical Journal,* reported treating 90 patients with various types of warts with vitamin A palmitate in a water dispersible form averaging 25,000 units daily for one week to six months. Cure rates of 50 to 100 percent were obtained in 79 patients. There were *no* total failures. Dr. Kuhn suggested in his reports that the vitamin A exerted an *anti-viral* action that has specific therapeutic usefulness in the suppression of hyperkeratosis, or warts.

Some authorities believe that a wart develops where there is a lack of vitamin A in the skin and that introducing the vitamin will bring the skin back to normal. Dr. Marvin Sandler, a podiatrist in Allentown, Pennsylvania, said that he has used an injection of vitamin A on patients with plantar warts with excellent results. Another Allentown podiatrist, Dr. Philip LeShay, said that he prescribes vitamin A systemically in conjunction with other measures in the treatment of warts on the feet.

In the July, 1959, issue of *Clinical Medicine,* two researchers reported on the results achieved by 119 physicians who, among them, treated 228 cases of plantar warts with an aqueous solution of vitamin A palmitate. Substantial benefits or complete cures were achieved in 208 of the 228 cases. In only one case did the warts reappear.

In a controlled study of 25 patients at the Jewish Hospital of Brooklyn, N.Y., Dr. Joel S. Freeman and his colleagues concluded that the incidence of permanent cures and permanent relief of symptoms is so high when vitamin A palmitate is used, that it is difficult to justify repeated paring and application of keratolytics (usually salicylic acids) and astringents unless vitamin A palmitate has been found to be ineffective. Vitamin A palmitate, Dr. Freeman noted, should be tried before resorting to less conservative methods such as surgery, radiation or stronger caustics.

The fact that both warts and malignancies are on the increase might indicate an increasing inability in the general population to manufacture antibodies. Could this inability be related to the increasing depletion of vitamin A in our foods? W. M. Beeson, Ph.D., of the Department of Animal Sciences at Purdue University warns that our vitamin A food sources are victims of synthetic nitrogen fertilizers. These compounds act on plants to limit the amount of vitamin A they contain.

Vitamin A is abundant in fats which most calorie-conscious people are avoiding, thus compounding their deficiencies. The reduction in intake can be made up, however, with low-calorie foods rich in A, such as pumpkin, carrots, spinach, kale, leaf broccoli, sweet potatoes, apricots, asparagus, parsley, olives, peaches, peas, green and red peppers. Liver of all kinds is rich in vitamin A and lower in calories than muscle meats.

Section 55
Avoiding Ailments of Teeth and Gums

257. Don't Ignore The Real Cause Of Tooth Decay

Surprising as it seems, the best available evidence indicates that those groups of people who have the best teeth in the world don't know what a toothbrush is, while those who have half a dozen perched above the bathroom sink are quite likely to wind up with a complete set of dentures.

Actually, the experts know perfectly well what causes tooth decay. Listen to what one of the leading researchers in the United States said at the convention of the American Association for the Advancement of Science (AAAS) in 1971: "Sucrose seems to have emerged as the prime villain in the dental caries story. From a great number of studies, we know this is one of the prime factors in estimating the cariogenic (cavity-causing) challenge." And this remark from another top researcher: "The major cause of tooth decay is what doctors used to call galloping consumption—the galloping consumption of sugar." Now those two statements would seem to be rather plain and clear: eating sugar is the most important cause of tooth decay, and it stands to reason, therefore, that if you don't want your teeth to rot, you shouldn't eat sugar.

Primitive Hawaiians Had Beautiful Teeth
But the message is even plainer than that: both scientists showed that compared to eliminating sugar intake, every other caries-preventing measure dwindles to insignificance. Dr. Harris J. Keene, Chief of the Epidemiology Division of the Naval Dental Research Institute at Great Lakes, Ill., told fellow scientists at the AAAS session in Philadelphia how the teeth of ancient Hawaiians compared to the teeth of the naval recruits he had seen over the years. The primitive teeth were found in the skeletal remains of Hawaiians who had lived several hundred years ago, before white men reached the islands. Naturally, these people had no toothpaste, with or without fluoride; no tooth-brushes (as we know them), manual or electric; no dental floss,

with or without wax; and no dentists, with or without the budget payment plan.

Nevertheless, nine out of 10 of these ancient Hawaiians under the age of 25 did not have a single cavity in their mouths, Dr. Keene reported. Among naval recruits tested at Great Lakes in 1970, however, more than 99 percent had decayed teeth!

Dr. Keene told all this to his audience in Philadelphia, but the message didn't carry very far. Scientists—unlike toothpaste manufacturers—don't put ads on TV, and TV executives don't produce documentaries proving that their sponsors' products are useless. It's no great wonder that most people are still in the dark about the most widespread disease in the world—tooth decay.

On the other hand, scientists themselves don't get very excited about the fact that diet is the key to dental health. Dr. Irwin D. Mandel, director of the Division of Preventive Dentistry at Columbia University, typified the attitude of modern researchers in the talk he gave at the dental science conclave in Philadelphia. He began by making the startling statement that in Southeast Asia, the caries rate is 0.5 percent, which means that one tooth in 200 has a cavity, while in Western countries like the U.S., the caries rate is 25 percent, or 50 times as much. He followed this with his remark about the "galloping consumption of sugar" and then left the subject altogether to spend the rest of his talk discussing the difficulties involved in chemically analyzing the difference between healthy teeth and carious teeth. Likewise, Dr. Keene, while also briefly mentioning the superb dental health of the ancient Hawaiians, spent most of his time reviewing possible factors involved in why one percent of Americans don't get cavities.

With no disrespect to either of these dedicated researchers, it's clear that they're much more interested in chemical complexities and statistical anomalies than they are in proclaiming to the American people that 90 percent of all tooth decay is preventable. Another reason why today's dental scientists aren't bubbling over with enthusiasm as a result of the ancient Hawaiian discoveries or the figures from Southeast Asia is that all this was known and fully documented many years ago. Some of it dates back to 1914. And yet, today, the facts are largely ignored by professionals and all but unknown by laymen.

The Facts Most People Don't Know

Here is some of what the public doesn't know about tooth decay, who gets it and why, as explained by Dr. Weston A. Price, dental researcher and physical anthropologist, in his 500-page classic, *Nutrition and Physical Degeneration,* first published in 1938. What he reported was based on his own personal examination of thousands of human beings in every corner of the world, not on professional doctrine, statistical manipulation, or animal experimentation.

In the early 1930's, Dr. Price went to Switzerland, and with the help of local authorities, began prying into mouths. In the high Alpine village of Ayer,he discovered that only 2.3 percent of all the teeth he examined were carious. This means that on the average, among any three people, there would be a total of about two cavities. Perhaps you think the Swiss are a hardy breed. Well, the people in Ayer are, but when Dr. Price went down the road to the nearby town of Vissoie, he discovered that the percentage of decayed teeth was 20.2, nearly ten times as much as in Ayer. The difference between the two towns? Ayer, Dr. Price observed, was isolated, and the people ate a diet largely restricted to whole rye bread, cheese, and raw milk. Vissoie, in contrast, was connected with a modern road, and the people had long given up chewy homemade bread in favor of fluffy white rolls and cakes. Instead of gulping down fresh raw milk, they sold it to milk chocolate manufacturers and used the profit to buy chocolate candies. Although Dr. Price saw the same contrast in many other Swiss towns, he was cautious about jumping to conclusions. Perhaps there was something unique about the Swiss situation.

So he traveled to the windswept Outer Hebrides Islands off the northwest coast of Scotland, all the way out to the Isle of Lewis. Examining the teeth of the children, he found that only 1.3 out of every hundred teeth showed signs of decay. And did they eat whole grain rye and raw milk, like the Swiss? Not at all. In fact, they barely knew what milk was, Dr. Price learned. Their diet consisted very largely of oats and codfish, especially the liver from the cod. But when Dr. Price went to Tarbert, the port city of the island, which had a commercial bakery selling all kinds of cakes, pies, tarts, pastries and refined wheat products, and where other commercial food was also available, the caries rate was a gross 32.4 percent.

Not content to draw conclusions from a study only of Europeans, Dr. Price chartered a plane and flew into the Stony River region of Alaska. In one small Eskimo settlement in this area, he examined a total of 288 teeth, and found that only one had been attacked by decay, or 0.3 percent. Moving on to the Nelson Island, another remote area, he examined 830 teeth in the mouths of 28 individuals, and again found only a single tooth that was decayed, or 0.1 percent. But when he went to the settlement of Crooked Creek, he found that of 216 teeth in the mouths of eight people, fully 18.9 percent showed decay. Here, as opposed to the other settlements, nearly everyone lived on "store grub"—all except one individual, and he was free of cavities. In the remote settlements where people lived exclusively on natural foods such as caribou meat, berries, kelp, ground nuts, fish, and flower blossoms preserved in seal oil, teeth were so healthy, Dr. Price noted, that even when they were worn down to the pulp by the habit of chewing leather, the teeth would grow new dentin to protect the pulp. This is almost never seen in "civilized" societies, Dr. Price noted.

Over and over again, in different parts of the world, Price found the same pattern. In Canadian Indians who lived on the likes of moose meat and berries, he found that only 0.16 percent of the teeth were decayed. At a settlement which had contact with white men, the rate shot up to 25.5 percent and in a full-fledged "frontier town," the rate was all of 40 percent, or about 240 times as much pathology as among those living in the "wild." This was especially cruel, Dr. Price observed, because the white men almost never brought a dentist to these outposts along with their white flour, jam, sugar, and chocolate. In some cases, because of the extreme agony of toothaches, natives were actually driven to suicide, which, like tooth decay, was often unknown before the arrival of the whites.

Early Indians Had No Cavities

And so it went as Price continued his epic dental survey. In Fiji, among groups that were still eating crabs, fish, and wild pigs, the decay rate was 0.42 percent. Those who ate a Western diet suffered with a rot rate of 30.1 percent. In Samoa, it was 0.3 percent versus 18.7 percent. On the other side of the world, 88 Masai were found to have only four carious teeth among them, and 21 Watusi had only three. In the United States, an examination of several hundred skulls of pre-Columbian Florida Indians in a museum revealed not one cavity in the lot, while fully 40 percent of the teeth of modern Seminole Indians are decayed.

Because Dr. Price did his research in so many different parts of the world, from the plains of Africa to the Arctic Circle, from the

Pacific Basin to the Swiss Alps, we can begin by tossing out the idea that there might be some special mineral in the water that these people are drinking. Because his subjects were racially different, we can also dispense with the notion that they might enjoy some special inherited immunity to dental caries. What about eating a special food? That's not it either, because a diet of taro and bird eggs is very different from one of dried fish and seal oil, which is very different from raw milk and whole grain rye. Yet people on all these diets enjoyed an extremely high measure of dental health, Dr. Price found.

What about "dental hygiene"? Were these people brushing their teeth on the sly, or maybe eating foods that scoured their teeth clean? Let Dr. Price answer that one: "Many primitive races have their teeth smeared with starchy foods almost constantly and make no effort whatsoever to clean their teeth. In spite of this they have no tooth decay."

Diet: The Inescapable Conclusion

That leaves us with the same inescapable conclusions which Dr. Price arrived at by the time he completed his field work in 1933. Namely, that eating a diet of natural, fresh foods provides nearly complete protection against tooth decay, while eating a diet of sweet, refined, processed and canned foods creates nearly complete vulnerability to tooth decay.

But it isn't merely the absence of sugar and baked goods that makes the diet of these primitive people so protective, Dr. Price found. In analyzing the widely varying diets he encountered in the cavity–free people, he discovered that all of them were very rich in vitamins A and D, and in the minerals calcium and phosphorus. This was no accident either, he insisted. The so-called primitive peoples, he argued, actually have a much better knowledge of food and its importance than highly civilized people.

The natural diet enjoyed by primitives does a lot more for them than prevent cavities, Dr. Price found. Just as their teeth are free of lesions, the arrangement of the teeth in their dental arches is of classical perfection. Crowded, misplaced teeth, so common today, and so lucrative for orthodontists, are all but unknown. Dr. Price put great stress upon the fact that these people, whatever their race, have uniformly broad faces with full, wide jaws, and that their teeth have plenty of room to grow. And he proved this assertion with scores of photographs taken in every corner of the world, showing the dazzling, perfectly aligned teeth of the nonsugar eaters. It's dramatically evident that the same good nutrition which protects their teeth also builds the quality and shape of facial bone that makes the perfect foundation for these teeth.

Dr. Price was still not content. He felt that he ought to be able to prove his findings experimentally. So, over a period of six years he put 50 people on specially supplemented diets which included large amounts of lean meat, bone marrow stews with lots of fresh vegetables, fresh juice, fish chowder, animal organs and rolls made from freshly ground whole grain wheat and served with yellow, high vitamin butter. Further supplementation was often given in the form of extra amounts of butter oil and fish liver oil. Since the diet of these people was not completely controlled, there was no way to absolutely remove all traces of sugar and refined foods from their diet, so we must assume that some of the 50, at least, indulged at times in these dental toxins. All 50 people in the test, including a number of teenagers, had a history of severe tooth decay. The results of Dr. Price's dietary regimen? After an average of three years, in the entire group of 50 people, there were only two new cavities. Furthermore, when some of these people went off the diets, they soon began to develop fresh cavities. Return to the diet, however, would immediately arrest their oral pathology.

Food Is 20 Times Better Than Fluoride

How does this dietary approach to oral health compare with the currently popular approach, emphasizing brushing, dental care, and above all, the addition of fluoride to drinking water? What is the caries rate among schoolchildren who have drunk nothing but fluoridated water since birth? In Philadelphia, when 330 five-year-olds from different sections of the city were examined in 1967, some 13 years after the city fluoridated, it was found that 41.8 percent had at least one cavity, and nearly one-quarter of those had six or more cavities. In 1965, of some 1,700 10-year-olds examined (11 years after fluoridation), 69.6 percent had cavities. This works out to a caries rate of 5.5 percent, or 15 to 20 times as much decay as Dr. Price found in the Eskimos, Africans, and Fijians. And yet, the same article which reported these results of fluoridation in the *Archives of Environmental Health*

(Vol. 8, No. 5) also declares that fluoridation "is undoubtedly the greatest single preventive procedure currently available to prevent dental caries." Between "experts" making declarations such as this, and cosmetic companies huckstering toothpaste on TV, it's no wonder so many of us live in a dream world when it comes to dental health.

258. Bone Meal For Sound Teeth

In November, 1971, fluoridation was banned in Sweden, after an investigation found that the claimed careful and intensive epidemiological studies that were supposed to have demonstrated its safety do not actually exist. Challenged by Professor Arvid Carlsson, a pharmacologist, to name any actual studies that had demonstrated that fluoridation is safe, dentists were unable to do so. The Swedish Parliament promptly forbade any further experimentation with the health of that country's citizens.

With the fluoridation question out of the way, the press became a great deal more interested in other ways to prevent tooth decay. They became aware that in their midst there was a scientist and agronomist of international stature, Dr. Alfred Aaslander, who since 1938 had raised three of his own children with such superb teeth that none of them had ever had a cavity. In addition, those children now had children of their own and none of them had ever had a cavity either.

Good heredity? Anything but. Both Dr. Aaslander and his wife had suffered from rampant dental caries as children and much of their motivation was simply to protect their own children from the same suffering they had endured.

Years before, Dr. Aaslander's studies had convinced him that when man gave up eating the bones of animals and fish, an important contribution to health-building nutrition was lost. Specifically, he discovered that bone meal is an ideal way to prevent tooth decay. Dr. Aaslander added it to his children's diet with spectacular results. But for many years, his findings were ignored.

While most of the Swedish dental profession was poohpoohing bone meal, one dentist, Dr. Eva Aronson, a dental consultant at a state clinic for children in Lund, was openminded enough to try giving bone meal to her own two children. Neither child developed a single cavity.

As a result, Dr. Aronson started recommending bone meal tablets to the mothers of the children whose teeth she cares for.

She was quoted in the prominent national newspaper, *Svenska Dagbladet*, as saying that since tooth enamel is kept healthy by using a mineral supplement and particularly bone meal, there is no sound reason why anyone should have tooth decay if it is administered from childhood. Moreover, the Swedish newspaper reported similar results obtained by dentists and other investigators in Norway and West Germany who also had sufficiently open minds to experiment with bone meal.

The Swedish public was convinced, and adults and children alike became regular consumers of the mineral supplement, hindered only by the difficulty of obtaining enough to satisfy the demand. Dr. Aaslander, at the age of 83, had finally become recognized as the discoverer of the most likely answer to date to the problem of tooth decay.

Here in his own words, is the full account of Dr. Aaslander's important research:

"There is a great similarity between tooth formation and the development of a plant. From a tiny seed the plant grows out of the soil from which it received a good many mineral nutrients, and the vigor and health of the plant are wholly dependent upon a sufficient supply of all the nutrients needed. Likewise, the tooth develops from a tiny embryo and grows out of the mandible, from which it receives a good many mineral nutrients, and the vigor and health of the tooth are wholly dependent upon the mineral supply. . . .

"Every one of the essential elements, even the trace elements, must be present in the soil in sufficient quantities and in a state available to the plant if it is to grow, and show a healthy growth. For instance, if boron is not present in sufficient quantities (and the need for a crop of 35 tons of sugar beets has been found to be around 260 grams of boron) the beets will develop a deficiency disease known as 'heart rot' which, incidentally, is very similar in appearance to dental caries. From the top of the beet a large black cavity develops down the center of the root. There are also many other diseases known to be caused by mineral deficiency and cured or prevented by minute doses of the lacking nutrient. . . .

"Although tooth formation has never, as far as is known, been treated in the light of plant nutrition, the importance of at least some of the tooth-forming elements has been stressed in terms of nutritional deficiency. The most remarkable case of interest in tooth nutrition has been shown regarding fluorine."

Healthy Teeth Need More Than Fluoride

"The intense interest in water fluoridation is incomprehensible from the plant-physiological point of view. The foundation of the movement must be an assumption that fluorine is the single trace element of importance for the formation of healthy teeth. But it would be extremely strange if in plant nutrition a large number of trace elements are essential, while in tooth formation only a single one should be active. In fact, at least two new trace elements have already been discovered that are essential for the development of teeth that are resistant to dental caries. . . . When vanadium and strontium were added to the feed given to rats and guinea pigs, the experimental animals were almost 100 percent free from dental caries after a period of 90 days. . . .

"In Bonn and other cities of this region more than 50 percent of the schoolchildren leave elementary schools at the age of 16 completely free from dental caries, whereas in Oslo almost 100 percent of the schoolchildren at the same age suffer from the disease. The diet is stated to be very similar in the two cities. In Oslo more fish is eaten and more milk drunk, while in Bonn the daily fare contains more meat, vegetables and sweet dessert. The chief difference between the cities was found to be the mineral content of the water supply. In Bonn the tap water contains considerable amounts of strontium and vanadium, while the tap water in Oslo is completely free from these trace elements.

"It is also pointed out that the fluorine content of the Bonn water is low, only .26 parts per million (p.p.m.) while the optimal content is stated to be 1 p.p.m. Thus an exceptionally good state of dental health has been demonstrated in Bonn in spite of a very low fluorine content but with a good supply of strontium and vanadium. It is evident that fluorine cannot be the one single trace element of importance for securing and maintaining healthy teeth. On the contrary, it has been admitted that in some districts in Scania, Sweden, where the fluorine content of the tap water is by nature optimal according to the common conception, not a single child has been found with teeth completely free from dental caries; only a reduction of the number of cavities has been demonstrated. The conclusion must be that fluoridation of the water supply cannot improve dental health where other trace elements are lacking—Liebig's law of the minimum. And we do not know how many trace elements are essential for the production and maintenance of teeth 100 percent immune against dental caries. Fluoridation must thus be regarded, from the nutritional point of view, as a very unsatisfactory method of combating dental caries. . . .

"It may be added that, according to analyses made by the writer, the fluorine content of the tap water in Stockholm is .30 p.p.m., compared with a content of .26 p.p.m. in the tap water in Bonn. In Stockholm practically 100 percent of the children have dental caries, while in Bonn more than 50 percent leave school without any trace of dental caries. It is evident that the fluorine content of the tap water does not govern the rate of dental caries.

"From the nutritional point of view, we must strive to attain a complete form of nourishment for the teeth, especially during the periods of tooth formation."

The Goal: Perfect Teeth For His Own Children

"The writer has been forced to try to prevent dental caries in children. As a boy around the turn of the century I suffered severely from toothache in spite of the fact that I grew up on a dairy farm and on a diet with plenty of milk and other home-produced foods commonly assumed to provide good teeth. The conclusion from the point of view of plant nutrition must be that the common diet is lacking in elements essential for the forma-tion of teeth resistant to dental caries. In 1938 my first child was born and it became a matter of paramount importance to me to save that child from the plague of my childhood, dental caries. The fact that my wife has, if possible, an even larger number of mended teeth than I have myself, gave added weight to the problem. Apparently, there was no hereditary resistance against dental caries to be expected. Our child's diet had to be better than that given to me in my childhood. Improvements in the organic nutrients of the diet did not seem possible to any vital degree; the desirable improvements in the diet had most proba-bly to lie in the field of its mineral nutrients.

"It was desirable to find a mineral supplement of such univer-sality that perfect teeth could be produced. . . .

"Bone meal must be such a universal mineral nutrient. The bulk of bone meal consists of tricalcium phosphate just as in the case of the teeth. In addition, bone meal contains a good many trace elements including fluorine, strontium and vanadium and probably all those essential for the teeth.

"The selection of bone meal as the universal tooth nutrient was aided by two observations.

"1. Bone meal is used, and has been used extensively for a long time, in the feed given to farm animals, especially pigs brought up on a feed consisting mainly of grain, potatoes and skim milk. Without bone meal such pigs often suffered attacks of osteomalacia (softening of the bone).

"2. Our forefathers used to eat bones—and they had perfect teeth. The bones eaten were those of small fish, mostly from the small Baltic herring which was—and in many places still is—a daily fare. In olden times the herring was grilled over the open fire on the hearth and eaten with head and tail, bones and all. It seems safe to conclude that this daily bone diet was a factor of decisive influence for the production of the perfect teeth of our forefathers. When this method of cooking fish disappeared with the open hearth, the decay of the teeth started with a vengeance."

Bone Meal Diet Starts Early

"In 1940, the bone meal period started for our first-born child. For our children born in 1941 and 1944 the bone meal diet started as soon as the mother's milk was supplemented with other foods, for instance, orange juice. The first dose was around 10 milligrams. It was increased steadily so that the daily dose at the age of two years was around 1.5 to 2 grams, a small teaspoonful. The bone meal has always been given mixed with fruit juices, the reason being twofold. In the first place, the fruit juice makes the bone meal more palatable and, secondly, the slightly acid juice was able to dissolve the bone meal to some extent. Thus the children have been given more or less soluble bone meal, which probably has faciliated its digestibility.... The result was perfect teeth, in spite of the fact that the diet for the later children was not so carefully planned as for the first-borne.... Toothbrushes have not been used more than once a day, in the evening before going to bed. No toothpaste has ever been used, only pure water. The experimental conditions have thus been in no way especially favorable for the production of teeth free from dental caries. In spite of this the teeth of the children have been and are of an exceptionally good quality....

"The excellent results of the bone meal diet must be due to the fact that bone meal contains all the nutrients that are essential for the complete nutrition of the teeth. In terms of plant nutrition, bone meal is a complete fertilizer for the growth of the teeth. The growing tooth—and perhaps also the full-grown tooth—is able to select from the complete nutrition any element that is needed under any conditions."

No Substitute For Natural Bone Meal

There is a subtle and highly effective scientific technique that is used over and over for the assassination of any unwelcome advance in science. It involves running seemingly objective experiments with nearly invisible but highly significant changes that assure they will not work properly. Such an experiment is reported in *Caries Research* (Vol. 6, No. 3, 1972) by three Swedish dental investigators, Gustasson, Stelling and Brunius.

These three investigators of high repute tested whether the inclusion of bone meal in the diet would have any effect on the incidence of caries in the golden hamster. It was a very careful test concluding that the only element in bone meal that could have a cariostatic effect is the calcium fluoride and that this is less effective than fluoridated water. Undoubtedly the study will be cited many times by dentists in many parts of the world as an argument for water fluoridation.

Here is the joker, however. Gustasson, Stelling and Brunius didn't use bone meal at all. They used a chemical mixture of calcium fluoride, hydroxyapatite and calcium carbonate. Hydroxyapatite is calcium phosphate. So they used calcium, phosphorus, calcium fluoride and calcium carbonate. No strontium. No magnesium. No molybdenum. None of the other trace elements that are found in bone meal and that Dr. Aaslander has pointed out are absolutely vital, even as traces, to complete tooth nutrition.

Naturally, their deficient synthetic mixture had little or no ability to improve the health of teeth. By labeling that mixture "artificial bone meal" however, they produced a study that will certainly be used often in the effort to prove Dr. Aaslander wrong and to claim that bone meal is of no value in tooth nutrition.

What they have actually succeeded in proving though, to the careful reader of the study, is that you cannot decide any particular element in bone meal is the important one and use that element alone to fight against tooth decay. You have to do precisely what Dr. Aaslander did—use the whole natural bone meal to nourish the teeth to their maximum health. The healthy tooth, it seems, is a better fighter against tooth decay than any chemical mixture from a laboratory.

259. Can Malocclusion Be Prevented?

The science of orthodontics is today, in this country, a flourishing branch of dentistry devoted to the prevention and correction of malocclusion of the teeth and "such other deformities and abnormalities as may be associated therewith." Orthodontists are patient, painstaking men who spend their days correcting, mostly by mechanical means, the serious defects in structure which result in malocclusion—common in American mouths, especially the mouths of children.

Malocclusion is defined in the medical dictionary as "occlusion of teeth in positions not conformable to anatomical rule." In other words, if your teeth do not meet in such a way as to give you a fully functioning "bite" as well as good appearance, you have malocclusion. When your "bite" is ineffective, when your teeth are growing so far out of line with one another and with the plane in which they function that you cannot use your teeth as you should—that is malocclusion.

Anatomical Causes Of Malocclusion

The condition of "baby" teeth is apparently of utmost importance. Not so many years ago it was generally believed that baby teeth were not too important and many parents paid little attention to cavities, missing teeth or teeth which came out, for "you'll soon get your permanent teeth and we'll take you to the dentist then."

Youngsters of five or six with missing teeth were proverbially cute and appealing. Such a viewpoint demonstrated a complete misunderstanding of what the role of "baby" teeth is. They are not there just so that young children can have something to chew with until their permanent teeth arrive. They are there to reserve space for the permanent teeth in a child's rapidly growing jaw. If a child loses a baby tooth, his jaw begins to close very rapidly around the space left by that tooth. Especially if a molar has been lost, there is every possibility that the permanent molar may not be able to erupt properly. It may come in crooked, it may interfere with teeth on either or both sides, or it may not erupt at all. In any case, there is a shortening of the arch of the jaw on that side which is bound to result in a disharmony in the child's bite in later years.

So the first rule for preventing malocclusion is to take a child to the orthodonist if any one of his baby teeth has been lost prematurely. The orthodontist has a mechanism called a "space maintainer" which will provide and maintain room for the later tooth.

The second warning of possible malocclusion is the prolonged retention of baby teeth. If they stay in too long, the permanent teeth trying to erupt beneath them may be deflected out of their proper course or may not erupt at all. This is particularly true in the case of the cuspids which, if unable to erupt at the proper time, may not grow out at all. Generally, the permanent teeth begin to replace the baby teeth at about the age of seven. Since the time varies with individual children, there may be doubt as to whether or not the permanent teeth are ready to erupt. X-rays are the most dependable way of knowing for sure.

A third hazard is the loss of a permanent tooth before the entire set of permanent teeth has grown in, for here again the space will tend to close rapidly, throwing out of line the teeth in that side of the jaw which are still coming through the gums. Of course, when any permanent tooth is lost, at any age, and not replaced, there may be resulting malocclusion, for the shape of the jaw is bound to change.

Another good reason for keeping baby teeth in good order is that if there should be unfilled cavities which are painful, the child may favor one side when he chews. This is certain to disturb the alignment of his jaws.

Extra teeth occasionally develop—that is, teeth which erupt where some other tooth should be. Even if they do not erupt, they may be present in the jaw and an X-ray will reveal them. If such a tooth is interfering with the normal teeth, it should be removed. If there are teeth which fail to come in at all, these too are likely to cause malocclusion and restorations should take their place.

Habits Which May Cause Malocclusion

Among habits which sometimes lead to malocclusion are these: mouth breathing, lip biting, thumb or finger sucking, incorrect swallowing, tongue biting or thrusting, pencil biting or nail biting. Bottle-feeding continued for too long a time can also result in serious malocclusion.

By some means or other, orthodontists have discovered that many people do not swallow correctly. In correct swallowing, the jaws and teeth are brought together and the tongue thrust against the sides of the teeth and palate. The tongue functions best during swallowing when its tip and sides are braced against the hard palate and teeth. In incorrect swallowing the tongue is braced against the lips, which eventually produces malocclusion.

The most interesting controversy among orthodontists is the question of whether malocclusion is caused by heredity or environment. Granted that bad habits may wreak havoc on tooth alignment, what about those youngsters who do not bite their lips, breathe through their mouths and so forth—why do they have teeth that do not meet in a perfect "bite"? Because one parent or both had this same trouble, says one school of orthodontists, and facial structure is hereditary. If a parent has a jaw so narrow that the full quota of teeth cannot erupt without crowding one another, then the child may possibly have just such a jaw, too. The other school of orthodontic thinking declares that heredity is not the whole answer, but that other factors in environment must be important, too. They are bent on finding out what these other factors are.

Primitive Foods Build Sound Jaws

According to Dr. Weston Price, D.D.S., whose book, *Nutrition and Physical Degeneration* is described in detail elsewhere in this section, diet is the most important environmental factor. Dr. Price visited Canada, Australia, Europe, South America and the South Sea islands, studying the mouths of primitive peoples in all these places who had never eaten modern, "civilized" foods. In some cases he also studied the children of these same people who had been eating store-bought food.

In his book, Dr. Price quoted Dr. Ernest A. Hooton of Harvard: "I firmly believe that the health of humanity is at stake and that, unless steps are taken to discover preventives of tooth infection and correctives of deformation, the course of human evolution will lead downward to extinction . . . The facts we must face are, in brief, that human teeth and the human mouth have become, possibly under the influence of civilization, the foci of infection that undermine the entire bodily health of the species and that degenerative tendencies in evolution have manifested themselves in modern man to such an extent that our jaws are too small for the teeth which they are supposed to accommodate, and that, as a consequence, these teeth erupt so irregularly that their fundamental efficiency is often entirely or nearly destroyed ... The dental practitioner should equip himself to become the agent of an intelligent control of human evolution, insofar as it is affected by diet. Let us go to the ignorant savage, consider his ways of eating, and be wise. Let us cease pretending that toothbrushes and toothpaste are any more important than shoe brushes and shoe polish. It is store food which has given us store teeth."

Dr. Price went on to say that orthodontists have ascribed malocclusion to the blending of racial stocks. Crowded teeth have been said to be due to the inheritance of the large teeth of one parent and the small bone formation of the other. But Dr. Price studied and photographed for his book hundreds of examples of young people whose diet was store-bought while that of their parents was primitive. In the course of this one generation, the bony structure of the children had degenerated to such a degree that cases of malocclusion were commonplace among these young folks, who lived in the same houses with their parents and grandparents whose jaw structures were flawless.

Dr. Price also showed in his book pictures of whole families of children of which one brother had eaten refined foods and suffered from malocclusion. Another brother in the same family had eaten unrefined foods and had perfect occlusion.

Preventing Malocclusion

How do you prevent malocclusion? If the malocclusion is threatening in an individual it is recommended that he or she see an orthodontist immediately. But if you are speaking in terms of planning a family of children who would not be subject to malocclusion, then a healthful diet for mother and father both, long before their children are born, and the same healthful diet for the children from the very day of their birth are recommended. You cannot, in today's America, eat a primitive diet. The very seeds you put into your garden bear the mark of civilization on them. But you can plan your meals so that a very minimum of processed food appears on your table. You can learn how to preserve most food value by proper cooking methods. You can serve quantities of raw food. You can decide that good health, sound teeth and strong, functioning bone structure are the most important things for you and your family.

260. How To Stop Grinding Your Teeth

There are thousands of people who wake every morning with stiff jaws after a night of grinding their teeth while they sleep. Spouses have been led to threaten divorce, and on occasion to seek one, in response to too many noisy and sleepless nights. In some, the habit is so out of control that the grinding goes on intermittently during the day.

Bruxism—tooth grinding—is more than an unpleasant habit. It is a prominent cause of tooth loss and of gum recession, both resulting from the loosening of the tooth in its socket that frequent grinding induces.

If your slumbers are constantly being interrupted by the gnashing sound of teeth that grind in the night and you have tried dentistry, psychiatry, stuffing your ears with cotton and stuffing the grinder's mouth with a wet towel, don't despair! It may well be, according to at least one research study, that the grinder doesn't need the dentist or tea and sympathy as much as he needs more calcium and pantothenic acid.

Bruxism—Too Harmful To Ignore

While many parents tend to consider bruxism as a temporary phase—something the child will grow out of—it is not a practice which should be ignored. A Swiss dental scientist, Peter Schaerer of Bern, has reported that persons who clench their teeth during sleep or during a "confrontation" can cause damage to the teeth, gingiva (gums), jaw joint, and muscles (*Journal of the American Dental Association*, January, 1971).

While the practice is usually associated with children (three out of every 20 gnash their molars out of line), adults, too, are adding to the nocturnal cacophony and their own gum problems. These grinding statistics were revealed by Dr. George R. Reding, Assistant Professor of Psychiatry at the University of Chicago, and Dr. John E. Robinson, Jr., Associate Professor in the Walter T. Zoller Dental Memorial Clinic of the same university. The two researchers have investigated nocturnal teeth-grinding by means of dental examination, interviews, and sleep laboratory techniques.

While psychiatrists, psychologists and dentists who have considered the problem of nocturnal teeth-grinders have often assumed it was associated with mental illness or emotional disturbance, according to Dr. Reding, there is no demonstrable evidence of such an association. Psychological tests of matched groups of grinders and non-grinders recruited among University of Chicago students gave no indication the grinders were more emotionally disturbed than the non-grinders (University of Chicago news release, February 13, 1968).

What then can be the force which makes children and adults persist in noisily and unconsciously causing damage to their teeth during sleep?

Tooth Gnashers Respond To Two Nutrients

According to evidence reported in the December, 1970 *Dental Survey*, by University of Alabama researchers E. Cheraskin, M.D., D.M.D. and W. M. Ringsdorf, Jr., D.M.D., M.S., bruxism is a nutritional problem that can be greatly ameliorated with increased dosages of calcium and pantothenic acid.

In order to explore the relationship between diet and nocturnal teeth gnashing, Drs. Cheraskin and Ringsdorf set up a multiple testing program for 91 dentists and their wives. Each one was asked to fill out an Oral Health Index Questionnaire in which one of the questions was, "Do you clench or grind your teeth or are you conscious of the way your teeth fit together, awake or asleep?" Each one was also asked to complete a questionnaire designed to reveal the nutrient content of his or her diet. Then the group listened to lectures on diet.

One year later, each participant again completed both questionnaires. By this technique it was possible to relate dietary habits to the practice of tooth grinding.

Of the 94 people studied, 58 (group 1) reported no bruxism at the first visit. On the second visit they reported a higher intake of protein, calcium, vitamins A, B_1, B_2, niacin, C, B_6, pantothenic acid, iodine and vitamin E. They again reported no tooth grinding at all on the second visit a year later.

There were five people established as group 2 who had not improved their nutrition at all and developed the habit of grinding their teeth during the course of the experimental period.

Sixteen people placed in group 3 were tooth grinders at the beginning of the study. These 16 increased their intake of calcium, vitamins A, C, pantothenic acid, iodine and vitamin E. Without any other change in life situations—without any deliberate effort—by the end of the year they were quiet sleepers—no longer disturbing their families' slumber with the sound of a nocturnal cement mixer. More important, they were not loosening their teeth in their sockets or tearing them away from their gums. The 15 people in group 4, who were tooth grinders before and remained tooth grinders, increased their intake of vitamins A, C, iodine and vitamin E.

What nutrients did group 3 get that group 4 did not get? *Calcium and pantothenic acid.*

But why should these two nutrients be involved in a phenomenon that disturbs the slumber of thousands of people every night of the year?

Nerves And Muscles Need Calcium

It is well known that calcium is vital to the strength of the bones. But nerves, muscles and various organs of the body also depend on a regular supply of calcium for their health. Calcium is used by the nerves, and indeed has been found by 1970 Nobel Laureate Sir Bernard Katz to be the key requirement for transportation of impulses along the nerves from one part of the body to another. It is urgently needed by muscles; lack of calcium will cause cramps or convulsions. What is a convulsion? A violent involuntary series of contractions of the voluntary muscles. What is bruxism? An involuntary movement of the muscles of the mouth bringing the teeth together in a grinding movement.

Of particular revelance therefore, Drs. Cheraskin and Ringsdorf point out, is the part played by calcium in muscle contractility and the preservation of the physiologic response of nerve tissue to stimulation.

Hence, it is noteworthy, they say, that "bruxism, a neuromuscular problem, should vanish in parallel with an increase in calcium consumption."

What about pantothenic acid? When a deficiency of this member of the vitamin B family is induced in volunteers, the symptoms include headache, fatigue, gastrointestinal disturbances, numbness in the extremities and both *muscle cramps and impaired motor coordination.*

Thus, the Alabama researchers point out, "it would appear to be of some note that in the subjects who stopped bruxing there was an increase in pantothenic acid intake." Pantothenic acid is known as the anti-stress vitamin.

Grinders Are Stress Victims

While, by psychiatric standards, tooth grinders are considered normal, Peter Schaerer, Swiss dental scientist, says that "the primary causes of bruxism seem to be changes in central nervous activity—as in sleep, in states of nervous tension, or in conflict situations."

Tooth grinders, then, are not candidates for the psychiatrist's couch. It's just that their stresses are showing—in the middle of the night. A good supply of pantothenic acid may be just what they need in order to "cope" with their stresses without disturbing the whole family.

261. Brush Properly To Save Your Teeth And Gums

In people past the age of 35, periodontal disease, a disease of the gums and supporting structure of the teeth, is by far the greatest cause of tooth loss. Its presence is marked by red, swollen gums that bleed, recede, and eventually become so weak and incompetent that they can no longer protect the bone that holds the teeth firmly in place.

Bacterial plaque in the mouth, often accompanied by tartar (deposits of calcium salts), has been identified as one of the chief agents in the development of periodontal disease. Composed of living microorganisms, this plaque is highly concentrated at the gum margin, where it is in constant contact with soft mouth tissue. If the bacteria can overcome the natural defense mechanisms of the host tissues, infection follows.

Brushing Technique Is Important

Brushing certainly can get rid of plaque, but only if it is done correctly. Many conscientious people follow the advice of a jingle that goes: "Brush your teeth the way they grow, down from above and up from below." This is a good rhyme but a poor way to brush your teeth.

Perhaps you use a medium or hard toothbrush and scrub the daylights out of your teeth, using a back-and-forth motion. A medium or hard brush is likely to scrub your gums right off your teeth, leaving you with gum recession, notches on your teeth and tooth sensitivity.

In 1948, Dr. Charles Bass, Dean Emeritus of Tulane University Medical School in New Orleans, developed a brushing technique that is being taught today to dental students as well as patients.

Curiously, Dr. Bass was a physician, not a dentist. He became interested in preventive dentistry for one reason—he had personal dental problems. Although he was brushing his teeth twice a day and seeing his dentist regularly, he was still getting cavities and his gums bled occasionally when he brushed them.

As a physician, Bass realized that bleeding from the epithelium is neither normal nor healthy. The fact that his gums were bleeding meant that the epithelium was broken and that germs could enter his system and infect the bone that supports the teeth.

Dr. Bass wondered if the toothbrush he was using had anything to do with his dental problems. Having several lenses around, he casually began looking at the bristles of his toothbrush under magnification. He suddenly realized that something was definitely wrong with conventional toothbrushes. Looking at the magnified bristle-ends, he noticed they had "sharp, rough corners." The points of the bristles looked to him just like miniature knives! No wonder his mouth was bleeding.

Soft, Flexible Brush Needed

Bass knew enough about dentistry to realize that germs that cause gum damage are lodged in the plaque at the gum line where the teeth and gums meet, and within the gum crevice— the shallow space between the gums and teeth. But when those sharp bristles were used to remove plaque from the gum line, they tended to scratch the delicate gum tissue or even puncture it, creating small holes. Furthermore, he discovered that it's difficult to push the thick bristles of a hard toothbrush into the gum crevice, which is normally a very narrow space.

Bass concluded that the right kind of toothbrush should have thin, flexible bristles that would be easy to put into the gum crevice to clean out plaque. The thinner bristles needed to be rounded off and polished at their ends, so that the filament tip would be smooth and not sharp. Bass' modifications resulted in a new brush head that was soft and flexible enough to bend when pressed against the gums.

After using such a brush, Bass declared: "The author maintains his own teeth and gums free from active dental disease. No hemorrhage occurs from his gums" (*Dental Items of Interest*, 70:697, 1948).

Bass recommended a toothbrush which has a plain, straight handle and is about six inches long. The brush head should be small in size, about an inch or less, with the bristles arranged in a straight line.

The toothbrush is one case in which something synthetic (nylon) is better than something natural. When a natural bristle is cut in the manufacturing process, it breaks off, leaving a rough or sharp-angled surface that is not easily rounded and polished, as is the case with nylon filaments. Nylon bristles also soften up under warm water, which is not true of natural bristles. There are many brushes on the market that are soft and have rounded, polished bristles, and are therefore useful and safe for removing plaque. The key words to remember are "soft", "rounded," and either "polished" or "satinized."

How To Brush The Bass Way

To brush the Bass way, hold the toothbrush horizontally and put the bristles directly into the crevice where your teeth meet your gums, pushing them in as far as possible, at about a 45 degree angle. Use firm pressure and wiggle the brush back and forth with short strokes. The base of the brush head will be moving much more than the tips of the bristles, which will remain nearly stationary. This action helps dislodge plaque, which is the whole point of the procedure.

Your gums may bleed when you first try this. If they do, it is either a sign that your gums are unhealthy or that you picked an improper toothbrush. If you continue to brush correctly with a proper brush, the bleeding should go away within five days, and your gums will toughen up.

To brush the biting surfaces of the teeth, place the bristles on top of the teeth, press down firmly, and vibrate the brush back and forth with short strokes.

The inside, or lingual (tongue side) surfaces, are brushed in a similar manner to the outside surfaces, except that you may find it easier to hold the brush in a vertical, rather than a horizontal position, especially in the front of the mouth, where the dental arch is curved. But the idea is still the same: push the tips of the bristles directly into the crevice where the teeth meet the gums, and then vigorously vibrate the brush so that plaque is cleaned out.

Flossing Is Also Important

It is impossible to get the brush into the interproximal surfaces between the teeth, unless you have large spaces there. Normally the teeth are touching each other. You will therefore need dental floss to get these interproximal surfaces clean.

Take out a three-foot piece of floss and wrap it around the middle finger of each hand. Then, using the first finger and thumb as a guide, gently ease the floss through the contact area between each tooth and insert the floss as far down as it will go between the gum and tooth. Be careful not to snap the floss through the contact area between the teeth as this might injure the gum. Instead, gently tease it through, by sawing it in and out as you carry the floss down to the gum.

Now hold the floss snugly around the tooth and bring it up and down several times. As the floss becomes ragged, wind it around one finger and off the other. This method removes plaque from between the teeth. This is an important area to keep clean every day, because most cavities and gum problems start in this area. Many people think that the purpose of using floss is to remove just the food that gets stuck between the teeth. These food particles may cause bad breath, but they do not cause cavities or gum disease. Plaque does. Even if you don't eat for a day, plaque will still accumulate in your mouth.

The important thing is to remove all your plaque by brushing and flossing properly at least once a day. Brushing after every meal is not necessary.

262. Calcium And Phosphorus To Prevent And Treat Periodontal Disease

Everyone knows that children need lots of calcium to build strong healthy teeth. But did you know that *you* need plenty of calcium, too, if you want to hold on to those teeth?

The right kind of oral hygiene is important in keeping the gums firm and strong enough to maintain their grasp on the teeth. But work in the laboratory and clinic shows there may be a deeper reason for tooth loss—as deep as the jawbone, to be exact.

While it's true that the teeth are supported by the gums, their roots are actually anchored in bony sockets on the crests of the jawbone. In advanced periodontal disease, these sockets shrink away from the teeth, and that is the main reason why 20 million Americans haven't got a single natural tooth left in their mouth.

Periodontal disease is slow and insidious. The first sign is usually tender, red and inflamed gums. As the gums recede from the neck of the tooth, pockets form below the gumline. The supporting alveolar bone, where the teeth attach to bony sockets in the jaw, is also affected and recedes away from the tooth roots. As the gums and bone retreat, more and more tooth is exposed: that's where the expression "long in the tooth" comes from.

While all this is going on, the teeth begin to loosen—first imperceptably, then quite noticeably. Eventually they are left with so little support that they fall out or have to be removed.

The most widely held view is that the direct cause of the bone recession is inflammation produced by bacteria which gained entrance through diseased gums. But there is another theory which says that the bone loss comes *first*, and the cause of the bone loss is poor nutrition, not poor oral hygiene.

Jawbone Shrinkage A Symptom Of Osteoporosis

When Lennart Krook, D.V.M., Ph.D., and Leo Lutwak, M.D., Ph.D., and other researchers at Cornell University examined the jaws and several other bones from recently deceased patients who had periodontal disease, they found evidence of osteolysis, a deep-seated bone resorption (*Cornell Veterinarian*, July, 1972). Here is where calcium plays a crucial role. Normally 99 percent of the calcium in the human body is found in the skeleton, while the remaining one percent circulates in the blood and other extracellular fluids. If the level in the blood should dip (as a result of a dietary calcium deficiency, for example) the blood must "borrow" some of this mineral from the bones.

In the cases that Cornell researchers examined, this "borrowing" had been going on for so long that the jawbones had lost considerable mass, and actually shrank. Other bones besides the jawbone were affected. "Bone loss caused by enhanced osteolysis was present in all bones from all subjects," the researchers reported. But, "The bone loss was most severe in the jawbones, then in ribs and vertebrae, and least in long bones (such as arms and legs)."

The researchers theorize that as the jawbone recedes, movement of the loosened teeth traumatizes adjacent gum tissue, causing inflammation and bleeding.

"It thus appears," they concluded, "that periodontal disease in man is probably a manifestation of generalized osteoporosis." Osteoporosis is the malady that makes bones porous, brittle and fracture-prone with advancing age, particularly in women. Too low an intake of calcium is a major contributing cause.

Teeth Gain Firmer Hold With Extra Calcium

What effect would extra calcium have on patients with periodontal disease? To find out, Drs. Krook, Lutwak and others selected ten patients—five men and five women—with ages ranging from 29 to 45 (*Cornell Veterinarian*, January, 1972).

Taking a nutritional background survey, the researchers discovered that nine of the ten patients had daily calcium intakes of only 400 milligrams or less. The Recommended Dietary Allowance for calcium for adult men and women is set at 800 mg. But the average intake of all ten patients was just 325 mg.—"a rather severe calcium deficiency," according to Dr. Krook and his colleagues.

For the next 180 days, the patients received 1,000 mg. of calcium a day in the form of calcium gluconolactate and calcium carbonate supplements. "All patients had gingivitis (gum inflammation) and bleeding at the start," the researchers noted. But after just six months of treatment, inflammation was improved in all cases and gone in three. Pockets along the roots of the teeth were recorded in eight patients before the study. In every case, pocket depth was reduced at the end of the treatment. Eight patients initially reported loose teeth. By the end of the study, tooth mobility was reduced in all but one. In one case, the teeth were now found to be completely firm in their foundations.

Even more impressive was what the investigators discovered when they examined X-rays of the patients' jaws. In seven of the ten cases, alveolar bone increased in amount and bony pockets along the roots of the teeth were partially filled in. *Healthy new bone had actually been deposited while the subjects were receiving additional calcium.*

Summing up their findings, the researchers concluded that "The clinical response to calcium therapy in periodontal disease was excellent. The radiologic examination showed that the osseous (bony) lesions are reversible. The improvement in amount of alveolar bone was remarkable, considering the relatively short period of treatment."

In still another study reported in the *Israel Journal of Medical Sciences* (7: 504-505, 1971), Drs. Lutwak, Krook and others found that calcium supplementation does more than reverse the effects of bone resorption by depositing new tissue on bone surfaces. It can even make the *interior* of existing bone denser and stronger. Ninety patients with mild periodontal disease were selected, and their jawbone density measured by a special technical process called photon densitometry. Then one group received a gram of calcium every day for 12 months, while another group received a placebo. At the end of this period, the placebo group showed no change in bone density. But those who took calcium supplements regularly showed a significant increase in bone density of approximately 12.5 percent.

Rx: 1,100 Mg. Of Calcium Plus Magnesium And Zinc

As a result of these and other experiments, Drs. Krook and Lutwak now believe that most adults need at least 1,100 mg. of calcium a day to protect against periodontal disease.

And if you're going to increase your calcium intake, you might want to consider magnesium and zinc supplements as well. "Because it is known that the requirement of magnesium and zinc increases with increased dietary calcium," the pair note, "we propose that treatment of periodontal disease should include, in addition to increased calcium intake, increases in magnesium and zinc."

Now we get down to the question of *how* you're going to increase your calcium intake. Drs. Lutwak and Krook point out that milk and milk products are the primary calcium source in the American diet. One quart of skim milk provides 1,200 mg. of calcium and about 950 mg. of phosphorus, which is a favorable ratio of these minerals. (Some foods contain much more phosphorus than calcium which seriously interferes with calcium absorption.) Brick, cheddar, parmesan and Swiss cheeses are also excellent sources of calcium. Three and a half ounces of cheddar, for example, contains 750 mg. of calcium and only 478 mg. of phosphorus. Cottage cheese, on the other hand, contains considerably more phosphorus than calcium.

If you eat a great deal of meat, you're fighting two calcium problems at the same time. First, beef has 22 times as much phosphorus as calcium. That kind of phosphorus excess means that only scant traces of the calcium from the meat are going to be absorbed into your system. Second, there is evidence indicating that large amounts of protein tend to wash calcium right out of your system (*Transactions of the New York Academy of Sciences*, April, 1974).

Whether man is "naturally" a carnivore or a vegetarian, or both, is open to discussion. Whatever your own opinion may be, Drs. Lutwak and Krook have explained that "Under natural conditions, carnivores take great care in balancing the calcium deficiency and phosphorus excess of meat by consuming bones. Two grams of fresh bone provides about 380 mg. of calcium and 190 mg. of phosphorus, and this excess of calcium in bone is enough to offset the phosphorus excess in 100 grams (3 1/2 ounces) of meat. When dogs are fed the left-over hamburger or commercially available '100 percent meat dog food,' skeletal disease results" (56th Annual Meeting of the Federation of American Societies for Experimental Biology, April, 1972).

In other words, a few grams of bone have enough calcium to balance the phosphorus in a typical serving of meat. For human beings, this can be accomplished by supplementing the normal diet with bone meal tablets or powder. Bone meal is made from the sterilized long bones of cattle, and contains more than twice as much calcium as phosphorus, along with traces of other elements needed for good bone growth. Another commonly-taken form of calcium supplement is calcium gluconate, which contains only calcium and no phosphorus.

A Nurse's Success Story

Many people already take calcium and other mineral supplements as part of their total health-building program. In March, 1975, a registered nurse from St. Louis reported that "Fifteen years ago, I received the diagnosis of osteoporosis of the anterior region of the lower jaw . . . . Though I improved my dietary calcium intake substantially over the years, X-rays continued to show little change in my bone condition. However, for about the past three years I have been taking bone meal and dolomite tablets, as well as A and D perles, twice daily. I was pleasantly surprised to learn that a recent dental film revealed almost complete recalcification of the area!"

What this registered nurse did for herself makes very good nutritional sense. She got extra calcium both from the bone meal and from the dolomite, but got magnesium in the dolomite as well. The vitamin D she took helped absorb the calcium and move it along to her bones, where it was needed.

The Unbeatable Combination

As important as good mineral nutrition is in holding on to your teeth, it shouldn't exclude the importance of oral hygiene. There is no question that the right techniques of brushing and plaque control help keep the gums healthy and prevent bacteria from attacking the underlying bone. If you use the Bass technique of brushing, as described in the preceding chapter, you are doing the best you can to protect your teeth and gums from an external point of view. It's something like applying fresh coats of paint to a house to prevent the underlying structures from being attacked by the elements.

But when you add calcium to your diet, you're protecting your teeth and gums from the inside as well. The combination of good oral hygiene and good nutrition is an unbeatable one for total oral health. Avoiding sweets, boosting calcium, and using the Bass technique should virtually guarantee that you and your precious teeth will remain in close company forever.

1185

263. Dentures Can't Help A Sick Mouth

Many new denture wearers, after untreated periodontal disease has necessitated the removal of their natural teeth, sadly discover that their troubles are just beginning. The same underlying mouth infection and inflammation that gradually robbed them of their teeth, now makes their new dentures too painful to wear. In despair, they put aside their uncomfortable, inefficient dentures and turn to a bland diet of overly refined foods, thus completing a vicious cycle. For the inevitable result of such a dietary adjustment—poor nutrition—is often one of the factors that led to their periodontal disease in the first place.

This is the unfortunate, and often preventable, chain of events outlined by Dr. Charles T. Peterson, D.D.S., in the *Pakistan Dental Review*, July, 1970. Because of his unorthodox approach—he considers the health of the whole mouth, instead of just filling cavities—the London, Ontario, dentist finds it difficult to get his views published in U.S. professional journals.

But it is hard to question the logic and urgency of his message: "Many people are in difficulty today because they have lost their teeth and are unable to wear dentures. Many of these problems have come about because of untreated periodontal disease that has destroyed the bone which should support the dentures. Fifty percent or more of people suffer from periodontal diseases, and if they have only sought treatment for 'holes in the teeth' they have trouble. . . ."

All too often, when the average dentist does come face to face with a case of advanced periodontal disease, he automatically pulls all the patient's teeth, replacing them immediately with dentures. He doesn't even begin to treat the root cause of the trouble—the underlying infection. Yet, he expects the artificial dentures to work satisfactorily, as if by some miracle the pain and discomfort will go away.

To such a dentist, Dr. Peterson offers the following warning: "Removing teeth does not necessarily clean up the infection in the bone tissues and the placing of dentures on top of infected tissues may only aggravate the condition."

Before letting a dentist talk you into having all your teeth extracted, you should ask yourself two questions. Should the mouth be treated, instead, for periodontal disease? And, if the teeth must still be pulled, what effect will their loss have on digestion and health?

Your Own Teeth Can Never Be Duplicated

Artificial dentures, no matter how carefully fitted, are a poor substitute for natural teeth. Dentures sitting on top of the jaw bone can never be as stable as teeth attached directly to the bone. Therefore, a hasty decision to have all teeth taken out may be regretted later, after the effects on the mouth and health in general are felt. Of course, then it is too late.

Teeth should be pulled only if it is absolutely necessary. If there is no alternative but to go ahead, any mouth infection which might be present should be treated and cleared up first. Otherwise, dentures will only bring more discomfort and the deterioration of tissue and bone will continue.

Tooth removal, or even a sore mouth, shouldn't be taken lightly. As Dr. Peterson warns, the effects may be far-reaching:

"No teeth should be removed from the mouth until the infection is under control. Infections from mouth tissues may affect the valves of the heart, produce serious toxins in the blood and secondary infections in the body.

"Never try to eliminate teeth because the mouth is sore. It may be a crucial sign of diabetes, anemia or even leukemia. Even if it is suggested that the teeth are causing your arthritis or stomach upset, be *certain* to make sure of the cause and correct it before having all the teeth removed.

"Consult an oral diagnostician interested in the health of your whole mouth. It may be that one tooth is the culprit or that the oral sepsis can be treated."

Denture Fit Is Important

When it comes to dentures, whether partial or complete, the Canadian dentist emphasizes the importance of proper construction and fit. There should be enough room left over for the tongue and other mouth tissues to function in their proper positions. The teeth of the upper and lower jaw should be placed in functional occlusion so that a properly-aligned, natural bite is obtained. By reproducing normal tooth anatomy as closely as possible, further breakdown of the jaw bone is avoided and the collection of food debris is kept to a minimum.

Dentures should be made to comply with the functional movement of the human jaw. "Apes chomp their food, man should grind his food in all movement of the jaw. Many dentures made just cause people to chomp," Dr. Peterson points out.

The discomfort, emotional aggravation and outright pain associated with inadequate dentures would be bad enough. But the long-range consequences for the denture wearer and his family are even more serious.

"It has been shown," says Dr. Peterson, "that sore mouth tissues are related to nutritional deficiencies and especially the lack of trace minerals. The lack of chewing ability with artificial dentures soon eliminates nutritious food for soft, bland, refined eating habits. The loss of teeth by the parents soon brings about a softy mushy diet for the whole family and the children suffer and do not develop strong teeth and jaw structures."

Chewing is good exercise. It is essential for healthy gums and teeth. But our modern diet of over-processed foods—soft white bread being one of the worst offenders—offers little opportunity to really bear down while chewing, even for the person with strong, natural teeth. We should all eat more foods of substance—raw vegetables, hard fruits, seeds and nuts—both for their nutritional value and the healthful workout they give our teeth. But many a suffering denture wearer couldn't eat such raw, fibrous foods even if he wanted to. Instead, he settles for poor nutrition.

Tips For Proper Cleansing

Finally, Dr. Peterson warns, perfunctory overnight cleaning of the dentures is no substitute for total mouth cleanliness. "Emphasis has been placed," he notes, "on the cleaning of the dentures rather than the importance of cleansing the mouth tissues ... when the teeth have been removed. The whole mouth can be cleaned and rinsed out with a quarter teaspoonful of salt and baking soda in a glass of water twice a day.

"Bleaching cleaner should not be used on artificial dentures as it removes the finish and weakens the denture material. In addition, bleach often remains on the denture and when placed in the mouth irritates the mouth tissues.

"Dentures can be placed in vinegar and water or a weak saline solution for half an hour or so, then cleansed with a brush and soap and water over a basin partly filled with water to act as a cushion against the dentures falling and cracking a tooth."

264. How To Rate Your Dentist

How would you rate your family dentist? Excellent, you say. A good man. His work is fast, painless and inexpensive.

You're glad you managed to find such an efficient, no-nonsense practitioner. Instead of that dentist down the street, who has to almost beg for patients. They say he's terribly expensive, a real "con-man" who prescribes unnecessary work, and a bungling amateur (he takes too long, even for the simplest job).

Worst of all, word is out that he's a painful dentist—even his routine scaling and cleanings cause some discomfort. No wonder patients avoid him like the plague. Funny thing though, you can't recall every hearing of anyone who had a tooth extracted by him.

What would you say if a person in the know, a respected dentist with more than 15 years experience, told you the latter was quite possibly the better man? That's exactly the point of a revealing book, *Dentistry and Its Victims* (St. Martin's Press, New York, 1970), written under the pseudonym "Paul Revere, D.D.S."

Bad Work Brings In More Money

It's not that some dentists don't know how to do competent work. It's just that bad work brings in a lot more money. The author has a collective name for these professional opportunists in their various guises—Dr. Poorwork.

Good dental service (not the Poorwork brand) can mean the difference between a person's keeping his natural teeth throughout his life and losing them prematurely to the ravages of decay or periodontal disease. People should not have to lose their teeth. "A person who gives his mouth good care," says the author, "should never lose important teeth, except, perhaps, in his later years." But Dr. Poorwork can make more money replacing teeth than filling them. After all, if a tooth is filled properly the first time, how can he expect to collect any subsequent fees?

If this "Dr. Revere" really knows what he's talking about, why does he hide behind a pen name? The answer can be found in the American Dental Association Code of Ethics—dedicated to guarding the welfare of the dental profession rather than the public. Under this official policy, any conscientious dentist who would stoop so low as to criticize the work of a colleague is subject to immediate discipline.

First-Rate Fillings Can't Be Hurried

The author couldn't help but notice the paradox. On the one hand was the ADA denying that an ethics problem existed, since all dentists maintain the same high standard. But in his own private practice, he observed that the "great majority" of patients coming to him for an initial examination had dental restorations which fell far below the licensing standards set by state boards.

Every dentist must demonstrate his competency—during dental school training, in earning a degree, and then in the state board examination. Yet here was work so far below the licensing standards it was disgraceful. The only way "Dr. Revere" could account for it was to assume that many Dr. Poorworks, trained and able to do better, were choosing to do shoddy work. And, obviously, the motive was money.

Take an ordinary silver filling as an example. On state board exams, young dentists are allotted three hours just to do one filling. Why? Because it takes that long to do a decent job. The dentist must completely remove all decay, extend the space to be filled to include all adjacent areas prone to decay in the future (the "extension for prevention" principle), line the area with insulation, allow for proper placement and condensation of the filling amalgam and trim the filling margins flush with the tooth surface.

Thus, as you can see, even a "simple" filling is quite a complicated process and it takes time. But "I know of many dentists today," says the author, "who in three hours, presume to stick in thirty such fillings."

Good Dentistry Sometimes Hurts

Why should any patient prefer such a dentist? Because most people want dentistry to be quick, painless and cheap. If they are in pain, they want immediate, stop-gap relief, with no postoperative discomfort or inconvenience. Dr. Poorwork's slipshod methods work fine for them, because they expect to lose some teeth over the years and won't blame their dentist when they do.

On the other hand, a conscientious dentist faces many obstacles. Deep, thorough drilling and proper scaling and cleaning can hurt. Nobody likes a painful dentist. It is harder for him to gain public acceptance and build up a profitable private practice. People consider him expensive and slow because he takes no shortcuts; yet, in the long run, his higher fees prove to be a great bargain.

Your dentist's attitude toward extracting teeth may be the best tipoff, if you suspect another Dr. Poorwork. Most decisions to go ahead and extract are downright wrong. A good dentist will do everything in his power to salvage a troublesome tooth, no matter how bad the pain of infection. If the root is periodontally sound, a tooth can nearly always be rebuilt from practically nothing.

Beware of the highly recommended "painless" extractor, "Dr. Revere" warns. Pulling a tooth is the easiest job in dentistry. It requires little skill or intelligence and, with anesthesia, it is supposed to be painless. "Remember, the good dentist . . . is only rarely called upon to extract a tooth, because he is in the business of saving his patients' teeth, not of squandering them."

Beware Of Mouth Care Misinformation

Disease of the gum and jaw bone claims more teeth than decay, but many dentists either don't recognize it until it's too late or neglect to treat it. Some apply gentian violet, a strong purple dye, to the gums. But as "Dr. Revere" notes, this has no medical effect whatsoever. "Its major value is its deep color. The patient, seeing his gums turn purple with the 'medication,' is led to believe that something is really being done for him, and indeed it is: his attention is being diverted from his complaint to his gruesomely stained gums."

Into the informational vacuum about periodontal disease, left unfilled by Dr. Poorwork, Madison Avenue gladly steps. Americans are urged to buy "kickier-tasting" toothpastes and miraculous mouthwashes to keep their mouths "clean and fresh." What the ads don't tell you, but "Dr. Revere's" book does, are the following plain facts:

—Teeth are not naturally white; they are yellowish. Any attempt to scrub them white with abrasive toothpastes can cause severe damage.

—The toothbrush, not the dentifrice, does most of the work in brushing.

—No mouthwash or toothpaste can cure halitosis ("bad breath"). "It is like putting perfume on garbage and living with it instead of making an effort to remove the garbage; this can be particularly poignant when the garbage is in one's own mouth."

—Commercial mouthwashes, when used consistently, destroy the natural chemical and bacteriological balance of the mouth, allowing disease to get out of hand. They kill off some microorganisms but allow the survivors to proliferate.

—Your mouth has a natural tendency to keep itself clean and in good health, if the saliva has a chance to do its job.

—Plain drinking water is the best mouthwash. A good rinsing after eating is a "simple, common, and effective, though under-rated" oral hygiene technique.

These are the facts. Yet, according to the author, "after years of watching television commercials for dental products, I cannot recall a single advertisement which, either directly or by implication, did not seek to mislead the viewer."

Does Your Dentist Pass Or Fail?

How can you avoid Dr. Poorwork? "Dr. Revere" has listed some things to watch for when evaluating your present dentist or selecting another:

Your dentist's initial examination should be careful and thorough. There should be a full explanation of the diagnosis, proposed treatment and cost. The health of the gums should not be overlooked. (Bleeding gums are not "normal.") Extractions should be considered only as a last resort.

If your dentist doesn't meet these criteria, perhaps you should consider a switch. Your sound teeth and gums are worth more than money, and they are worth the time to have them cared for properly. Your dentist, if he is a good one, will feel exactly the same way.

Section 56
Tetany

265. The Mineral-Imbalance Disease

There is a strong similarity between the symptoms of an anxiety attack and the early symptoms of tetany (a disease characterized by fatigue and nervousness) resulting from calcium deficiency. This was the conclusion of two psychiatrists, Ferris Pitts, Jr., and James McClure, after completing a historic study (*New England Journal of Medicine*, December 21, 1967) showing how nervous symptoms can be physically produced. They decided to conduct a further test under double-blind conditions trying out the administration of lactic acid on both normal people and anxiety patients. In some cases, calcium ions were added to the lactic acid, making the compound, calcium lactate.

They found that the lactate alone led to anxiety attacks in 13 out of 14 anxiety subjects within a minute or two after the infusion started, and also in two of the 10 normal subjects. One of the normal subjects described his physical symptoms as "Palpitations, tightness-lump in the throat, trouble breathing, shuddering sensation all over, can't stop shaking feeling . . . I'm very apprehensive and jumpy." But when calcium lactate was used, the anxiety symptoms for the most part did not occur.

The study goes a long way toward establishing an identity between anxiety and calcium deficiency tetany. The authors speculate that in a healthy nervous system calcium combines with lactate around the sensitive endings of the nerves, preventing the acid from irritating the nervous system. But if too much lactate is produced because of an error in the glucose metabolism, or if there is insufficient calcium available to perform its neutralizing role, the result is anxiety which may or may not culminate in tetany, depending on how acute and how persistent the calcium deficiency is.

This study is important because it has demonstrated that the presence of calcium in sufficient quantity will prevent attacks of anxiety. It appears that anyone who is troubled by even mild attacks of anxiety ought to be able to help his condition by taking a daily supplement of bone meal. Bone meal, which is the pulverized long bones of beef cattle, contains all the bone minerals, with calcium predominant. But in addition to the calcium it also contains phosphorus, magnesium, and other trace minerals that aid the body in the proper absorption and use of its calcium. The only other nutrient necessary to make certain that the calcium in bone meal is put to good use is vitamin D. You can get bone meal tablets with vitamin D already added to them, or preferably you can secure your vitamin D from a capsule of either halibut or cod liver oil.

Tetany is one of the most common and least recognized conditions afflicting womankind. It is a great deceiver. Thorough physical examinations, all sorts of detailed analyses and X-ray studies may reveal absolutely nothing wrong, says the French publication, *Ici Paris* (February 15, 1971). The doctor gives his patient a reassuring pat and tells her kindly there is absolutely nothing wrong with her *physically*.

But, while tetany is a condition which can easily escape diagnosis, there is a way to determine its presence. It is so simple that doctors do not even think about it. Just tap lightly on the lower part of the face with a reflex hammer. This kind of tap, if a woman has tetany, will cause her to draw her lips into a position which resembles the mouth of a carp.

There are other small clues to the condition. The enamel of the teeth tends to deteriorate; white spots appear on the fingernails, which have ridges and tend to split; the hair becomes brittle and more of it appears on the comb and hairbrush. The subject feels as if insects were crawling under her skin. At unpredictable times she may feel an obstruction in her throat as if unable to swallow. Sometimes she feels unaccountably dizzy, almost faint.

Because of the contraction of the muscles caused by tetany, sometimes the hands have a tendency to bend inwards, giving the aspect of what is known medically as "obstetrician's hand." While this stiffness is not painful, it does persist. It can also affect the feet and the face and the carp mouth can become permanent.

All these sensations are related to the bone-deep fatigue which is with the victim constantly. They are all manifestations of a condition called spasmophilia. The motor nerves show an abnormal sensitivity to stimulation and the patient shows a tendency to spasms and sometimes convulsions.

What causes it? A lack of magnesium or a lack of calcium or an imbalance in the controls which regulate the proportions of calcium, magnesium and phosphorus in the blood and in the cells. The nervous system and the parathyroid glands are involved in this regulation.

Trouble with the bowels or kidneys can trigger the condition. Diarrhea causes a big loss of many nutrients including calcium and magnesium. If the kidneys are not functioning properly, they do not act as a proper filter and thus cannot maintain the right proportion of calcium, magnesium and phosphorus. Wouldn't urine and blood analyses reveal the condition? No. Urine and blood analyses do not reveal anything because they do not give an accurate reading of these proportions. In order to get such data, it would be necessary to measure the amounts of magnesium and phosphorus which exist in the cells and then tabulate the flow in and out of the cells. This is practically impossible, says the French publication.

In most cases, careful attention to nutrition is all that is needed to bring back that old-time vitality. The nutrients most needed are calcium and magnesium. Vitamin D is indispensable, too, to promote absorption of the minerals. As a matter of fact, it has been found that spasmophilia or tetany has a tendency to become worse at the end of winter because of the low stores of vitamin D in the body at that time.

Even Babies Can Suffer From Tetany

For half a century now, doctors have been baffled by a strange illness developing in some newborn babies. The birth occurs without complications. The infant is healthy and strong. But three to six days later he develops an attack of tetany, a potentially serious disease in which the infant suffers muscular twitching, cramps and convulsions. Sometimes stridor, an infantile respiratory spasm, also occurs.

According to Drs. Thomas E. Oppe and David Redstone of St. Mary's Hospital Medical School in London, tetany has been occurring with far greater frequency in recent years than ever before. Writing in the May 18, 1968 issue of *The Lancet*, the physicians said, "In the maternity units under our supervision, tetany presented (occurred) most often in otherwise healthy and vigorous babies born at term who have been artifically fed."

Once that fact was discovered, a solution was in sight. Since babies who are breast-fed do not develop tetany, cow's milk must either contain or lack a factor which causes the problem. Ordinary cow's milk is low in calcium, compared to breast milk—but not low enough to cause the disease.

Drs. Oppe and Redstone discovered, however, that cow's milk is extremely high in phosphorus. Human milk is quite low in that mineral. From that point, the solution was obvious to anyone with any knowledge of how calcium and phosphorus interact in the body.

According to Franklin C. McLean, Ph.D., M.D., writing in the January, 1969 issue of *The Journal of the American Medical Women's Association*, phosphate and calcium molecules are bound together by another substance—perhaps several others—to form the bones and teeth. That's why both are necessary for good health.

But the ratios of these minerals in the body should be about one part phosphorus to two and a half calcium. The reason it is important to maintain those levels is that, like it or not, the binding process continues to go on even after the body's need for healthy bones and teeth have been met. As long as the calcium levels generously exceed the phosphorus levels, there is always enough calcium left to perform the other crucial functions it has in the body—including those which prevent tetany. But once the condition reverses and the phosphorus is more plentiful than the calcium, a deficiency of utilizable calcium develops.

That happens no matter how much calcium is in the diet if the phosphorus is too plentiful!

And that is what happened to the babies fed ordinary milk, for cow's milk contains 91 milligrams of phosphorus per every 100 milliliters. Compare that to breast milk which contains 16 milligrams.

Human milk is both lower in phosphorus and higher in calcium than cow's milk. And that's why tetany, a growing problem among bottle-fed infants, is unheard of among those who are breast-fed.

The thing to remember is that as long as your calcium levels generously exceed your phosphorus levels, there will always be enough calcium left to perform other crucial functions in the body. That is why bone meal is an excellent source of calcium. It contains more calcium than phosphorus and includes many trace minerals that are essential to the utilization process, including some magnesium.

Section 57
Tonsillitis

266. You Need Those "Unnecessary" Tonsils

266. You Need Those "Unnecessary" Tonsils

The tonsils often fall victim to unnecessary surgery. For years, mildly swollen or inflamed tonsils, and even healthy ones, have been removed in a misguided attempt to prevent future throat infections and colds. Although a tonsillectomy may be the necessary last resort in serious cases of tonsillitis, there is evidence that we should do everything we can to hold on to these organs as long as possible.

The body's lymphatic system, of which the tonsils are a part, is relatively unknown. One thing that is known about it, however, is that it plays a big part in the body's defense against invading organisms.

Lymphoid tissues, which appear in the appendix, in the thymus, spleen and tonsils are coming to be recognized as important interceptors of infection. It is significant that lymphoid tissues collect in the tonsils and that the number of lymph follicles gradually increases to a peak between the ages of 10 and 20. After 30, there is an abrupt reduction to less than half the number of follicles, tapering off to a trace after age 60. This phenomenon suggests that the body's major threats from infectious diseases occur in early life.

Tonsillectomy Linked To Hodgkin's Disease
The child who has his tonsils removed is 2.9 times more likely to develop Hodgkin's disease later in life than a child who does not undergo a tonsillectomy, three American medical researchers reported in the British journal, *The Lancet*, in 1971.

Hodgkin's disease is a painless, progressive and fatal enlargement of the lymph nodes, spleen and general lymphoid tissues, often beginning in the neck and spreading throughout the body. In its final stages, it may spread to the lungs, flooding them with lymph.

Aware of previous evidence that appendectomy increases the risk of subsequent Hodgkin's disease, Nicholas Vianna, Peter Greenwald and J.N.P. Davies supervised a survey—conducted in all 25 hospitals in Nassau and Suffolk counties, New York—involving 109 patients with Hodgkin's disease and 109 controls. Through interviews and the study of medical records, they found that the two groups differed significantly in their histories of prior tonsillectomy. Of the 109 diseased patients, 67 had undergone tonsillectomies; only 43 of the controls had had their tonsils removed.

These findings led the trio to theorize that surgical removal of lymphoid tissue (such as the tonsils and appendix) facilitates the onset of Hodgkin's disease by removing some sort of protective barrier.

If this hypothesis is correct, surgeons would be advised to think twice before performing unnecessary or marginally-justified tonsillectomies—a not uncommon practice in light of medical statistics indicating that the United States has the world's highest surgery rate. The researchers noted that "in our society, tonsillectomy is performed more commonly on children from the more affluent homes." This suggests that ability to pay may be the critical factor in deciding whose tonsils are removed—and when.

Tonsils Help Fight Colds

For many years, it was fashionable to assume that diseased tonsils in children were at the root of the cold problem. However, as we have seen, tonsils have the function of channelling disease away from the system, not infecting it. In spite of the large number of tonsillectomies performed on children, no effect on disposition to future colds has been observed. An article in the *Journal of the American Medical Association* (February 8, 1958) noted that more people who had kept their tonsils were able to avoid colds than those who had had them removed. In a survey of London families, with regard to the problem of respiratory infections, it was reported (*British Medical Journal*, January 18, 1958) that comparisons showed a slightly greater tendency toward catching colds in children whose tonsils had been removed. Obviously, a good set of tonsils can be considered a strong asset.

Another doctor who has appealed to his colleagues to be less hasty in removing the tonsils of young children believes the practice cuts down the secretion of polio virus antibodies. As reported in the *Journal of the American Medical Association* (May, 1970), Pearay L. Ogra, M.D., told the American Pediatric

Society, "I would be very careful about doing tonsillectomies in children under eight years of age."

Dr. Ogra stated that tonsillectomies may actually leave the children more vulnerable to all kinds of infection, not just polio. "The operation reduces the antibody content of the nasopharynx and this allows the virus to multiply. It has been shown that polio virus can pass directly from nasopharynx to the brain and this may be true of other neurotropic viruses (those which attack nerve tissue)."

In studying 40 children before and after tonsillectomy, the doctor found that, "The mean antibody levels decreased three to fourfold, and individual titers (in this case, measures of strength of the antibody levels) in several children dropped four to eightfold. Four children who had appreciable levels of polio virus antibody in the nasopharynx before tonsillectomy failed to demonstrate any antibody activity there after the operation.

"The antibody levels have remained decreased for as long as eight months," he added.

A Role For Tonsils In Avoiding Multiple Sclerosis?

Doctor David C. Poskanzer of Harvard Medical School's Departments of Preventive Medicine and Neurology, has suggested that tonsillectomies may be implicated in multiple sclerosis, a disease of the nervous system. Reporting in *The Lancet* (December 18, 1965), he said that incidence of prior tonsillectomy was compared in 240 multiple sclerosis patients, their spouses and brothers and sisters closest in age. Results showed that patients had a "significantly higher" tonsillectomy rate than either comparison group.

Dr. Poskanzer suggested that some infective agent (germ or virus) originating outside the body plays a role in the causation of multiple sclerosis. It may well be active in childhood many years before the development of the disease. And the lymphoid system—which includes tonsils, adenoids and appendix—could be our first line of defense.

Section 58
Toxemia of
Pregnancy

267. Poor Nutrition Leads To Risky Pregnancy

Toxemia, a condition which manifests itself in late pregnancy, is responsible for one third of all maternal deaths and for some 30,000 still births or neonatal deaths each year in this country. This disease which is characterized by soaring blood pressure, headache, fever, albumin in the urine and edema is essentially a disturbance of the metabolism. There are two forms of toxemia of pregnancy, pre-eclampsia and eclampsia, the latter being more advanced and far more dangerous. In addition to the symptoms listed above, eclampsia has the potential for convulsions, coma and even death of the mother, the fetus or both. It can also be responsible for low birth-weight or retardation in the child.

The slight, normal swelling of extremities that occurs during most pregnancies is not to be confused with toxemia. The swelling in pre-eclampsia is far more pronounced.

The causes of this scourge of pregnancy have long been debated. But the evidence is mounting that it is basically due to a nutritional deficiency.

It is interesting to note, for instance, that the two states with the highest maternal mortality rates from toxemia—Mississippi and South Carolina—are the same states which have the lowest per capita income and the lowest nutritional standards. In 1972, the rate of mothers dying from toxemia per 100,000 of live births was 6.2 nationwide, while in Mississippi it was 30.2 and in South Carolina, 20.3. These statistics caused Nicholson J. Eastman, M.D., Professor Emeritus, Department of Obstetrics, Johns Hopkins, (and the man who has trained many of the OB professors who are now chairmen of departments in medical schools) to comment:

"The geographic distribution of toxemia pregnancy in the United States, when correlated with per capita of family income, indicates that environmental factors associated with low income play an important role in the etiology of this condition. It strikes me as very convincing evidence that malnutrition plays an important, possibly the most important part in the etiology of the toxemias."

California obstetrician and gynecologist Dr. Tom Brewer has long been outspoken in his plea for preventing metabolic toxemia by means of proper nutrition. "Metabolic toxemia of late pregnancy," says Dr. Brewer, "is preventable socially by the elimination of poverty, and medically by sound nutritional advice, the avoidance of salt restrictions, and the elimination of diuretic agents." Dr. Brewer has waged a long battle against the proponents of low salt diets and minimum weight gains for pregnant women. In the past twelve years he has done much research to back up his belief that toxemia is totally preventable with our present knowledge.

Of more than 5,000 cases treated in Dr. Brewer's clinic, not one mother has suffered convulsions, a symptom of toxemia. The low birth-weight rate in his three clinics is less than three percent compared with the national average of seven percent.

The clinic is the base from which Dr. Brewer is documenting the relationship between malnutrition, toxemia, and damaged babies. He operated a clinic for a year at General Hospital in San Francisco in 1962, then left to open one in Contra Costa County as clinical physician.

Once a week he gives the nutrition story to a new group of mothers-to-be, and after this, they see him once a month till the eighth month, then weekly for a checkup. He gives them the ABC's of nutrition in easy-to-understand vocabulary and, through questions, involves them. He explains simply that to have a healthy baby it's vital to eat food containing high grade protein. Basically, it's a diet of non-fat milk—a quart a day—dried or skimmed; two eggs; green leafy vegetables; yellow vegetables; soybeans; whole wheat bread; fruit or juice; meat or fish; cheese; a baked potato. Each patient gets vitamin and mineral supplements, and the importance of taking them religiously is drilled into them in follow-up visits.

He's confident that if doctors everywhere were telling their patients the truth about what to eat and what not to eat, "the impact would be staggering."

During the lecture Dr. Brewer emphasizes his objection to soft drinks and starchy foods. At a given point he lowers the boom on the diuretics (water pills) and amphetamines and tells the women they can have all the salt their bodies seem to demand during pregnancy. He also tells them not to worry about swelling hands and ankles; it's normal except in the cases of starvation diets. He refutes the theory that a mother's weight should not go more than 15 or 20 pounds above normal during pregnancy. Even if you go to 50 or 60 pounds, he says, "it won't hurt you. The average weight-gain of a healthy mother is 32 pounds; on a balanced, adequate diet you don't gain too much."

The weight bugaboo developed because some fat women have trouble at childbirth, Dr. Brewer insists. "You can gain weight from eating a good diet or you can gain weight eating a bad diet. It isn't the pounds that count, it's the quality of food you eat."

Anyone familiar with the traditional low-salt diet syndrome will be startled by this doctor's observations: "Millions of women are told not to eat salt during pregnancy. But that's wrong advice. A pregnant woman needs salt just as a pregnant animal does to remain in good health." He then explains that since salt is stored only in the blood and in the fluid outside the cells, it leaves the body if a person perspires. A study in England by Margaret Robinson revealed that mothers on low-salt diets often developed leg cramps, and addition of salt to the diet relieved the condition.

The water pill, which came out in 1958, is condemned by Dr. Brewer. How do they affect the body? According to Dr. Brewer, "It's a drug that poisons the kidneys, makes more water and salt begin to pour out of the kidney, more than the body thinks should come out. It's an interference with Nature. In many clinics, a woman gaining more than the doctor thinks she should, is put on a 1,200-1,500 calorie low-salt diet and then when she starts having normal physiologic edema he brings out the water pills. If she's well nourished, it may not hurt her too much, but if the woman is malnourished and he gives her the water pills, it really becomes difficult."

Equally taboo with the nutrition-minded California M.D. are "diet pills" such as the amphetamines. "Don't take them, they're not healthy for you or your unborn baby. Every drug you take passes quickly from the placenta or afterbirth over into the baby's bloodstream and body. Amphetamines are given to kill the hungry mother's appetite. They also give her an unnatural boost. They relieve depression, make her work seem to go smoother, make her feel she is living a healthier life even though she is not getting enough to eat. But the drug goes right over through the placenta into the baby, and there's a little baby hopped up on drugs. Then when the babies are born we wonder why they're hyperactive, why they have so much trouble. Their metabolism is starved."

During four years of research at Jackson Memorial Hospital in Miami, Dr. Brewer produced scientific evidence that toxemia is directly caused by malnutrition adversely affecting the liver, and that liver dysfunction results in such abnormalities as edema, arterial hypertension, etc.

Often called the watchdog of the gastrointestinal tract, the liver makes albumin, and toxemia patients have low serum albumin. As the albumin level falls, the water and salt from the blood leak out into the spaces between cells creating pathological edema, and the body swells. Dr. Brewer fed his patients albumin intravenously and the swelling subsided.

Another function of the liver is to conjugate and excrete through bile and kidneys the excess female hormones produced in large quantities by the placenta during pregnancy. When its ability to detoxify is impeded by malnutrition, the hormones are not eliminated from the body and accumulate in abnormal quantity.

Dr. Brewer emphasizes that when a pregnant mother is receiving a high quality protein diet, liver dysfunction and the resulting toxemia do not occur. The thrust of his research was on providing patients with high quality protein diets.

Good nutrition, particularly an adequate protein intake, helps support another mechanism that enables the pregnant woman to cope successfully with potentially toxic hormone levels. High estrogen levels, according to Dr. K. J. Catt, author of *An A.B.C. of Endocrinology*, stimulate the synthesis of several proteins by the liver. Among these are proteins that bind with various hormones. "The sex-hormone-binding-globulin," he writes, "is sharply increased and probably minimizes the level of free estrogen in circulation." In other words, while bound to the special protein, estrogen is preserved in large quantities and available for its necessary functions in pregnancy, but much of it is not circulating in a free state to disrupt general body function.

Hormones of various endocrine glands are affected by estrogen levels of pregnancy. According to endocrinologist Dr. Charles Lloyd (in *Textbook of Endocrinology*, W. B. Saunders), the thyroid's hormone, thyroxin, is synthesized in increased quantities—so much so that it can reach levels customarily associated with thyrotoxicosis. This is the disease of racing metabolism and (frequently) bulging eyes caused by an overactive thyroid.

Toxemia Of Pregnancy

The glucocorticoid hormones of the adrenal cortex—such as cortisone—also reach high levels. But in both cases, Dr. Lloyd notes, the stepped-up consumption of fowl, fish, eggs, milk, and cheese provide all the essential amino acids that the body must have to build its own protein molecules.

Besides the glucocorticoids of the adrenal cortex—hormones that regulate metabolism of proteins, carbohydrates, and fats—there's another adrenal hormone concerned with regulation of salt and water balance. It's called aldosterone, and its production increases during pregnancy. Apparently the extra supply is not rendered inert by any hormone-binding protein. According to Dr. Lloyd: "It has been suggested that this rise in aldosterone level may play a role in the production of salt and water retention which is so frequent in late pregnancy."

Aldosterone stimulates the kidneys to retain salt. Water is retained, also, because of the body's need to keep in balance the salt concentration in the serum, intercellular fluid, and within the cells (osmosis).

When, in the normal progress of pregnancy, body mechanisms go to work to hang on to available salt, we see that pregnancy has a stepped-up requirement for this mineral.

Apparently the anti-salt regime originally was tried out because an exaggerated edema (fluid retention in the tissues) is one of the symptoms of toxemia of pregnancy. Because edema is accompanied by weight gain, strict "weight control" became a part of the treatment package.

Dr. Marshall Lindheimer, of the University of Chicago, brought much the same message to a recent meeting of the Chicago and Illinois State Medical Societies (reported in *Family Practice News*, May 1, 1972). Retention of salt and fluid in pregnancy, he said, brings about what "seems to be a physiological hypervolemia"—that is, a normal benign high volume of blood. He warned that salt restriction can be harmful.

Failure to retain salt and water may actually be a cause of toxemia of pregnancy. There is evidence, Dr. Brewer reports, that the high blood pressure of toxemia may be a result of the body's attempt to compensate for a falling blood volume. A postmortem report on deaths from this disease in Bangkok revealed that the women's adrenal glands that produce aldosterone had been overworking. In other words, the bodies of these women had been desperately fighting to conserve salt and increase their water retention and blood volume.

To prevent hypovolemia in pregnancy—that is, low blood volume—both dietary protein and dietary salt are vital, Dr. Brewer stresses.

"Classical obstetrical thought considers 'excess weight gain' from over-eating a possible *cause* of toxemia of pregnancy which remains a major cause of maternal and fetal deaths throughout the world. The *quality* of the obese pregnant woman's diet is totally ignored. There is no longer any question that the obese woman with adequate supplies of essential nutrients in pregnancy will escape having toxemia. It is the malnourished obese woman, the woman lacking essential nutrients, who develops this disorder. Researchers Tracy and Miller in 1969 reported 48 'massive obese' pregnant women with weights reaching 250 pounds or more. Twenty-eight showed no evidence of metabolic toxemia; obviously obesity, per se, does not *cause* toxemia.

"The irrationality and hazards of limiting 'total weight gain' in human pregnancy can be understood in the light of this background. If an arbitrary limit of 20 pounds is set, the healthy pregnant women with access to good foods reaches the limit by the 30th week of gestation. She then is often told to starve herself (and her fetus) during the last 10 weeks during which the fetal demands for essential nutrients, particularly proteins, are rapidly increasing. There are also increased metabolic demands on the maternal liver for conjugating and excreting placental steroids. This function is dependent on adequate supplies of essential amino acids. There is no longer a rational basis for use of 'weight control' and starvation diets in human prenatal care."

Dr. Brewer has support from some well known figures in medicine.

Professor Jean Mayer of the Harvard School of Public Health, Department of Nutrition, wrote Dr. Brewer on Aug. 17, 1971, that "I have always agreed with you on the importance of the role of good nutrition in preventing complications of pregnancy."

Dr. Brewer admits there are problems which can arise for the pregnant woman that make eating a good diet seem impossible. The three problems that follow are the most common and Dr. Brewer presents easy solutions:

1. Nausea and vomiting. Many women have morning sickness in early pregnancy that passes away in a few weeks, but some women have nausea and vomiting throughout pregnancy severe enough to interfere with a good diet. Many pregnant women begin to have heartburn, indigestion, nausea and vomiting when

they're about six or seven months along. If any of these symptoms come up, the doctor should be informed because it is important to have this balanced diet right up to the day of labor.

2. Crowded stomach. During the last month of pregnancy, as the baby is getting larger, the expectant mother may find that her stomach doesn't hold as much as before. The solution to this problem is to eat six smaller meals during the day and even a snack if she wakes up in the middle of the night.

3. Dieting. If a woman is a little overweight she may be put on a special diet for plump women. But she still needs the quart of milk, two eggs, lean meat, vegetables and fruit every day no matter what anyone tells her. The baby inside can't afford to diet.

The late Prof. B. S. Platt of London's School of Tropical Medicine and a leading nutrition scientist worked for years on the thesis that protein-calorie deficiency during pregnancy leads to low birth weight and central nervous system-damaged offspring. His studies were on beagle dogs since he was loathe to starve pregnant women to see if he could produce defective human infants with CNS damage. He made a short movie of some of these puppies who manifested all forms of neurological dysfunction seen in human children from "hyperactivity" and spasticity, to cerebral palsy and epilepsy.

Dr. Roger Williams pointed out in his book *Nutrition Against Disease* that "If all prospective human mothers could be fed as expertly as prospective animal mothers in laboratories, most sterility, spontaneous abortions, stillbirths, and premature births would disappear; the birth of deformed and mentally retarded babies would be largely a thing of the past."

The important thing to remember: a pregnant woman is not just "eating for two." During pregnancy, her endocrine system has greater nutritional demands than at any other time of life. She must take in the extra nutrients that will keep her hormones operating smoothly and safely 24 hours a day.

Section 59
Tuberculosis

268. TB Is Still With Us

268. TB Is Still With Us

The Greek physician Hippocrates first gave tuberculosis the descriptive name *phthisis*, meaning "to waste away." This appellation, along with the term *consumption*, stuck until the discovery in the late 1800's of the *tubercle bacillus*, the organism which causes the disease.

The acute form of tuberculosis, which often afflicted children, was called *galloping consumption*, because its progress was so rapid and severe, particularly in children.

During the late nineteenth and early twentieth centuries, the sanatorium formed the basis of tuberculosis treatment. Patients "taking the cure" were required to eat large meals and get plenty of rest and fresh air. All demanding activity was strictly forbidden to the sanatorium dweller. A stay in the sanatorium could last from a few months to several years, depending on the individual's progress.

In 1882, Robert Koch first isolated the *tubercle bacillus*, but it was not until 1924 that the first vaccine was developed. Since that time, the incidence of new cases has dropped steadily, except during the world wars, but the disease is still far from being completely eradicated.

Who Gets Tuberculosis?
The vast majority of Americans are no longer even vaguely threatened by tuberculosis. For most of us, tuberculosis is a deadly ghost of the past, and thankfully so. But this idyllic state is not world-wide; indeed, it is not even nation-wide. Right here in America there are still thousands of men and women suffering from TB. In 1973, some 31,000 new active cases were reported in the United States. And tuberculosis remains a serious health problem in many developing countries, where resources for its detection and treatment are limited.

A high incidence of tuberculosis is associated with such factors as high population densities (the highest rates of new cases are found in large cities), low living standards and inadequate nutrition, in addition to contact with persons having active cases of the illness.

During the 1950's, a quiet torpor settled on American TB control. The disease, people believed, was safely gone. But in the early 1960's, the news media once again reported TB—not its lingering presence, but an alarming return. In the impoverished areas of America, where resistance to infection was as low as the malnutrition rate was high, TB was making a startling comeback. Re-emergence was not among the middle class, but among the urban poor, chiefly among blacks who had migrated from the South.

Symptoms Of TB

Tuberculosis can affect any tissue of the body, but usually attacks the lungs, causing nodules and cavities, and eventual scarring of the lung tissue. It may seem at first to be a simple respiratory ailment, and it is often mistaken for chronic bronchitis. But as the illness progresses, the following symptoms generally appear: dry cough, periods of breathlessness, slight fever accompanied by sweating in the night, extreme fatigue from everyday activities, loss of weight, loss of appetite, especially in the morning and finally coughing of blood-stained sputum.

Sometimes the illness appears with no warning signs. In 10 percent of cases, the patient suddenly coughs up blood when seemingly in perfect health.

How TB Is Spread

Once inside the body, the *tubercle bacillus* may remain dormant for a long time, until a weakening of the body's resistance gives the bacillus a chance to multiply. When enough bacilli are present, the symptoms of tuberculosis appear and the disease becomes active. Although over a quarter of the population carries some *tubercle bacilli* in the body, only a small percentage ever develops active TB.

The disease is also carried by cows, and the bacilli can be transmitted through the unpasteurized milk of infected cows.

Testing For TB

With the rise in tuberculosis cases during World War II, the need arose for a quick, efficient way to test for the disease. The primary objective was to identify tuberculosis in its early stages and isolate those infected in the hope of arresting and possibly curing the illness.

The solution was to modify conventional X-ray equipment so it could be transported to places within easy access of the general population. The chest X-ray seemed ideal—it was cheap, fast and simple to operate. Results are immediate and no follow-up period is needed, as there is for the skin testing method. The chest X-ray has been widely used, and is still in service today.

Unfortunately, this method of tuberculosis screening has several important drawbacks which have caused many health agencies to question its desirability in recent years. The amount of radiation to which the chest X-ray exposes a person is 10 times the amount received from the diagnostic X-ray used to locate broken bones and other injuries. Also, the X-ray can only identify the disease in its active stage, when the cavities and scarring are visible in the lungs. The presence of inactive *tubercle bacilli* in the body, from which a person might develop active TB, is not detected by the X-ray. Therefore, many potential cases of tuberculosis can go unidentified.

The only other type of test for tuberculosis is the skin test. There are several kinds of skin tests, but basically, the procedure consists of injecting a small amount of a tuberculin solution under the skin of the forearm and checking for a reaction a few days later. A small hard patch of several raised bumps will develop on the arm. If they remain small, the test is considered negative, but if they exceed a certain size, the test is positive.

The skin test also has its drawbacks. Since the procedure is rather involved, and follow-up is necessary to determine results, the test is not feasible for mass screening, especially in developing countries with limited personnel and resources. Further, the skin test will detect people who have *tubercle bacilli* in their bodies, but cannot show whether the organisms are active or inactive. A positive skin test must be followed by further testing to determine the severity of the disease.

A child who has been exposed to an adult with active tuberculosis must continue to have a negative skin test for at least 10 weeks after his last contact with the infected person, before he is considered free of infection.

Treating Tuberculosis

When a person tests positive, he begins treatment. If his case is inactive, he is given drugs to prevent him from developing active tuberculosis. If his case is already active, he must undergo full treatment, and will probably have to spend some time in the hospital.

Modern methods of treatment center around drugs, apparently

the only means known for eliminating the *tubercle bacilli* from the body.

The first step toward contemporary methods of treatment was taken in 1921, when the first TB vaccine, called BCG after its discoverers, Calmette and Guerin, appeared on the medical scene. A patient was inoculated with *tubercle bacilli* (taken from a cow or a potato) that were no longer virulent. His body developed antibodies to fight the invading germ and he became immune to the disease. The vaccine seemed to work initially, but it had many bad features.

BCG eliminated the chance of detecting tuberculosis with conventional tests because the person inoculated with the vaccine appeared to have TB. The vaccine was of no use to people already infected. And because BCG was made from what is called a "mixed culture" of bacilli, rather than a "pure" culture, no two batches were exactly the same. Sometimes the vaccine was too weak, and could not cause immunity, and sometimes it was too strong, and inoculees came down with TB.

As research continued, BCG was abandoned in favor of newer and more effective drugs.

The cornerstone of tuberculosis treatment today is a drug called isoniazid, or INH. Other drugs, such as PAS, streptomycin and ethambutol are also used in some cases. The goal of drug therapy is first, to make the patient non-contagious and second, to eliminate the bacilli from his body.

Isoniazid is used both for patients with active TB, and for those who have only been exposed to the disease. Members of a patient's family, even though they test negative, are usually given isoniazid for a year to prevent them from contracting TB. Sometimes, people may be diagnosed as tuberculous and put on drugs on the basis of a single X-ray, without further corroborating evidence that they harbor active bacilli in their bodies.

Isoniazid therapy is apparently effective in wiping out tuberculosis in those suffering from it, but the drug causes several undesirable and sometimes dangerous side effects.

Sensitive persons can develop liver disease during isoniazid therapy. Liver damage can range from slight to severe and even fatal. In most cases, the possibility of developing liver disease cannot be predicted before it occurs. Symptoms of liver damage include fatigue, loss of appetite and a general "unwell" feeling. Urine will be dark, and the skin or eyeballs may appear jaundiced. If an isoniazid patient notices any of these signs, he must discontinue using the drug and have treatment for the liver disease.

Isoniazid is structurally related to the B vitamins niacin and pyridoxine (B_6). Because it interferes with the metabolism of pyridoxine, peripheral neuritis (an inflammation of nerve endings) is a common side effect. This aggravating condition produces sensations of tingling, burning, numbness and weakness in the muscles. A study performed at the University of Hawaii and reported in *The American Journal of Clinical Nutrition* in May, 1974, showed that supplementing the diets of isoniazid patients with pyridoxine relieved the symptoms of peripheral neuritis.

The study further indicated that subjects being treated with isoniazid were deficient in B_6, and even a control group of normal healthy individuals was on the borderline of deficiency. The researchers concluded that persons being treated with isoniazid need pyridoxine supplementation to prevent B_6 deficiency.

It doesn't seem that even our modern drug treatments will be able to make tuberculosis truly a disease of the past. In addition to causing harmful side effects, the drugs simply don't reach many TB victims, especially the elderly, and those in crowded, low-income areas. Many of these people are missed in mass TB screening programs, and rarely see a doctor. And should they be aware that they are suffering from tuberculosis, the required hospital stay and costly drugs are often unaffordable. Also, those on isoniazid must be motivated and supervised to continue taking the drug throughout the long course of treatment, which can run from one to two years.

Problems In Diagnosis

The misdiagnosis of tuberculosis as various other ailments contributes to its persistence. A study conducted at two hospitals in Belfast (*British Medical Journal*, January 19, 1974), showed that many cases of tuberculosis had been overlooked in middle-aged and elderly hospital patients because they were suffering from another acute illness at the same time, or because the TB was misdiagnosed.

Researchers found that tuberculosis was sometimes wrongly diagnosed as chronic bronchitis or carcinomatosis (widespread cancer), and abnormalities evident in chest X-rays were often disregarded. Also, since most of the patients studied who were found to have tuberculosis also had other illnesses, no TB tests were performed even though symptoms were present.

The findings of this study illustrate yet another pitfall in tuberculosis treatment. Since many medical people (as well as the general public) believe the disease to be rare, symptoms may be overlooked and the disease allowed to go untreated. In such a situation, there is great danger that *tubercle bacilli* will be transmitted to hospital personnel attending the patient, as well as to members of the patient's family, without anyone realizing it.

The Role Of Nutrition

Improvement of nutrition formed the basis of the old sanatorium treatment for tuberculosis. Huge quantities of milk were prescribed for the "consumptive," or tubercular patient. The method of "force feeding," getting the patient as fat as possible, led one doctor to stuff his patient with 16 raw eggs, 29 glasses of milk, a pound of raw beefsteak, bacon and potatoes. Although doctors in those days didn't know about specific nutrients and what they contribute to the health of the body, they did know that most TB patients were frail and underweight. The goal of treatment was first to isolate the contagious patient, and then to build up his physical strength by having him eat several large meals each day. Patients were also to get lots of rest, and most sanatoria had several mandatory rest periods throughout the day.

As we now know, inadequate diet predisposes us to disease. When people are frankly malnourished, or even when minor deficiencies of important nutrients occur, the body's defenses are weakened and unable to fight off disease organisms. When a disease such as tuberculosis does attack, it is much more virulent, spreads more rapidly and can recur more readily in an undernourished person.

In *Postgraduate Medicine* (December, 1971), Harvard nutritionist Dr. Jean Mayer discusses the role of nutrition in tuberculosis. He cites evidence gathered during the two world wars that among undernourished people in blockaded cities and in prison camps, the incidence of tuberculosis rose sharply. In peacetime, when the quality but not the caloric value of the diets of Norwegian navy personnel was improved, incidence of tuberculosis declined.

Tuberculosis

Dr. Mayer states that although faulty diet cannot be regarded as a major cause of tuberculosis, poor nutrition inhibits the production of antibodies to fight the disease. A balanced diet can certainly help increase the body's resistance to *tubercle bacilli*, and reduce the chances of developing an active case of TB.

Section 60
Ulcers

269. What Is An Ulcer?

Your digestive system produces strong acids and juices that are designed to help break down the food you eat so that its components can be used to nourish the body. The lining of the healthy stomach is marvelously resistant to these juices and is not affected by their caustic nature. In ulcer patients, this defense of the stomach's lining against stomach acids has broken down somehow, so that, even when the ulcer patient's stomach is empty of food, the digestive juices pour forth and work away at his stomach lining as though it were food. The continued irritation of this now-delicate area soon produces a sore, which we know by the name of ulcer.

It is easy to become confused by the terminology commonly used by doctors in discussing ulcers. The bewildered patient's family cringes as his duodenal, gastric or peptic ulcer is discussed. Surely it would help them to know that all gastrointestinal ulcers are termed "peptic." The gastric type is usually the most serious and actually occurs in the stomach lining. A duodenal ulcer occurs in the duodenum, the short tube through which the stomach empties. Duodenal ulcers, the less dangerous type, are the most common.

Usually an ulcer responds to treatment, at least for a time. When it does not, there is a danger that it will "perforate," that is, it will eat through the stomach wall, allowing the contents of the stomach to leak into the abdominal cavity. When this happens, immediate surgery to mend the opening is essential.

A "hemorrhaging ulcer" is one which has penetrated a blood vessel, causing it to bleed into the digestive tract. The victim is likely to have the frightening experience of vomiting blood, or, if the ulcer is further down, and the bleeding is less severe, blood may appear in the stool.

Another ulcer complication is "obstruction," the result of scar tissue from a healed ulcer which has spread into passageways between the stomach and the duodenum, blocking the movement of food.

What Is An Ulcer?

The symptoms of ulcers can vary from headaches to choking sensations to low back pains and to itching. When pain does occur in the stomach, a person often charges it off to some dietary indiscretion. Finally, the pain becomes so intense as to be clearly recognizable as an ulcer, and a hasty trip to the doctor is in order.

270. Do Emotions Play A Role In Ulcers?

Whether or not the emotions play a role in the cause of ulcers has always been an open medical question, since no objective tests have ever shown a definite cause and effect relationship. However, several researchers now maintain that increased daily pressures in business and society are responsible for the growing number of ulcer patients, now numbering 10 to 12 percent of the United States' population.

The ulcer victims come from all the social classes, with men, for some unknown reason, apparently much more susceptible to ulcers than women. Ulcers were once pictured as an affliction of the so-called "executive set." But several medical researchers state that anyone who is subjected to a great deal of stress is a prime candidate. According to *Psychosomatics: How Your Emotions Can Damage Your Health* by Howard and Martha Lewis (The Viking Press, 1972), the frustrating situations of daily life which constantly demand that the individual make important decisions are often the cause of stress, and can cause many illnesses, including ulcers. "In one study fully 86 percent of ulcerative colitis patients had a well-defined and serious life crisis in the six months before they became ill. These included job changes, moving to a new home, death in the family, and other upsetting situations," they reported.

In the mid-1960's, Dr. Sidney Cobb, then a professor at the University of Michigan, studied the health of blue-collar workers at a Detroit paint plant who had received a two year advance notice in 1963 that their company would close down and that they would lose their jobs, according to an article in the *Medical World News* (March 24, 1975). For many of these men it also meant the end of a 20 year career and the frustration of learning a new skill (if they were lucky enough to find one) and literally starting life all over again. Observing signs of other illnesses as well, once the plant was ready to shut down, Dr. Cobb noticed that "symptoms of peptic ulcer were 'unduly common around the time of termination.'" He was also surprised to find that the wives of three workers were hospitalized with peptic ulcers within two months of the plant's closing.

Dr. James P. Henry, professor of physiology at the University of California School of Medicine, regarded the findings of Dr. Cobb as typical of the effects of stress. In regard to coping with the ill effects of stress upon ulcers, Dr. Henry advised keeping one's composure simply by being practical about anxiety-causing drugs. "Drop the analeptic drugs like caffeine. Don't drink coffee. The point is, if a patient is going up the curve of unavoidable stress, then at all costs advise him to keep the avoidable stresses down." (*Medical World News*, March 27, 1975).

Encountering stress is almost inevitable in this day and age. Therefore it is wise to take preventive measures against the potential effects of day to day stress, such as ulcers. The best course is to maintain a strong body through good nutrition, and to eliminate intake of any items which can create stress, such as certain drugs, alcohol and all caffeine-containing products.

271. Types Of Ulcers And Their Causes

Ulcerative Colitis

Once a doctor has diagnosed a case of ulcerative colitis, a chronic ulceration of the colon, his problems are just beginning as he attempts to find a cause for the illness. He may have to pick his way through scores of technical papers that blame things like curtailed breast feedings, emotional frustrations, and allergenic diets, among many other possibilities. The next problem is to decide whether to keep the patient in bed, prescribe cortisone suppositories, advise psychiatric help, operate, or take something out of the diet—all recognized treatments for ulcerative colitis. In official medical texts ulcerative colitis is of "unknown etiology" (cause), and "there is no specific course of therapy."

Drs. Ralph Wright and S. C. Truelove, reporting in the *British Medical Journal* (July 17, 1965), stated that after controlled experiments they came to believe that milk is a major offender in the development of ulcerative colitis, and taking it out of the diet, they said, may be a simple and effective treatment for many patients.

The test was triggered by repeated suggestions in medical literature that ulcerative colitis is involved with food allergy. Cow's milk was always a strong suspect, along with wheat, tomatoes, oranges, potatoes, and eggs in that order. But the reports that appeared never involved the scientifically desirable controlled therapeutic trials. Drs. Wright and Truelove decided to make such a test.

A group of 77 patients suffering from attacks of ulcerative colitis was divided into three dietary categories: milk-free diet; gluten-free plus milk-free diet; and a control group on a "dummy" diet. The patients were required to keep strictly to the diet for a year and to have monthly checkups. In addition to the diet, all the patients received the standard medical treatment for ulcerative colitis. This way any changes in the individual groups could be directly associated with diet.

On the milk-free, low roughage diet, all milk and milk products, including cheese and powdered milk, were eliminated. The gluten-free plus milk-free diet was a modification of the gluten-free diet used in the hospital to treat celiac-type diseases. Patients on the dummy diet were told (largely for appearances) to eliminate such items of diet as fried foods, condiments and ice cream. In particular they were advised to consume milk and milk products liberally.

Of the 77 patients, those on the gluten-free plus milk-free diet had to be eliminated from the test, because they were unable to maintain strict adherence to the diet. The comparison was made then between the patients on the milk-free diet and those on the dummy diet. Ten patients on a milk-free diet remained well for the year compared with five on a dummy diet. Three other patients had relapses and were withdrawn from trial on the milk-free group compared with eight who had relapses in the control group.

"From our figures," the authors stated, "the best estimate appears to be that a milk-free diet is beneficial to about one in five patients with ulcerative colitis, with a suggestion that the proportion may be higher in patients in their first attack of the disease." It should be noted that all of the patients included in the test were receiving standard medical care at the same time. In spite of this, twice the number of patients on the milk-free diet were symptom-free for a year compared with those on the dummy diet.

Some of the patients included in the test had previously responded well to a milk-free diet, and had relapses when milk was reintroduced. One of these, a married woman of 35, said she was symptom-free for three and a half years on a milk-free diet and relapsed six weeks after milk was reintroduced. She returned to the milk-free diet from 1960 to 1962 and stayed well. When she joined the present trial, she fell into the dummy-diet group and relapsed three times in rapid succession before she had to withdraw from the trial after eight months. She went back to a milk-free diet, and since then has been entirely well for the 21 months that followed.

Another of the patients in the test, a woman age 37, was put on a milk-free diet in 1955 after a three-year period of repeated attacks. From then on she remained well on a milk-free diet, but twice relapsed when milk was deliberately reintroduced. When she was admitted to the present trial, she fell into the milk-free group and the relapse responded swiftly to the no-milk treatment. She remained well through the one-year trial period and also during the year which followed. She has refused to use any milk in her diet again.

No one would deliberately chance a return bout with ulcerative colitis. It involves abdominal pain and diarrhea which is profuse, frequent and bloody. Stools are characterized by mucus and pus. Weight loss may be severe. Fever and a general feeling of discomfort usually associated with anemia and malnutrition are common symptoms. Anyone suffering from ulcerative colitis processes food through the digestive tract so rapidly that he gains little of the nourishment from it.

Because ulcerative colitis tends to occur in a familial pattern, the suggestion that diet plays a part in its development is especially reasonable. One thing common to most families is the type of food served. People become used to certain types of food served at the table week after week, and they carry these preferences with them into married life and pass them on to the next generation. If you come from a milk-drinking, bread-eating family, it is likely that your children will also take to these foods.

Typical Victim
Many writers have pointed out the psychological characteristics which ulcerative colitis victims have in common. They tend to be dependent, sensitive, insecure, fearful and submissive. Some physicians believe that ulcerative colitis may be the result of failure to meet a challenge, or it might occur after an outburst of emotion in people who are prone to this weakness. None of us has much control over the emotional make-up we were born with, which might predispose us to ulcerative colitis, but we can take the precaution of eating sensibly. The best protection an individual has against ulcerative colitis is a healthful diet.

Of course the last measure in the treatment of ulcerative colitis is radical surgery. It is known that ulcerative colitis of long duration can turn into cancer in a small percentage of cases. For this reason an effective treatment is extremely important.

If you have ulcerative colitis, be certain that your doctor includes a test for allergy to milk, wheat and other foods as part of his diagnosis. It may save you from the complications of a serious illness whose treatment is admittedly a medical guessing game.

Esophageal Ulcers
Another type of ulcer and one that is becoming increasingly more common, is the esophageal ulcer. The walls of your stomach are

coated with a thick mucous coating as a protection against the powerful stomach acids, but the walls of your esophagus (the tube connecting the throat to the stomach) are not. And when the stomach acids touch the walls of the esophagus, it stimulates the nerve ending there—an extremely painful condition—and can cause an ulcer.

Gastric juices, except during regurgitation, are normally never in your esophagus, but during a certain type of hiatal hernia, the diaphragm is too high and part of the esophagus can be easily trapped in the abdomen when the stomach muscles are displaced.

The best way to prevent an esophageal ulcer is simply to prevent the conditions that allow the hiatal hernia to form. A hiatal hernia is formed by the loosening of muscles in the area of the diaphragm which allows the stomach muscles to break through. Your eating habits and your physical condition have a significant effect. If you stuff yourself at meals, drink too much or let yourself become overweight, you put unnecessary strain on the diaphragm by bloating your stomach. Naturally your stomach will try to push through because of the pressure of expansion.

The symptoms are not always easy to recognize, and when they do appear, it's not hard to mistake them for something else. Dr. T. W. Challis of Queen's University, Kingston, Ontario, estimates that about half of the poeple whose hiatal hernias were discovered accidentally had no signs of the problem. But if you suffer from any of the symptoms, you should certainly nurture suspicions. It's best to have it diagnosed early, because waiting can lead to complications, including infections and hemorrhaging of the esophagus. Also, irritation of the esophagus by the stomach acids can cause a spasm or involuntary contraction of the muscles there, producing pain that is quite similar to that caused by a heart attack.

Aspirin Causes Ulcers

While all the bland diets in the world will not help to reduce or eliminate ulcers, a simple decision to avoid the use of aspirin and aspirin-containing drugs, as well as corticosteroids, will go a long way toward eliminating this painful and serious disease.

Aspirin (chemically known as salicylic acid) was easily the wonder drug of yesteryear. But even then, the irritation and damage it caused to the membranes lining the mouth, gullet and stomach made medical men reluctant to prescribe it. By 1876, doctors found a way to cut down on some of the damage to the stomach wall by replacing the hydrogen ion that made the original salicylic acid so irritating with sodium. This created a new complication, an obnoxious sweetish taste. It took another 20 years before Felix Hofmann, a Bayer chemist, accomplished the successful acetylation of salicylic acid, giving us the overwhelming American favorite with sales exceeding 400 million dollars a year.

In the early days, patients were warned to dissolve the aspirin tablets in "a little sugar water flavored with two drops of lemon juice." Otherwise, the tablets would have disintegrated slowly and unevenly in the stomach, bringing lumps of acetylsalicylic acid into contact with the stomach wall, with damaging results. Although modern aspirin tablets are designed for quick dissolution, an article in the *Scientific American* (Nov., 1963) reported that ". . . a real risk remains, as indicated by the gastrointestinal bleeding in some individuals that can follow the taking of aspirin and by the fact that acetylsalicylic acid and its chemical relatives can produce a stomach ulcer in rats, even when these drugs are injected under the skin rather than swallowed. In some people aspirin induces an allergic hypersensitivity; thereafter a small dose has been known to provoke a fatal reaction." It is estimated that about five percent of this country's population has some allergy to aspirin.

These findings were later corroborated by the studies of such researchers as Dr. Elliot L. Sagall, M.D., director of medical education for the American Trial Lawyers Association, who reported that "Aspirin is potentially capable of inducing severe gastric upset, acute ulceration of gastric and duodenal mucous membrane, aggravation of pre-existent or latent gastric and duodenal peptic ulcer, initiation of fresh ulceration, and precipitation of chronic or acute massive gastroduodenal hemorrhage . . ." (*Trial*, March, 1969).

Aspirin often aggravates bleeding in people who don't realize that they have an ulcer, according to Dr. J. Donald Ostrow of the University of Pennsylvania, who testified at the Senate Subcommittee Hearing on Monopoly in June, 1973, that one out of 10 Americans develop a peptic ulcer during his lifetime, sometimes without knowing it and sometimes with ulcer pain accompanied by a headache. When these ulcer or potential ulcer victims take aspirin for their headaches, reported Dr. Ostrow, they can further damage the stomach lining and precipitate gastrointestinal bleeding.

If you must keep aspirin in the house, you should put it with your "calculated risk" remedies. And remember that aspirin comes in many cloaks. Common preparations containing acetyl-salicylic acid include: Anacin, Anahist, APC compound, Ascriptin, Aspergum, Bufferin, Coricidin, Darvon compound, Dristan, Edrisal, Empirin, Excedrin, Fiorinal, Phensal, Pyrroxate, Sine-off, Trigesic, Vanquish and Zactirin, Cope, Novahistine, Tranco-gesic, Panalgesic, Percobarb, Percodan, Persistin, Pabi-rin, Kengesin, Measurin, Ecotrin, Daprisal, Cirin, Cama Inlay-Tabs, Buff-A Comp, Ascodeen and many other compounds.

Aspirin, of course, does have its uses. It does reduce pain and inflammation and it does bring down fever. But what we don't realize is that we pay a price—sometimes a very high one—for these favors.

Steroid Ulcers

When cortisone and the other steroids were introduced as treatments for rheumatoid arthritis, doctors never suspected the trouble they were getting into. Gradually it became clear that relief was only temporary, and the side-effects so serious and far-reaching that indiscriminate use of these drugs for treating chronic disease was both unwise and dangerous. One of the major side-effects is the "steroid ulcer."

In a discussion of this very special type of ulcer, Dr. R. Menguy, writing in the *American Journal of Digestive Diseases* (December, 1967), said, "Steroid ulcers appear to have certain characteristics which differentiate them from the ordinary 'garden variety' of peptic ulcer." Their most dangerous characteristic is their lack of symptoms. They often appear without the usual manifestations of ulcer distress —no pain, no digestive discomfort, no warning blood. Add the fact that these ulcers have a high incidence of hemorrhage and perforation, and it is clear that a steroid ulcer can be extremely dangerous.

Dr. Menguy noted that patients receive large doses of steroids under circumstances other than rheumatism—certain collagen diseases, for graft rejection and skin disease. Many of them develop ulcers. Dr. Menguy also stated that adrenal cortico-steroids frequently caused ulcers in experimental animals.

However, for some people, the pain and immobility caused by

arthritis can only be alleviated by the use of certain steroid drugs. If the patient is willing to risk the dangers of the drug to obtain some relief, then he should also take some vitamin B_{12}. Three Rumanian researchers reported in the *Archives Internationales de Pharmacodynamie et de Therapie* (Sept., 1965) that vitamin B_{12} neutralized the ulcer-causing effect of cortisone in experimental animals. Drs. Hadnagy, Biro and Kelemen discovered that B_{12} actually fought cortisone in certain ways. Sometimes B_{12} improves glucose tolerance in patients using cortisone; where cortisone inhibits the regeneration of the liver in rats, vitamin B_{12} stimulates this regeneration and can counteract the damaging effect of the cortisone.

Surprisingly, the Rumanian experiments showed that ulcers are brought on by cortisone only in certain parts of the stomach. In the forestomach cortisone actually prevented the development of ulcers; but, in the glandular (pyloric) portion of the stomach, the size of the ulcers was greater, and the number almost doubled in hydrocortisone-treated animals compared with the controls. However, B_{12} proved capable of neutralizing this ulcer-causing effect of hydrocortisone, even in the most susceptible part of the stomach.

The three researchers found that cortisone inhibits the mucus secretion of the stomach lining. This mucus ordinarily protects the stomach lining against the digestive action of the gastric juices. Thus, it is possible that cortisone causes ulcers because it cuts down on protective mucus secretions. The cortisone ulcer might also be due to a selective poisonous effect cortisone has on the cells, while vitamin B_{12} encourages orderly breakdown and replacement. Cortisone also tends to destroy protein while B_{12} builds it.

Why does cortisone cause trouble only in the pyloric area of the stomach? Ulcers that occur in the forestomach usually result from some inflammation. Cortisone acts to soothe inflammations. The mechanism involved in forming pyloric ulcers is not the same and inflammatory reactions do not play a part. These Rumanian scientists believed that B_{12} could reverse whatever metabolic changes are brought about by cortisone in the pyloric area, and that this is how B_{12} provides protection.

When the doctors suspected that vitamin B_{12} not only counteracted the ulcer-causing effects of cortisone, but also appeared to reduce the formation of the ulcers from other causes, they decided to examine the effects of B_{12} further. As they expected,

B_{12} treated rats, made ulcer-prone by fasting, had a lower number of gastric perforations (ulcers) than the group that did not get B_{12}. This was true in both parts of the stomach, the pyloric section and the forestomach. "We find that vitamin B-treated animals showed a larger percentage (36 percent) of ulcer-free cases than in the control group (24 percent)," reported the researchers.

Coffee, Smoking And Alcohol Dangerous To Stomach

Your common sense should tell you to avoid such stomach irritants as alcohol, smoking and products containing caffeine. The substances, almost all ulcer experts agree, are potential causes of new ulcers and will aggravate any already present.

Alcohol is not only a local irritant that can eat away vulnerable parts of your stomach lining, but it also depletes the body of tissue building nutrients such as the B complex vitamins. It also strips the body of other vital nutrients.

For more than half a century, biostatisticians dismissed the correlation between cigarette smoking and ulcers as coincidental. But in 1971, Dr. Eugene Jacobson, chairman of the Department of Physiology at the University of Oklahoma, announced that he and his colleagues had "the first demonstration of what we feel might be the direct link." Dr. Jacobson said, according to a report in *Medical World News* (June 4, 1971), that laboratory studies with test animals had shown that nicotine in the blood was "lifting protection from the duodenum by inhibiting pancreatic and bilary buffering secretions," while at the same time increasing the output of gastric juices.

Caffeine products, especially coffee, are known to cause an increased flow of the digestive juices, which are responsible for continued irritation of the stomach lining. It stands to reason that any person who saturates his stomach with six to eight cups of coffee a day is needlessly coating the stomach with these acids on a regular basis. But coffee is not the only beverage that contains the ulcer producing caffeine. It is true that coffee contains more of the chemical than other beverages—about 100-150 milligrams per cup. But caffeine is also found in tea (67 milligrams per cup), chocolate (68 milligrams per cup) and cola drinks (32 milligrams per 8 oz. cup). If you are suffering from an ulcer, it is extremely important that you eliminate these beverages from your diet.

272. Is There An Ulcer Diet?

Traditional Diets Won't Help

Despite the fact that the medical profession has recognized ulcers as a major health problem for quite some time, no one knows exactly what causes them. Intense emotions have been blamed, yet we are aware that even the mildest persons can be stricken by ulcers. Even though, statistically, men are more prone to ulcers than women, there is no clearcut way to identify those who will get an ulcer and those who will not, since people with every imaginable type of personality have suffered from them.

And when it comes to curing ulcers, there have been just as many variations. At first it was believed that only the surgeon's knife could "cure" an ulcer. Then, it was chemical treatments; in some instances, even attempts to freeze them. But the most traditional therapy has been the bland diet liberally laced with milk and cream.

Doctors have been using a milk-based bland diet (Sippy Diet) for so long that many people think that milk has some magical quality which soothes and heals any number of gastric ailments, not to mention stomach ulcers. But while many doctors still use bland diets, medical leaders have long known that the Sippy Diet—designed by Chicago doctor Bertram W. Sippy more than a half-century ago—is of no value in the treatment of gastric ulcers, except, of course, immediately following surgery.

The Sippy Diet consists of milk-sodden foods whose primary function is to inhibit the action of the gastric juices or at least to neutralize them. A daily meal regimen consists of small portions of prescribed foods taken at frequent intervals. Hourly intakes of milk and cream are recommended, theoretically providing a constant drip of milk into the stomach to counteract the effect of gastric acids. Also on the forbidden list, at the direction of most physicians, are raw fruits and vegetables, even though there is no evidence that these foods actually aggravate ulcers.

Though milk may have a palliative effect on the pain of ulcers, there is little evidence that it actually heals them. In *The*

American Journal of Clinical Nutrition (February, 1969), Dr. Douglas W. Piper described studies showing that an ulcer patient would have to drink almost a quart of milk every hour to neutralize the gastric juices which aggravate an ulcer.

Medical World News (June 23, 1972) reported on this country's first controlled study of the effects of bland diet therapy on ulcer patients. A group of 50 duodenal ulcer patients eating a traditional bland diet was compared with another group of duodenal ulcer patients who were fed the standard hospital diet. After an initial in-hospital study of 21 days, with controlled outpatient studies of more than a year, the researchers concluded: "Our data show that duodenal ulcers in humans heal as rapidly with a regular diet as with a restricted diet. In addition, X-ray recurrences of duodenal ulcer were not more frequent while the patient was following a regular unrestricted diet during a one-year follow-up."

A Sensible Diet

Although most doctors know that bland diets have no bearing on the treatment of an ulcer, many still routinely prescribe them to patients. Ironically, some patients are disappointed when the doctor doesn't do so!

But if bland diets have been found ineffectual, what can be done? The advice of a group of British surgeons, which was reported in the *Drug and Therapeutic Bulletin* (January 20, 1967), suggested a sound common sense approach to diet therapy. Instead of looking for universal remedies to peptic ulcers, they say each person should trust his own reactions. In other words, if you find that a certain food disagrees with you or causes discomfort, stop eating that particular food. An ulcer patient should never eat an abundance of food at any one meal, but should take snacks on and off. That way there is always a little bit of food in the stomach for the digestive acids to work on. And besides, if you eat large amounts of food often, it conditions your stomach to secrete large amounts of acids to digest the food. In other words, eat what you want, when you want, but limit yourself in terms of quantity. This group of British physicians agrees that while ulcer patients generally are able to eat all types of foods, fried foods appear to be more than the stomach can handle. So for all ulcer patients, as well as for people who are not afflicted with an ulcer, avoiding fried foods is advisable.

The Natural Diet Therapy

The ulcer cliche revolves around too much hard work, the anxiety of our age, too many highly spiced foods, too few meals at irregular times, and the list goes on. However, Dr. T. L. Cleave, a noted British physician, rejects these standard theories. In his book, *Peptic Ulcer, Causation, Prevention and Arrest* (John Wright and Sons Ltd., Bristol, 1962) he asserted that the cause of ulcers can be found in what we have done to our foods by processing essential protein out of them. When there is no protein to be broken down by the gastric juices, they spend their power on the stomach lining, and an ulcer results when the lining can no longer stand the onslaught.

Dr. Cleave believes that the lack of proper nutrition is responsible for the enormous number of peptic ulcers found throughout the world today.

Concerning stress, Dr. Cleave cites several instances in which stress was unusually prevalent, yet the persons involved emerged with no signs of ulcers. Such trying times as the period of rule in Germany before Stalingrad, or that period of time when thousands of prisoners were held in Tokyo during many months in which the city was almost annihilated, were instances when people emerged free from ulcer symptoms. Why? During these trying times people had very little to eat, and what they did eat consisted of items such as raw turnips and potatoes taken directly from the fields. There was no cooking or refining of these foods, thus retaining all the essential minerals so necessary for good health.

"Natural instincts should be allowed to play on natural foods." By natural instinct, Dr. Cleave is referring to the instincts involved in choosing meal patterns and the food that is eaten. By natural foods, Dr. Cleave is speaking of all foods, whether cooked or raw, as long as the foods have not been subjected to any refining processes.

He feels that people should eat natural foods and eat them only when they are really hungry. Eating just for the sake of eating or because food happens to be available, then perhaps depriving yourself of food when you are really hungry, does much more harm than good for an individual. By not eating when one is hungry, the peristaltic action and gastric juices build up and have no new food to work on. The acidity of the stomach reaches an unusually high level, thus subjecting the stomach to long exposures of these juices. The membranes lining the stomach are then irritated by these juices, thus providing a conducive atmosphere for starting an ulcer.

There is no need whatsoever for this to occur. If an individual satisfies his appetite, he will be combining foods in a most natural way. Dr. Cleave feels that there is no need to refrain from eating special food combinations, nor is there any need to refrain from drinking with meals. He states, "Whatever a person wishes to eat or drink under the dictates of natural appetite, will be healthful for him."

If the question of just what natural foods are should still have you puzzled, Dr. Cleave makes it as clear as can be: "The unnatural foods mostly consist of refined carbohydrates and fall into two groups: (1) food containing white flour (or other processed cereals, such as polished rice), and all the pastry, cakes, cookies, macaroni and other foods made from white flour; (2) foods consisting of the ordinary white or brown sugar sold in grocery stores, or containing it, as in chocolate, candies, ice creams and other confections."

Dr. Cleave's recommendations are as simple as that. Eat natural foods, and eat them when you're hungry only, and the bleak prospect of an ulcer which so many Americans must face, can indeed be avoided.

273. Nutrients Fight Ulcers

Vitamin E And Ulcers

Researchers in California discovered that when mice are subjected to stress, those given large amounts of vitamin E developed far fewer and less serious ulcers than those who received nothing but a standard "good" diet. Writing in *The American Journal of Clinical Nutrition*, (Sept., 1972), Jon A. Kangas, Ph.D., K. Michael Schmidt, Ph.D., and George F. Solomon, M.D., explained that they divided rats into two groups of 12 each. The first received 50 mg. of a vitamin E solution twice daily while the second received a fluid similar to the vitamin E, but lacking the vitamin.

Special cages were built with clean plastic dividers running down the center. The dividers effectively kept the rats from their food and water but made sure that they could see it sitting there, just out of reach. The rats were permitted access to the food only once a day. Just as the constant crush of business with its high pressure gives men ulcers, the agony of seeing the food and water just out of reach gave ulcers to the rats.

After 12 days of this routine, the rats were meticulously autopsied. A panel of three pathologists then determined that the rats who didn't get vitamin E had stomach ulcers of a very strong intensity, rated 3.42 on a four-point scale. Those given vitamin E had ulcer ratings of only 1.92, far lower than the other group, or, simply, the unsupplemented rats developed 78 percent more ulceration.

"It was clearly demonstrated," said the authors, "that vitamin E in large doses administered at the beginning of and during a period of stress effectively retarded the production of stomach ulceration." Further: "It is possible that, because vitamin E has significant prophylactic properties in relation to the formation of ulcers, it may also facilitate the treatment of established ulcers. Further research in this area is indicated."

Vitamin A Is Also An Anti-Ulcer Specific

The three researchers theorized that the protective potency of vitamin E may be related to its antioxidant properties—that is, its ability to prevent bodily substances from combining chemically with oxygen compounds and thereby being degraded. But besides the general protection afforded to the tissues of the gastrointestinal system, vitamin E has a very specific protective relationship with vitamin A.

The synergistic effect of vitamin E with vitamin A was observed as long ago as 1946, when J. L. Jensen published in *Science* (103, 586) his findings that alpha-tocopherol or vitamin E prevented stomach ulcers in rats receiving very low amounts of vitamin A.

In 1947, a kind of follow-up to this experiment was reported by T. L. Harris and associates (*Proceedings of the Society for Experimental Biology and Medicine*, March, 1947). This time, the researchers wanted to see what would happen when vitamin A was given in ample amounts, and the amount of vitamin E varied. Forty young male rats were first placed on a diet deficient in both vitamins A and E, which is known to produce ulcers. After two weeks, supplementation was begun of all rats with 300 units of vitamin A daily. But only half the rats were also given vitamin E. Seven weeks later, the animals were sacrificed and examined for stomach lesions. Fifty percent of the rats on the high-A, low-E diet had one or more ulcers in the forestomach. But not a single animal in the group which had received the vitamin E had any ulcers!

As dramatic as this finding was, it comes as no surprise to anyone familiar with the basic physiology of vitamins A and E. Vitamin A is crucial to the health of the mucous membranes which line the body's cavities, the throat, nose, sinuses, middle ear, lungs, gall bladder and urinary bladder. When there is adequate vitamin A, these membranes continuously secrete a liquid or mucus which covers the cells and protects them from bacteria, acids and other environmental assaults. Vitamin E, in sparing vitamin A, assures an adequate supply of protective mucus for the epithelial cells.

Actually, the relationship between these two vitamins is a little more complicated than that. When Harris and his colleagues performed further experiments with these two vitamins, they came to the conclusion that vitamin A deficiency by itself does not produce ulcers. Nor can vitamin A, even in high doses, prevent ulcers in animals under stress, they reported. This in turn led them to the conclusion that "the action of tocopherol (vitamin E) cannot be explained simply as a sparing of vitamin A in the gastrointestinal tract." In other words, vitamin E by itself affords an important kind of protection—as was reported in the California study.

But later studies in human beings indicate that vitamin A, by itself, is also able to "single-handedly" fight the ulceration process. Dr. Neil Hutcher of the Medical College of Virginia reported in 1971 (*Medical World News,* Oct. 29) that vitamin A helped heal ulcers brought on in people undergoing steroid treatment. Steroids—adrenocorticotropin and corticosteroids—are believed to help cause ulcers by lowering the gastric defense mechanisms. This means that the surface epithelial cells are not renewed at the proper rate. Therefore, mucus production lags, according to Dr. Hutcher. He and his associates believe vitamin A retards ulcer formation by actually stimulating the epithelial cells to reproduce normally, with the ultimate result being increased mucus production.

There now exists clear-cut evidence that vitamin A works to save the stomach lining in the face of the worst kind of stress. Dr. Chernov and his associates, Dr. Harry W. Hale, Jr. and Dr. MacDonald Wood, undertook a two-part study of patients suffering from stress due to severe injuries in order to determine serum vitamin A levels after injury and to determine whether the prophylactic administration of vitamin A would prevent the formation of stress ulcers.

As reported in *Medical World News* (January 7, 1972), they first measured serum vitamin A levels in 35 severely stressed patients at the time of admission and every two to three days during their hospital stay. These included patients with burns of more than 25 percent of the body's surface and patients with major injuries of two or more organ systems. It was found that vitamin A levels in the serum fell dramatically in 29 of the 35 patients in the first group within 24 to 72 hours after admission. The majority of these patients required massive doses of parenteral vitamin A just to raise the serum levels to normal.

In the second part of the study, 36 similarly stressed patients were selected to test the prophylactic value of parenteral vitamin A in preventing stress ulcers. Those patients selected for treatment received 10,000 to 400,000 I.U.'s of a water soluble vitamin A preparation daily. In every other respect their care was the same as that of the control group. This part of the study proved that vitamin A can prevent or minimize the formation of stress ulcers. Evidence of these ulcers was seen in 15 of 22 untreated patients, or 69 percent. Serious upper gastrointestinal bleeding developed in 14 of these patients, massive in seven, and one patient was found at autopsy to have a perforated ulcer.

Of the 14 patients treated with massive doses of parenteral vitamin A, however, upper gastrointestinal bleeding occurred in only two. One of these patients had been so severely injured that he suffered bleeding from many parts of his body including the gastrointestinal tract.

Dr. Chernov's study has tremendous significance for all of us. It points out the highly important role that vitamin A can play in almost every type of disease condition, since any disease is a stress on the body.

The severely injured patient goes into a catabolic state (destructive metabolism) and exhibits a high degree of protein deficiency, Dr. Chernov pointed out. "The sudden and marked depletion of vitamin A is directly related to the corresponding depression of the serum protein, and particularly that fragment of the serum protein involved in transport of vitamin A," he said.

"As a result of this sudden depletion of the serum vitamin A, we believe that the mucous cells are adversely affected and begin to undergo autolysis (dissolution) and failure to replicate normally. This results initially in the development of superficial mucosal erosions followed later by frank ulceration and hemorrhage."

Now that we know how very vital vitamin A is, the big question is how much? What is the optimal dose to insure us of an adequate supply under all conditions? This is a very personal question because each one of us has different needs. People who smoke or live in highly polluted areas need more than others. People who must be in the company of people who smoke have an increased need for vitamin A. People who have lost vitamin A through pneumonia or nephritis or any stress situation will most surely need more than the average.

Vitamin C Therapy

More than a quarter of a century ago, researchers in Great Britain discovered that injections with vitamin C proved therapeutic in the treatment of peptic ulcers. Dr. B. A. Meyer of London and his colleague, Dr. J. I. Orgel, reported in the *Medical World News* (February 15, 1950) that ulcer patients had a noticeable deficiency of vitamin C. Dr. Meyer mentioned four case histories of ulcer patients where extremely low levels of vitamin C were found. "Sub-clinical scurvy" was the name given to such deficiencies. In other words, these people had scurvy—not enough to have put them to bed or have brought fatal consequences—but enough to have caused some of the symptoms of scurvy.

There are three reasons for the condition of vitamin C deficiency in ulcer patients, Dr. Meyer stated. First, the diet for ulcer patients usually consists of little or no fresh fruits or vegetables. The original bland ulcer diet—the "Sippy Diet"—contained only five milligrams of vitamin C per day for the first week and 15 milligrams per day in the fourth week, when other foods were gradually introduced. A satisfactory intake should be around 70 milligrams a day, said Dr. Meyer. Far more than that would be even better, since we are surrounded every day by so many substances that use up the relatively small amounts of vitamin C most of us get in our foods.

Individuals on other kinds of diets can suffer from this same difficulty. Ulcerative colitis patients are usually placed on "bland" diets. Such diets are bound to be short on vitamin C. Since this vitamin is essential for the process of healing, it becomes apparent why ulcers in the colon are slow to heal. We know that this important vitamin is necessary for the sound and rapid healing of wounds, since it is necessary for the formation of intercellular material. Its deficiency has been shown to cause a marked decrease in the tensile strength of wounds. When there is inadequate formation of the intercellular material, or collagen, the cells remain immature and blood vessels do not easily penetrate the poorly developed granulation tissue.

A blender is the answer for the person who wants fresh raw foods without irritating fibers. Even the toughest vegetables can be blended into a soft mass or (with the addition of a little water) a fine drink.

The second reason for a condition of near-scurvy in ulcer patients is that there is defective absorption of the vitamin by the intestines. Vitamin C is not well absorbed in other ailments involving abnormal bowel conditions, for example, ulcerative colitis, or constipation, which is relieved by daily cathartics.

The third reason for ulcer patients being short on vitamin C is, said Dr. Meyer, a derangement of vitamin C metabolism. Absorption is improved by the presence of the bioflavonoids, substances which usually occur with vitamin C in fruits and vegetables.

It seems, then, that the typical ulcer patient is short on vitamin C, cannot absorb it properly through his digestive tract and has trouble using it after it is absorbed, unless it is accompanied by the bioflavonoids. Injections of vitamin C directly into the bloodstream should solve the problem. Apparently there is no risk of any unpleasant aftereffects from vitamin C injections.

Dr. Meyer's ulcer patients treated with injections of vitamin C had these results: Prompt relief of symptoms; no necessity for rest in bed or absence from work; no dietary restrictions; no toxic effects; and a general tonic effect which was apparent in most cases.

Comfrey: A Plant That Treats Ulcers

Comfrey has a long and rich history as a medicinal herb, especially in the treatment of stomach ulcers. Early medical physicians knew of its bone-knitting and wound-healing properties. The 16th century volume of Turner's *Herball* (1568) states that the roots of comfrey "are good if they be broken and dronken for them that spitte blood and are bursten."

The British physician Charles J. Macalister of Lancaster, England, was the first to specify the healing component of the comfrey plant—allantoin. After systematically testing the plant in clinical studies and investigating its chemical composition, he presented his early findings in the *British Medical Journal* and later (1936) published a full account in the booklet, *Narrative of an Investigation Concerning an Ancient Medieval Remedy and Its Modern Utilities*. Since that time, allantoin has become part of the pharmacological arsenal. The *Merck Index of Chemicals and Drugs* identifies allantoin as "used topically in suppurating wounds and resistant ulcers to stimulate the growth of healthy tissue; has also been given internally for gastric ulcer."

The comfrey leaves contain vitamins A, C, E, and B vitamins—and not only the usual B complex of vegetation but also B_{12}, the anti-anemia vitamin characteristically found only in meat products, most notably in liver. Because its roots dig down deep into the subsoil, comfrey also is a rich source of the trace minerals so lacking in the average American diet. And its protein content is high, with a good percentage of four of protein's essential amino acids, including methionine which most vegetable proteins lack.

Prevention With Comfrey

For its vitamin, mineral, and protein content alone, comfrey must be regarded as a healthful food, but its allantoin content gives it an extra value not only for treating such conditions as gastrointestinal ulcers but also for preventing their development. Allantoin's ability to stimulate leucocytic activity also puts this plant high on the list of protective foods. When you take a comfrey tea break instead of a coffee break, you are increasing your body's own self-defense against invading microorganisms.

Though Dr. Macalister discovered allantoin in comfrey and further proved allantoin's healing power and introduced it as a pharmaceutical agent to the medical world, allantoin itself was not an unknown substance to the chemists and biologists of that day. It was first discovered in animals and gained its name from the fact that it was found in the fetal allantoic fluid—the allantois being a sac-like appendage to the embryo, its blood vessels forming the important pathways for the circulation of blood between the fetus and the placenta (and thence to the mother). Allantoin has also been found in a variety of plants (though comfrey is the richest source known), and, as Dr. Macalister pointed out, its distribution in plant life (as in animal life) is related to growth, either active or potential. Specifically, in the comfrey plant it is most highly concentrated in the root (from which the growing leaves can draw) and in the terminal buds.

A native of Europe, comfrey can now be found growing wild from Newfoundland to Maryland. You can grow this perennial plant yourself, make your own home remedy and your own home health food from start to finish. Of course, you can also buy comfrey at a health store, either as chopped roots or dried tea leaves.

Alfalfa

After years of misery from stomach ulcers, Dr. Stanley Slinger, a poultry specialist at the Ontario Agricultural College in Ontario, Canada, tried alfalfa tea, and he has had no trouble since. The tea was able to accomplish what surgery and stomach freezing could not.

He told a 1964 Convention of the American Dehydrators Association at Fort Lauderdale, Florida, that many people have been eating and drinking alfalfa for years, just for general health. Dr. Slinger took a tablespoonful of ground dehydrated alfalfa dissolved in a glass of water once a day. From the very first dose he had almost immediate relief. Dr. Slinger admitted that he did not know why alfalfa provided relief for him and several of his friends suffering from ulcers, but he theorized that it could have been what scientists refer to as "certain unidentified factors" in the hay.

The amazing nutritional values in alfalfa may explain it. It has 8,000 international units of vitamin A in every 100 grams; this compares favorably with vitamin A-rich apricots (7,500 units) and beef liver (9,000 units). Vitamin A is important in maintaining membranes, including the stomach lining. Alfalfa is also a good source of pyridoxine, one of the rarer B vitamins. It contains notable amounts of vitamin E, whose great importance as a catalyst for other nutrients and for the health of muscles and heart is well known. In fact, alfalfa is regarded as one of the most reliable sources of vitamin E for grass-eating animals.

Alfalfa is also a rich source of rutin, one of the bioflavonoids. In the *American Journal of Gastroenterology* (July, 1958) Doctors Samuel Weiss, Jerome Weiss and Bernard Weiss described remarkable success with bioflavonoids in treating 36 cases of bleeding duodenal ulcers. The doctors used no other medication but a bioflavonoid compound in capsule form administered orally at the rate of three to nine capsules per day. Aside from this only a change in diet was prescribed.

All of the 36 ulcer cases treated in this way responded with a return to normal of the mucous membrane and duodenal contour. This healing usually took place in a period of 12 to 22 days and was confirmed by means of X-ray examinations.

If you already have an ulcer, ask your doctor about trying alfalfa. You can get it as meal which you can use in the kitchen, in tablets, or as seeds or leaves, which you can make into tea.

Raw Foods Fight Ulcers

A therapeutic nutrient, known as vitamin U or vitamin 21, was reported to cure ulcers in a diet therapy program proposed by Russian scientist Dr. E. M. Vermel. The report appeared in the Russian publication *Clinical Medicine* (4, 23-25, 1960). Dr. Vermel, at the time the article was written, was affiliated with the Institute for Research into Medicinal Plants of the USSR Academy of Sciences.

What is vitamin U? No one is certain. It is something that is contained in cabbage juice, which is the food that Professor Vermel said has been used most successfully to treat ulcers. The most conspicuous constituent of cabbage juice is methionine, an amino acid, which is believed to play an active role in the curative properties of cabbage juice. But tests employing purified methionine against ulcers have been uniformly unsuccessful. And many cases of ulcers have been cured by the raw juice of vegetables other than the cabbage, juice that does not contain any substantial amount of methionine. Therefore it is clear that vitamin U is some still unidentified factor present in fresh, raw vegetables and contained in greater quantity in the cabbage than in any other vegetable.

Dr. Vermel mentioned the studies of Dr. Garnett Cheney, a Stanford University researcher and doctor, who discovered and announced the cabbage juice treatment for both peptic and duodenal ulcers in 1949. He confirmed this in later studies published in *California Medicine* in 1954 and 1956. In his 1956 study, Dr. Cheney reported on treating 26 ulcer sufferers with concentrated cabbage juice. Twenty-four made a complete recovery in three to four weeks' time, while in a control group of 19 receiving conventional milk diet therapy, only six recovered.

Dr. Cheney's experimental investigations were repeated and checked in Italy in 1955 and 1956 in no less than six different places. Three Bulgarian investigators each independently carried on the same work in 1958. There were also investigative checks in Poland and in Switzerland. All confirmed that in at least 85 percent of cases treatment with concentrated or desiccated cabbage juice could bring about not only a remission in symptoms but radiologically proven disappearance of a stomach ulcer in three to four weeks' time.

Reviewing the literature, Professor Vermel found that more than 500 cases had been reported as cured by vitamin U therapy. And still, as he stated, nobody yet knows what vitamin U is. Some of its characteristics, he said, have been established. It is a substance which is destroyed by heat, is fat soluble, and is oxidized easily. It is not harmed, however, by refrigeration or by low heat desiccation. Its success in therapy also depends, obviously, on how much of it is present in the vegetables whose juices are used.

Professor Vermel speculated that the mode of action of vitamin U is probably that of supplying a nutrient necessary for the formation of sufficient mucus to protect the lining of the stomach. In other words, he stated, an ulcer is very possibly a deficiency disease arising because the patient has not eaten enough raw vegetables or the vegetables have been grown in such a way that they lack sufficient vitamin U in their content.

Section 61
Varicose Veins

274. More Than Just A Cosmetic Problem

274. More Than Just A Cosmetic Problem

Varicose veins are not confined to women, but they seem to afflict more women than men. Varicosities are *not* a mere cosmetic problem. The walls of the veins may become inflamed in a condition known as phlebitis. A dark red solid mass of fibrin and blood cells may plug the vein up in a more serious condition known as thrombophlebitis. The danger here is that the clot may break loose from the wall of the vein and be swept along to the lungs or heart, where it may obstruct a crucial blood vessel and precipitate a heart attack. Varicosities of long duration are often accompanied by ugly, itching eczema and ulcerations which can become so large as to involve the entire leg structure, even down to the bone.

These complications of varicose veins are found more frequently in the aged than the young, and in many cases, according to Philip H. Rakov, M.D., of the Department of Surgery at the State University of New York at Syracuse, the diagnosis is difficult because the varicosities are not always visible or discoverable by touch (*Geriatrics*, August, 1970).

Result Of Impaired Blood Circulation

For some women the trouble seems to stem from the fact that during childbirth, pressure from the baby's emerging head distorts veins in the pelvic area which drain blood from the legs. As a result, blood tends to back up in the veins of the legs, disabling the venous valves whose job it is to fight the effects of gravity by preventing blood from lying stagnant in the veins or even slipping backwards when it should be pumped back to the heart. With these valves disabled, it is more difficult for the blood to run up the legs, and the result is that the veins stretch and expand under the increased pressure, making swift return of the blood even more difficult.

Following childbirth, a woman usually rests in bed for several days and thereafter "takes things easy for a while." This aggravates the problem considerably, because even under normal

1246

conditions, the veins depend on muscle contractions in the legs to force the blood upwards. The longer the period of immobilization, the greater tendency there is for the leg veins to become distended and incapacitated. And frequently, there is a period of constipation before and after childbirth, as a result of pressure on the lower bowel. But as waste matter collects in the colon, still more pressure is exerted on the portal vein, further retarding the return of venous blood from the lower extremities.

The result of all this—at least the most immediate and obvious result—is the development of varicose veins. But the unsightly blue cords popping out of the calves and ankles are only a superficial sign of deeper distress. That's because the veins that run near the surface of the skin normally transport only a small fraction of the venous blood. It is the veins deep inside the leg muscles which are designed to carry about 80 to 90 percent of the returning blood up and out of the legs. And it is these deep veins which are first affected by pressure against the large pelvic veins which they feed. What you are seeing in visible varicosities is nature's way of bypassing or at least easing the burden of invisible varicosities deep within the leg. Unfortunately, the superficial veins are all too often disabled themselves as they are forced to carry this extra burden.

Exercise Opens The Blood Channels

Exercise is important in preventing varicose veins. Since varicose veins are caused by residue deposits of clotting blood within the vein interiors, it stands to reason that anything that will keep blood pulsing through the circulatory channels of the blood system is extremely important.

Dr. T. K. Scobie, a physician from Ottawa, Canada, noted in a story in the *Toronto Star* (April 26, 1974) that jogging, cycling, hiking and other sports should reduce an individual's susceptibility to varicose legs. But if you are unable to partake in some of these strenuous exercises, other less exacting forms of exercise can be employed, even just plain walking or keeping your leg muscles firm with isometric exercise and massage.

Bran And Varicose Veins

The daily use of a bran supplement to prevent diverticulosis, a painful disease of the lower bowel, is also recommended for the prevention of varicose veins. The use of bran was the focal point of research by Dr. C. Latto and colleagues of the Royal Berkshire

Varicose Veins

Hospital of Reading, England. In *The Lancet* (May 19, 1973), in an article entitled "Diverticular Disease and Varicose Veins," they noted they began their investigation because of a hypothesis put forward by several other physicians that diverticular disease and varicose veins are only different manifestations of the same underlying problem—a low-residue diet. British doctors who have served long periods in Africa have noted that Africans eating a bulky diet are almost completely free of diverticular disease—and almost never get varicose veins.

So the Reading physicians examined several groups of patients to see just who had varicose veins. They found that of those patients who had diverticular disease (confirmed during surgery), 74 percent had varicose veins. In contrast, only 16 percent of randomly selected outpatients had varicose veins. When another group of non-diverticular patients who were closely matched for age and sex with those who did have diverticular disease were examined, 33 percent were found to have varicose veins. In other words, people with diverticular disease are more than twice as likely to have varicose veins as other people who are the same age and sex.

The physicians went on to cite several possible explanations for the association of these two ailments. They said that the raised pressure created within the colon as the muscles contract with abnormal strength to expel too-small stools "is known to be transmitted down the leg veins after the valves become incompetent." Dr. Denis Burkitt, a noted researcher into the causes of diverticular disease, believes that this pressure on the veins passing through the pelvis causes a back-up of blood flow and is most likely the cause of the *initial* failure of the valves. Dr. Latto and his colleagues agree that Burkitt's explanation for the creation of varicose veins makes more sense than any other they had heard.

There is no special amount of bran which is appropriate for everyone to take. Some people require several tablespoons a day; others as little as two or three teaspoons. When you add bran to your diet, begin with the smallest amount, and slowly increase it until the desired effect becomes evident.

The kind of bran used by medical men in these studies is unprocessed bran, plain and simple, without sugar and without additives of any kind. It is a perfectly natural food substance which, until the last century or so, was eaten in ample quantities by a large portion of mankind. It is not really so much a dietary supplement as it is a dietary *restorative*. That is why diverticulitis was not even mentioned in medical textbooks until after World War I. Since then, it has become "increasingly common" (*Canadian Medical Journal*, Vol. 105, Aug. 7, 1971), not just because of the removal of bran from bread, but because of the replacement of other fibrous carbohydrates in the diet by refined foods—especially sugar.

Relief From Support Hose

Not so very long ago people who suffered from circulatory problems of the legs were forced out of sheer necessity to bandage their legs in wraps which looked very much like the old Army puttees. Today's elastic stockings are a far cry from the surgical support hose doctors used to prescribe for edema, phlebitis and varicose veins. And they give far better and longer lasting support, according to medical research.

In the late 1960's Dr. Arthur J. Heather, Medical Director of the Delaware Curative Workshop in Wilmington, Delaware, tested the effectiveness of several commercial brands of sheer hose containing spandex elastic fibers on women patients who had developed peripheral edema (swollen ankles) and secondary venous complications (varicose veins). The 12 women in the study ranged in age from 31 to 93, and all of them objected to the unattractiveness of surgical support hose or bandages and refused to wear them for any extended period of time.

To treat their edema and prevent it from getting worse, these women were provided with various brands of cosmetically sheer, commercial support hose. The women preferred a degree of sheerness that resembled dress hose, but objected to extremely high sheerness that failed to hide their swollen veins and blemishes.

On the basis of these cosmetic considerations and supportive requirements, brands of commercial support hose containing 10% to 24% elastic yarn were selected. The women were instructed to wear the support hosiery regularly. At the beginning of the study and at periodic intervals, legs were photographed against a blackboard marked in squares, and their volume measured by the Archimedian water-displacement principle. (A tank was filled with water to an overflow spout. After immersing the leg in the tank, foot and leg volume was determined by measuring the volume of the water that overflowed from the spout.)

The results proved that elastic stockings can, for one thing, do a great service for legs that are heavy because of poor circulation. Not only was pain reduced, but a large part of the swelling was also reduced. Calf circumference in some legs went down as much as 1-7/8 inches. Leg volume went down as much as 1070 milliliters.

While these size reductions would delight the vanity of any woman, by far the more notable benefits were recorded in the lessening of pain and fatigue.

One patient who had suffered a compound fracture of the left femur and lacerations of the calf muscles, and complained that her legs ached and were heavy before treatment, reported that her "legs feel better" after wearing the elastic stockings. Another woman who had experienced a cerebral thrombosis and whose legs ached and felt heavy before treatment reported that her "leg feels good" after treatment. Other women reported less swelling and less fatigue.

In all cases, except one, decrease in leg volume was accompanied by a decrease or elimination of pain and discomfort, and even in the single exception, swelling began to subside at the conclusion of the study.

Varicose Veins And Chair Sitting

Remember in the third grade when the teacher would insist that you sit up straight at your desk? Why did you have to sit so straight, you wondered, and why were those chairs so hard? Probably the teacher was trying to instill some superficial sense of discipline in you, but what she was really doing, according to Dr. Colin James Alexander of New Zealand, was priming you to develop varicose veins.

That's what you get, said Dr. Alexander in the *British Medical Journal,* in the spring of 1972, from permitting the edge of a chair to press against the blood vessels in your stationary thighs year after year. This isn't the kind of thing you can prove in a laboratory, but Dr. Alexander is convinced. In primitive peoples, who sit on the ground, varicose veins are rare. But among Westerners, who sit on chairs, the ailment is common in every group of people.

Dr. Alexander, an anatomist, explained that pressure is greatest on the leg veins when you're standing, but because most of us move about, the effect isn't that bad. However, chair-sitting results in constant pressure, which Dr. Alexander measured as being more than twice that of ground-sitting, and this pressure is what makes for varicose veins.

If Dr. Alexander is right, varicose veins are preventable if we can learn to spend time reading, sewing, or conversing while cross-legged or sprawled on a pillow-scattered carpet. Some schools are getting rid of chairs in favor of open, carpeted areas to increase the child's sense of freedom. The architects may not know it, but they're also improving the child's blood circulation.

Vitamin E And Varicose Veins

Along with lots of exercise, a minimum of chair sitting and diet that contains plenty of bulk foods, vitamin E can be of significant help, both as a preventive measure and as a treatment for varicose veins.

The pioneers in vitamin E therapy are Doctors Evan and Wilfrid Shute, of the world-famous Shute Foundation in London, Ontario, Canada. The Shute brothers are best known for their work in treating cardiovascular disease, but the beneficial action of vitamin E in the veins is for all practical purposes identical to its action in the arteries. And as we have seen, a blood clot which tears loose from a vein in the leg is as dangerous as one in an artery, and can easily bring about a heart attack. So the use of vitamin E for phlebitis is very intimately associated with its use in controlling heart disease.

Specifically, Dr. Evan Shute on June 6, 1958, told the Second World Congress of Obstetrics and Gynecology in Montreal, Canada, that in a group of 166 patients, all of whom had chronic phlebitis, 32 patients got excellent or complete relief, 79 cases good relief, 20 cases moderate relief, and 35 cases light relief after treatment with vitamin E. Most of these patients had suffered from 1 to 5 years and some of them had had phlebitis for longer than 6 years.

One man of 47 had suffered for 6 years with the usual swelling and soreness. He was given 300 mg. and later 400 mg. of vitamin E daily. The trouble in one of his legs cleared four days after the dosage was raised to 400 mg. At his last visit he could walk half a mile each day and there was no tenderness in his leg. His feet swelled very slightly and ached slightly on rare occasions.

Dr. Shute went on to explain to his colleagues why vitamin E should have such a striking beneficial effect on all these patients. Vitamin E, he said, "produces collateral circulation about the obstructed deep veins by calling into play the unused networks of veins lying in wait for emergency utilization. We have such venous reserves just as we have reserves of brain, lung and liver. Alpha tocopherol (the most active part of vitamin E) mobilizes them. It does more. It has the unique power of enabling tissues to utilize oxygen better and hence the devitalized and congested leg tissues of the chronic phlebitic who is given alpha tocopherol are receiving the equivalent of more oxygen." Alpha tocopherol, he has stated elsewhere, also has a clear-cut fibrinolytic (fibrin dissolving) potency. This ability eliminates internal blood clots while interfering only slightly or not at all with the clotting of blood to seal a wound.

More results achieved using vitamin E for impaired circulation of the legs are reported by Dr. Wilfrid Shute in his book *Vitamin E For Ailing and Healthy Hearts* (Pyramid House, 1969), which he wrote with Harald J. Taub. Dr. Shute writes "we have treated patients with varicose veins, with and without previous surgery, with gratifying results. However, the reasons for treatment have not been to shrink the varicosities but to reduce the symptoms. The distended and torturous veins cause a chronic venous stasis which produces edema, stabbing and aching pain, and, if severe enough and prolonged enough, indolent ulceration, overgrowth of connective tissue, and occasionally, hemorrhages or ecchymosis, leakage of blood under the skin."

Here is one case which Dr. Shute presents: A woman, age 65, had varicose veins in both legs since her first pregnancy. For four years there had been marked discoloration of both ankles and the lower halves of both legs aggravated by the development of varicose eczema and an episode of infection which set in as a result of the woman's scratching. This woman, who lived on a western prairie farm in Canada, had 16 children, and by the time she saw Dr. Shute, her legs bothered her constantly, with severe cramping in bed.

On alpha tocopherol, Dr. Shute writes, "these varicose veins of nearly 50 years' duration aggravated by numerous pregnancies, not only ceased to cause symptoms of venous stasis but diminished greatly in size. She now wears her normal nylon stockings and has a nice pair of legs, just like her eight daughters."

Here is another case: A 35-year-old woman developed varicose veins with her first pregnancy 15 years before she saw Dr. Shute. With her second child, she had a thrombophlebitis while in the hospital. Both legs ached continuously, especially as the day progressed. On alpha tocopherol therapy her legs ceased to bother her in three months.

Another one of Dr. Shute's patients came to him in August of 1960, after having suffered from varicose veins for some 30 years. She had phlebitis in both legs in 1935 and an acute thrombus in 1960. There was swelling of feet and ankles during the last 20 years, and in the last two years both legs had become badly discolored with "a dead heavy feeling in them."

On 300 units of alpha tocopherol a day, the aching was all gone in six weeks. But when she decreased her dose, her legs started to ache again. On 600 units a day, her legs ceased to bother her at all, Dr. Shute reported.

The Shute brothers are both the pioneers and leaders of research and therapy using vitamin E for improving circulation, but they are not the only ones who have reported success using alpha tocopherol for circulatory diseases of the legs. *Arizona Medicine* (16: 100, 1959) carried an article by Dr. R. F. Bock, concluding that post-operative and post-partum thrombophlebitis responded well to 1,100 units of alpha tocopherol per day. Usually, Bock reported, the patient notices subjective improvement in 12 to 24 hours, while clinical results are apparent in 24 to 48 hours.

Varicose ulcers are also cured by alpha tocopherol, according to Dr. Bock. It can be used prior to surgery as a preventive against dangerous blood clots, and is characterized as safer and just as effective as the drugs dicumarol and heparin and is never accompanied with hemorrhage complications. Bock saw no side effects from alpha tocopherol use.

Dr. Wilfrid Shute has reported on many cases of varicose ulcers helped with vitamin E. One case he mentions in his *Vitamin E for Ailing and Healthy Hearts* is that of a woman who had an ulcer on the right leg which almost completely girdled the lower third of that limb, while the ulcer on the left leg was equally wide but even larger, extending beyond the natural crease between the foot and ankle into the upper part of the foot. After a course of treatment with oral vitamin E and vitamin E ointment, the ulcers healed, for the first time in 13 years.

Equally dramatic is the evidence reported by Marcus T. Block, M.D., in *Clinical Medicine* (January, 1953). Dr. Block, who used vitamin E to combat a number of skin ailments, many of them associated with impaired circulation, saw one case of severe ulcer of some 20 years' duration which was healed within two weeks after treatment with vitamin E. Dr. Block also gave vitamin E to 25 patients suffering from eczema and ulcers associated specifically with varicose veins. In 18 cases, the results were excellent; in four cases, good, and in three cases, poor. The average amount of vitamin E taken by these patients was about 150 milligrams a day.

Section 62 Venereal Diseases

275. V.D.—The Silent Epidemic

275. V.D.—The Silent Epidemic

The relaxed sexual mores, the breakdown of the family unit, the advent of the pill and ignorance of the seriousness of untreated venereal disease have combined to thwart the efforts of health agencies to prevent or bring to early treatment sexually transmitted diseases. Venereal disease reached epidemic proportions in the early 1970's, when young people, including a high percentage of teenagers, comprised about half of the victims of V.D.

Failure to recognize symptoms is a major contributor to the number of cases of untreated disease. The U.S. Public Health Department estimates 500,000 Americans are walking around unaware that they have syphilis. Those who suspect that they have been exposed to a venereal disease should immediately go to a V.D. clinic for help. These clinics exist in most major cities and treatment is either free or the fee is nominal.

Venereal diseases fall into two major categories—those that manifest themselves in the form of lesions, spots or swelling and those that begin with a genital discharge.

The following are in the first category:

Syphilis—This is the most serious of the venereal diseases. If syphilis remains untreated, it can result in a breakdown of body tissues, deterioration of bones, mental disorders, heart problems, blindness and even death. The disease is generally characterized by genital ulcers, although the ulcers may erupt on or in the mouth. These sores appear two to four weeks after exposure. The standard treatment, which consists of a series of penicillin injections given every four hours for a number of weeks, should begin as soon as those symptoms appear. Since many people are extremely allergic to penicillin, tetracycline or erythromycin are often used instead.

World Health (May, 1975) reported a new experimental vaccine which has proved effective in treating syphilitic rabbits. However, the serious side effects must be eliminated before the vaccine can be tested on humans.

If syphilis is to be eradicated, all cases have to be recognized and brought to treatment. Many of those cases could be detected in the course of routine dental examinations.

Approximately two-thirds to three-fourths of all extragenital chancres are seen in the area of the mouth, a majority on the lips and tongue, says William J. Brown, M.D., Chief of the Venereal Disease Branch, Communicable Disease Center, Atlanta, Georgia. These chancres are often accompanied by palpable, non-tender lymph nodes under the jaw. However, chancres may be so slight as to be almost unnoticeable. Such lesions are highly infectious, and will disappear completely in time with or without treatment, but the disease remains active within the body (*Journal of American Dental Hygienists Association,* 3rd Quarter, 1965).

During the secondary stage of the disease, from about ten weeks to two years after infection, split papules are often visible at the corner of the mouth. On the mucous membrane of the inner cheek and tongue there may be mucous patches which take the form of minute erosions covered with a thin, grayish exudate.

Late syphilis also may be manifest through involvement of the tongue and hard palate. The patient may not be infectious at this point but he needs treatment to avoid tragic consequences. One such sign is a completely bald and denuded tongue, devoid of all papilae, frequently with areas of leukoplakia.

Sometimes the dental hygienist who routinely cleans teeth is in a better position than the dentist to observe these signs suggesting syphilitic infection. She should discreetly request examination by the dentist immediately, so that the patient may be referred to a physician, Dr. Brown suggests.

Here is an area in which the dentist can and should perform a valuable service. If he will take the trouble to familiarize himself with all the stigmata of this dread disease and conscientiously report every case, he can do more perhaps than any other medical practitioner in the battle to wipe out syphilis.

Chancroid (soft sore)—The many ulcers which erupt on the genitals are extremely painful as is the accompanying swelling. This disease, which used to be widespread is now quite rare, thanks to the improved hygiene of the last century. When it does occur it is readily controlled with sulphonamide.

Herpes genitalis—This herpes virus, closely related to the virus which causes cold sores, presents itself in clusters of small blisters on the genitals. This is the second most common venereal disease in the United States and while it can be controlled and rendered inactive, once it is acquired the virus remains in the system indefinitely.

It is strongly suspected of being a principal cause of cancer of the cervix if it remains unchecked, according to *World Health*.

Numerous drug preparations are used by physicians to treat the ailment including iododeoxyuridine which is applied topically.

In the *Medical Tribune* (November 13, 1974), Dr. Te-Wen Chang, a Tufts University virologist, reported 70 percent of 35 subjects suffering from herpes genitalis were treated successfully with a combination of methylene blue and light exposure. Methylene blue is a germicide that was used in the 19th century for infections of the intestines and the urinary tract.

Venereal warts—These pink warts do not appear for many weeks after the exposure has taken place. They are generally not serious and are treated topically except in stubborn cases where they are cauterized.

The following are venereal diseases characterized by a genital discharge:

Gonorrhea—The most prevalent of all the venereal diseases, gonorrhea usually shows its symptoms of painful urination and a pus-like discharge within a week of exposure.

This disease, which used to result in sterility, blindness, arthritis and other serious diseases is now cured in most cases by a single shot of penicillin. It is easy to become reinfected, however, unless both sexual partners are treated.

Many antibiotics and sulfa drugs are effective in treating gonorrhea patients who are allergic to penicillin.

Non-gonococcal urethritis—This is easily recognizable only in males, and manifests itself by a genital discharge. Since it does not readily respond to penicillin, it is generally treated with oral doses of tetracycline.

Candidiasis (thrush)—A common female complaint, this cheese-like, vaginal discharge is treated with vaginal suppositories for a period of two to three weeks. The infection, which is usually accompanied by soreness and itching, is a recurring one. Anyone who is susceptible would be well-advised not to wear nylon underwear as it seems to encourage the problem.

Trichomoniasis—This vaginal discharge is caused by a parasite which can be carried by a male and transmitted to his sexual partner. It is advisable for both the male and female to be treated with metronidazole or nimorazole for a period of about one week.

Although penicillin seems to be a panacea for those who contract venereal disease, its frequent use is resulting in a lowering of its effectiveness.

"At the present time," reports a Canadian physician, "there is an urgent need for a satisfactory substitute for penicillin in the treatment of gonorrhea." According to Dr. C. R. Amies of Toronto, the disease has developed an increasing resistance to penicillin throughout the course of a recently concluded eight-year study (*Canadian Medical Association Journal*, January 7, 1967).

We are fortunate that modern science has developed effective treatments for many of the venereal diseases that crippled and killed their victims in the past. But it is regrettable that these treatments are so hard on the rest of the body. Antibiotics and sulfa drugs are hard on the body's intestinal flora, the liver and on the B vitamins. Patients undergoing extensive treatment for venereal disease should reinforce their supply of these nutrients with such foods as yogurt, brewer's yeast, wheat germ and organ meats.

Section 63
Weight
Problems

276. Overweight And Obesity

A long time ago it was stylish and a mark of success to be fat. A man took pride in his wife's double chin—it meant he was a good provider. That was when man had to depend on a seasonal and precarious supply of food. Since there was no refrigerator-freezer in which to safely store food, man stored fat on his body and mobilized it in time of need. In spite of the attempt to store fat for the lean years, obesity was not an overriding problem in those early days.

Today, it is no longer stylish or advantageous to be fat. Man stores his food in freezers and has access to well-supplied markets summer and winter. But today obesity *is* an overriding problem. Besides being unattractive and uncomfortable, it has become a matter of considerable concern to the medical profession.

Actuary tables reveal that mortality is one-third higher in those who are 10 percent overweight. For those 20 percent or more overweight, the mortality rate jumps to nearly one half higher.

Figures on expectation of life, gathered by the Metropolitan Life Insurance Company, provide much evidence of the adverse effects of overweight. For example, men 45 years of age of medium height and frame who weigh 170 pounds—which is about average—have a life expectancy that is one and one-half years less than that for men of comparable build who weigh 150 pounds. Those who weigh 200 pounds, or 35 pounds above the average, can expect to live four years less than the men weighing 150 pounds.

Cardiovascular and kidney diseases account in large measure for the high mortality among overweight men. Cerebral hemorrhage and other vascular disorders of the central nervous system account for 50 percent of the increase in mortality. Mortality from diabetes among overweight men is more than twice that for standard risks. Mortality from pneumonia, influenza and even cancer are higher among the overweight.

Some non-fatal illnesses are made worse by overweight. An arthritic, for instance, if he is obese, moves around very little. This lack of movement makes his arthritic condition worse. The diabetic who loses weight often improves dramatically. Obese patients face much greater risk when they undergo surgical procedures.

There is no longer any doubt that weight control is one of the most effective measures available to prevent or delay the onset of the major degenerative diseases and to extend the length of active life.

Among teenage girls, obesity can have a serious effect upon personality. The obese adolescent develops attitudes and neuroses similar to those of minority groups who are subjected to intense prejudice.

These attitudes are quite different from those observed in teenagers of normal weight or in persons who become obese during adulthood, Dr. Jean Mayer, of Harvard University School of Public Health, has noted (*Postgraduate Medicine*, May, 1972).

Obesity in children which develops before the age of 10 or after the age of 16 is the kind which persists and presents a continual girth problem throughout adulthood. But overweight which develops just before the onset of puberty may be merely an exaggeration of a normal physiologic process and is often self correcting in the next few years. A proper psychological approach is particularly important with obese children and adolescents. Such dangerous syndromes as *anorexia nervosa* (a loss of appetite or refusal to eat) sometimes occur as consequences of a tactless treatment for obesity, or even because of insulting references.

Overweight Or Obese?

Overweight is not the same as obesity. A college football player may be overweight but seldom obese. On the other hand, an executive who gets very little exercise can be obese without being markedly overweight. Obesity can be determined by the measurement of skin fold thickness. The physician uses calipers to measure skin fold thickness. You have only to examine your body in a mirror. If you don't like the folds of excess flesh you see around your abdomen, thighs, chin, and arms, then face the fact that you are obese. Moderate degrees of overweight do not necessarily mean obesity. But if you're very much overweight, then the chances are that you are also obese.

There are two kinds of obesity. One type, called hypercellular obesity, is due to an increased number of fat cells. The other kind is hypertrophic obesity, in which the fat cells have become enlarged. When obesity begins in adult life, it is usually the hypertropic variety. Hypercellular obesity almost invariably begins in childhood. Dieting will reduce the size of individual fat cells, but the number of the fat cells one possesses remains constant. These fat cells tend to become filled with fat very easily. The overproduction of fat cells characteristic of obese people can be detected as early as age two, and once this hypercellularity is established, nothing is able to change it, Dr. Jerome L. Knittle, of Mt. Sinai School of Medicine, New York, told the meeting of the American College of Physicians in the summer of 1974 (*Internal Medicine News*, vol. 7 #12, June 15, 1974). Treating obesity, he said, means treating the entire family unit, not just the fat adults.

There is some evidence, Dr. George A. Bray, of Harbor General Hospital, Torrence, California, noted that those who become fat as adults, as opposed to those who have always been fat, may be at increased risk of hypertension and diabetes. And in some cases, it may be better to remain fat than to endure the adverse effects that result when one's weight fluctuates like a yo-yo (*Internal Medicine News*, June 15, 1974).

While physicians express many viewpoints as to the cause of obesity, all agree that it is a hazard to health.

Some Causes Of Overweight

"The obese state in its simplest form represents an imbalance between caloric intake and caloric expenditure," wrote Dr. George Bray in the May, 1972 issue of *Postgraduate Medicine.* "The available evidence," he continued, "suggests that most obesity in most instances represents a combination of increased food intake and decreased energy expenditure."

Here is a rock-bottom fact you can't dispute. You may say, quite truthfully, that you eat no more than your next door neighbor and certainly move about as much as he does—so how come he's lean and you're heavy? Given your individual metabolic pattern, you're taking in more food than you're burning up. The inevitable consequence is storage of the excess food as fat.

This double cause of obesity demands a double approach to its cure—less food and more exercise. Increased exercise, said Dr. Bray, is of equal importance to restricted food intake. "Indeed," he added, "in my clinical experience the most striking examples of prolonged weight loss have been seen in grossly obese patients who voluntarily undertook regular and vigorous exercises."

The most important word to stress here is "regular." Your first objective must be to increase your physical activity on a regular basis. However much or little you presently exercise, you want to do more.

Another theory on the prevalence of obesity today concerns the widespread reliance on an over-refined, high-carbohydrate diet. "The extreme commonness of obesity in Western countries may be related to the fact that most dietary carbohydrate is refined and fiber-depleted," says Dr. K. W. Heaton of the Bristol Royal Infirmary in Bristol, England (*The Lancet*, December 22, 1973).

Food fiber, which is stripped almost completely from white flour during milling and totally removed from sugar during refining, requires more chewing and thus slows down the intake of food, especially of sugars. Chewing also promotes a feeling of satiety because it stimulates secretions of saliva and gastric juices which distend the stomach and promote the sensation of being full.

Dr. Heaton feels that a primary cause of overweight is not so much consumption of too much food, but consumption of an "abnormal type of food." There has been a pronounced fall in the consumption of starchy staple foods like whole grain cereals and whole potatoes, and a pronounced rise in the consumption of refined sugars. "Whole, unrefined plant foods contain their natural fiber intact, whereas refined foods are invariably depleted of fiber."

In simplest terms, then, another basic approach to weight loss should be to eliminate everything from your diet that is not a whole, nutritious, non-processed, natural food. In addition to food energy (primarily provided by carbohydrates and made available as glucose in the bloodstream), your body constantly needs protein, fats, minerals and vitamins in optimum amounts to participate in body processes and to repair and renew body cells. When you eat whole foods, you can be pretty confident that you're getting necessary nutrients and not "empty" calories.

And don't avoid the processed commercial products, then over-process food in your own kitchen. Where skins are edible in vegetables and fruits, leave them on—if you can be sure the produce wasn't sprayed with insecticides. Keep cooking time to a minimum. Boil, broil or bake rather than fry; frying is destructive to nutrients, not to mention fattening.

Poultry, meats, eggs, whole grain products, vegetables and fruits, fresh or frozen fish, natural cheeses—do your own thing with these good whole foods. Don't buy them in "convenience" packages all gooped up with sauces and starchy paddings that rob you of nutrients and pile on the calories.

Is It Glandular?

Dr. Roger J. Williams, in his book, *Nutrition Against Disease* (Pitman, 1971), cites a disordered appestat mechanism as another cause of obesity. The mechanism which controls the appestat is located in the hypothalamus, a small gland situated in the brain. When this gland is not functioning properly, you don't know when to start eating or when to stop. You don't know when you're hungry—you don't know when you're full. You may eat compulsively and continually, and obesity is the usual result.

In the hypothalamus gland there are two food consumption mechanisms. One is the hunger center, the other the satiety center. Experimental damage in the region of the cells designated as the hunger center (ventromedian), results in an increased food intake in animals. All of these animals become obese as a result of this damage. They do eventually reach a plateau where food intake levels off and they tend to maintain themselves, but at an obese level.

If, however, experimental damage is inflicted to the area of the hypothalamus where the *satiety* center is located, the animal loses his desire to eat and will starve unless force fed.

The appestat, then, is a double-acting mechanism. On a regular basis, if the appestat performs correctly, a person's intake of food will be exactly what it should be.

How do these appetite controls go out of order? Dr. Williams thinks it is possible that an impaired appestat mechanism can be induced even before birth, by poor prenatal nutrition. This does not have to be a permanent handicap. Through improved nutrition, training and exercise, one can control the situation and restore his appestat to healthy function. No obese individual is beyond help.

Dr. Williams suggests frequent consumption of small amounts of food. Nibble—don't gorge. When five subjects were studied at the Ohio State University Health Center, gorging increased the cholesterol and phospholipid levels and nibbling had the opposite effect. In four cases, the gorging was accompanied by some gain in weight. Nibblers lost weight. The results point out the foolhardy practice of trying to lose weight by eating one big meal a day.

Many doctors and family members too, tend to scold the overweight person about overeating; they warn, threaten, cajole, coax and shame him, but to no avail. Many times, this kind of treatment has the opposite effect. The overweight person will seek comfort in food. When he is depressed or feels like an utter failure, or if he is ashamed of his silhouette, he turns to food for solace. And his weight balloons even more.

Dr. Jean Mayer, the Harvard nutritionist, says that attributing overweight to overeating "is hardly more illuminating than ascribing alcoholism to overdrinking."

Low Blood Sugar Can Make You Fat

Overweight people are probably not born with the metabolic derangement known as hypoglycemia (low blood sugar), but years of overloading the bloodstream with carbohydrates can cause the condition doctors now recognize as "reactive hypoglycemia." This means that periodically the level of sugar in the bloodstream takes a nose dive. It gets much too low for such fundamental requirements as mental alertness, energy, or even general well being and health. Every time a person's blood sugar takes this kind of a dip, he gets a panic message from the brain demanding more sugar immediately. He may reach in desperation for a candy bar, a soda, or a cup of coffee with lots of sugar in it. *But, taking more sugar merely perpetuates the merry-go-round.*

It is estimated that nine out of ten overweight people suffer from this kind of reactive hypoglycemia. They can be tired, miserable and hungry all the time—and still gain weight.

Starve And Gain Weight

It may seem like a paradox that while one is starving he is gaining weight. But it does happen. A disordered metabolism may drive sugar out of your bloodstream where it is needed into the tissues where it is converted into fat.

The process starts in a subsection of the pancreas called the Islets of Langerhans, the function of which is to manufacture insulin. The purpose of insulin is to remove surplus glucose from the bloodstream, a very important and sometimes life-saving function. Diabetic coma is the result of too little insulin (and, therefore, too much sugar) in the blood.

Instead of manufacturing *too little* as is the case with diabetes, when one has hypoglycemia, he manufactures *too much* insulin. The insulin keeps not only the surplus but also the required sugar out of the blood and, like the sorcerer's apprentice, keeps carrying it into the cells. This means that the brain, which uses sugar (glucose) as its food, is not getting enough. So it sends out distress signals.

The patient feels a desperate craving for sweets; he eats a candy bar, secretes too much insulin, and the sugar is driven right into his tissue cells where it is converted into fat. After a short period of relief, his brain is again getting too little sugar. In a very real sense, he is simultaneously starving and getting fatter. When this cycle occurs for no organic cause other than poor food habits, it is known as *reactive hypoglycemia.*

This kind of hypoglycemia is self perpetuating. With every dietary sin, a victim gets more desperate, more hungry and more obese.

The good news is that this condition is reversible. With a change of diet, the hypoglycemic can experience a metamorphosis. He will enjoy new vitality and he will lose weight.

Low blood sugar patients can break the hypoglycemic cycle and get their metabolism back to normal by following several basic guidelines. These suggestions also provide an effective system of weight loss for over-weight people who don't have low blood sugar:

1. Avoid sugar. *The net effect of consuming sugar is a drop in blood sugar.* What the hypoglycemic must do is keep his blood sugar *up.* For a while, this means avoiding all sugars—even natural ones which occur in fruits (especially dried), honey, maple syrup, molasses and, of course, all products made with sugar. He should use no grape juice, prune juice, cocktails, wines, cordials, or beer. No sugar in beverages. For a day or two, he may find this kind of abstinence quite difficult. But if he perseveres, this kind of sugar deprivation will force his body to convert fat into glucose and will help to normalize his blood sugar metabolism. Then his appestat can once more begin to function properly, and his battle is half won.

2. The obese person should always take the time to enjoy a hearty, high-protein breakfast that includes eggs, meat or

fish. This kind of breakfast does not overload the blood with sugar but sends the glucose first to the liver which, when it is functioning efficiently, doles out the sugar allowance as it is needed, thus preventing overloading and subsequent bankruptcy of sugar in the bloodstream. The working girl's typical breakfast of coffee and a sweet roll is absolutely out.

3. Take frequent meals—five or six small ones instead of having three large ones. By eating frequently you eat less each time so that instead of having three wide upward and downward swings in blood sugar level, you will have six or seven small ones. In time the level will tend to smooth out. Small meals minimize conversion of food into fat and frequent meals make hunger very improbable.

4. Include some fat in your diet. Fats have satiety value that keeps the hunger pangs away, and also help to stoke the fires which burn body fat. Fat in the diet does not mean fat on the hips. A few years ago, doctors were advising "no fat" diets for the overweight, but we are now seeing the danger of omitting fats from the diet. For one thing, vitamin A, being fat soluble and always closely associated with animal fat, is either poorly absorbed or cannot be absorbed at all, without fats. Therefore, a diet low in fat means low vitamin A utility, and decreased resistance to infection.

Fats act on the metabolism of the body to improve combustion of the food that is eaten. In the book *Eat Fat And Grow Slim* (Collins of Canada), Dr. Richard Macharness of London cites detailed medical experiments with three different diets of equal caloric value, which found the high fat diet removed excess weight fastest. When one uses the polyunsaturated fats, there should be an increase in the intake of vitamin E in the diet to prevent rancidity. It's a good idea to pierce a few vitamin E capsules and express the contents into a bottle of polyunsaturated oil. The vitamin E which is present in oils in their original state is removed from the oil by processing. When it is lacking the oils tend to become rancid.

5. Eliminate salt at the table and all highly-salted foods. Salt in the body encourages the retention of fluid in the tissues. Your body needs only about a gram of salt a day, but most of us consume ten times that much. Avoid foods that are

prepared with large amounts of salt like olives, pickles, relishes, smoked foods, salted nuts, pretzels and potato chips.

6. Since most unwise snacking is done in the evening, it is a good idea to retire before one succumbs to the impulse to snack. This habit will contribute to a better appetite in the morning, and a good high-protein breakfast will be most welcome. Calories consumed in the morning are more readily converted into energy than calories consumed before bedtime.

7. A good supply of natural vitamins is necessary to good metabolism and to a sense of well-being. The vitamin B's are necessary to the assimilation of carbohydrates. Some of the B vitamins (B_6 for instance) are catalysts for enzymes which help the body to utilize proteins more efficiently. To this extent they help to satisfy some of the hidden hungers which can force one to unwise nibbling. Thiamine (vitamin B_1) is absolutely necessary to marshal the energy in food. When thiamine is lacking, carbohydrates cannot be properly utilized by the body. This is one reason why a person can eat enough to get fat but still never have any energy.

   Good sources of thiamine are brown rice, nutritional yeast (use it in soups, stews and as a mid-morning broth) and sunflower seeds which can be eaten out of hand, in salads, and taken to work to provide a healthy snack. Desiccated liver, nutritional yeast and wheat germ provide all the B vitamins in a good balance.

8. It is most unwise to substitute artificially sweetened foods for the sugared variety. The goal is to retrain the taste buds so that one no longer experiences a craving for something sweet. Besides, since the object is to build good health, one should avoid all synthetic substances which are generally suspect in that regard.

9. Don't skip meals. This is a common practice among the overweight. It makes them feel virtuous, but it is most unwise. When a meal is missed, so much stored fat pours into the bloodstream that the fat content in the blood often rises to six times above the normal. This can be dangerous for the heart. The object of a diet program is to melt body fat, but slowly.

10. Include some lecithin in your diet. It helps to burn body

fat, and it helps one feel well-fed on less food. It also contributes to the symmetry of a figure that is heavy in spots. When one first takes lecithin, it appears to work in reverse because it raises the level of fat in the blood. But this is only because it tends to pull fat deposits out of other parts of the body and concentrate them in the blood where the fat is burned chemically by normal body processes. Lecithin helps the body to utilize the oil-soluble vitamins (A—which strengthens the mucous membranes, thus building resistance to infections; vitamin E, which gives every cell better utilization of oxygen; vitamin D, which helps in the utilization of calcium; and vitamin K, which is so important to the coagulation of blood).

Because lecithin dissolves fat, it is a tool for using cholesterol—sometimes dangerous lipid manufactured in your body whether you eat fats or not. Some diets on which people lose weight successfully are dangerously low in lecithin-containing oils (lecithin is removed from commercial oils in the processing). These diets can lead to cholesterol build-ups that bring about such complications as gallstones, eczema, nervousness and atherosclerosis.

11. *Start an exercise program and stay with it.* Dr. Warren Guild, of Peter Bent Brigham Hospital in Boston, stresses the importance of physical fitness achieved with regular exercise and suggests four rules for a program. (1) it must be fun; anything involving willpower has a short life span; willpower itself lasts only two weeks and is soluble in alcohol; (2) it must be inexpensive; (3) it should be something that can be done all year round; (4) it should allow for convenient scheduling. "Contrary to opinion," Dr. Guild says, "exercise can actually cut down the appetite." He suggests a 30 minute work out before supper or the heaviest meal of the day (*This Week in Massachusetts Public Health* February 25, 1963). When you exercise, you eat less but enjoy it more. Vigorous walking is one of the best forms of exercise and is one activity which fits the four criteria set down by Dr. Guild.

If you stay with this regimen, you'll lose excess weight and feel much more energetic.

277. Underweight Is A Problem, Too!

People who are underweight have been getting the short end of the editorial stick. You can hardly pick up a magazine that doesn't promise a new diet for melting the solid flesh. But you'll need a divining rod to find an article on how to gain weight. Yet there are many people whose problem is "How do I fill out my bikini?" "How do I regain the weight I lost in the hospital?" "How can I put some weight on my skinny kids?"

People who are fighting the urge to indulge in strawberry shortcake, banana splits and sour cream on baked potatoes, think that skinnies should get down on their boney knees and thank God. But, if you are the gaunt one who has been trying to flesh out your bones, you know that putting it on can be harder than taking it of.

A Metropolitan Life Insurance study revealed that nearly one-fourth of all men under 40 years of age and a slightly smaller proportion of those over 40, are at least 19 percent under average weight.

Strange as it may seem, there are more women than men who just don't have enough fat to support their abdominal organs and pad their bones attractively. As much as 29 percent of women in their twenties are considered underweight. And in spite of all the *avoirdupois* you see at the beaches, 35 percent of all women in their thirties don't have the flesh to hold up a bikini. Even though middle age has been characterized as "fat and fortyish," almost one-third of all women over 40 should be going to a weight gaining club.

Quite a few of these skinnies simply went overboard on low-calorie diets, lost their capacity for food along with their sex appeal, and can't gain an ounce.

For some unfortunate souls, the desire to lose weight is so intense that they become victims of an emotional disorder called *anorexia nervosa*. This ailment is characterized by a lack of appetite so extreme that the person becomes physically unable to eat, and literally wastes away.

It is believed that the emotional trauma impairs pituitary function which, in turn, interferes with normal growth patterns and the menstrual cycle. Victims of *anorexia nervosa,* usually teenage girls, show abnormal patterns of growth hormone and have irregular menstrual periods. The illness can only be reversed when the emotional block is overcome. Psychotherapy alone may help, but if the illness is advanced, the patient must also be hospitalized and fed intravenously to save her life.

Bear in mind, there is a difference between being attractively slender and too thin or emaciated looking. If your weight is a little under what the charts mandate for your age and height, if you feel great, look terrific and have lots of pep, then you must be doing something right. In fact, the odds are on your side that you will live to a healthy old age, untroubled by high blood pressure, diabetes, or some of the other problems that plague the overweight.

But, male or female, if you lack endurance, or look so frail that no one would ask you to open a jar of soybeans, then you are what doctors call the "asthenic" type. Chances are you tire quickly, you are easily driven up a wall, you are high strung and nervous and have a predisposition to many ailments. Some extra weight would do you a world of good.

To put on the pounds where they belong and at the same time improve your health, stamina, and zest for life, observe these simple guidelines:

1. Be careful not to eat the banana split and highly-refined starch diet in an attempt to add pounds.
2. Eat the right natural foods and supplements for a balanced diet and proper nutrition.
3. Avoid burning extra calories haphazardly. Relax.
4. Exercise carefully to distribute your new weight where it counts. Don't overdo the exercise or you'll revert to Mr. Thinman.

At one time the theory was that, since sweets and starches make people fat, these foods should help a thin person to flesh out his bones. It doesn't work that way. Sweets and starches rob the appetite and displace the foods that really count. The high protein diet, so favored by the overweight person to help him lose weight, can also help to normalize the figure of the person who is underweight. The best weight gaining diets include lots of protein and high-calorie foods which supply valuable nutrients along with the calories.

Weight Problems

You should not try to put on weight by gorging yourself with lots of refined cereals, pure starch foods like noodles, spaghetti, macaroni, cake or pie, or foods that are high in refined sugar like candy, ice cream and so forth. Put the emphasis on meat, fish, fowl, eggs, cheese and vegetables—especially the unrefined starchy vegetables like potatoes and sweet potatoes—as well as salads dressed with lots of good vegetable oil. Be sure that you eat three big, nutritious meals every day and enjoy wholesome snacks between meals and at bedtime.

Look for the calories that come in small packages. Cheese, salad oils, butter and nuts furnish many calories but don't take up much room. Snack on nuts and seeds. They are a superb source of natural fat and are so handy to take along with you to work, shopping, to the theater, to the park. Because they are high in protein, minerals, and the B vitamins, as well as fat, they help to regulate your blood sugar. Pound for pound, nuts and seeds supply more calories than virtually any other natural food. Take advantage of these delicious little prize packages which deliver a nutritional wallop without making you feel overstuffed. By simply adding about a half cup of nuts (about 400 calories) to your daily diet you can put on almost a pound a week.

Other weight-gaining foods that are powerhouses of good nutrients and easy to eat are:

Avocados—half of a 10-ounce fruit gives you 185 calories.

Dates—a half cup of dates gives you 245 calories.

Raisins—a half cup is 230 calories.

Prune Juice—200 calories to an 8-ounce glass.

Sweet Potatoes—155 calories for a medium as compared to 90 calories for a medium white potato.

Mayonnaise—1 tablespoon is 100 calories.

Blackstrap Molasses—40 calories, and lots of blood-building iron for a mere tablespoon.

Butter—100 calories to a tablespoon.

Sour Cream—445 calories per cup.

All of these foods can easily be added to your diet without taxing your stomach's capacity. Avocados can enhance your salad. So can mayonnaise. Dates or raisins or nuts can be added to your fruit salad. Enjoy a sweet potato with a pat of butter—delicious! Add a big dollop of sour cream to your white potato. If you're on a yogurt kick, try adding a little sour cream to the yogurt. Try a tablespoon of blackstrap molasses in hot milk as your morning beverage. Down your vitamin supplements with fruit juice instead of water. And take the whole alphabet of vitamins. They will help you utilize your nutrients more efficiently.

Desiccated liver and brewer's yeast should figure prominently among your supplements. They supply the full spectrum of B vitamins which perk up your appetite, your digestion and your metabolism. Rice bran, too, is a good source of B vitamins and minerals; use rice bran and wheat germ liberally on your cereals and in all your baked goods, in chopped meat mixtures and casseroles.

Granola made with oats, raisins, dates, wheat germ, rice bran, soy grits and nuts provide a most delicious dish for excellent nutrients and calories. Try blackstrap molasses and raw honey for a little sweetness and forget the sugar. This is a great breakfast treat for kids who need to gain weight. Make sure that your skinny children don't fill up on the dry cereals.

If your appetite is good, you are eating well, and still not gaining weight, it might be that you are hyperactive. You could be wasting nervous and muscular energy, and burning up more calories than you can consume.

If you are the type who never relaxes, never gets enough sleep, always has a million and one things to do and no time to do them, keep telling yourself to take it easy. Don't rush. Everything gets done in due time. Whatever you do, do it with the least possible expenditure of nervous energy. Try making a little list of the things you can put off till tomorrow or next year.

This does not mean that you should neglect an exercise program. A daily exercise program will serve as a release of tension so that you will be better able to relax and enjoy your sleep, thus burning up fewer calories in the long run. But, don't overdo it. Don't get overtired.

Another decided value of exercise is that the weight you do gain goes on where you want it instead of thickening your waistline and hips.

Usually, a program of exercise, adequate rest, and a high-protein, high-calorie diet of good nutritional foods will lead to a weight that is normal for you—neither too heavy nor too thin.

Index

Index

Index

Index

Cerumen. See *Earwax.*
Cervix, cancer of, 300-302
Chain smoking, allergy and, 17
Chancroid, 1257
Chemicals, birth defects and, 193-197
  cancer producing, 252
Chicken pox, shingles and, 1093
Childbirth, depression following, vitamin B$_{12}$
  for, 584
Children, autistic, communicating with, 559
  megavitamin therapy for, 559-563
  blindness in, 680
  brain disorders in, megavitamin therapy for,
    549
  deformities in, thalidomide and, 193
  diarrhea in, carrots for, 474-476
  disturbed, megavitamin therapy for, 552-555
    niacin need in, 553
    pellagra in, 554
  hyperactive, drug therapy for, 610, 612
    learning disabilities in, 610
    megavitamin therapy for, 610-613
  iron deficiency in, 43
  myopia prevention in, 678-679
  retarded, vitamin E for, 597-599
  shoes for, 712-713
Chlorine, in water, dangers of, 894
Chlorosis, in teenage girls, 45
Chocolate, addiction to, allergy in, 17
  allergic reactions to, 28
    frequency of, 29
  as stimulant, 29
  health dangers of, 28-30
  substitute for, 30
  theobromine in, 29
Cholesterol, arteriosclerosis and, 899
  atherosclerosis and, 899
  diet and, 898-899
  ear problems and, 508-509
  excess, vitamin C and, 901-904
  functions of, 900
  gallstones and, 747-748
  heart disease and, 898-900
    in women, 918
  in arteries, reduction of, 903-913
  inner ear problems and, 508-509
  need for, 899
  plasma levels of, water hardness and, 885
  serum, 816
Choline, deficiency of, cirrhosis of liver and,
    1022-1024
  in muscular dystrophy, 1057
Chromium, deficiency of, 460-461
  in brewer's yeast, 458
  in insulin function, 459
  sources of, 461
Chromosome test, for hermaphroditism, 198
Chromosomes, deletion of, 185
  ionizing radiation injury to, 184
  types of, 199
Circulation, of blood, vitamin E and, 395-400
Cirrhosis of liver, 1016
  alcohol and, 1024

causes of, 1021
choline deficiency in, 1022-1024
mortality in, 1021
symptoms of, 1022
treatment of, 1024
Claudication, intermittent, 813
  vitamin E and, 396
Climate, asthma and, 132-136
Clofibrate, vitamin E and, 852-853
Clostridium perfringens, food poisoning and,
  736
Cocoa, health dangers of, 28-30
Coenzyme A, 83
Cold, heart disease and, 926-927
Cold sores, See *Fever blisters.*
Colds, air pollution and, 410
  chilling and, 421
  dry air and, 424-427
  in babies, antibiotics in, 428-430
  milk free diet in, 431
  moist air and, 424-427
  prevention of, 422
  preventive measures in, 407
  smoking and, 409
  summer, 414
  vaccines for, 406
  vitamin A and, 408
  vitamin C and, 411-420
    dosages in, 413, 415-417
  weather and, 421-423
  wheat germ in, 417-420
Colitis, 480
  ulcerative, 1224-1226
Collagen degeneration, in slipped intervertebral disc, 141
Comedones, and acne, 1108
Comfrey, in ulcer prevention, 1241-1242
Congestive heart failure, 813
  abdominal pain and swelling in, 846
  breathing difficulties in, 847
  malnutrition and, 846
  vitamin therapy in, 847
Conjunctivitis, calcium for, 671-673
  symptoms of, 671
  types of, 671
  vernal, vitamin deficiency in, 672
  vitamin D for, 671-673
Constipation, and urinary tract infections, 440
  bowel habits and, 447
  causes of, 438
  diet and, 442
  disease-related, 438-440
  habitual, 437
    causes of, 441-443
  in cardiac patients, 439
  in children, 439-440
  laxatives and, 436, 441
  prevention of, blackstrap molasses in, 446
    bran in, 444-446
    fruits in, 446
    living habits and, 447
  straining in, heart disease and, 922-924
    dangers of, 923

Index

Index

fluid intake in, 661
incidence of, 644, 659
smoking and, 661
stimulants and, 660
sugar metabolism and, 659
symptoms of, 657
types of, 659
vision loss and, 658
vitamin C therapy for, 661-664
Glucose, and lactic acid, 575
Gluten, intolerance to, hereditary, 98
and rheumatoid arthritis, 97-99
makeup of, 97
Glyoxylide, in cancer treatment, 367-370
Goiter, endemic, iodine deficiency in, 754
exophthalmic, 753
iodine deficiency in, 753
toxic, 753
vitamin A deficiency and, 755-756
water pollution and, 754-755
Gonorrhea, 1258
Gout, treatment of, cherries in, 107-112
drugs in, 108
uric acid in, 109
Granulomas, of fingers, talc and, 267
Grippe. See *Influenza*.

H

Hair, graying of, nutrition and, 771
growth of, 758
diet for, 759
healthiness of, 758-759
herbal colorings for, 772
loss of, diffuse cyclic, 763
malnutrition and, 759
mineral analysis of, in mental disease, 568
transplant of, 761
Hair dyes, cancer and, 770-771
Hair follicle, 758
Halitosis, causes of, 162-165
garlic odor in, 163
hydrochloric acid and, 163
mucin and, 164
toothbrushing and, 162
Hallucinations, auditory, 529
vitamin B₃ in, 569
Handedness, stuttering and, 605
Hay fever, antihistamine for, 774-775
causes of, 774
drugs for, side effects of, 774-775
histamine and, 774-777
honey for, 785, 786
injections for, effectiveness of, 786-787
Headache, acupuncture for, 803-806
air pollution and, 795
aspirin and, 791
causes of, 790
low blood sugar and, 795
migraine, causes of, 797, 801
classic and nonclassic, 797
eating habits and, 800-801
heredity in, 797
vitamin B deficiency in, 798
vitamin therapy for, 799-800

neck muscle contraction and, 792-794
tension, 790, 791-795
in women, 792
relief from, 793-795
Hearing aid, choosing of, 530-534
need for, 530-531
types of, 532
wearing of, 534
Hearing loss. See also *Deafness*.
behavior and, 538
causes of, 502-503
gradual, aging and, 506-509
noise exposure in, 506
hearing aid and, 530-531
high fat diet and, 508
incidence of, 502
loud music and, 516-517
noise protection and, 510-515
signs of, 513
temporary, noise and, 511
tests of, 531
vitamins for, 507
Heart. See also entries under *Cardiac, Cardiovascular,* and *Coronary.*
enlarged, 815
fatty, 815
health of, calcium and, 869-870
exercise for, 934-936, 942-945
magnesium in, 869-870, 876-879
potassium in, 871-875
normal, heart disease symptoms in, 823-826
palpitations of, 824
Heart attack, atherosclerosis and, 191
emergency action in, 845
polarizing therapy for, 860
vitamin C for, 858-863
rationale for, 861-863
water mineral content and, 883-886
Heart disease, anxiety neuroses and, 825
cadmium and, 888
chlorinated water and, 894-897
cholesterol and, 898-900
cold-weather protection for, 926-927
constipation and, 439, 922-924
heat and, 927-929
in children, causes of, 914
incidence of, 914
vitamin B deficiency and, 916
vitamin C deficiency and, 916
in the obese, 929
in women, age factor in, 918
cholesterol and, 919-920
incidence of, 917
nutrition and, 921
sugar and salt in, 920-921
incidence of, 898
magnesium and, 877-879, 886
mortality and, 898
personality groups and, 818-822
personality testing and, 819-822
pulse in, 938-939
specific gravity and, 937-938
sugar and, 857

Index

Index

Index

Index

Index

intermittent claudication and, 396
leg ulcers and, 395
miscarriage and, 1028
muscular dystrophy and, 1058
open heart surgery and, 851
retarded children and, 597-599
storage of, hypolipidemic drugs and, 852-853
ulcers and, 1236
varicose veins and, 1251-1254
Vitamin E deficiency anemia, 48-52
"Vitamin U," in ulcer treatment, 1243-1244
Vitiligo, symptoms of, 1149
treatment of, B complex vitamins in, 1150-1151
hydrochloric acid in, 1149

W

Walking, benefits of, 936, 942, 944-945
foot disorders and, 711
heart action in, 934
Warts, treatment of, 1152-1153
venereal, 1258
Water, cadmium/zinc ratio in, 888-889
chlorinated, arteriosclerosis and, 896
atherosclerosis and, 894-896
effects of, 896-897
heart disease and, 894-897
copper/zinc ratio in, 889-890
hard vs. soft, heart disease and, 883-886
hardness of, cancer and, 886
kidney disease and, 886
testing for, 892
mineral content of, heart attack and, 883-886
soft, toxins in, 887

nutritional protection, 892-893
Water fluoridation, cancer and, 257
Weather, colds and, 421-423
Weight control, birth defects and, 177
in diabetes, 455
Weight lifting, rules for, 958-959
Wheat, allergy to, 18
Wheat flour, bronchitis and, 245
Wheat sensitivity, alcoholism and, 12-13
Whooping cough, 388
vitamin C for, 723
Women, baldness in, 762-763
headache in, migraine, 802
tension, 792
iron deficiency anemia in, 45
needs of, iron as, 44
Worms, 491-492

X

X-rays, cancer and, 259

Y

Yellow food dye, asthma and, 27
Yogurt, diarrhea and, 472
fever blisters and, 1115-1120

Z

Zinc, deficiency of, 1090
dietary, 1080
periodontal protection and, 1183-1184
prostate levels of, 1077
sexual health and, 1078
sinus protection and, 1103-1104